Peripheral Vascular Disease

A CLINICAL APPROACH

Peripheral Vascular Disease

A CLINICAL APPROACH

Carlos Meña, MD, FACC, FSCAI

Associate Professor of Medicine – Cardiology
Director Cardiac Catheterization Laboratories
Director Vascular Medicine & Endovascular Fellowship
Yale New Haven Hospital
New Haven, Connecticut

Sasanka Jayasuriya, MBBS, FACC, FASE, RPVI, FSCAI

Assistant Professor of Medicine
Section of Cardiovascular Medicine
Yale School of Medicine
New Haven, Connecticut

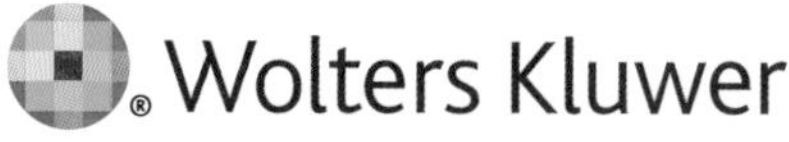

Philadelphia • Baltimore • New York • London
Buenos Aires • Hong Kong • Sydney • Tokyo

Acquisitions Editor: Sharon Zinner
Development Editor: Ashley Fischer
Editorial Coordinator: Lindsay Ries
Production Project Manager: Bridgett Dougherty, David Saltzberg
Design Coordinator: Stephen Druding
Manufacturing Coordinator: Beth Welsh
Prepress Vendor: TNQ Technologies

9 8 7 6 5 4 3 2 1

Printed in China (or the United States of America)

Library of Congress Cataloging-in-Publication Data

Names: Mena, Carlos (Carlos I. Mena-Hurtado) editor. | Jayasuriya, Sasanka, editor.
Title: Peripheral vascular disease : a clinical approach / edited by Carlos Mena, Sasanka Jayasuriya.
Other titles: Peripheral vascular disease (Mena)
Description: Philadelphia : Wolters Kluwer, [2020]
Identifiers: LCCN 2019017152 | ISBN 9781496349408 (paperback)
Subjects: | MESH: Peripheral Vascular Diseases–therapy | Endovascular Procedures–methods
Classification: LCC RC694 | NLM WG 505 | DDC 616.1/31–dc23
LC record available at https://lccn.loc.gov/2019017152

shop.lww.com

CCS0519

Contributors

Mahmoud Abdelghany, MD
Fellow in Cardiovascular Medicine,
Yale New Haven Hospital,
New Haven, Connecticut

S. Elissa Altin, MD
Assistant Professor
Division of Cardiology
Yale University School of Medicine
New Haven, Connecticut

Herbert D. Aronow, MD, MPH
Director of Interventional Cardiology
Division of Cardiovascular Medicine
Warren Alpert Medical School of Brown University
Lifespan Cardiovascular Institute
Providence, Rhode Island

Jeremy D. Asnes, MD
Associate Professor
Department of Pediatrics
Yale School of Medicine
New Haven, Connecticut

Robert R. Attaran, MD, FACC, FASE, FSCAI, RPVI
Assistant Professor Cardiovascular Medicine
Director, Venous Disorders Program
Yale New Haven Hospital
New Haven, Connecticut

Afsha Aurshina, MBBS
Resident, Department of Surgery
Yale University School of Medicine
New Haven, Connecticut

William L. Bennett, MD, PhD
Assistant Professor
Department of Cardiology
Ochsner Clinic Foundation
New Orleans, Louisiana

Kurt Bjorkman, MD
Chief Resident
Department of Pediatrics
Yale-New Haven Children's Hospital
Yale School of Medicine
New Haven, Connecticut

Peter A. Blume, DPM, FACFAS
Medical Director/HVC/Ambulatory Surgery
Yale New Haven Health Systems
Assistant Clinical Professor Of Surgery
Anesthesia and Cardiology
Yale School of Medicine
New Haven, Connecticut

Fouad Chouairi, BS
Department of Neurosurgery
Yale University School of Medicine
New Haven, Connecticut

Stacy Chu, MD
Department of Neurology
Yale University School of Medicine
New Haven, Connecticut

Branden Cord, MD, PhD
Department of Neurosurgery
Yale University School of Medicine
New Haven, Connecticut

Bennett Cua, MD, FACC
Cardiologist
Mission Viejo, California

John A. Elefteriades, MD, PhD (hon)
William W.L. Glenn Professor of Surgery
Director, Aortic Institute at Yale-New Haven
Yale Medicine Department of Surgery
New Haven, Connecticut

Young Erben, MD
Senior Associate Consultant
Mayo Clinic Florida
Jacksonville, Florida

Wassim H. Fares, MD, MSc
Senior Clinical Leader
Clinical Development
Actelion Clinical Research
Actelion Pharmaceuticals Inc
A Janssen Pharmaceutical Company of Johnson & Johnson
Allschwil, Switzerland

Senthilraj Ganeshan, MD
Clinical Cardiology Fellow
Division of Cardiology
Yale University School of Medicine
New Haven, Connecticut

Michael I. Gazes, DPM, MPH, FACFAOM, AACFAS
Yale New Haven Foot & Ankle Surgeons / Northeast Medical Group
Department of Pediatric Surgery
Yale New Haven Hospital
Clinical Instructor, Department of Medicine
Yale School of Medicine
New Haven, Connecticut

Andrew M. Goldsweig, MD
Assistant Professor
Division of Cardiovascular Medicine
University of Nebraska Medical Center
Omaha, Nebraska

Anton A. Gryaznov, MD, PhD
Resident, Aortic Institute at Yale-New Haven Hospital
Yale University School of Medicine
New Haven, Connecticut

Eileen M. Harder, MD
Resident Physician
Department of Internal Medicine
Yale University
New Haven, Connecticut

Ahmed Harhash, MBBCh
Cardiovascular Fellow
Department of Cardiology
University of Arizona
Tucson, Arizona

Faisal Hasan, MD
Associate Clinical Professor of Medicine
Heart and Vascular Institute
Cleveland Clinic Abu Dhabi
Abu Dhabi, United Arab Emirates

Khwaja Yousuf Hasan, MBBS
Associate Staff Physician
Heart and Vascular Institute
Cleveland Clinic Abu Dhabi
Abu Dhabi, United Arab Emirates

Ryan M. Hebert, MD
Assistant Professor
Department of Neurosurgery
Yale University School of Medicine
New Haven, Connecticut

Sasanka Jayasuriya, MBBS, FACC, FASE, RPVI, FSCAI
Assistant Professor of Medicine
Section of Cardiovascular Medicine
Yale School of Medicine
New Haven, Connecticut

Qurat-ul-Aini Jelani, MD
Peripheral Vascular Interventional Fellow
Division of Cardiology
Department of Medicine
Yale University School of Medicine
New Haven, Connecticut

Michele H. Johnson, MD, FACR, FASER
Professor, Department of Radiology and Biomedical Imaging and Neurosurgery
Director, Interventional Neuroradiology
Yale University School of Medicine
New Haven, Connecticut

Andrew Koo, BS
Department of Neurosurgery
Yale University School of Medicine
New Haven, Connecticut

Kwan S. Lee, MBBCh
Associate Professor of Medicine
Department of Cardiology
University of Arizona
Tucson, Arizona

Anna Lynn, BS
Department of Neurosurgery
Yale University School of Medicine
New Haven, Connecticut

Wei-Guo Ma, MD
Visiting Attending
Yale University School of Medicine
New Haven, Connecticut;
Associate Professor
Department of Cardiovascular Surgery,
Beijing Anzhen Hospital of Capital Medical University
Beijing, China

Charles Matouk, MD, FRCS(C)
Associate Professor of Neurosurgery and of Radiology & Biomedical Imaging
Section Chief, Neurovascular Surgery
Director, Endovascular Neurosurgery Fellowship
Yale University/Yale-New Haven Hospital
New Haven, Connecticut

Carlos Meña, MD, FACC, FSCAI
Associate Professor of Medicine – Cardiology
Director Cardiac Catheterization Laboratories
Director Vascular Medicine & Endovascular Fellowship
Yale New Haven Hospital
New Haven, Connecticut

Michael Mercier, BA
Department of Neurosurgery
Yale University School of Medicine
New Haven, Connecticut

Sameh Mohareb, MD
Fellow in Cardiology
Department of Cardiology
Ochsner Clinic Foundation
New Orleans, Louisiana

Sameer Nagpal, MD
Interventional Cardiology Fellow
Department of Cardiovascular Medicine
Yale University School of Medicine
New Haven, CT

Reshma Narula, MD
Assistant Professor of Neurology
Yale University School of Medicine
New Haven, Connecticut

Rishi Panchal, DO
Peripheral Vascular Interventional Fellow
Yale-New Haven Hospital
New Haven, Connecticut

Chandni Patel, MD
Pediatric Cardiology Fellow
Department of Pediatrics
Yale University
New Haven, Connecticut

Imaad Razzaque, MD
Interventional Cardiology Fellow
Department of Medicine
Tulane University School of Medicine
New Orleans, Louisiana

Ayman Saeyeldin, MD
Resident, Aortic Institute at Yale-New Haven Hospital
Yale University School of Medicine
New Haven, Connecticut

Mamadou L. Sanogo, MD
Assistant Professor of Radiology
University of Michigan
Division of Vascular and Interventional Radiology
Ann Arbor, Michigan

John F. Setaro, MD, FACC, FSCAI
Associate Professor of Medicine
Director, Cardiovascular Disease Prevention Center
Attending Physician, Adult Cardiac Catheterization Laboratory
Section of Cardiovascular Medicine
Yale University School of Medicine and Yale New-Haven Hospital
New Haven, Connecticut

Samit M. Shah, MD, PhD
Clinical Fellow
Division of Cardiovascular Medicine
Yale University School of Medicine
New Haven, Connecticut

Madhan Shanmugasundaram, MD, FACC, FSCAI
Assistant Professor of Medicine
University of Arizona College of Medicine
Tucson, Arizona

M. Abigail Simmons, MD
Post-Doctoral Fellow
Adult Congenital Heart Disease Department of Internal Medicine
Section of Cardiovascular Medicine
Yale University School of Medicine
New Haven, Connecticut

Atul Singla, MD
Assistant Professor
Section of Cardiology/Department of Medicine
Tulane University School of Medicine
Southeast Louisiana Veterans Health Care System
New Orleans, Louisiana

Samuel Sommaruga, MD
Geneva University Hospital
Geneva, Switzerland

Bauer E. Sumpio, MD, PhD
Professor
Department of Surgery, Radiology and Medicine
Yale University
New Haven, Connecticut

Tze-Woei Tan, MBBS
Assistant Professor of Surgery
Department of Vascular Surgery
University of Arizona
Tucson, Arizona

Camilo A. Velasquez, MD
Resident, Aortic Institute at Yale-New Haven Hospital
Yale University School of Medicine
New Haven, Connecticut

Chiranjiv S. Virk, MD
Assistant Professor
Department of Surgery
Section Chief Vascular Surgery
Louisiana State University
Shreveport, Louisiana

Gabriella Wilson, MD
Clinical Medicine Resident
Department of Internal Medicine
Yale University School of Medicine
New Haven, Connecticut

Mohammad A. Zafar, MD
Resident, Aortic Institute at Yale-New Haven Hospital
Yale University School of Medicine
New Haven, Connecticut

Bulat Ziganshin, MD, PhD
Associate Research Scientist in Surgery
Yale University
New Haven, Connecticut

Preface

This book is written for endovascular operators to summarize the current indications, techniques, and data in endovascular intervention. The goal is to present this information in a succinct and comprehensive "easy to follow" format.

We recognize the field of endovascular intervention is rapidly evolving. This could be a field, which has the highest turnover of equipment—different new technologies are gaining popularity with supportive data; however, older techniques are filed away in the archives of history, at times to resurface in common practice.

We have made a comprehensive effort to present to you a snapshot of contemporaneous practices at the time this book is in print. Chapters have an outline format to ensure ease of following the content. Each chapter also begins with bulleted "Key Points" list, created by the authors and editors, that highlights critical topics discussed in the chapter.

This guide does not in any way substitute adequate training and a through knowledge of endovascular interventions. We recommend that societal current guidelines and practices be closely followed.

We hope you enjoy this book and it adds to your strengths in caring for the highly complex patient population with vascular disease!

Carlos Meña, MD, FACC, FSCAI
Sasanka Jayasuriya, MBBS, FACC, FASE, RPVI, FSCAI

Contents

CHAPTER 1

History of Endovascular Intervention, Fluoroscopy, Basics of Angiography, Contrast, Patient Selection, and Informed Consent

Andrew M. Goldsweig, MD and
Herbert D. Aronow, MD, MPH

Key Points

- Major landmarks in the history of endovascular intervention include the discovery of X-rays by Röntgen, the synthesis of nonionic contrast media by Almén, the development of angioplasty by Grüntzig, and the first use of vascular stents by Puel and Sigwart.
- Fluoroscopic systems generate X-rays via Bremsstrahlung. After passing through a patient, these X-rays initiate a cascade of energy transfers that ultimately converts the signal into an electronic digital image.
- X-ray exposure causes DNA mutations that may result in deterministic effects (ie, tissue damage) as well as stochastic effects (ie, malignancy).
- Each vascular territory and intervention is best imaged from specific angulations. Endovascular intervention relies heavily upon digital subtraction imaging (DSA).
- Contrast agents are ionic or nonionic iodine-containing molecules that attenuate X-rays. Risks associated with contrast agents include contrast-induced acute kidney injury (CI-AKI) and hypersensitivity reactions.
- Patient selection for endovascular procedures relies upon history, physical examination, noninvasive imaging, and guidelines for each vascular territory (when available), and should incorporate patient preference. Patients and providers must discuss the risks, benefits, and alternatives of a procedure during the preprocedural informed consent process.

I. Introduction

Endovascular intervention offers effective, minimally invasive therapy for many diseases of the peripheral arteries and veins. Now four decades old, the field of endovascular intervention continues to see explosive growth and rapid development of new, advanced technologies. This chapter introduces the basics of endovascular intervention, beginning with a review of the major landmarks and pioneers in the development of fluoroscopy and angiography. An understanding of the fundamentals of X-ray imaging is necessary to all endovascular operators, as is an appreciation for the risks of working with radiation. Effective angiography requires knowledge of optimal technique and contrast use. Finally, procedural specialists must carefully select which patients may benefit from endovascular intervention and review with these patients the risks, benefits, and alternatives of the planned procedures. Expertise in fluoroscopy and angiography coupled with appropriate patient selection provides the basis for successful endovascular intervention.

II. History of Fluoroscopy and Angiography

The modern era of medical imaging began on November 8, 1895, when German physicist Wilhelm Conrad Röntgen first produced X-rays and generated an image of his wife Anna's hand on a barium platinocyanide screen (Fig. 1.1).[1] For his discovery, Röntgen was awarded the first Nobel Prize in Physics in 1901. Within a year of Röntgen's invention,

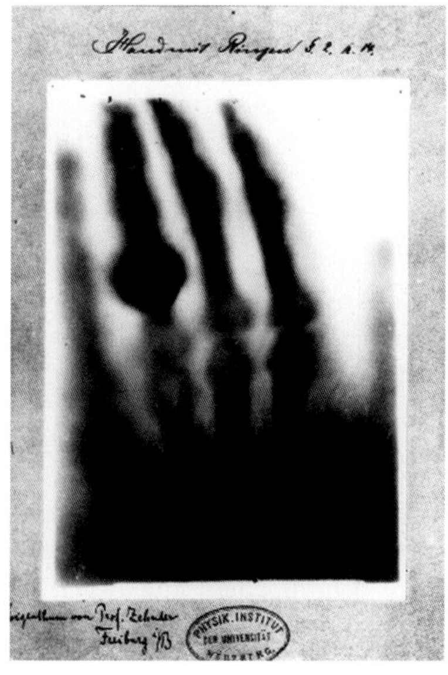

FIGURE 1.1: Röntgen's first X-ray image of his wife Anna's hand.

Thomas Edison developed the first fluoroscope in 1896 before abandoning X-ray research owing to the dangers associated with radiation exposure.[2] Also in 1896, Austrians Eduard Haschek and Otto Lindenthal dissolved bismuth, lead, and barium salts in oil to perform the first angiogram in an amputated hand (Fig. 1.2).[3]

A. **In Vivo Imaging: Limitations and Advances** Initially, the toxicity of radiopaque substances limited in vivo imaging. Earl Osborne, a syphilologist working at Mayo Clinic, accidentally discovered radiocontrast when he noted that the urinary tracts of syphilis patients treated with oral sodium iodide agents were radiopaque.[4] In 1919, Argentine Carlos Heuser performed the first vascular study in a living human by injecting dilute potassium iodide into a vein on the dorsum of a patient's hand and following the bolus to the heart fluoroscopically.[5] In Munich, Berberich and Hirsch obtained the first femoral venogram in 1923 by infusing a solution of aqueous 20% strontium bromide. Soon after, in 1924, Brooks pioneered intraarterial injection of sodium iodide to obtain the first clinical femoral arteriogram.[6] Egas Moniz, a French neurologist, initiated carotid and intracranial angiograpy in 1927 as a means to localized intracranial tumors by their characteristic vasculature.[7] For his contributions, he was awarded the 1949 Nobel Prize in Physiology or Medicine.

Early inorganic contrast agents were highly toxic and principally used experimentally. However, in the late 1920s, with the advent of new, organic, iodine-containing radiocontrast media, clinical angiography began to develop rapidly. While searching for new syphilis remedies in Berlin, Binz and Rath developed the first water-soluble iodinated pyridine contrast called Selectran Neutral.[8] In 1933, Swick and Wallingford synthesized para-aminoiodohippuric acid with three iodine atoms per molecule, Hippuran, heralding the dawn of the modern era of polyiodinated contrast agents.[9] Ionic contrast media with higher iodine content and improved water solubility proliferated over the ensuing decades; however, the quest for less toxic media continued. Swedish radiologist Torsten Almén pioneered nonionic contrast media in 1969 with monomeric metrizamide (Amipaque); he remained at the forefront of the field with

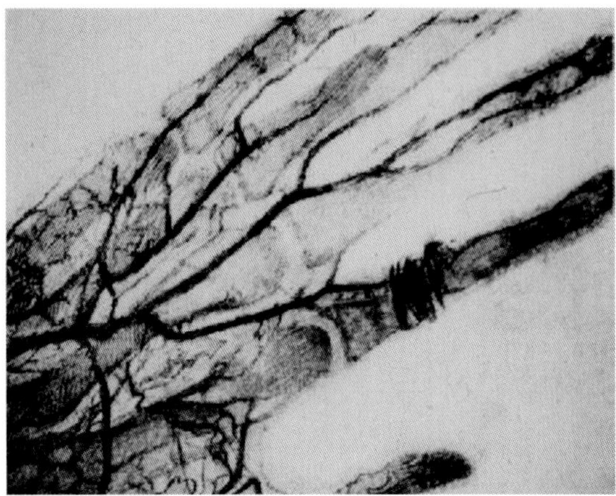

FIGURE 1.2: Haschek's and Lindenthal's first angiogram of a cadaveric hand.

the 1982 release of the low-osmolar monomer iohexol (Omnipaque) and the 1993 introduction of the iso-osmolar dimer iodixanol (Visipaque).[10]

Concomitant to these advances in contrast media, procedural advances permitted expanded use of angiography. In 1929, a Berlin surgical resident named Werner Forssmann inserted a urinary catheter through his own basilic vein to visualize his right ventricle.[11] Although he lost his job for the stunt, he was awarded the Nobel Prize in 1956 for his contribution. In 1953, Swedish radiologist Ivar Seldinger described guidewire technique that allowed reliable access to any major artery or vein.[12] Selective angiography was soon performed in every vascular territory. Notably, however, the first selective coronary angiogram obtained by Sones at the Cleveland Clinic on October 30, 1958 was performed inadvertently during aortography when the catheter landed in the right coronary artery.[13]

B. **Transcatheter Vascular Intervention** Transcatheter vascular intervention began in 1964 when Dotter and Judkins used rigid, Teflon-coated catheters to dilate 11 femoral and popliteal stenoses.[14] Soon after, Fogarty described catheter aspiration of arterial thrombus.[15] Using homemade equipment, Andreas Grüntzig performed the first iliac double-lumen balloon angioplasty on January 23, 1975 at University Hospital in Zurich[16] and reported the first coronary angioplasty on September 16, 1977.[17] Ten years later in Toulouse, Jacques Puel reported the first clinical use of a self-expanding coronary stent on March 28, 1986.[18] Puel and Ulrich Sigwart of Lausanne reported the first ileofemoral self-expanding stents in 1987.[19] Later that year, Julio Palmaz and Richard Schatz implanted the first balloon-expandable peripheral and coronary stents.[20] Adjunctive endovascular tools soon followed including intravascular ultrasound (IVUS) in 1988[21] and coronary rotational atherectomy in 1989.[22] The last 25 years have seen a proliferation of devices too numerous to recount including drug-eluting stents, drug-coated balloons, lesion crossing devices, luminal reentry devices, and additional atherectomy modalities.

III. Fluoroscopy

Fluoroscopic X-ray imaging guides almost all endovascular intervention. Numerous models of imaging equipment are available, but all rely on the same fundamental mechanism. Inside a vacuum tube, a voltage potential (kVp) is applied between cathode coils and a rapidly spinning tungsten anode. This potential results in a current (mA) of electrons bombarding the anode. Ninety-nine percent of the energy generated by this circuit is released as heat. The anode spins rapidly to dissipate this heat, and the high melting point of tungsten makes this element the preferred anode material.

As electrons fly through the anode, a small minority pass close enough to a positively charged tungsten nucleus to be magnetically deflected and slowed. The energy from this change in electron velocity is released as an X-ray; this phenomenon is called Bremsstrahlung, German for “braking radiation.” The energy of these X-rays increases logarithmically with increasing kVp due to the increased velocity of the electrons. The Bremsstrahlung X-ray beam is shaped by a collimator, a lead block with holes that only allows passage of X-rays in the intended direction of the beam, reducing scatter. Copper and aluminum filters remove low-energy X-rays that do not contribute to imaging.

The patient’s body attenuates X-rays in proportion to each tissue’s density and component atomic weights (“Z”). Unattenuated X-rays pass through the patient to generate images. In a traditional digital imaging system, these X-rays strike a panel of input phosphors, which convert the X-ray energy into light. This light in turn strikes a panel of photocathodes, causing the release of electrons into an image intensifier, which increases their energy by applying a voltage potential. These electrons are absorbed by an output phosphor, which emits light that is detected by a silicon array charge-coupled device (CCD). The analog signal from the CCD is relayed to a video camera and converted by an analog-digital converter into a digital video signal (Fig. 1.3).

In newer flat panel systems, light from the input phosphor strikes photodiodes, releasing electrons. These electrons are detected directly by a thin film transistor array, which produces an analog signal that is converted into a digital video. By avoiding a second conversion from electron signal to light, the flat panel provides higher image resolution than the traditional image intensifies. The very newest systems may employ amorphous selenium instead of an input phosphor. Amorphous selenium can convert X-rays directly into electrons, bypassing both traditional light conversion steps.

Digital acquisition permits adjustment of image rendering for several purposes. Automatic image brightness feedback modulates the kVp and mA to optimize imaging. Frame rate can be increased when necessary to capture rapidly moving objects and decreased to minimize X-ray exposure. DSA records an initial image and subtracts that image as a mask from all subsequent frames: the result is exclusion of radiopaque structures and display of only the moving angiographic contrast column.

IV. Radiation

Ionizing radiation such as X-rays causes single- and double-strand breaks in deoxyribonucleic acid (DNA).

A. **Patients** Patients undergoing fluoroscopically guided procedures may be acutely exposed to significant doses of radiation. In the days to weeks following exposure, DNA damage may cause dose-dependent deterministic effects including skin erythema, epilation, and cataracts[23] at doses as low as 2-5 Gy. Exposure of 10-50 Gy may cause life-threatening hematopoetic, gastrointestinal, and cerebrovascular syndromes.[24]

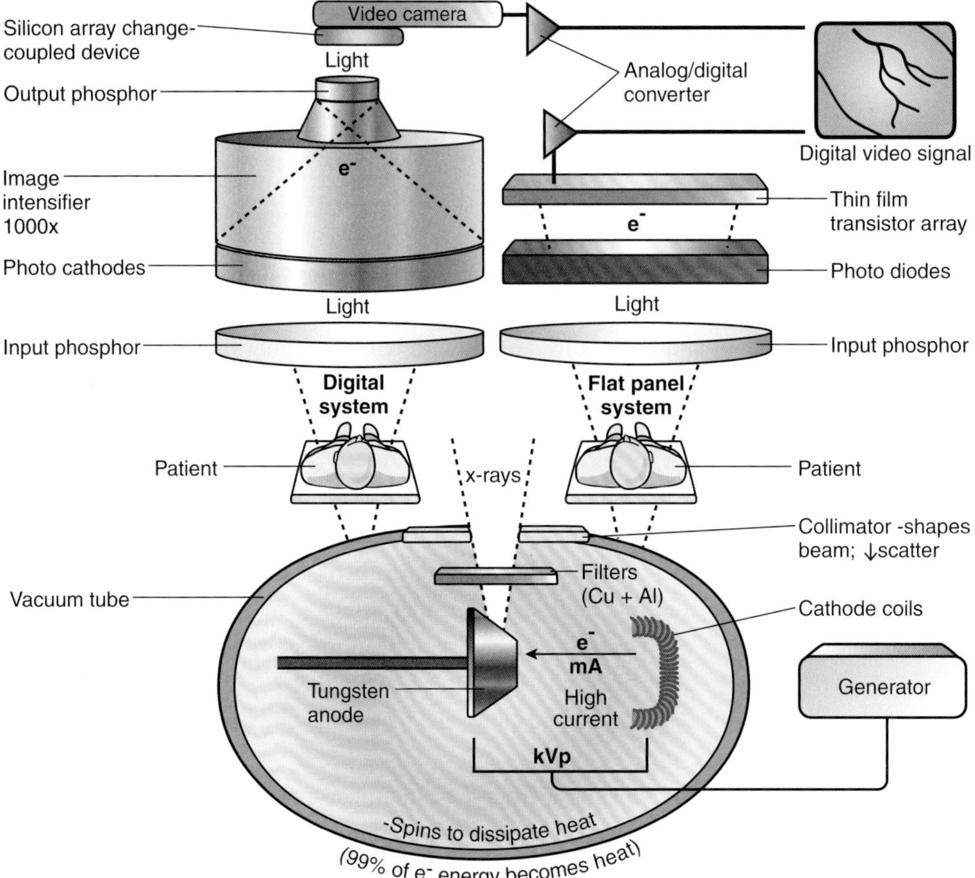

FIGURE 1.3: Schematic diagram of traditional image intensifier and flat panel system.

B. **Operators** Procedural operators are chronically exposed to scatter radiation. Both patients and operators are at stochastic risk for malignancy. The risk of malignancy is not precisely dose-dependent but follows a linear nonthreshold model. Similarly, DNA damage to reproductive tissues may result in fetal malformations and childhood malignancies. The United States Nuclear Regulatory Commission limits the annual whole-body doses of radiation users to 50 millisieverts (mSv) with specific limits of 150 mSv to the lens of the eye and 500 mSv to the skin of the extremities. Pregnant individuals must keep their exposure below 5 mSv during the duration of pregnancy.

C. **Procedural X-ray Dosage** Several modifiable factors affect the procedural X-ray dosage. Operators may reduce radiation exposure to patients and themselves by minimizing fluoroscopy time, frame rate, magnification, source-to-image distance, DSA imaging, and steep angulation, while maximizing beam filtration and collimation, shielding of radiation-sensitive tissues, and personal distance from the X-ray source.

V. Angiography

X-ray angiography of intravascular contrast defines the vascular anatomy as a basis for endovascular intervention. Angiography is used to demonstrate lesion location, morphology, severity, and collateralization as well as the lesion's effect on blood flow. Additionally, angiography can detect vessel abnormalities such as dissection, thrombosis, and calcification. High-quality angiography is essential to guide safe and effective endovascular intervention and can facilitate decisions regarding appropriateness.

A. Angiographers

1. Angiographers must ensure appropriate catheter selection, contrast administration, and fluoroscopy parameters.
2. Angiographers must also know which imaging projections are ideal in each clinical situation (Table 1.1; Fig. 1.4).
   a. Vessels should ideally be visualized in multiple planes perpendicular to the imaging surface, although in practice, each vascular territory is canonically imaged in a particular projection.
      i. The aortic arch is visualized at approximately 30° in the left anterior oblique (LAO) projection.
      ii. Carotid angiography is performed at approximately 30° in the ipsilateral projection and in the lateral projection; subclavian angiography is performed at approximately 30° in the ipsilateral and contralateral projections. Intracranial vessels are imaged at approximately 20° cranial anteroposterior (AP) and in the lateral projection.

Table 1.1. Optimal Imaging Projection by Vascular Territory

Vascular Territory	Optimal Imaging Projection
Aortic arch	LAO 30°
Carotid arteries	Ipsilateral 30°
	Lateral
Subclavian arteries	Ipsilateral 30°
	Contralateral 30°
Intracranial arteries	AP cranial 20°
	Lateral
Descending aorta	Flat AP
Renal arteries	LAO 20°
Common and external iliac arteries	Contralateral 30°
Common and superficial femoral arteries	Ipsilateral 30°
Tibial and peroneal arteries	Flat AP
	Ipsilateral 30°
Pedal arteries	Lateral

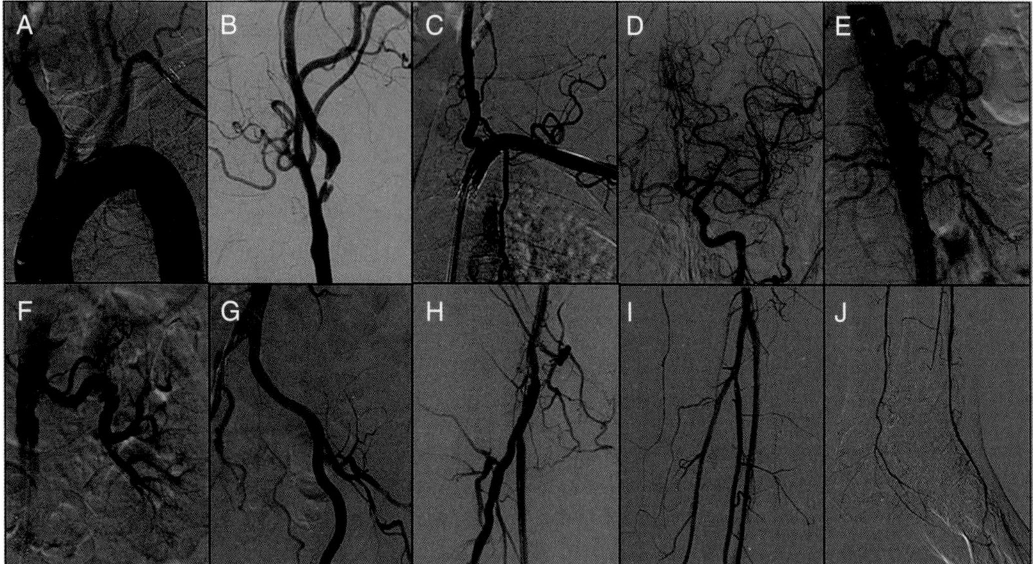

FIGURE 1.4: Selected angiograms at optimal imaging projections. A, LAO (left anterior oblique) 30° image of aortic arch. B, LAO 30° image of left common, internal, and external carotid arteries with high-grade internal carotid stenosis. C, RAO (right anterior oblique) 30° image of left subclavian and vertebral arteries with patent subclavian stent. D, AP (anteroposterior) cranial 20° image of left internal carotid and intracranial arteries. E, Flat AP image of descending aorta and mesenteric arteries. F, LAO 20° image of left renal artery with fibromuscular dysplasia. G, RAO 30° image of left common and external iliac arteries. H, RAO 30° image of right common femoral, superficial femoral, and profunda femoris arteries. I, LAO 30° image of left posterior tibial, peroneal, and anterior tibial arteries. J, Left lateral image of left posterior tibial and dorsalis pedis arteries and pedal arch.

iii. The descending aorta is visualized in the flat AP projection, although a 20° LAO projection is ideal for demonstrating the renal artery origins.

iv. Common iliac artery distal bifurcations are best seen from approximately 30° contralateral oblique views, whereas the common femoral artery bifurcations are seen best with approximately 30° of ipsilateral oblique angulation.

v. Tibial and peroneal vessels may be imaged in either the AP or ipsilateral 30° oblique projections.

b. Pedal angiography is usually performed laterally.

B. Peripheral Vascular Angiography and Intervention

1. Several digital imaging modes are used for peripheral vascular angiography and intervention.
    a. Standard low-dose fluoroscopy at 7.5-15 frames per second is used for catheter and wire manipulation to minimize patient and operator radiation exposure, especially given the frequently long fluoroscopy time during complicated procedures.
    b. High-resolution cine angiography at 15-30 frames per second, the staple for coronary intervention, is seldom used in the peripheral space.
    c. DSA is the staple of peripheral vascular imaging to permit vessel visualization despite the presence of adjacent radiopaque bones and high-velocity blood flow.

2. The degree of vessel stenosis is reported as a percentage lumen diameter reduction compared with a normal adjacent segment without an intervening bifurcation.
   a. Quantitative angiography uses digital calipers to make precise vascular measurements, normalized to a reference of known size such as a catheter.
      i. Digital imaging systems also frequently include a roadmap feature, which superimposes onto a fluoroscopic image a partially transparent mask of a previously recorded image. This feature allows manipulation of endovascular tools without recurrent contrast injection for visualization of the vascular anatomy.
   b. When angiography alone is inadequate to provide optimal vessel or lesion visualization, intravascular imaging techniques (eg, IVUS or optical coherence tomography) can be used to facilitate diagnostic or therapeutic peripheral vascular procedures).

VI. Contrast

A. **Modern Radiocontrast Agents** Modern radiocontrast agents are water-soluble compounds carrying tri-iodinate benzene rings. Iodine attenuates X-rays, so vessel opacification is a function of contrast flow and the concentration of iodine. Older, ionic contrasts carry a carboxyl group and a sodium cation, resulting in two active osmolar moieties. These agents include the monomer diatrizoate (Hypaque), with three iodine atoms on 1 benzene ring, as well as the dimer ioxaglate (Hexabrix), with six iodine atoms on two benzene rings linked by amide groups. Newer, nonionic contrasts contain only one active osmolar moiety and carry numerous hydroxyl groups to improve solubility at the expense of increased viscosity. These agents include the monomer iohexol (Omnipaque), with three iodine atoms on one benzene ring, as well as the dimer iodixanol (Visipaque), with six iodine atoms on two benzene rings linked by amine groups (Fig. 1.5).

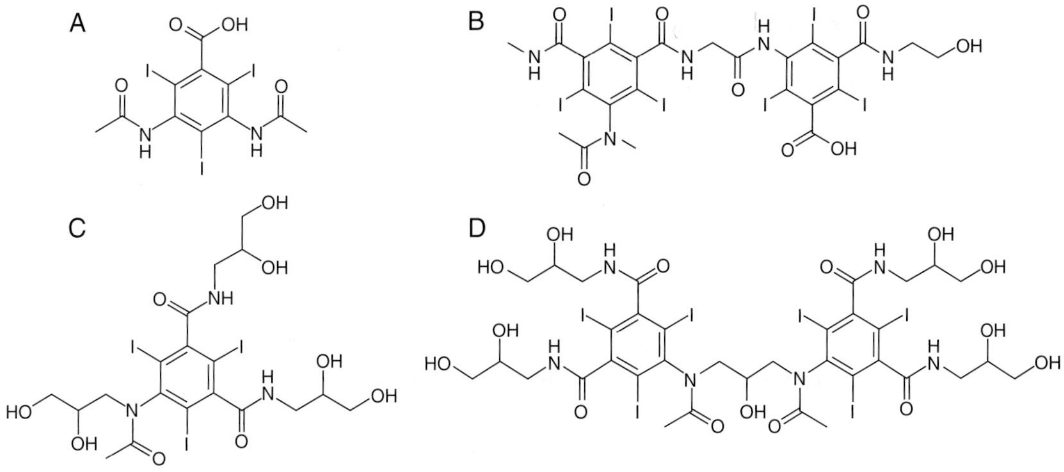

FIGURE 1.5: Molecular structure of several common contrast agents. A, Diatrizoate (Hypaque). B, Ioxaglate (Hexabrix). C, Iohexol (Omnipaque). D, Iodixanol (Visipaque).

B. Adverse Effects

1. **Common Adverse Effects** The most common adverse effects of contrast media include contrast-induced acute kidney injury (CI-AKI) and hypersensitivity reactions. CI-AKI is most commonly defined as a 25% increase in serum creatinine or an increase of ≥0.5 mg/dL within 72 hours of contrast administration, although other definitions are employed.[25] Although the exact pathophysiology is unclear, contrast media are known to be directly nephrotoxic. Risk factors for CI-AKI include ionic contrast, chronic kidney disease, diabetes, advanced age, low body-mass index, congestive heart failure, prior cerebrovascular disease, prior PCI, acute coronary syndrome at presentation, dehydration, anemia, hypertension, cardiogenic shock, balloon pump use, cardiac arrest, and concomitant use of other nephrotoxic agents (eg, nonsteroidal anti-inflammatory drugs, angiotensin converting enzyme inhibitors, diuretics).[26–28]
   a. The risk of CI-AKI is minimized if the administered contrast volume in mL is less than two to three times the patient's glomerular filtration rate.[29] In addition to minimization of contrast dosage, the risk of CI-AKI may also be mitigated by adequate pre-, intra-, and postprocedural intravenous hydration to increase urine volume and contrast clearance[30] as well as through use of low-osmolar contrast agents. All isotonic fluids appear to convey similar protection; fluids containing sodium bicarbonate provide no advantage over normal saline. No evidence or current guidelines support the use of N-acetylcysteine to prevent nephrotoxicity.
   b. Hypersensitivity reactions of varying severity may occur as a result of contrast exposure. These are mast cell–mediated reactions with a spectrum of presentations from simple urticaria to complicated anaphylactoid reactions including vasodilation, circulatory collapse, angioedema, and bronchospasm. Risk factors for hypersensitivity reactions include high osmolar and ionic contrasts, atopy, asthma, advanced age, and female gender. Contrast hypersensitivity is not IgE-mediated anaphylaxis and is entirely unrelated to shellfish allergy, which is an IgE-mediated reaction to a tropomyosin protein antigen. Patients with prior contrast hypersensitivity or a strong atopic history may be premedicated with steroids and antihistamines.
2. **Less Common Adverse Effects** Several other less common adverse effects have been associated with contrast exposure.
   a. A delayed hypersensitivity presenting with rash and fever 24-48 hours after exposure is mediated by IgA and IgE; this self-limited reaction is particularly associated with nonionic, dimeric agents. Also, a high osmolar load and significant volume of contrast may expand the intravascular space, leading to volume overload. Contrast extravasation into a nondistendable space may cause compartment syndrome. Contrast-related sialadenitis called iodine mumps and iodine-induced hyperthyroidism are rarely observed.

b. CO_2 angiography avoids most adverse effects associated with contrast including CI-AKI and hypersensitivity. Also, the low viscosity of CO_2 permits better filling of collateral branches than iodinated contrast. Extreme caution must be used to prevent air contamination: given the concern for air embolism, CO_2 angiography is only indicated in the lower extremities and should never be used in coronary, thoracic, or cerebral vascular procedures.[31]

VII. Patient Selection and Consent

A. **Patient Selection** Patient selection for endovascular procedures is an individualized process dependent upon consideration of multiple factors. A thorough history of symptoms and comorbidities is critical. A comprehensive physical examination should include assessment of associated pulses and supplied tissues. Initial diagnosis of lower extremity peripheral artery disease should be performed by ankle-brachial index, sequential limb pressures, and pulse-volume recording or Doppler waveforms. Further disease characterization may be performed by Duplex ultrasonography or by CT, MR, or invasive angiography when revascularization is being contemplated.

1. **Lower Extremity Intervention** Appropriate symptoms include lifestyle-limiting claudication, ischemic rest pain, nonhealing ulceration, or gangrene. Asymptomatic stenosis of a surgical graft detected on surveillance imaging may also be an indication for intervention.[32] Life expectancy and medical comorbidities must also be considered. Additionally, the likelihood of successful endovascular intervention depends heavily upon the lesion anatomy including accessibility, length, and calcification.

2. **Upper Extremity Intervention** Nonquantitative criteria similar to those for the lower extremity apply. Further indications for upper extremity intervention include symptomatic subclavian steal phenomenon due to retrograde vertebral artery flow as well as compromised flow into an internal mammary coronary artery bypass graft in the setting of ischemic coronary symptoms.

3. **Carotid Artery Stenosis** Carotid endarterectomy (CEA) reduces the stroke rate by 25%-50% for symptomatic patients with >70% stenosis by noninvasive imaging or >50% stenosis by invasive angiography[33,34] as well as for asymptomatic patients with >60% stenosis by noninvasive imaging.[35,36] Both CEA and carotid artery stenting (CAS) pose similar composite risks of stroke, death, and myocardial infarction in symptomatic and asymptomatic patients and yield identical stroke risk reduction over time.[37,38] CAS is indicated as an alternative to CEA for symptomatic or asymptomatic patients.[39]

4. **Acute Ischemic Stroke** Endovascular therapy is safe and efficacious. Patients with acute ischemic stroke are eligible for endovascular therapy with a stent retriever device if they have a prestroke modified Rankin Score of 0-1, received guideline-driven intravenous tissue plasminogen activator (tPA) with 4.5 hours of symptom onset, have acute occlusion of the internal carotid or proximal middle cerebral artery (M1), National Institute of Health Stroke Scale ≥6, Alberta stroke program early CT score (ASPECTS) ≥6, and begin procedural therapy within 6 hours of symptom onset.[40]

5. **Renal Artery Stenosis** For patients with hemodynamically significant renal artery stenosis, multisociety guidelines recommend renal artery stenting in the presence of hypertension refractory to maximally tolerated doses of three antihypertensive agents including a diuretic, inability to tolerate antihypertensive agents, hypertension before age 30 years, and unexplained pulmonary edema or heart failure.[41] Hemodynamic significance may be defined by stenosis ≥70% lumen diameter, a peak translesional gradient of ≥20 mm Hg, a mean gradient ≥10 mm Hg, resting fractional flow reserve of <0.9, or IVUS minimum luminal area of <7.8 mm^2. Patients with significant bilateral disease or a solitary kidney may be considered for intervention even in the absence of clinical symptoms, especially in the presence of chronic renal failure. Balloon angioplasty rather than balloon-expandable stenting may be employed for medically refractory symptoms of fibromuscular dysplasia in the setting of favorable anatomy.

6. **Mesenteric Artery Stenosis** Mesenteric artery stenosis can cause symptoms of chronic mesenteric ischemia; stenoses must usually be present in at least two of the three major splanchnic arteries, the celiac trunk, the superior mesenteric artery, and the inferior mesenteric artery. In most cases, ostial or proximal atherosclerotic lesions are responsible for the ischemia, and these lesions are amenable to endovascular intervention. Rarely, fibromuscular disease may cause more distal stenoses, which cannot be intervened upon.

7. **Abdominal Aortic Aneurysms** Endovascular aneurysm repair (EVAR) may be performed to reduce the risk of rupture or thromboembolism. Indications for EVAR include symptoms (typically abdominal or back pain, embolic phenomena) at any diameter, an aneurysm diameter of ≥5.5 cm regardless of symptoms, or expansion by >5 mm over 6 months.[42] Anatomic criteria for EVAR include normal aortic neck length of at least 1 cm without severe angulation, healthy common or external iliac artery landing zones of at least 15 mm, and common femoral artery diameter adequate to accommodate a 14 French sheath. Thoracic EVAR (TEVAR) is indicated for patients with descending thoracic aortic aneurysms ≥2 times the diameter of the adjacent aorta with at least 2 cm of normal landing zone both proximally and distally.[43] Reported off-label uses of TEVAR include traumatic aortic rupture, focal penetrating ulcer, and descending thoracic aortic dissection. Patients with connective tissue disorders are poor TEVAR candidates because of the high likelihood of further aortic degeneration.

8. **Deep Venous Thrombosis** Catheter-directed thrombolysis (CDT) is indicated in patients with ileofemoral thrombus, symptom duration <14 days, good functional status, life expectancy ≥1 year, and low bleeding risk. For pulmonary embolism, there is some evidence to support low-dose CDT over full-dose systemic thrombolytic therapy. In patients with shock, high bleeding risk, or failed systemic thrombolysis, catheter-assisted thrombus removal is recommended.[44]

B. **Informed Consent** Before any endovascular procedure, a health care provider must inform a competent patient or surrogate about the details of the planned procedure, expected benefits, potential risks, and reasonable alternatives. The provider should answer relevant questions, assess the individual's understanding, and ultimately allow the individual to accept or decline to procedure. For medicolegal clarity, this informed consent process is documented with the patient's or surrogate's signature on a document indicating his or her understanding and acceptance of the information presented by the provider. For a child, consent must be given by the parents, but the child should also assent if capable of comprehending some information about the intended procedure. The informed consent requirement may only be waived in cases of emergency when delay to obtain consent may jeopardize the patient's health.[45]

Suggested Readings

1. Nickoloff EL. AAPM/RSNA physics tutorial for residents: physics of flat-panel fluoroscopy systems: Survey of modern fluoroscopy imaging: flat-panel detectors versus image intensifiers and more. *Radiographics.* 2011;31(2):591-602.[46]
2. Limacher MC, Douglas PS, Germano G, et al. ACC expert consensus document. Radiation safety in the practice of cardiology. American College of Cardiology. *J Am Coll Cardiol.* 1998;31(4):892-913.[24]
3. Wennberg PW. Approach to the patient with peripheral arterial disease. *Circulation.* 2013;128(20):2241-2250.[47]
4. Thukkani AK, Kinlay S. Endovascular intervention for peripheral artery disease. *Circ Res.* 2015;116(9):1599-1613.[48]

References

1. Röntgen WC. On a new kind of rays. *Science.* 1896;3(59):227-231.
2. Tselos GD. New Jersey's Thomas Edison and the fluoroscope. *N J Med.* 1995;92(11):731-733.
3. Haschek E, Lindenthal O. A contribution to the practical use of the photography according to Roentgen. *Wien Klin.* 1896;9:63-64.
4. Osborne ED, Sutherland CG, Scholl AJ, Rowntree LG. Roentgenography of the urinary tract during excretion of sodium iodide. *JAMA.* 1923;80:368-373.
5. Heuser C. Pieloradiografía con ioduro potásico y las inyecciones intravenosas de ioduro potásico en radiografia. *Radiología.* 1919. (Sessions at the Argentine Medical Association, April 24, 1919).
6. Brooks B. Intraarterial injection of sodium iodide. *JAMA.* 1924;82:1016.
7. Moniz E. L'encephalographie arterielle, son importance dans la localization destemeurs cerebrales. *Rev Neurol.* 1927;2:72-89.
8. Binz A, Rath C. Uber biochemische eigenschaftern von Derivaten des Pyridins und Chinolins. *Biochem Ztschr.* 1928;(203):218.
9. Swick M. Excretion urography with particular reference to a newly developed compund: sodium ortho-iodohippurate. *JAMA.* 1933;101(24):1853-1857.
10. Nyman U, Ekberg O, Aspelin P. Torsten Almén (1931–2016): the father of non-ionic iodine contrast media. *Acta Radiol.* 2016;57(9):1072-1078.
11. Sette P, Dorizzi RM, Azzini AM. Vascular access: an historical perspective from Sir William Harvey to the 1956 Nobel prize to André F. Cournand, Werner Forssmann, and Dickinson W. Richards. *J Vasc Access.* 2012;13(2):137-144.
12. Seldinger SI. Catheter replacement of the needle in percutaneous arteriography; a new technique. *Acta Radiol.* 1953;39(5):368-376.

13. Sones FM, Shirey EK. Cine coronary arteriography. *Mod Concepts Cardiovasc Dis*. 1962;31:735-738.
14. Dotter CT, Judkins MP. Transluminal treatment of arteriosclerotic obstruction. Description of a new technic and a preliminary report of its application. *Circulation*. 1964;30:654-670.
15. Fogarty TJ, Cranley JJ. Catheter technic for arterial embolectomy. *Ann Surg*. 1965;161:325-330.
16. Grüntzig A. Percutaneous recanalisation of chronic arterial occlusions (Dotter principle) with a new double lumen dilatation catheter (author's transl). *Rofo*. 1976;124(1):80-86.
17. Gruntzig A. Transluminal dilatation of coronary-artery stenosis. *Lancet*. 1978;1(8058):263.
18. Puel J, Joffre F, Rousseau H, et al. Self-expanding coronary endoprosthesis in the prevention of restenosis following transluminal angioplasty. Preliminary clinical study. *Arch Mal Coeur Vaiss*. 1987;80(8):1311-1312.
19. Sigwart U, Puel J, Mirkovitch V, Joffre F, Kappenberger L. Intravascular stents to prevent occlusion and restenosis after transluminal angioplasty. *N Engl J Med*. 1987;316(12):701-706.
20. Roguin A. Stent: the man and word behind the coronary metal prosthesis. *Circ Cardiovasc Interv*. 2011;4(2):206-209.
21. White NW, Yock PG. Intravascular ultrasound: catheter-based Doppler and two-dimensional imaging. *Cardiol Clin*. 1989;7(3):525-536.
22. Fourrier JL, Bertrand ME, Auth DC, Lablanche JM, Gommeaux A, Brunetaud JM. Percutaneous coronary rotational angioplasty in humans: preliminary report. *J Am Coll Cardiol*. 1989;14(5):1278-1282.
23. Ainsbury EA, Bouffler SD, Dörr W, et al. Radiation cataractogenesis: a review of recent studies. *Radiat Res*. 2009;172(1):1-9.
24. Limacher MC, Douglas PS, Germano G, et al. ACC expert consensus document. Radiation safety in the practice of cardiology. American College of Cardiology. *J Am Coll Cardiol*. 1998;31(4):892-913.
25. Slocum NK, Grossman PM, Moscucci M, et al. The changing definition of contrast-induced nephropathy and its clinical implications: insights from the Blue Cross Blue Shield of Michigan Cardiovascular Consortium (BMC2). *Am Heart J*. 2012;163(5):829-834.
26. Tsai TT, Patel UD, Chang TI, et al. Validated contemporary risk model of acute kidney injury in patients undergoing percutaneous coronary interventions: insights from the National Cardiovascular Data Registry Cath-PCI Registry. *J Am Heart Assoc*. 2014;3(6):e001380.
27. Gurm HS, Seth M, Kooiman J, Share D. A novel tool for reliable and accurate prediction of renal complications in patients undergoing percutaneous coronary intervention. *J Am Coll Cardiol*. 2013;61(22):2242-2248.
28. Solomon R. Contrast-induced acute kidney injury (CIAKI). *Radiol Clin North Am*. 2009;47(5):783-788.
29. Gurm HS, Dixon SR, Smith DE, et al. Renal function-based contrast dosing to define safe limits of radiographic contrast media in patients undergoing percutaneous coronary interventions. *J Am Coll Cardiol*. 2011;58(9):907-914.
30. Brar SS, Aharonian V, Mansukhani P, et al. Haemodynamic-guided fluid administration for the prevention of contrast-induced acute kidney injury: the POSEIDON randomised controlled trial. *Lancet*. 2014;383(9931):1814-1823.
31. Cho KJ. Carbon dioxide angiography: scientific principles and practice. *Vasc Specialist Int*. 2015;31(3):67-80.
32. Cronenwett JL, Johnston KW. *Rutherford's Vascular Surgery*. 7th ed. Saunders; 2010.
33. Ferguson GG, Eliasziw M, Barr HW, et al. The North American symptomatic carotid endarterectomy trial: surgical results in 1415 patients. *Stroke*. 1999;30(9):1751-1758.
34. Randomised trial of endarterectomy for recently symptomatic carotid stenosis: final results of the MRC European Carotid Surgery Trial (ECST). *Lancet*. 1998;351(9113):1379-1387.
35. Halliday A, Harrison M, Hayter E, et al. 10-year stroke prevention after successful carotid endarterectomy for asymptomatic stenosis (ACST-1): a multicentre randomised trial. *Lancet*. 2010;376(9746):1074-1084.
36. Endarterectomy for asymptomatic carotid artery stenosis. Executive Committee for the Asymptomatic Carotid Atherosclerosis Study. *JAMA*. 1995;273(18):1421-1428.
37. Brott TG, Howard G, Roubin GS, et al. Long-term results of stenting versus endarterectomy for carotid-artery stenosis. *N Engl J Med*. 2016;374(11):1021-1031.
38. Gurm HS, Yadav JS, Fayad P, et al. Long-term results of carotid stenting versus endarterectomy in high-risk patients. *N Engl J Med*. 2008;358(15):1572-1579.

39. Brott TG, Halperin JL, Abbara S, et al. 2011 ASA/ACCF/AHA/AANN/AANS/ACR/ASNR/CNS/SAIP/SCAI/SIR/SNIS/SVM/SVS guideline on the management of patients with extracranial carotid and vertebral artery disease: a report of the American College of Cardiology Foundation/American Heart Association Task Force on Practice Guidelines, and the American Stroke Association, American Association of Neuroscience Nurses, American Association of Neurological Surgeons, American College of Radiology, American Society of Neuroradiology, Congress of Neurological Surgeons, Society of Atherosclerosis Imaging and Prevention, Society for Cardiovascular Angiography and Interventions, Society of Interventional Radiology, Society of NeuroInterventional Surgery, Society for Vascular Medicine, and Society for Vascular Surgery. *J Am Coll Cardiol.* 2011;57(8):e16-94.
40. Powers WJ, Derdeyn CP, Biller J, et al. 2015 American Heart Association/American Stroke Association focused update of the 2013 guidelines for the early management of patients with acute ischemic stroke regarding endovascular treatment: a guideline for healthcare professionals from the American Heart Association/American Stroke Association. *Stroke.* 2015;46:3020-3035. doi:10.1161/STR.0000000000000074.
41. Hirsch AT, Haskal ZJ, Hertzer NR, et al. ACC/AHA 2005 Practice Guidelines for the management of patients with peripheral arterial disease (lower extremity, renal, mesenteric, and abdominal aortic): a collaborative report from the American Association for Vascular Surgery/Society for Vascular Surgery, Society for Cardiovascular Angiography and Interventions, Society for Vascular Medicine and Biology, Society of Interventional Radiology, and the ACC/AHA Task Force on Practice Guidelines (Writing Committee to Develop Guidelines for the Management of Patients With Peripheral Arterial Disease): endorsed by the American Association of Cardiovascular and Pulmonary Rehabilitation; National Heart, Lung, and Blood Institute; Society for Vascular Nursing; TransAtlantic Inter-Society Consensus; and Vascular Disease Foundation. *Circulation.* 2006;113(11):e463-e654.
42. Chaikof EL, Brewster DC, Dalman RL, et al. SVS practice guidelines for the care of patients with an abdominal aortic aneurysm: executive summary. *J Vasc Surg.* 2009;50(4):880-896.
43. Bavaria JE, Appoo JJ, Makaroun MS, et al. Endovascular stent grafting versus open surgical repair of descending thoracic aortic aneurysms in low-risk patients: a multicenter comparative trial. *J Thorac Cardiovasc Surg.* 2007;133(2):369-377.
44. Kearon C, Akl EA, Ornelas J, et al. Antithrombotic therapy for VTE disease: CHEST guideline and expert panel report. *Chest.* 2016;149(2):315-352.
45. Appelbaum PS. Clinical practice. Assessment of patients' competence to consent to treatment. *N Engl J Med.* 2007;357(18):1834-1840.
46. Nickoloff EL. AAPM/RSNA physics tutorial for residents: physics of flat-panel fluoroscopy systems: Survey of modern fluoroscopy imaging: flat-panel detectors versus image intensifiers and more. *Radiographics.* 2011;31(2):591-602.
47. Wennberg PW. Approach to the patient with peripheral arterial disease. *Circulation.* 2013;128(20):2241-2250.
48. Thukkani AK, Kinlay S. Endovascular intervention for peripheral artery disease. *Circ Res.* 2015;116(9):1599-1613.

CHAPTER 2

Acute Stroke Intervention

Ryan M. Hebert, MD, Fouad Chouairi, BS, Branden Cord, MD, PhD, Samuel Sommaruga, MD, Michael Mercier, BA, Anna Lynn, BS, Andrew Koo, BS, Stacy Chu, MD, and Charles Matouk, MD, FRCS(C)

Key Points

- An occlusion in major blood vessels at the base of the skull supplying the brain (paired internal and vertebral arteries) as well as their proximal intracranial branches (anterior cerebral artery, middle cerebral artery, and basilar artery) is referred to as an LVO (large vessel occlusion).
- It is estimated that LVOs account for at least 10%-15% of all acute ischemic strokes.
- Mechanical thrombectomy for anterior circulation LVOs is now standard of care for patients presenting within 6 hours of stroke onset but in select cases can be of value up to 24 hours since the event.

I. Introduction

In 2015, five clinical trials were published that established mechanical thrombectomy as a new standard of care in the management of large vessel occlusions (LVOs) of the brain.[1-5] These studies and those that followed forever changed the paradigm of acute stoke management from solely focused on the timely administration of intravenous (IV) thrombolytics to emergent interventional revascularization.[6-9] This is a watershed moment in acute stroke care. The stroke community is currently reorganizing triage protocols so that as many people as possible can benefit from this lifesaving intervention.

This chapter will provide a brief review of stroke epidemiology and pathophysiology, clinical trials data, and mechanical revascularization strategies for the nonexpert interventionist. The focus will be on the subset of acute ischemic strokes potentially amenable to mechanical revascularization, ie, LVOs.

II. Acute Stroke 101

A. Stroke Epidemiology

1. The definition of stroke is an acute-onset loss of neurological function (typically focal) that results from a vascular etiology. There are two main types of strokes: (1) **ischemic** (resulting from an obstruction within a brain blood vessel) and (2) **hemorrhagic** (resulting from vessel rupture). Ischemic stroke is far more common (accounting for 87% of all stroke cases) and is the topic of this review.[10]

2. Stroke is a common disease. Every year in the United States, approximately 800,000 people will have a stroke. More than three-fourth of these cases will be first presentations, and nearly 20% will suffer a second stroke within 4 years.[11,12]

3. Stroke is a leading cause of death and disability. It is the 5th leading cause of death behind heart disease, cancer, chronic lower respiratory disease, and accidents (unintentional injuries). Every 4 minutes, someone in the United States dies of a stroke, accounting for 130,000 deaths per year (or 1 in 20 deaths overall). Because stroke

often takes people out of the workforce, it represents a tremendous societal cost estimated at 34 billion dollars per year.[13]

4. Often, the largest stroke syndromes with the worst clinical outcomes result from a major blood vessel in the brain being occluded. These major blood vessels are the vessels at the base of the skull supplying the brain (paired internal and vertebral arteries) as well as their proximal intracranial branches (anterior cerebral artery, middle cerebral artery, and basilar artery). A blockage in any of these vessels is referred to as an LVO. It is estimated that LVOs account for 10%-15% of all acute ischemic strokes.[14,15] It is these ischemic stroke patients who are potentially candidates for mechanical revascularization.

B. Stroke Pathophysiology

1. In acute ischemic stroke, if a territory of the brain is solely supplied by a single-end vessel, then occlusion of the vessel will result in brain infarction within a very short period of time. This most-at-risk brain territory is referred to as the **ischemic core.** Just outside of this core area is an area of the brain that experiences decreased, but somewhat maintained, cerebral blood flow (CBF) because of arterial collaterals. This area is referred to as the **penumbra.** Average CBF in a healthy adult is around 50 mL/100 g/min. Cellular function is perturbed in areas where CBF drops to 15-20 mL/100 g/min. Cells in this penumbral region may survive for several hours before irreversible cell death, ie, cerebral infarction, ensues. CBF <10 mL/100 g/min produces failure of cellular ionic gradients. If flow is not improved, cell death occurs in less than 60 minutes.[16] An important clinical correlate of this basic stroke pathophysiology is that a clinician at the bedside cannot determine whether a patient with an acute ischemic stroke, eg, acute-onset hemiplegia, has a penumbral (reversible) or core (irreversible) neurological deficit.

2. Although time plays a significant role in stroke pathophysiology, it is not the only factor. The brain is supplied by a robust network of arterial collaterals, primarily arising from the circle of Willis (COW). The COW is supplied anteriorly by the internal carotid arteries (anterior circulation) and posteriorly by the vertebrobasilar system (posterior circulation). A complete COW is found in less than 50% of people. An incomplete COW has been associated with increased stroke risk.[17] COW facilitates leptomeningeal collateralization between the middle cerebral artery (MCA), anterior cerebral artery (ACA) and posterior cerebral artery (PCA) territories. Some patients have good collateral circulations, others do not. It is the strength of these collaterals that helps define, in large part, the size of the ischemic core and penumbra. A second important clinical correlate is that the penumbral area is dynamic in space and time. For example, blood pressure augmentation may better support brain tissue supplied by a collateral network for a longer period of time, effectively increasing the size of the penumbra. Collateral status can be assessed noninvasively and has been correlated to stroke outcome.[18,19]

3. **Noninvasive Imaging of "At-Risk Brain"—Clinical Assessment of Ischemic Core, Penumbra, and Collateral Circulation**
   a. Patients being evaluated for stroke universally undergo noncontrast computed tomography (NCCT) of the brain. This is primarily used to identify hemorrhagic stroke for intravenous tissue plasminogen activator (IV tPA) exclusion. NCCT is also useful in identifying early ischemic parenchymal changes. The Alberta Stroke Program Early CT (ASPECT) Score is a popular method to quantify anterior circulation early ischemic change (EIC) on computed tomography (CT) to predict the outcome after IV thrombolysis. In this scoring system, 7 points are assigned to the MCA territory and 3 to subcortical structures. The scoring system starts at 10. Each region showing EIC accounts for a 1-point deduction. Lower ASPECT Scores were associated with poor outcomes after IV tPA.[20]
   b. CT angiography (CTA) is an extremely useful diagnostic tool and establishes the diagnosis of LVO. In addition, it provides the interventionist with valuable technical information about the aortic arch, vessel tortuosity, and carotid bifurcation disease. CTA of the head also provides important information about collateral blood flow to the territory at risk. Several studies have shown that good collaterals on CTA are predictors of good outcome after mechanical thrombectomy.[18,21]
   c. CT perfusion is performed by intravenously administering a bolus of contrast and using serial CT scans to follow the contrast bolus through the intracranial circulation. This imaging technique provides estimates of CBF, mean transit time (MTT), time-to-peak (TTP), and cerebral blood volume (CBV). Decreased CBF and CBV reflect the ischemic core, ie, irreversibly injured (nonsalvageable) brain. The penumbra is demonstrated as a region of brain with preserved CBV and increased MTT (or TTP).[22-27]
   d. MRI (magnetic resonance imaging) is more sensitive than CT for detecting cerebral ischemia and infarction. Diffusion-weighted imaging (DWI) can detect ischemic changes within 5-10 minutes of symptom onset. T2-weighted sequences identify subacute infarction 6-24 hours after ictus. Hyperintensity on DWI is the best imaging correlate of the ischemic core.[28,29]
   e. There is vigorous debate regarding utilization of CT perfusion and MRI in the evaluation and triage of acute ischemic stroke. Both have been shown to increase time to puncture and are not associated with improved outcomes. However, in certain scenarios, both provide invaluable data that aid in complex clinical decision-making.[30]

III. Intravenous Tissue Plasminogen Activator—Long-Time Standard of Care and Important Limitations

A. **NINDS and ECASS** In 1995, the National Institute of Neurological Disorders and Stroke (NINDS) published a paper in the *New England Journal of Medicine* supporting the efficacy of IV recombinant tissue plasminogen activator (tPA) in the setting of acute stroke.[31] Their results failed to show a statistically significant, clinical improvement or resolution of stroke symptoms at 24 hours. However, at 3 months, there was a statistical, clinical improvement in the IV tPA group compared with placebo. This clinical improvement was realized despite an increase in the rate of symptomatic intracerebral hemorrhage (6% vs 0.6%). These results were confirmed by the European Cooperative Acute Stroke Study (ECASS) that also extended the time window in which IV tPA could be administered (4.5 hours after stroke onset).[32] These studies established the first effective treatment for acute ischemic stroke and defined a new standard of care.

B. Intravenous Tissue Plasminogen Activator for Ischemic Stroke Limitations

1. **A narrow therapeutic window.** The narrow window from stroke onset to administration of IV tPA means that most patients arrive in hospital too late to receive the medication. Approximately one-fourth of patients have so-called "wake up" strokes of uncertain time of onset and are therefore ineligible to receive IV tPA. On average, only 7% of patients presenting with acute ischemic stroke receive IV tPA.[33-37]
2. **Limited efficacy for LVOs and large stroke syndromes.** In 2006, Smith et al. reported on a consecutive series of patients with large stroke syndromes and LVOs.[38] They divided their study population into two groups: one group in which IV tPA achieved recanalization and another with persistent vessel occlusion. The group in which recanalization was achieved, albeit much smaller than the group with persistent occlusion, realized much better clinical outcomes. These data are consistent with other reports demonstrating poor recanalization rates for internal carotid artery (ICA) terminus and basilar artery occlusions.[39]
3. **Increased rate of systemic hemorrhage.** The administration of a systemic thrombolytic excludes an important segment of patients on oral anticoagulants or director factor Xa inhibitors; recent neurosurgery, stroke, head trauma, or other major surgery; and history of intracranial hemorrhage.[37]

IV. Intra-arterial Thrombolytics, First-Generation Mechanical Thrombectomy Devices, and Failed Clinical Trials

A. **PROACT I, PROACT II, IMS Trials** Given the limited efficacy of IV tPA, especially for patients with large stroke syndromes and LVOs, intra-arterial (IA) administration of thrombolytics was studied. In 1998, the Prolyse in Acute Cerebral Thromboembolism (PROACT) trial compared recombinant pro-urokinase with placebo (IV heparin) for MCA occlusion.[40] Recanalization and hemorrhage were more common in patients receiving pro-urokinase, with only recanalization reaching statistical significance. PROACT II aimed to prove clinical efficacy by comparing modified Rankin scores at 90 days of patients receiving pro-urokinase versus placebo.[41] Recanalization in the treatment arm was 66% compared with 18% in the placebo group. Modified Rankin Score (mRS) less than or equal to 2, ie, favorable outcome, at 90 days was 40% in the treatment arm compared with 25% in the placebo arm. Symptomatic intracranial hemorrhage (ICH) was 10% in the treatment arm compared with 2% in the placebo arm. It is important to note that none of the patients in PROACT I or II received IV tPA. The Interventional Management of Stroke (IMS) trial was a single-armed, safety, and feasibility study of

IV tPA plus IA tPA.[42] In addition to 0.6 mg/kg of IV tPA, patients received a 2 mg IA bolus of tPA into and beyond the clot. A total of 22 mg of tPA was given over 2 hours. Treatment was stopped if TIMI 3 recanalization was achieved before 2 hours. Compared with historical NINDS placebo–treated patients, IA-treated patients in IMS had significantly better outcomes at 3 months. IMS II confirmed these findings.[43]

B. **MERCI Trial** In 2005, the MERCI trial was conducted to evaluate the safety and efficacy of the Merci retriever device for mechanical thrombectomy in patients ineligible for IV tPA.[44] The Merci retriever is a preshaped, tapered, helical device consisting of 5 loops. The described procedure consisted of placing a 9-French balloon guide catheter (BGC) into the carotid artery. A microcatheter was navigated through the thrombus. The Merci device was deployed across the thrombus. The BGC was inflated, suction applied, and the Merci device rotated five times. The device and microcatheter were then retrieved in unison.[45] Results of the MERCI trial were promising. The MERCI device alone led to a recanalization rate of 54%, while recanalization rates for MERCI plus IV tPA was 69%.[46,47] Complication rates were 10% for symptomatic ICH (4% higher than IV tPA alone) and 10% for vessel perforation.[47,48]

C. **SYNTHESIS, IMS-III, and MR RESCUE: 2013 Trials**

1. In 2013, three trials were published in the *New England Journal of Medicine* comparing IV tPA with endovascular therapy for acute ischemic stroke.[49-51] SYNTHESIS randomized patients to IV alteplase or endovascular therapy. Noncontrast CT was the only imaging modality used for screening. Intervention occurred within 6 hours of stroke onset. If no occlusion was present on angiography, alteplase was administered to the presumed vascular territory. If occlusion was seen on angiography, the endovascular device used for clot retrieval was at the discretion of the interventionist. Of the 109 patients in the interventional group, only 56 were treated with a device. There was no difference in mRS at 3 months between the interventional group and the IV alteplase group. In addition, interventional treatment delayed therapy by one hour.[49]

2. IMS-III was the largest of the 2013 trials enrolling 656 participants.[50] Patients were required to have a baseline NIHSS of 10 or greater, ie, large stroke syndromes. All patients received IV tPA within 3 hours of stroke onset. Patients randomized to the interventional arm received treatment within 5 hours of symptom onset. Treatment had to be completed before 7 hours of stroke onset. Although CTA was used in the latter part of the study, most patients were randomized to intervention without proving a LVO. Intervention was primarily microcatheter-based administration of IA tPA. The Merci device was used in 28.4% of the interventional group. The Solitaire stent retriever was available toward the end of the study and only used in 1.5% of study patients.[52] There was not a significant difference in independent outcomes between the interventional group and the IV tPA group. A major deficiency of the IMS-III study was that CTA was not utilized to randomize patients between treatment groups. A subgroup analysis of the IMS-III subjects with a proven large

vessel occlusion revealed a statistically significant difference in the rate of 24-hour recanalization. There was also a trend toward improved functional independence.[53]

3. Mechanical Retrieval and Recanalization of Stroke Clots Using Embolectomy (MR RESCUE) randomized patients to mechanical thrombectomy versus medical therapy based on a documented LVO after IV tPA and "favorable penumbral pattern."[51] A "favorable penumbral pattern" was defined as a core infarct volume less than 90 mL and a predicted infarct of 70% or less of the territory at risk. Mechanical thrombectomy was initiated within 8 hours of onset. There was no significant difference in mRS at 90 days between the groups. Interestingly, revascularization measured on day 7 by MRA or CTA was not different between the 2 groups. Interestingly, the patients who had a favorable penumbral pattern 3 hours after onset had better outcomes, regardless of treatment arm. This supports the hypothesis that collateral status is an important predictor of stroke outcome. The 2013 trials were marred by a number of suboptimal conditions. Patient selection was poor. Indeed, most of the studies did not confirm an LVO before randomization! Study conclusions were inappropriately generalized to mechanical thrombectomy as a concept even though IA administration of thrombolytics was the dominant form of endovascular therapy. Finally, early generation devices were inefficient and, simply put, had poor recanalization rates.

V. MR CLEAN and the Emergence of a New Standard of Care

In 2015, five clinical trials were published which studied mechanical thrombectomy in the era or improved patient selection and second-generation mechanical thrombectomy devices, ie, stent retrievers.[1-5]

A. **MR CLEAN Trial** The Multicenter Randomized Clinical Trial of Endovascular Treatment for Acute Ischemic Stroke in the Netherlands (MR CLEAN) was the first of these trials to be reported.[1] 500 patients with CTA-confirmed LVOs of the distal ICA or proximal MCA were randomized to IV tPA plus mechanical thrombectomy within 6 hours of stroke onset or IV tPA alone. Mechanical thrombectomy was performed with a stent retriever in 97.4% of the interventions. A favorable outcome, defined as mRS 0-2 at 90 days, was achieved in 33% of the interventional group, compared with 19% of the IV tPA–alone group. There was no significant difference in ICH or 90-day mortality.

B. **ESCAPE Trial** The Endovascular treatment for Small Core and Anterior circulation Proximal occlusion with Emphasis on minimizing CT to recanalization times (ESCAPE) trial sought to enroll 500 patients but stopped at 316 owing to efficacy.[3] Patients had an ASPECTS greater than or equal to 6. CTA confirmed an LVO of the anterior circulation. Intervention had to be started within 12 hours of stroke onset. In the intervention arm, 53% of patients achieved a good outcome, measured by an mRS 0-2 at 90 days, compared with only 29% of the medical arm. A stent retriever was used in 86% of cases. There was no difference in ICH. Mortality was reduced in the interventional arm.

C. **EXTEND-IA Trial** The Extending the Time for Thrombolysis in Emergency Neurological Deficits—Intra-Arterial (EXTEND-IA) trial randomized patients with ICA or MCA occlusions to IV tPA plus mechanical thrombectomy, using the Solitaire revascularization device (a stent retriever, Medtronic Neurovascular), versus IV tPA alone.[2] Perfusion imaging using RAPID software was used in all subjects. CT perfusion inclusion criteria consisted of mismatch ratio >1.2, absolute mismatch volume >10 mL, and ischemic core volume <70 mL. There were two primary outcomes: reperfusion of the vascular territory at 24 hours (measured by percentage reduction in the perfusion lesion volume) and 8-point improvement in NIHSS (or NIHSS 0-1) at day 3. The trial was stopped early (after enrollment of 70 patients) owing to the results of MR CLEAN. Median reperfusion at 24 hours was 100%. Neurologic improvement occurred in 80% of the mechanical thrombectomy group compared with 37% of the IV tPA group.

D. **SWIFT PRIME and REVASCAT Trials** The Solitaire with the Intention for Thrombectomy as Primary Endovascular Treatment for Acute Ischemic Stroke (SWIFT PRIME) compared IV tPA alone with IV tPA with stent retriever mechanical thrombectomy in patients with LVO presenting within 6 hours of symptom onset.[5] Perfusion imaging was used in 158 of 196 patients (83 of the interventional group) to screen patients. The trial was stopped early owing to efficacy. The chance of having an mRS 0-2 was 60% in the stent retriever group compared with 35% treated with IV tPA alone. The number needed to treat was 2.6. At the same time SWIFT PRIME was published, the Randomized Trial of Revascularization with Solitaire FR Device versus Best Medical Therapy in the Treatment of Acute Stroke Due to Anterior Circulation Large Vessel Occlusion Presenting within 8 hours of Symptom Onset (REVASCAT) trial reported its outcomes after closing the trial early due to the positive results of MR CLEAN.[4] Again, patients with known LVO assigned to the interventional group were more likely to be independent at 90 days compared to the patients receiving IV tPA alone. Infarct volume at 24 hours was smaller in the interventional group (16.3 mL) versus the medical group (38.6 mL).

Taken together, the 2015 stent retriever trials defined a new standard of care for acute ischemic stroke secondary to anterior circulation LVOs. MR CLEAN and ESCAPE showed a benefit from mechanical thrombectomy even in patients older than 80 years. Patients with large stroke syndromes as measured by NIHSS (SWIFT PRIME >17, ESCAPE >20, MR CLEAN >20) also showed benefit.

VI. The Number of Patients Eligible for Mechanical Thrombectomy Continues to Increase

A. **Posterior Circulation Strokes/Acute Basilar Occlusion** continues to increase including posterior circulation strokes/acute basilar occlusion. With the exception of a handful of patients in IMS III and SYNTHESIS, the 2015 mechanical thrombectomy trials studied anterior circulation LVOs. In part, this reflects the exceptionally high morbidity and mortality of acute basilar artery occlusion (80%-90%) without intervention. Most interventionists are reluctant to offer aggressive treatment given the grave natural history. A majority of reports in the literature support this philosophy. It is unlikely that a randomized clinical trial will ever be performed to answer this question conclusively.[54,55]

B. Extending the Therapeutic Window for Mechanical Thrombectomy

1. **Mechanical Thrombectomy for Anterior Circulation** Mechanical thrombectomy for anterior circulation LVOs is now standard of care for patients presenting within 6 hours of stroke onset. Although time is an important factor, collateral vascular networks are also important in predicting risk of stroke completion. Indeed, two recent trials—DAWN and DEFUSE-3—have extended the therapeutic window for mechanical thrombectomy to 16-24 hours from last known well in carefully selected patients with evidence of good collateral circulations.[7,8]

C. Chasing More Distal Clots While the major mechanical thrombectomy trials focused on major branch occlusions of the COW, more distal clots can also result in disproportionately large, disabling strokes. Growing evidence suggests that chasing more distal clots may be of substantial benefit when facing a potentially large, or disabling, stroke syndrome, eg, aphasia.[56]

D. Example Cases From Yale New Haven Hospital (YNHH)

Case 1

A 65-year-old man with multiple cardiovascular risk factors suddenly develops left-sided hemiplegia and dysarthria consistent with a large right MCA syndrome (NIHSS 17). He is emergently transferred to YNHH where a CT of the head demonstrates no evidence of intracerebral hemorrhage and minimal EICs. Because he is within 4.5 hours of symptom onset and he has no contraindications, IV tPA is administered. A CTA confirms a proximal R MCA occlusion, and the patient is taken emergently for mechanical thrombectomy. He is an "MR CLEAN" patient, similar to those enrolled in the 2015 clinical trials (Fig. 2.1).

The procedure is performed under conscious sedation. An 8F short sheath is inserted at the right groin. A 6F long sheath is positioned in the proximal R common carotid artery. Under roadmap guidance, the proximal right MCA occlusion is crossed with a 027 microcatheter navigated over a soft 014 microguidewire. A 068 reperfusion catheter is positioned at the face of the clot. A stent retriever is deployed across the occlusion, the microcatheter withdrawn, and the reperfusion catheter placed on pump suction. After several minutes, the reperfusion catheter and stent retriever are withdrawn in unison. Clot fragments are demonstrated on the stent retriever and within the reperfusion catheter. Control runs demonstrate complete revascularization after "one pass." Time from groin puncture to revascularization = 16 minutes.

Clinical examination on the angiography table confirms a rapidly improving examination result. One day after the procedure, he had nearly full strength on his left side with mild, persistent dysarthria. At his 3-month follow-up, he had made a near-complete clinical recovery.

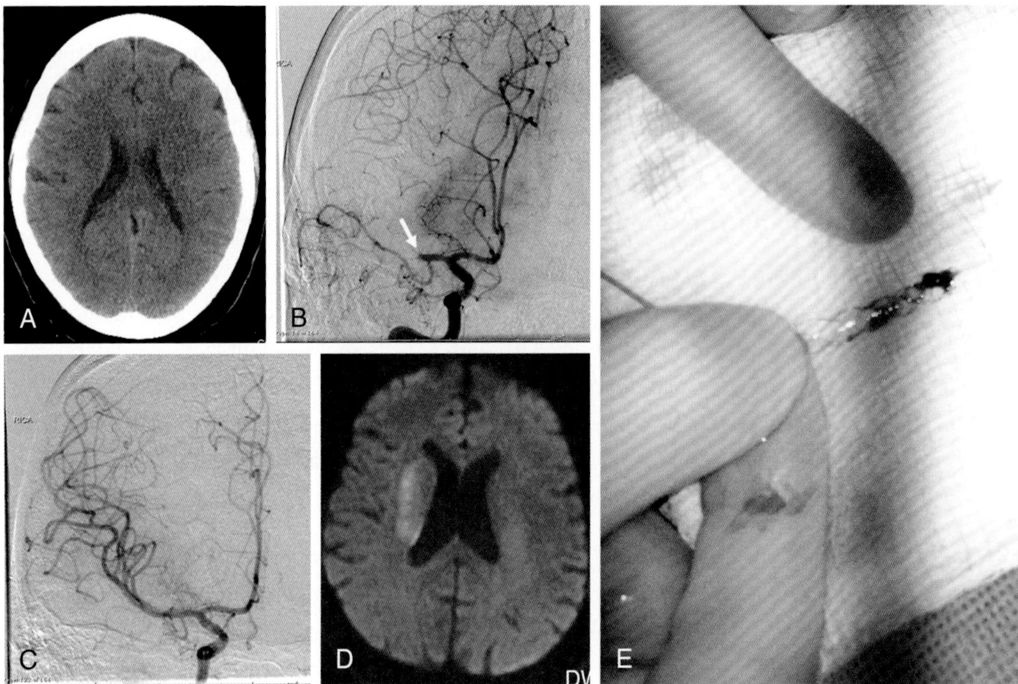

FIGURE 2.1: A, Normal noncontrast head CT. B, AP projection of a right internal carotid artery injection revealing a mid-M1 occlusion. C, Frontal projection of a right internal carotid artery injection after thrombectomy showing recanalization of the right MCA. D, MRI DWI sequence demonstrating final stroke burden. E, Stent retriever with clot.

Case 2

A 75-year-old man with atrial fibrillation (not on anticoagulation) was found slumped over the steering wheel of his car. He was last seen normal 8 hours ago after dropping his granddaughter off at school. He is emergently transferred to YNHH. Clinical examination reveals a large left MCA stroke syndrome (NIHSS 22) characterized by right-sided hemiplegia and global aphasia. A CT of the head demonstrates no evidence of intracerebral hemorrhage and minimal EICs. Because he is more than 8 hours from symptom onset, IV tPA is not administered. A CTA confirms a proximal L MCA occlusion. A hyperacute MRI demonstrates a small ischemic core and large territory at risk. He is taken emergently for mechanical thrombectomy (Fig. 2.2).

Again, the procedure is performed under conscious sedation. Two "passes" are required of a stent retriever used in conjunction with a large-bore reperfusion catheter placed on pump suction at the face of the clot. Clot fragments are retrieved on the stent retriever and within the reperfusion catheter. Control runs demonstrate near-complete revascularization. Time from groin puncture to revascularization = 34 minutes.

Clinical examination on the angiography table confirms a slowly improving examination result. By the next morning, he has definitely improved right-sided strength and can answer simple questions correctly. At his 3-month follow-up, he has made a near-complete motor recovery and has persistent, mild word-finding difficulty.

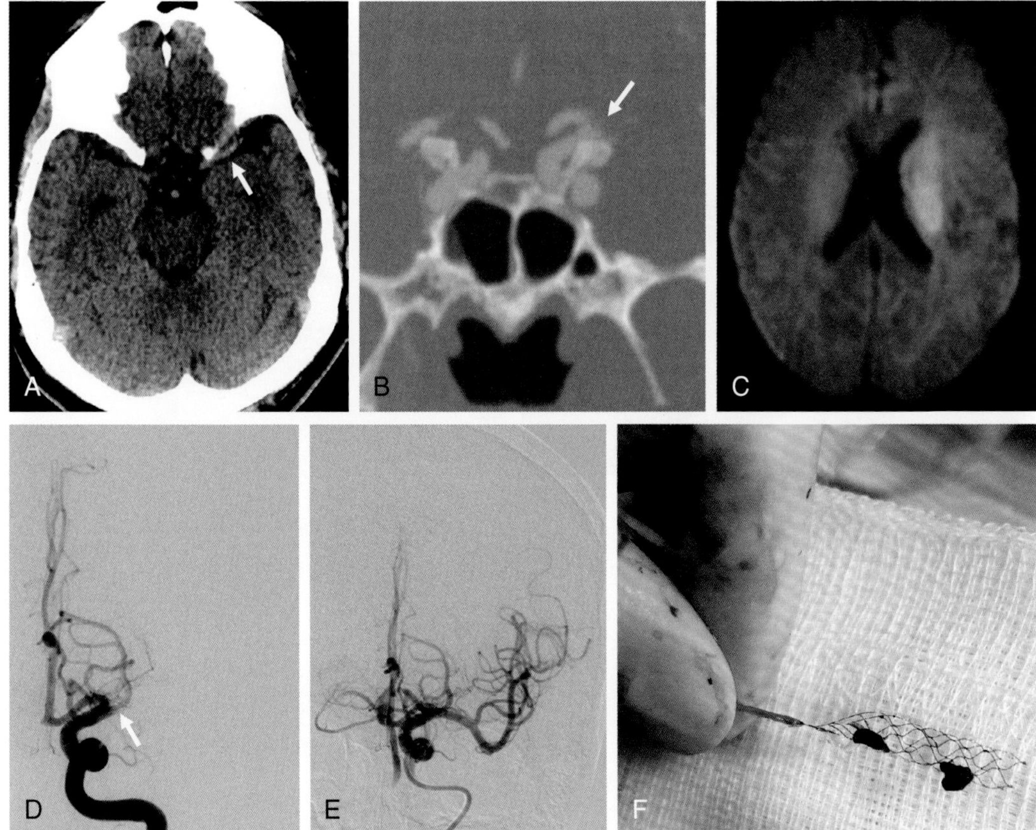

FIGURE 2.2: A, Noncontrast head CT revealing a hyperdense left MCA sign. B, Coronal CTA revealing proximal occlusion of the left M1 segment. C, Hyperacute MRI demonstrating small core infarct. D, Frontal projection angiogram confirming proximal M1 occlusion. E, Frontal projection after thrombectomy revealing recanalization. F, Stent retriever with clot.

Case 3

A 43-year-old woman with a history of prior strokes presents to an outside emergency room with vague complaints of vertigo, nausea and vomiting, and tingling in her arms. Several hours later she develops hearing loss and double vision. A CT of the head demonstrates nil acute. Several hours later she suddenly becomes unresponsive with extensor posturing (NIHSS 33). She is intubated for airway protection. A repeat CT of the head again demonstrates nil acute, but a CTA shows an acute basilar artery occlusion. Although acute basilar artery occlusions were not well studied in the 2015 (or subsequent) clinical trials, it portends a grave prognosis without aggressive intervention. She is transferred to YNHH for mechanical thrombectomy more than 16 hours after symptom onset (Fig. 2.3).

A single pass is performed with a stent retriever alone. Clot fragments are retrieved on the stent retriever. Control runs demonstrate near-complete revascularization. Time from groin puncture to revascularization = 18 minutes.

Three days later, she has a markedly improved clinical examination with normal level of consciousness, right-greater-than-left-sided weakness, and double vision. At her 3-month follow-up, she is ambulating independently and caring for herself. Prism glasses help with persistent double vision.

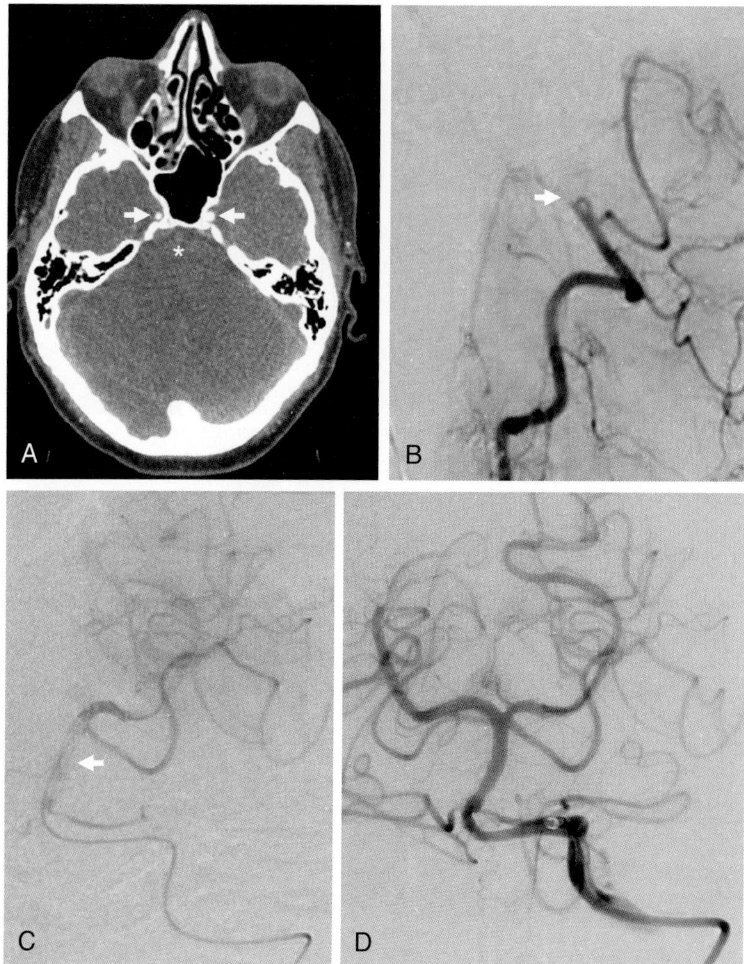

FIGURE 2.3: A, CTA demonstrating opacification of the bilateral internal carotid arteries without opacification of the basilar artery. B, Lateral projection angiogram revealing basilar summit occlusion. C, Frontal projection angiogram performed through the microcatheter placed distal to the occlusion revealing a patent right posterior cerebral artery distal to the clot. D, Frontal projection angiogram performed after thrombectomy revealing recanalization of the posterior circulation after thrombectomy.

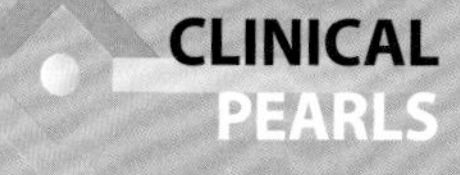

- A clinician at the bedside cannot determine whether a patient with an acute ischemic stroke, eg, acute-onset hemiplegia, has a penumbral (reversible) or core (irreversible) neurological deficit.
- Although not essential for triage and evaluation of *every* acute stroke patients, perfusion imaging provides invaluable data in complex clinical decision-making and may be of substantial benefit when the diagnosis of stroke is in doubt or late in the therapeutic window.
- The 2015 stent retriever trials defined a new standard of care for acute ischemic stroke secondary to anterior circulation LVOs.

Suggested Readings

1. Campbell BCV, Donnan GA, Lees KR, et al. Endovascular stent thrombectomy: the new standard of care for large vessel ischaemic stroke. *Lancet Neurol.* 2015;14:846-854.
2. Goyal M, Menon BK, van Zwam WH, et al. Endovascular thrombectomy after large-vessel ischaemic stroke: a meta-analysis of individual patient data from five randomised trials. *Lancet.* 2016;387:1723-1731.

References

1. Berkhemer OA, Fransen PS, Beumer D, et al. A randomized trial of intraarterial treatment for acute ischemic stroke. *N Engl J Med.* 2015;372:11-20.
2. Campbell BC, Mitchell PJ, Kleinig TJ, et al. Endovascular therapy for ischemic stroke with perfusion-imaging selection. *N Engl J Med.* 2015;372:1009-1018.
3. Goyal M, Demchuk AM, Menon BK, et al. Randomized assessment of rapid endovascular treatment of ischemic stroke. *N Engl J Med.* 2015;372:1019-1030.
4. Jovin TG, Chamorro A, Cobo E, et al. Thrombectomy within 8 hours after symptom onset in ischemic stroke. *N Engl J Med.* 2015;372:2296-2306.
5. Saver JL, Goyal M, Bonafe A, et al. Stent-retriever thrombectomy after intravenous t-PA vs. t-PA alone in stroke. *N Engl J Med.* 2015;372:2285-2295.
6. Goyal M, Menon BK, van Zwam WH, et al. Endovascular thrombectomy after large-vessel ischaemic stroke: a meta-analysis of individual patient data from five randomised trials. *Lancet.* 2016;387:1723-1731.
7. Nogueira RG, Jadhav AP, Haussen DC, et al. Thrombectomy 6 to 24 hours after stroke with a mismatch between deficit and infarct. *N Engl J Med.* 2018;378:11-21.
8. Albers GW, Marks MP, Kemp S, et al. Thrombectomy for stroke at 6 to 16 hours with selection by perfusion imaging. *N Engl J Med.* 2018;378:708-718.
9. Campbell BCV, Donnan GA, Lees KR, et al. Endovascular stent thrombectomy: the new standard of care for large vessel ischaemic stroke. *Lancet Neurol.* 2015;14:846-854.
10. Sacco RL, Kasner SE, Broderick JP, et al. An updated definition of stroke for the 21st century: a statement for healthcare professionals from the American Heart Association/American Stroke Association. *Stroke.* 2013;44:2064-2089.
11. Writing Group M, Mozaffarian D, Benjamin EJ, et al. Executive summary: heart disease and stroke statistics–2016 update: a report from the American Heart Association. *Circulation.* 2016;133:447-454.
12. Feng W, Hendry RM, Adams RJ. Risk of recurrent stroke, myocardial infarction, or death in hospitalized stroke patients. *Neurology.* 2010;74:588-593.
13. Benjamin EJ, Virani SS, Callaway CW, et al. Heart disease and stroke statistics-2018 update: a report from the American Heart Association. *Circulation.* 2018;137:e67-e492.
14. Smith WS, Lev MH, English JD, et al. Significance of large vessel intracranial occlusion causing acute ischemic stroke and TIA. *Stroke.* 2009;40:3834-3840.
15. Rai AT, Seldon AE, Boo S, et al. A population-based incidence of acute large vessel occlusions and thrombectomy eligible patients indicates significant potential for growth of endovascular stroke therapy in the USA. *J Neurointerv Surg.* 2017;9:722-726.
16. Astrup J, Siesjo BK, Symon L. Thresholds in cerebral ischemia – the ischemic penumbra. *Stroke.* 1981;12:723-725.
17. Krabbe-Hartkamp MJ, van der Grond J, de Leeuw FE, et al. Circle of Willis: morphologic variation on three-dimensional time-of-flight MR angiograms. *Radiology.* 1998;207:103-111.
18. Miteff F, Levi CR, Bateman GA, et al. The independent predictive utility of computed tomography angiographic collateral status in acute ischaemic stroke. *Brain.* 2009;132:2231-2238.
19. Silvestrini M, Altamura C, Cerqua R, et al. Early activation of intracranial collateral vessels influences the outcome of spontaneous internal carotid artery dissection. *Stroke.* 2011;42:139-143.

20. Barber PA, Demchuk AM, Zhang J, et al. Validity and reliability of a quantitative computed tomography score in predicting outcome of hyperacute stroke before thrombolytic therapy. ASPECTS Study Group. Alberta stroke programme early CT score. *Lancet*. 2000;355:1670-1674.
21. Menon BK, Smith EE, Modi J, et al. Regional leptomeningeal score on CT angiography predicts clinical and imaging outcomes in patients with acute anterior circulation occlusions. *AJNR Am J Neuroradiol*. 2011;32:1640-1645.
22. d'Esterre CD, Roversi G, Padroni M, et al. CT perfusion cerebral blood volume does not always predict infarct core in acute ischemic stroke. *Neurol Sci*. 2015;36:1777-1783.
23. Hatazawa J, Shimosegawa E, Toyoshima H, et al. Cerebral blood volume in acute brain infarction: a combined study with dynamic susceptibility contrast MRI and 99mTc-HMPAO-SPECT. *Stroke*. 1999;30:800-806.
24. Murphy BD, Fox AJ, Lee DH, et al. Identification of penumbra and infarct in acute ischemic stroke using computed tomography perfusion-derived blood flow and blood volume measurements. *Stroke*. 2006;37:1771-1777.
25. Heiss WD. Flow thresholds of functional and morphological damage of brain tissue. *Stroke*. 1983;14:329-331.
26. Lui YW, Tang ER, Allmendinger AM, et al. Evaluation of CT perfusion in the setting of cerebral ischemia: patterns and pitfalls. *AJNR Am J Neuroradiol*. 2010;31:1552-1563.
27. Campbell BC, Weir L, Desmond PM, et al. CT perfusion improves diagnostic accuracy and confidence in acute ischaemic stroke. *J Neurol Neurosurg Psychiatry*. 2013;84:613-618.
28. Birenbaum D, Bancroft LW, Felsberg GJ. Imaging in acute stroke. *West J Emerg Med*. 2011;12:67-76.
29. van Everdingen KJ, van der Grond J, Kappelle LJ, et al. Diffusion-weighted magnetic resonance imaging in acute stroke. *Stroke*. 1998;29:1783-1790.
30. Palaniswami M, Yan B. Mechanical thrombectomy is now the gold standard for acute ischemic stroke: implications for routine clinical practice. *Interv Neurol*. 2015;4:18-29.
31. National Institute of Neurological Disorders and Stroke rt PASSG. Tissue plasminogen activator for acute ischemic stroke. *N Engl J Med*. 1995;333:1581-1587.
32. Hacke W, Kaste M, Bluhmki E, et al. Thrombolysis with alteplase 3 to 4.5 hours after acute ischemic stroke. *N Engl J Med*. 2008;359:1317-1329.
33. Marler JR, Tilley BC, Lu M, et al. Early stroke treatment associated with better outcome: the NINDS rt-PA stroke study. *Neurology*. 2000;55:1649-1655.
34. Fink JN, Kumar S, Horkan C, et al. The stroke patient who woke up: clinical and radiological features, including diffusion and perfusion MRI. *Stroke*. 2002;33:988-993.
35. Kleindorfer D, Kissela B, Schneider A, et al. Eligibility for recombinant tissue plasminogen activator in acute ischemic stroke: a population-based study. *Stroke*. 2004;35:e27-e29.
36. Reeves MJ, Arora S, Broderick JP, et al. Acute stroke care in the US: results from 4 pilot prototypes of the Paul Coverdell national acute stroke registry. *Stroke*. 2005;36:1232-1240.
37. Schwamm LH, Ali SF, Reeves MJ, et al. Temporal trends in patient characteristics and treatment with intravenous thrombolysis among acute ischemic stroke patients at get with the guidelines-stroke hospitals. *Circ Cardiovasc Qual Outcomes*. 2013;6:543-549.
38. Smith WS, Tsao JW, Billings ME, et al. Prognostic significance of angiographically confirmed large vessel intracranial occlusion in patients presenting with acute brain ischemia. *Neurocrit Care*. 2006;4:14-17.
39. Bhatia R, Hill MD, Shobha N, et al. Low rates of acute recanalization with intravenous recombinant tissue plasminogen activator in ischemic stroke: real-world experience and a call for action. *Stroke*. 2010;41:2254-2258.
40. del Zoppo GJ, Higashida RT, Furlan AJ, et al. PROACT: a phase II randomized trial of recombinant pro-urokinase by direct arterial delivery in acute middle cerebral artery stroke. PROACT Investigators. Prolyse in acute cerebral thromboembolism. *Stroke*. 1998;29:4-11.
41. Furlan A, Higashida R, Wechsler L, et al. Intra-arterial prourokinase for acute ischemic stroke. The PROACT II study: a randomized controlled trial. Prolyse in acute cerebral thromboembolism. *JAMA*. 1999;282:2003-2011.

42. Gwak MS, Yang M, Hahm TS, et al. Effect of cryoanalgesia combined with intravenous continuous analgesia in thoracotomy patients. *J Korean Med Sci.* 2004;19:74-78.
43. Investigators IIT. The interventional management of stroke (IMS) II study. *Stroke.* 2007;38:2127-2135.
44. Smith WS, Sung G, Starkman S, et al. Safety and efficacy of mechanical embolectomy in acute ischemic stroke: results of the MERCI trial. *Stroke.* 2005;36:1432-1438.
45. Gobin YP, Starkman S, Duckwiler GR, et al. MERCI 1: a phase 1 study of mechanical embolus removal in cerebral ischemia. *Stroke.* 2004;35:2848-2854.
46. Smith WS. Safety of mechanical thrombectomy and intravenous tissue plasminogen activator in acute ischemic stroke. Results of the multi mechanical embolus removal in cerebral ischemia (MERCI) trial, part I. *AJNR Am J Neuroradiol.* 2006;27:1177-1182.
47. Smith WS, Sung G, Saver J, et al. Mechanical thrombectomy for acute ischemic stroke: final results of the multi MERCI trial. *Stroke.* 2008;39:1205-1212.
48. Nogueira RG, Lutsep HL, Gupta R, et al. Trevo versus Merci retrievers for thrombectomy revascularisation of large vessel occlusions in acute ischaemic stroke (TREVO 2): a randomised trial. *Lancet.* 2012;380:1231-1240.
49. Ciccone A, Valvassori L, Nichelatti M, et al. Endovascular treatment for acute ischemic stroke. *N Engl J Med.* 2013;368:904-913.
50. Broderick JP, Palesch YY, Demchuk AM, et al. Endovascular therapy after intravenous t-PA versus t-PA alone for stroke. *N Engl J Med.* 2013;368:893-903.
51. Kidwell CS, Jahan R, Gornbein J, et al. A trial of imaging selection and endovascular treatment for ischemic stroke. *N Engl J Med.* 2013;368:914-923.
52. Badhiwala JH, Nassiri F, Alhazzani W, et al. Endovascular thrombectomy for acute ischemic stroke: a meta-analysis. *JAMA.* 2015;314:1832-1843.
53. Demchuk AM, Goyal M, Yeatts SD, et al. Recanalization and clinical outcome of occlusion sites at baseline CT angiography in the interventional management of stroke III trial. *Radiology.* 2014;273:202-210.
54. Schonewille WJ, Wijman CA, Michel P, et al. Treatment and outcomes of acute basilar artery occlusion in the Basilar Artery International Cooperation Study (BASICS): a prospective registry study. *Lancet Neurol.* 2009;8:724-730.
55. Yeung JT, Matouk CC, Bulsara KR, et al. Endovascular revascularization for basilar artery occlusion. *Interv Neurol.* 2015;3:31-40.
56. Sarraj A, Sangha N, Hussain MS, et al. Endovascular therapy for acute ischemic stroke with occlusion of the middle cerebral artery M2 segment. *JAMA Neurol.* 2016;73:1291-1296.

CHAPTER 3

Cervical Carotid and Vertebral Disease

Reshma Narula, MD, Samit M. Shah, MD, PhD, Mamadou L. Sanogo, MD, and Michele H. Johnson, MD, FACR, FASER

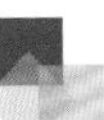

Key Points

- Review imaging options for assessment of the cervical vasculature.
- Recognize common pathologies that affect the cervical carotid and/or vertebral arteries.
- Review the indications, risks, and benefits of carotid artery stenting and neuroprotection options.

I. Introduction

Imaging assessment of the extracranial carotid artery includes a variety of cross-sectional and catheter-based techniques with different advantages, disadvantages, risks, and benefits. Cost, the need for iodinated contrast, radiation dose, imaging-modality–related limitations, and contraindications must be considered. Familiarity with features of each imaging modality is important for confidently selecting the best modality for an individual patient and suspected disease process.

A. Ultrasound

1. Duplex ultrasound (DUS) of the cervical carotid arteries is the mainstay for noninvasive evaluation of carotid stenosis (Fig. 3.1).[1]
2. DUS is low-cost and readily accessible and provides both anatomic and flow velocity information that each reflect the hemodynamic degree of stenosis and morphological characteristics of atherosclerotic plaque.
3. DUS is less useful for evaluation of the vertebral arteries because of the intraosseous course of the vertebral arteries through the foramina transversarium.
   a. Soft, friable plaque, calcified plaque, and ulcerated plaque each have characteristic appearances on anatomic ultrasound.
   b. Flow velocities and wave tracings are helpful, in determining both the degree of stenosis and the degree of flow alteration in any given patient.

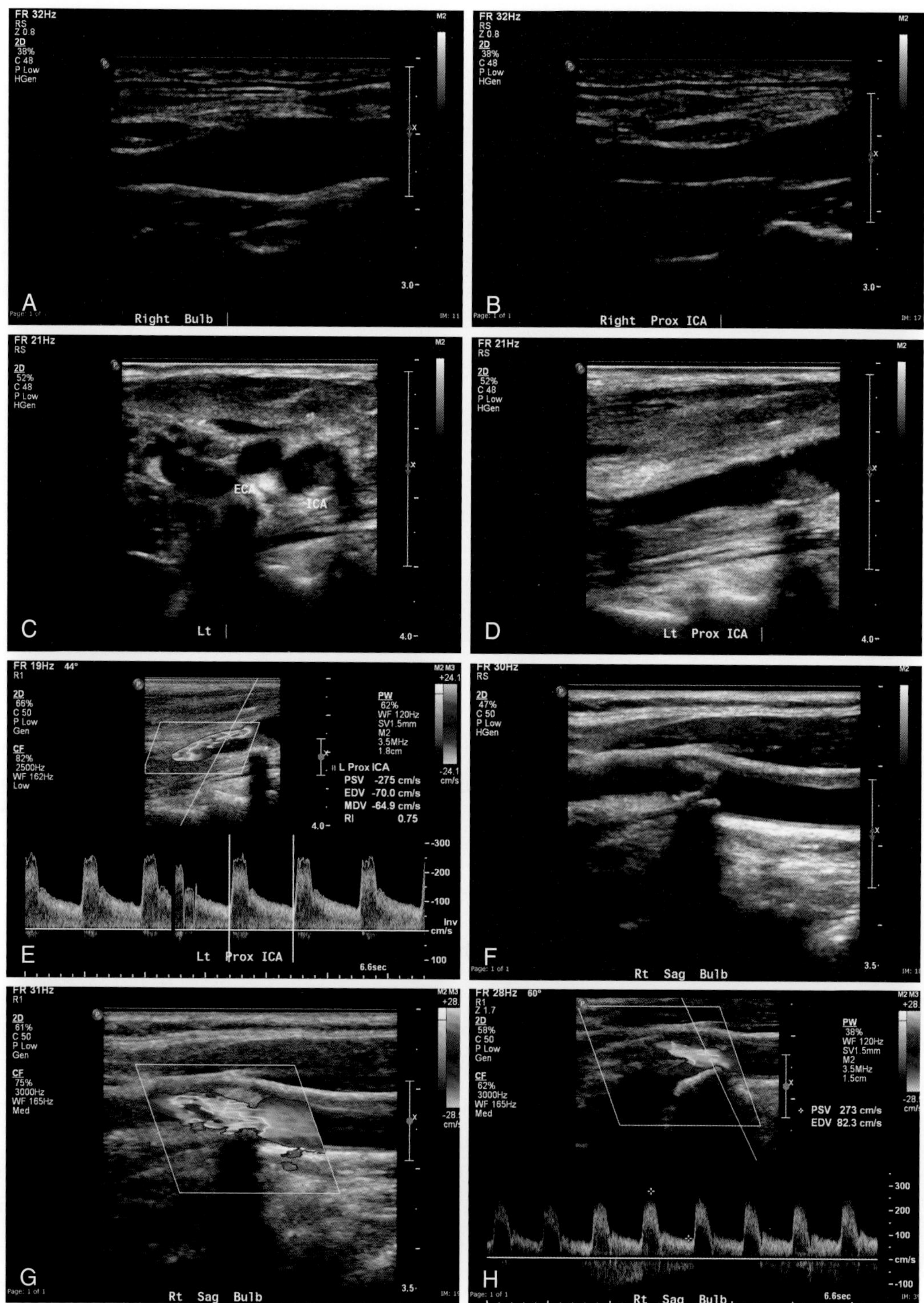

FIGURE 3.1: Carotid Ultrasound (DUS). A, Normal carotid bulb. B, Normal proximal internal carotid artery (ICA). C-E, Left carotid stenosis. Transverse and sagittal DUS images at the carotid bifurcation demonstrate soft plaque within the ICA. F-H, Right carotid bruit. DUS demonstrates the carotid bulb with calcified shadowing atherosclerotic plaque in the ICA. Peak systolic velocity at the bulb is 273 cm/s suggestive of >70% stenosis. Case courtesy of Dr. Gowthaman Gunabushanam.

4. DUS assessment can be limited when the patient has significant calcifications at the carotid bifurcation as well as in patients who are large in size with a "short neck" or in whom the carotid bifurcation is high—above the mandibular angle, making access to the carotid bifurcation difficult.

B. Computed Tomographic Angiography

1. Computed tomographic angiography (CTA) has become the primary cross-sectional imaging modality for suspected anatomic lesions of the extracranial carotid and vertebral arteries including clinical settings such as trauma, stable atherosclerosis, and stroke (Fig. 3.2).[2]

2. Ionizing radiation and iodinated contrast are both required.

3. Modern CT scanners acquire excellent images while minimizing contrast and radiation dosages.
   a. Most commonly, conventional CTA includes static images performed in the arterial phase with filming of the head and neck with the same contrast bolus. In practice, reconstruction protocols vary, but generally include axial, coronal, sagittal, and oblique images with or without 3D volume rendered or vessel tracking imaging.
   b. Application of dual energy techniques for CTA acquisition allows for automated bone removal and plaque characterization using the different energy spectrum for evaluation.[3]
   c. Newer time-resolved or multiphasic CTA with rapid sequential imaging allows for visible depiction of flow within the vessel, analogous to digital subtraction angiography.[4]

4. CT perfusion techniques may be adjunctive in the assessment of the significance of carotid stenosis or the significance of an intracranial stenosis.[5]

C. Magnetic Resonance Angiography

1. Magnetic resonance angiography (MRA) time-of-flight imaging has the advantages of requiring no ionizing radiation and no intravenous contrast administration to obtain imaging of the carotid artery (Fig. 3.3).[6]

2. There are some patients who cannot undergo MRI or who may require special monitoring (ie, pacemakers or implanted cardioverter-defibrillators).
   a. Metallic oral implants (including clips and dental hardware) may create significant imaging artifacts at the level of the carotid arteries, precluding adequate vessel evaluation.

3. Noncontrast time-of-flight MRA is an excellent screening tool for cervical or intracranial vascular disease but has the significant disadvantage that a high-grade stenosis may appear as an occlusion unless contrast MRA is employed.

4. Contrast MRA improves the visualization of a tiny residual vascular lumen, permitting accurate differentiation of high-grade stenosis versus occlusion.

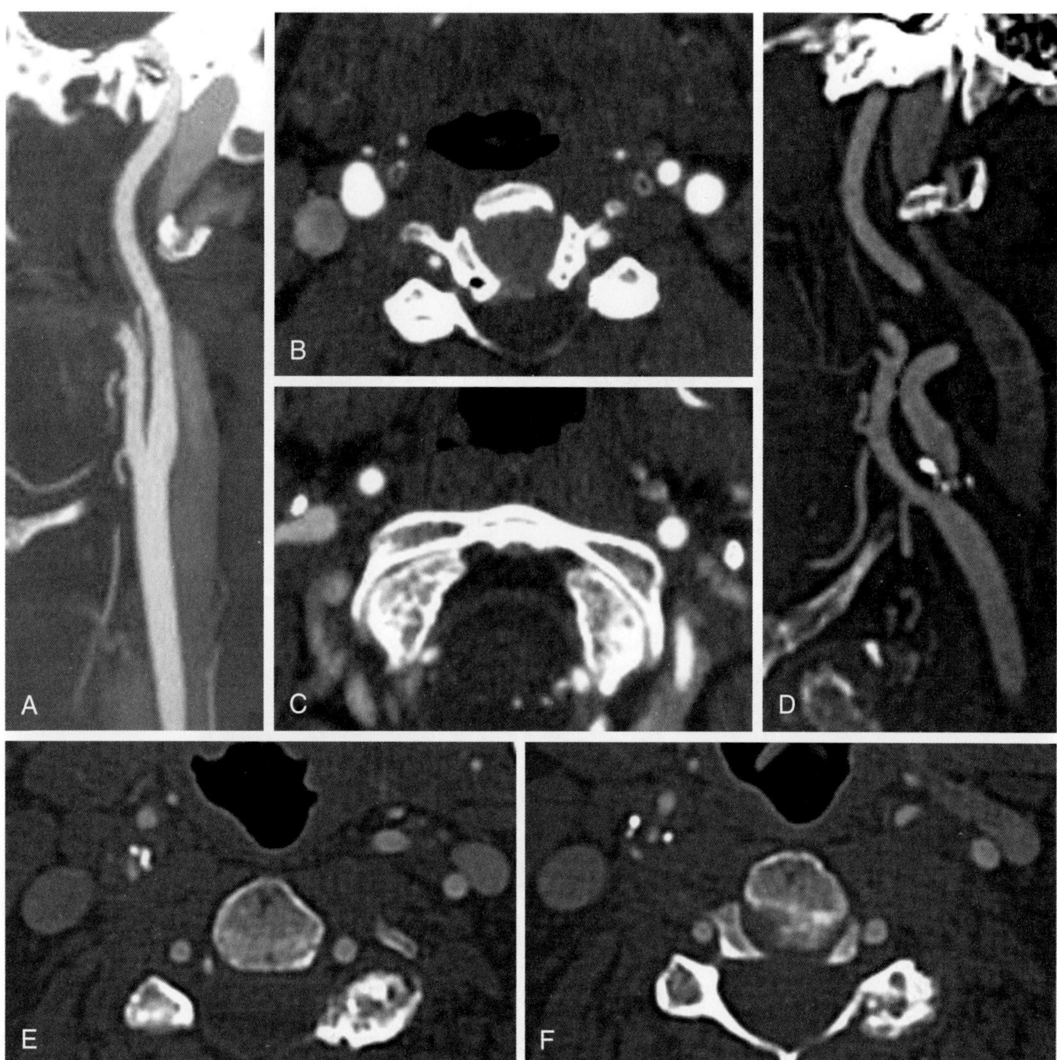

FIGURE 3.2: Computed tomographic angiography (CTA). A, Sagittal CTA of normal carotid bifurcation. B, Axial CTA demonstrates the carotid bulb on the right and the internal and external carotid arteries on the left. C, Axial CTA through the upper cervical carotid arteries bilaterally. D, Sagittal CTA demonstrates high-grade calcific stenosis. E and F, Sequential axial CTA images illustrate mixed calcified and noncalcified plaque and the marked right internal carotid artery stenosis. G and H, CTA of the left carotid artery viewed in the inverted format demonstrates the calcific plaque as black and mild luminal irregularity without hemodynamically significant stenosis. The 3D volume rendered images with vessel tracking and axial segmentation are helpful for assessment of the character of the plaque and the degree of stenosis. I and J, In contrast, on the right, there is a long segment but lesser narrowing than on the left, and the plaque is composed of both calcified and noncalcified plaque, which may be more friable and carry higher risk of distal embolization. Plaque characterization as well as anatomic features of the target lesion will influence treatment decisions.

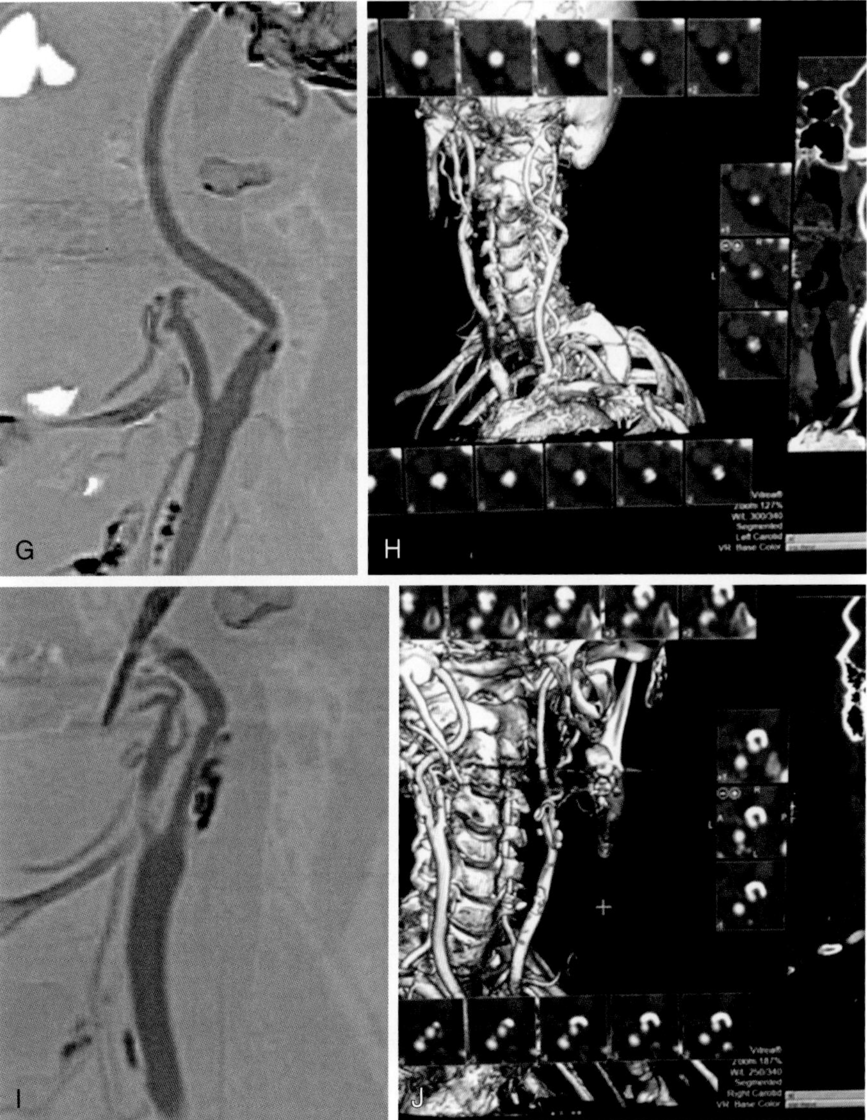

FIGURE 3.2 Cont'd

5. MRA predominantly images the lumen of the vessel; however, evaluation of source images may allow for plaque characterization, particularly when thin section high-resolution imaging algorithms are applied.
   a. Such thin section high-resolution imaging algorithms are referred to as vessel wall imaging or black blood imaging and are the subject of current research.[7,8]
6. Time-resolved MRA techniques are also useful primarily for assessment of arteriovenous shunting and fistulous lesions. These are less commonly employed for cervical vascular disease.

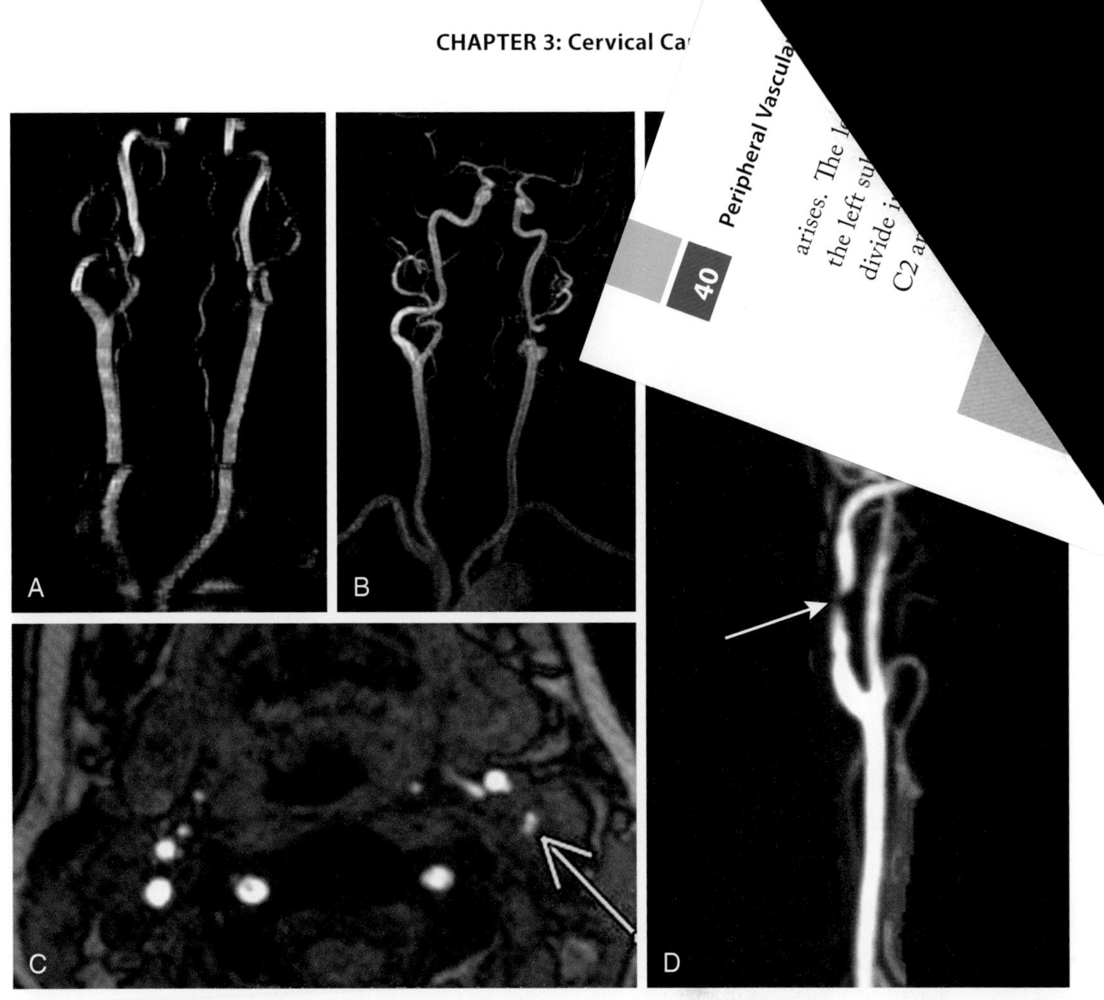

FIGURE 3.3: Magnetic resonance angiography (MRA). A, Time-of-flight (TOF) noncontrast MRA demonstrates the vasculature, which is better resolved on the postcontrast MRA series (B). C and D, Carotid stenosis (arrow) is best evaluated on the postcontrast axial source image and the MIP (maximum intensity projection) reconstruction.

D. Digital Subtraction Angiography

1. Digital subtraction angiography (DSA) utilizes conventional x-ray with digital acquisition of images in rapid sequence during intra-arterial injection of contrast.
   a. This provides high-resolution, time-resolved vascular imaging with both anatomic delineation and real-time physiologic depiction of flow dynamics (Fig. 3.4).
2. DSA is an invasive technique requiring catheter access usually via femoral, radial, or brachial routes, although direct carotid access may be employed in select cases.
3. Rotational digital acquisition permits creation of 3D volume rendered images. DSA remains the gold standard for DUS, CTA, and MRI/MRA.[9]

II. Cervical Carotid and Vertebral Disease

Evaluation of cervical extracranial vascular disease begins with the vessel origins from the aortic arch. The innominate artery arises from the aortic arch and divides into the right common carotid artery and the right subclavian artery, from which the right vertebral artery

ft common carotid artery arises as the next branch from the arch and finally
bclavian, which gives rise to the left vertebral artery. The common carotid arteries
nto internal and external carotid arteries in the mid cervical region usually between
d C6, and the level may vary from one side to the other. The vertebral arteries proceed

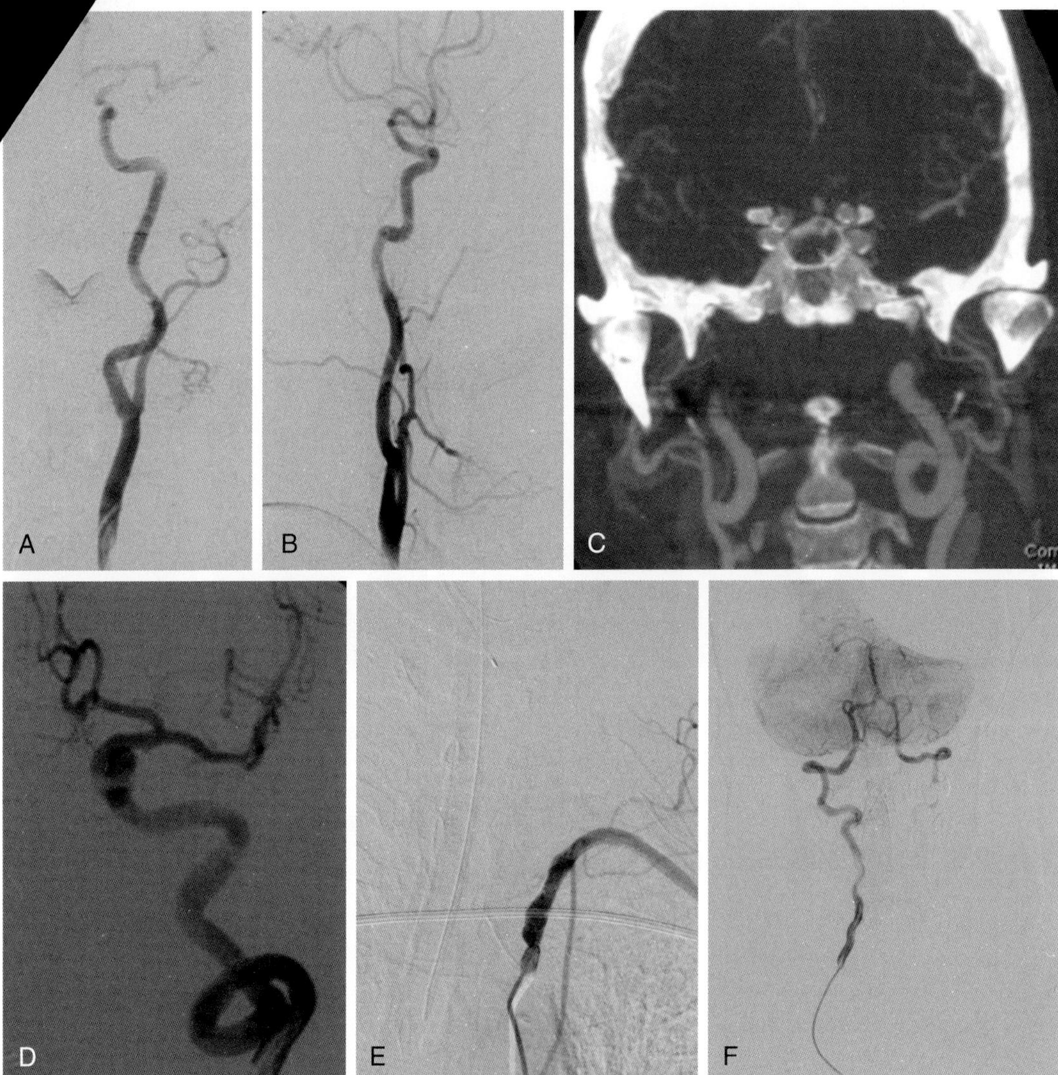

FIGURE 3.4: Digital subtraction angiography (DSA). A and B, AP oblique and lateral DSA of the common carotid artery demonstrate a normal configuration in this young adult patient. C and D, The cervical internal carotid artery may be tortuous with hairpin or 360° loops, which are easily appreciated on CTA but may be difficult to navigate when carotid stenting or intracranial intervention are contemplated. E, This 65-year-old patient presented with hand claudication and subclavian stenosis was demonstrated. F and G, DSA with injection of the right vertebral artery in the arterial and venous phases demonstrates retrograde flow in the left vertebral artery with faint filling of the subclavian artery—subclavian steal phenomenon. H, Following transfemoral left subclavian stent placement, the vertebral artery was preserved and antegrade flow restored.

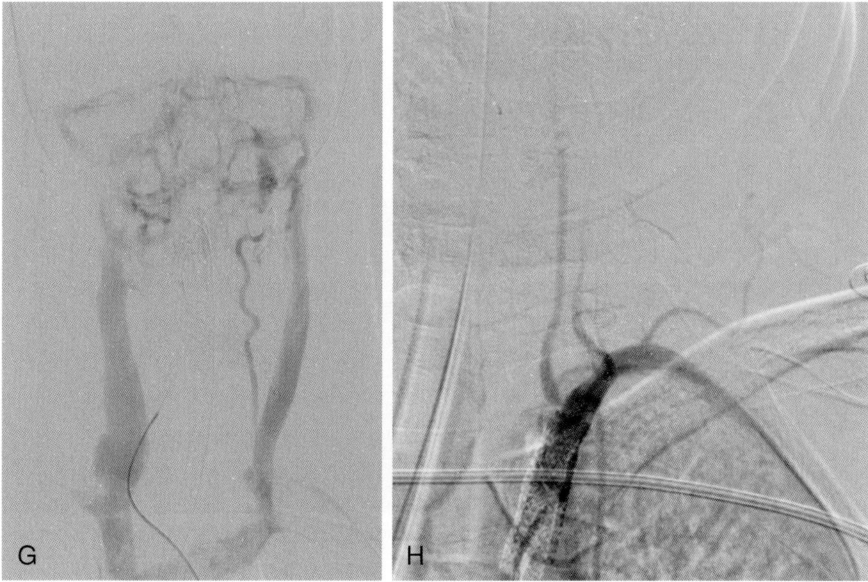

FIGURE 3.4 Cont'd

cranially, traversing the foramen transversarium of the cervical vertebra extending to the C2 level and around the arch of C1 until the arteries enter the dura at the foramen magnum and join to form the basilar artery superiorly[10] (Fig. 3.5; Table 3.1).

III. Atherosclerotic Disease

A. Causes of Ischemic Stroke

1. Extracranial carotid artery disease is one of the leading causes of ischemic stroke accounting for approximately 10% of all ischemic strokes.
2. Carotid artery revascularization in the setting of extracranial atherosclerotic disease, with either carotid endarterectomy (CEA) or carotid artery stenting (CAS), is now well-established treatment for symptomatic and asymptomatic carotid atherosclerotic disease in specific patients.[11]
3. As not every patient with extracranial carotid artery atherosclerotic disease carries the same risk of future stroke, key risk factors should be considered to determine which specific patients should be revascularized.

B. Risk Factors

1. Major risk factors include the degree of stenosis and characteristics of the plaque seen within the artery.
2. Other patient-specific characteristics include age, gender, and comorbid medical conditions.

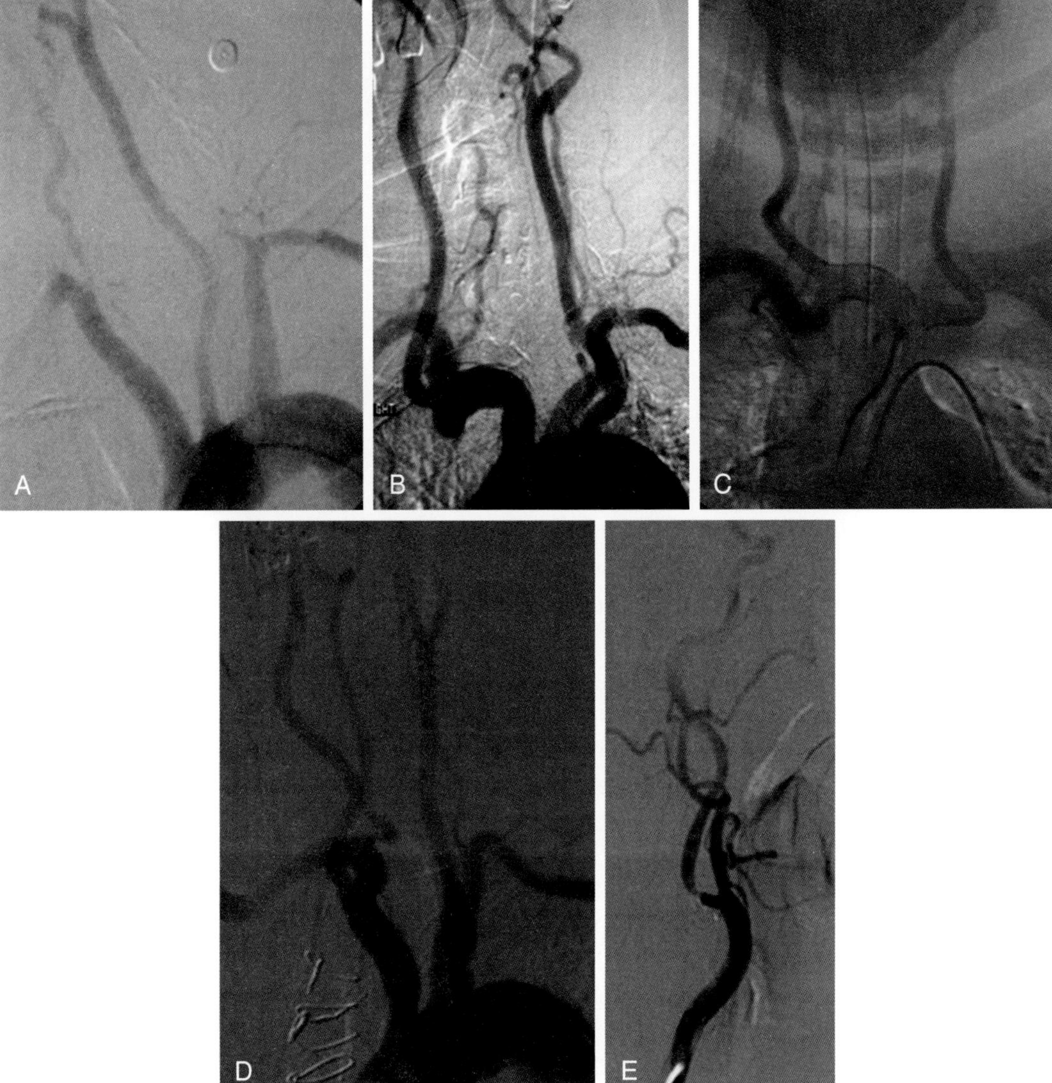

FIGURE 3.5: Arch Anatomy. A, Normal arch configuration. B, More tortuous great vessels in this elderly patient may make interventions more challenging. Note the left vertebral artery arises directly from the aortic arch. C, A common origin of the innominate and left common carotid arteries may require a recurve catheter for navigation as in this case. D and E, This patient was scheduled for a right carotid stent; however, the hostile arch and the acute reverse curve of the internal carotid stenosis led the operator to abandon this approach for carotid endarterectomy.

TABLE 3.1.	Aortic Arch Classification
Type I	Great vessels arising from the top of the arch
Type II	Great vessels arising between the parallel planes delineated by the outer and inner curves of the arch
Type III	Great vessels arising caudal to the inner surface of the arch or of the ascending aorta

C. Modality for Revascularization

1. The choice of modality for revascularization is based on a combination of these key risk factors and anatomic considerations.
2. We review recent trial evidence surrounding carotid revascularization in both symptomatic and asymptomatic carotid artery disease, and the data supporting patient selection for each modality.
3. A few definitions are important to know to understand and compare the trial data.

D. Defining Carotid Artery Stenosis

1. In the North American Symptomatic Carotid Endarterectomy Trial (NASCET), a uniform method for measurement of percentage carotid stenosis at angiography was defined by comparing the minimal residual lumen at the level of the stenotic lesion with the diameter of the more distal internal carotid artery at which the walls of the artery first become parallel (beyond any poststenotic dilatation).
2. The following formula is used: Degree of stenosis = $(1-A/B) \times 100\%$.
   a. A is the diameter at the point of maximum stenosis and B is the diameter of the arterial segment distal to the stenosis where the walls first become parallel.[12]
   b. This method of measurement has been adapted to CT angiography.
   c. It is routinely used to define carotid stenosis in current and ongoing trials. Bartlett et al 2006 proposed using the narrowest measurement of the lumen in millimeters stating that an absolute measurement of 1.3 mm corresponded to 70% stenosis by NASCET criteria and 2.2 mm to 50%[13] (Fig. 3.6).

E. Symptomatic Versus Asymptomatic Extracranial Carotid Stenosis

1. **Symptomatic** extracranial carotid artery stenosis is defined as an atherosclerotic lesion of at least 50% stenosis proximal to the vascular territory that corresponds to the patient's clinical symptomatology (stroke or transient ischemic attack) and/or the anatomic location of the infarct on imaging.
2. Atherosclerotic stenosis of the carotid artery may result in ischemic symptoms secondary to hypoperfusion or embolization.
3. **Asymptomatic** extracranial carotid artery stenosis is defined as an atherosclerotic lesion of at least 50% stenosis without clinical or imaging evidence of stroke.
4. Currently, it is recommended that best medical management should be implemented immediately in both symptomatic and asymptomatic atherosclerotic carotid disease whenever it is first discovered.[14,15]
   a. Best medical management involves vascular risk factor modification and includes aggressive control of hypertension, hyperlipidemia, diabetes mellitus, smoking cessation, and initiation of an antiplatelet agent.[16]

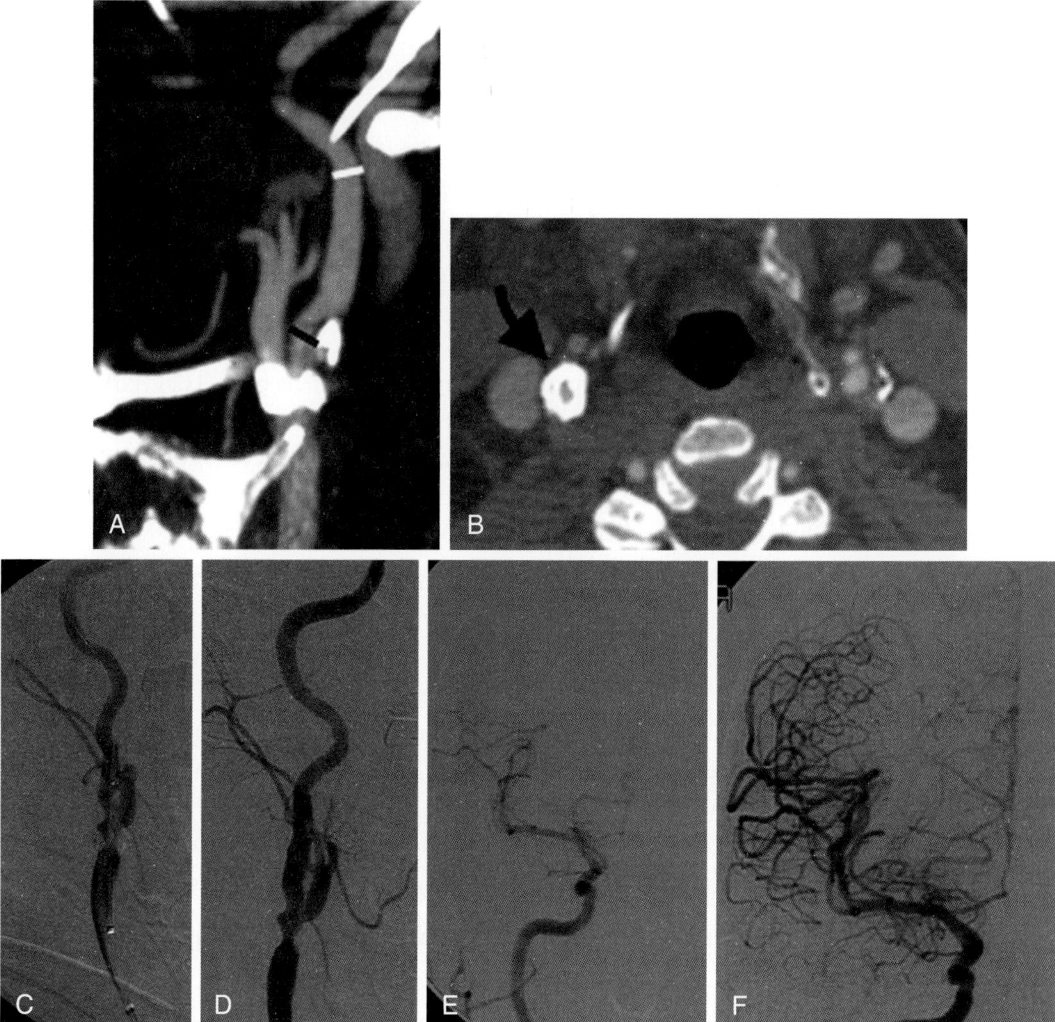

FIGURE 3.6: Digital subtraction angiography (DSA) and Computed tomographic angiography (CTA) with NASCET measurements. A, NASCET measurements on CTA minimal luminal diameter (black line) compared with the straight portion of the internal carotid artery beyond any poststenotic dilatation (white line). B, With heavy calcification (black arrow), absolute measurement in mm may be preferable. C and D, This patient had symptoms referable to reduced cerebral perfusion. Pre- and poststent cervical images demonstrate residual stenosis due to the heavy calcific plaque. E and F, Cerebral DSA pre- and poststent show remarkable improvement on perfusion on the right and his symptoms improved.

IV. Revascularization in Extracranial Carotid Artery Stenosis

A. Evidence

1. There is substantial evidence to support revascularization for symptomatic extracranial carotid artery disease. Many large randomized trials including the *European Carotid Surgery Trial (ECST), the NASCET,* and the *US Department of Veteran Affairs Cooperative Study Program (CSP)* showed superiority of carotid endarterectomy with best medical management over best medical management alone for symptomatic, high-grade carotid artery stenosis.[12,17,18]

2. Patients included in these studies were those with greater than 70% carotid artery stenosis on angiography and who had ipsilateral ischemic strokes, monocular blindness, or symptoms of a transient ischemic attack.
3. A pooled analysis from these trials showed that the rate of 30-day stroke risk was lower in the surgical group compared with the medical group.
4. The NASCET study specifically showed that the number needed to treat with carotid endarterectomy was six for patients with symptomatic high-grade carotid artery stenosis.
5. The studies also showed that for patients with less than 50% stenosis of the carotid artery, surgery did not significantly lower the future stroke risk.
6. For surgical patients with 50%-69% stenosis in the NASCET study, there was only moderate benefit to reduce stroke risk, as the rate of ipsilateral stroke was 15.7% in those surgically treated compared with 22.2% in the medical group.[12]

B. **Benefits** Both carotid endarterectomy and carotid artery stenting have been shown to be beneficial in the setting of significant stenosis of the extracranial carotid artery in the setting of atherosclerotic disease.

C. **Trials and Studies**

1. **SAPPHIRE** The first trial, **Stenting and Angioplasty with Protection in Patients with High Risk of Endarterectomy (SAPPHIRE) trial** showed noninferiority of carotid artery stenting compared with carotid endarterectomy.[19]
2. **CREST** Subsequently, the **Carotid Revascularization Endarterectomy versus Stenting Trial (CREST)** randomly assigned patients with symptomatic or asymptomatic carotid stenosis to undergo either carotid artery stenting or carotid endarterectomy.[11]
   a. The primary composite endpoint was stroke, myocardial infarction, or death from any cause during the periprocedural period or any ipsilateral stroke within 4 years after randomization.
   b. The results of this trial showed that the risks did not differ significantly between the carotid artery stenting group and the carotid endarterectomy group.
   c. Because of the results of this trial, carotid artery stenting emerged as one of the primary treatments for carotid artery atherosclerotic disease in select patients.
3. **ACES** The **Asymptomatic Carotid Emboli Study (ACES)** demonstrated that there was a higher risk of ipsilateral stroke risk with embolic signals on transcranial Doppler (TCD) ultrasound than in those without, suggesting that patients with asymptomatic carotid disease should undergo TCD to evaluate for microemboli.[20]
4. **Endarterectomy for Asymptomatic Carotid Stenosis Study** Revascularization for asymptomatic carotid disease was studied in the **Endarterectomy for Asymptomatic Carotid Stenosis Study.**[21,22]
   a. This study was a large-scale study, including 1662 patients, and compared carotid endarterectomy with best medical management with best medical management alone. CT angiography was used to identify patients with greater than 60% stenosis of the extracranial carotid artery, using the NASCET Criteria for measurement of carotid stenosis.

b. Patients were randomly assigned to either surgery plus best medical management or medical management alone.
c. A composite primary outcome of stroke or death occurring in the perioperative period and ipsilateral cerebral infarction was used.
d. This study was stopped early, given evidence of a clear benefit in the carotid endarterectomy group.
e. These data were further supported by the **Asymptomatic Carotid Surgery Trial (ACST).**[23]

5. These studies are not thought to be generalizable to modern clinical practice because optimal medical therapy has improved in the current era as compared with the time of these studies (2004-2010).[24,25]

6. Furthermore, operators selected for these trials were carefully screened and generally had lower complication rates than what was seen in the general nonstudy surgeon population.

7. Currently, there are no definitive guidelines for revascularization for asymptomatic extracranial carotid stenosis.
a. However, based on data from these studies and clinical practice, it is reasonable to consider revascularization in asymptomatic patients with greater than 70%-80% stenosis in the following types of patients:
1. Patients whose carotid artery stenosis continues to progress rapidly despite best medical management
2. Patients who have evidence of microemboli with TCD
3. Patients with a low potential for periprocedural complications
b. This topic is being further investigated in the *Carotid Revascularization and Medical Management for Asymptomatic Carotid Stenosis (CREST-2)* study, which is comparing best medical management alone with carotid endarterectomy or carotid artery stenting.[26]

V. Patient Factors Influencing Revascularization

A. NASCET

1. The *NASCET* also showed that patient characteristics including age, gender, and comorbid medical conditions should strongly influence the type of revascularization procedure that a patient with carotid artery disease should undergo.

2. Notably, NASCET showed that women with symptomatic carotid stenosis were more likely to have unfavorable outcome including carotid artery restenosis, surgical mortality, and neurologic morbidity with carotid artery stenting.[12]

B. CREST

1. Nearly a decade later, the *CREST* provided further evidence regarding specific patient characteristics that should influence the choice of revascularization method.

2. CREST showed that during the periprocedural period, there was a higher risk of stroke with carotid artery stenting and a higher risk of myocardial infarction with carotid endarterectomy.
   a. Therefore, patients with significant comorbid coronary artery disease or other cardiovascular conditions may be better candidates for CAS rather than CEA.[11]

3. The study also supported prior data that patient age should be factored into the procedural selection because younger patients, less than 70 years, were shown to have better outcomes with CAS whereas older patients may have had better outcomes with CEA.
   a. There may be a higher risk of stroke with CAS in very elderly patients because of acquired anatomical obstacles such as vascular tortuosity, calcifications, and/or tandem stenoses.
   b. In general, CAS is preferred in patients with severe comorbid medical condition and those with anatomic features that would make surgery difficult, including prior neck surgery or radiation therapy, restenosis after prior carotid endarterectomy, contralateral carotid occlusion, or surgically inaccessible lesions.[27]

VI. Timing of Revascularization

A. Trials and Trends

1. Timing of carotid artery revascularization in patients with ischemic stroke remains very important. Review of subgroup analyses from two large randomized clinical trials, the *European Carotid Surgery Trial (ECST)* and the *NASCET*, looked at the timing for optimal benefit of carotid endarterectomy for patients with ischemic stroke thought to be secondary to high-grade symptomatic extracranial carotid artery disease.

2. There was a trend toward benefit with CEA within 2 weeks of symptoms compared with patients who had delayed procedures.[12,28]
   a. The degree of benefit of the procedure appeared to diminish with time, especially if CEA was delayed beyond 12 weeks.

3. There are many factors to consider that should influence the timing of carotid revascularization for symptomatic patients including infarct size (as larger ischemic strokes may have a higher risk for reperfusion injury and hemorrhagic transformation) and complicating comorbidities and medical factors such as infection or hemodynamic instability.
   a. In medically stable patients with relatively minor ischemic strokes or transient ischemic attacks thought to be secondary to high-grade ipsilateral carotid artery stenosis, revascularization should occur within 2 weeks of symptom onset.
   b. However, in patients with other complicating factors, it would be reasonable to delay the procedure up to 12 weeks to medically stabilize the patient prior to revascularization.

B. Restenosis After Carotid Endarterectomy or Carotid Artery Stenting

1. Restenosis after CEA or CAS is typically asymptomatic and detected by surveillance imaging.
2. The risk of restenosis after carotid intervention was evaluated in the ACAS trial as defined as a recurrent stenosis of 60% or greater.
   a. The risk of restenosis was most likely in the first 18 months following surgery (7.9%) and declined steadily afterward (1.9% at 42 months).[21] CREST showed that approximately 6% of patients had a risk of restenosis greater than 70% in the first 24 months with either CEA or CAS.[29]
   b. In CREST, independent predictors of restenosis included diabetes mellitus, hypertension, and female gender. Smoking was an independent predictor of restenosis in the CEA group but not in the CAS group.
   c. Given the low incidence of restenosis after revascularization, there are no standard guidelines regarding repeat follow-up imaging in these patients.[11]
3. It is reasonable to follow patients annually with DUS for the first 2 years following revascularization, especially in patients with comorbid conditions of smoking, diabetes mellitus, hypertension, or female gender.

C. Intracranial Large Artery Atherosclerotic Disease

1. Intracranial large artery atherosclerosis of the carotid and vertebral arteries represents a leading cause of ischemic stroke.
2. There are limited data regarding treatment of intercranial large artery atherosclerosis.
   a. Stenting and Aggressive Medical Management for Preventing Recurrent stroke in Intracranial Stenosis (SAMMPRIS) Study enrolled 451 patients and compared optimal medical therapy with percutaneous angioplasty and stenting for the prevention of recurrent stroke in patients with symptomatic intracranial large artery, intracranial carotid, or intracranial vertebral artery atherosclerosis.[30]
      i. Medical therapy consisted of dual antiplatelet therapy (aspirin 325 mg per day and clopidogrel 75 mg per day), aggressive blood pressure control of less than 140 mm Hg and lipid control with an LDL less than 70 mg/dL, and enrollment in a lifestyle modification program.
      ii. The study was terminated early because of a higher 30-day rate of stroke and death in the percutaneous transluminal angioplasty and stenting arm.
      iii. There was a statistically significant difference in stroke or death, and the primary endpoint of stroke or death occurred in 5.8% of the medical therapy arm and 14.7% of the angioplasty/stenting arm.
      iv. This study ultimately showed that percutaneous stenting is not safe or effective for treatment of patients who experience a transient ischemic attack or ischemic stroke attributable to large artery intracranial disease.
      v. Based on the medical therapy that was used in this study, if there is severe stenosis of a large intracranial artery (of greater than 50%) with symptomatic

disease, it is reasonable to place the patient on aspirin and clopidogrel for 90 days in addition to high-intensity statin therapy with blood pressure control with a goal systolic less than 140 mm Hg.

b. The Warfarin-Aspirin Symptomatic Intracranial Disease Study (WASID) evaluated 569 patients and compared warfarin with aspirin following transient ischemic attack or ischemic stroke attributable to intracranial stenosis of the internal carotid artery, middle cerebral artery, vertebral artery, or basilar artery.[31]
   i. The study was stopped early because of higher rates of death and major hemorrhage in the warfarin arm.
   ii. Thus, based on this study, aspirin 325 mg per day is preferred to warfarin for the treatment of symptomatic large artery intracranial stenosis and secondary prevention of ischemic stroke.
   iii. The long-term follow-up did show that patients with a mean systolic blood pressure less than 140 mm Hg and an LDL less than 100 mg/dL had a lower risk of recurrent stroke.

D. Extracranial Symptomatic Vertebral Artery Disease

1. Extracranial symptomatic vertebral artery disease is a known cause of posterior circulation ischemic infarcts.

2. Treatment options for this disease are limited, and the current mainstay treatment is medical management.

3. One of the most recent studies that studied this was the Vertebral Artery Stenting Trial (VAST), which evaluated patients with recent transient ischemic attack or minor stroke associated with vertebral artery stenosis of at least 50%.[32]
   a. This study evaluated both intra- and extracranial vertebral artery disease.
   b. Patients were randomly assigned to either stenting plus optimal medical therapy or optimal medical therapy alone. The trial was ultimately stopped early because of regulatory requirements.
   c. From the analysis of the patients who were enrolled, the authors concluded that stenting of symptomatic vertebral artery stenosis was associated with an increased risk of major periprocedural vascular complication and the risk of recurrent strokes in the medical management group was low.
   d. However, current guidelines suggest that for recurrent disease vertebral artery stenting, or open procedures such as vertebral endarterectomy or transposition, may be considered in select patients who have recurrent ischemic strokes despite best medical management.[33,34]

VII. Additional Disorders of the Extracranial Vasculature

A. Fibromuscular Dysplasia

1. Fibromuscular dysplasia (FMD) is a disorder of the medial layer of the vasculature that manifests in an altered appearance of the normal vessel luminal contour.

2. The vessel may demonstrate a thin concentric smooth-walled narrowing, a "string of beads" appearance, or irregular narrowing and may be vulnerable to dissection, occlusion, or pseudoaneurysm formation.
3. Each of these may become a source of emboli causing TIA or stroke.[35]
4. FMD can be seen in the cervical carotid arteries and cervical vertebral arteries and is commonly seen in the renal arteries.
5. There is an association between FMD and intracranial aneurysms. Angioplasty with or without stenting has been employed for treatment of FMD-related carotid stenosis (Fig. 3.7).

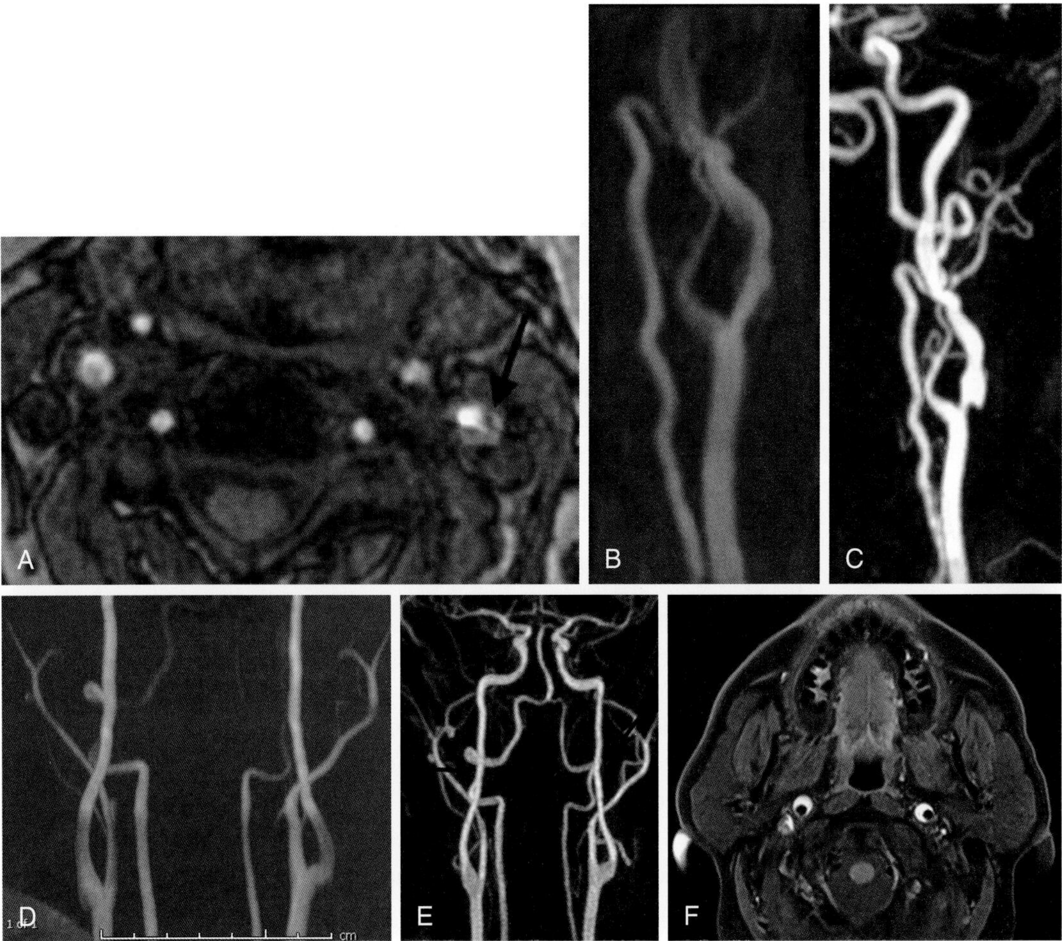

FIGURE 3.7: Fibromuscular dysplasia (FMD) and spontaneous dissection. A, Axial source contrast MRA demonstrated heterogeneous signal (arrow) surrounding the internal carotid artery (ICA) lumen. B, Noncontrast TOF MRA shows irregularity of the ICA lumen. C, The contrast MIP (maximum intensity projection) MRA image better depicts the degree of narrowing and better depicts the features of FMD. D, TOF MIP noncontrast MRA shows minimal luminal irregularity of the ICAs, left > right. E, This is better seen on the contrast MRA MIP image (arrows). F, The best and most reliable is the axial T1 fat saturation image showing intramural hemorrhage in the setting of bilateral ICA dissections.

B. Traumatic Cervical Vascular Injury

1. Cervical vascular injury can be divided into blunt and penetrating trauma.
2. CTA has been the mainstay of vascular evaluation in the setting of facial/mandibular fractures and cervical spine fractures as it can efficiently interrogate both primary and secondary pathologic lesions.
3. When focusing predominantly on blunt cerebrovascular injury, the cervical vessels (carotid and vertebral) may demonstrate dissection, with associated luminal compromise, vessel occlusion (acute or subacute), or pseudoaneurysm formation (often a delayed sequelae of dissection)[36] (Fig. 3.8).
4. Frank vessel rupture is more unusual with blunt cervical injury and is more commonly seen in association with cervical malignancies or infection (Fig. 3.9).

VIII. Techniques for Carotid and Vertebral Intervention

Femoral access is the most common access route for CAS; however, radial, brachial, and direct carotid access may be employed in specific patients to facilitate safe access or traverse an anatomically challenging artic arch. Femoral arterial access has been presented in an earlier chapter. A brief description of radial and direct carotid access (percutaneous and via cutdown) can be found in the sections that follow.

A. Radial Access for Carotid Stenosis

1. Peripheral arterial access technique was first introduced by Sven Ivar Seldinger in 1959.[37]
   a. Two decades later, the introduction of vascular sheaths made peripheral access more appealing by decreasing the need for repeated vascular access during percutaneous vascular procedures.
   b. Two main arterial accesses are commonly used for most percutaneous carotid artery interventions: the common femoral artery and radial artery.
   c. Direct carotid access is preserved for selective patients.
2. Lucien Campeau at the Montreal Heart Institute first described transradial access for diagnostic angiography of the coronary arteries in 1989, as a safer alternative to brachial or axillary access.[38]
   a. The transradial access was subsequently, successfully used for percutaneous interventions, including the first transradial coronary angioplasty by Kiemeneij in 1992 and coronary stenting in 1993.[39]
   b. The use of transradial access technique has significantly expanded in recent years accounting for 1 in 6 percutaneous coronary interventions (PCIs) in the United States.[40]
3. Although, there is abundant literature on the transradial coronary angiography, data are emerging on transradial access for cerebral angiography and stenting for carotid stenosis.

a. A multicenter randomized study has by Ruzsa et al, has shown the transradial approach for carotid stenting to be safe and with no difference in total procedure and fluoroscopic time.[41]

   i. The radiation dose was higher, while hospitalization was shorter for radial approach when compared with transfemoral approach.

b. A meta-analysis of randomized by Ferrante et al found transradial PCI to be associated with fewer vascular complications and a lower rate of major bleeding and death.[42]

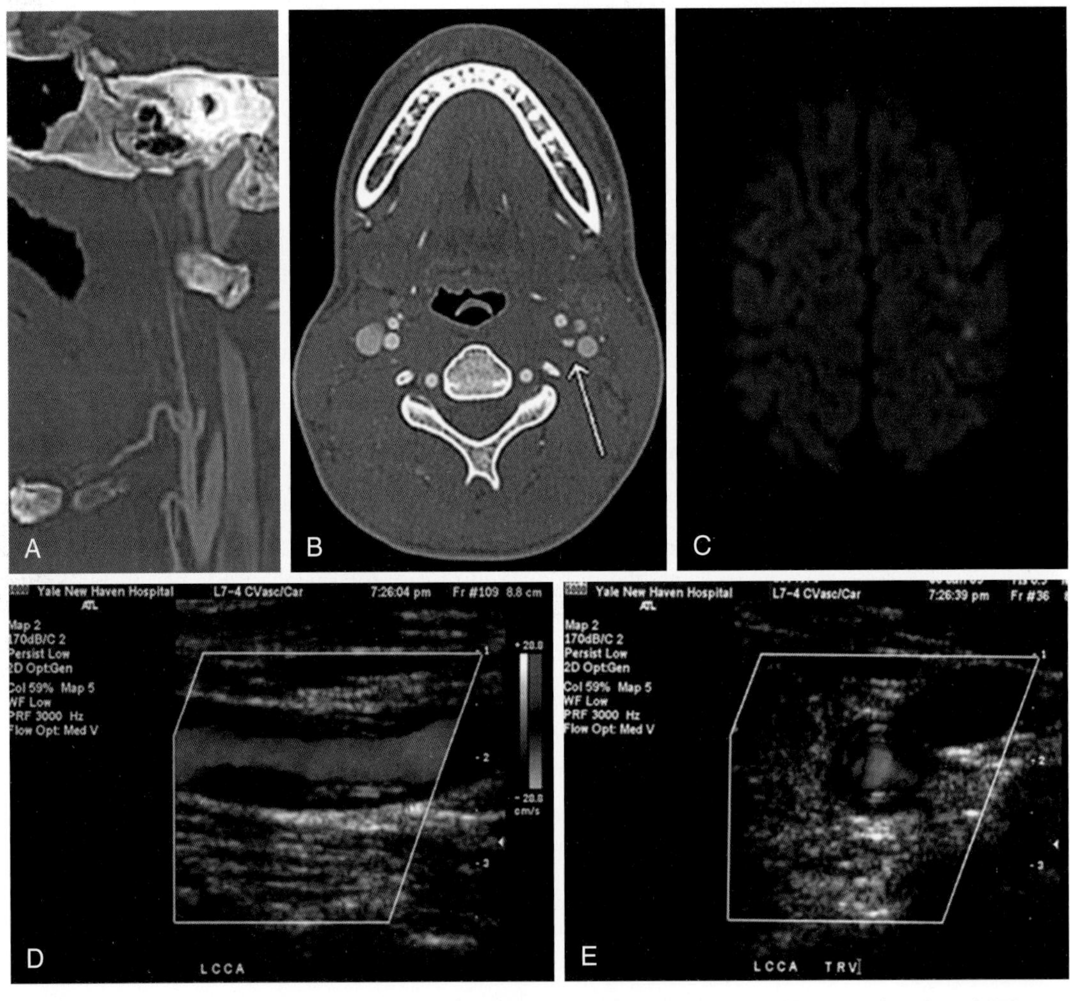

FIGURE 3.8: Traumatic dissection, pseudo-occlusion, pseudoaneurysm. A and B, Sagittal and axial CTA demonstrate an internal carotid artery dissection in this adolescent hit in the neck with a lacrosse ball. Note the luminal deformity on the axial view (arrow). C, Diffusion weighted MRI shows multiple foci of restricted diffusion consistent with distal embolization and stroke. D and E, Longitudinal and transverse ultrasound images of the common carotid artery show marked wall thickening and luminal compromise in this patient who was in a motor vehicle collision and had a seat belt mark on her neck. F and G, DSA demonstrates ragged appearance and narrowing of the common carotid artery. This was successfully treated with covered stents. H and I, This 95-year-old patient presented with an expanding neck mass, and US with color Doppler demonstrates a carotid pseudoaneurysm (PSA). J and K, DSA shows the PSA and the appearance following covered stent placement.

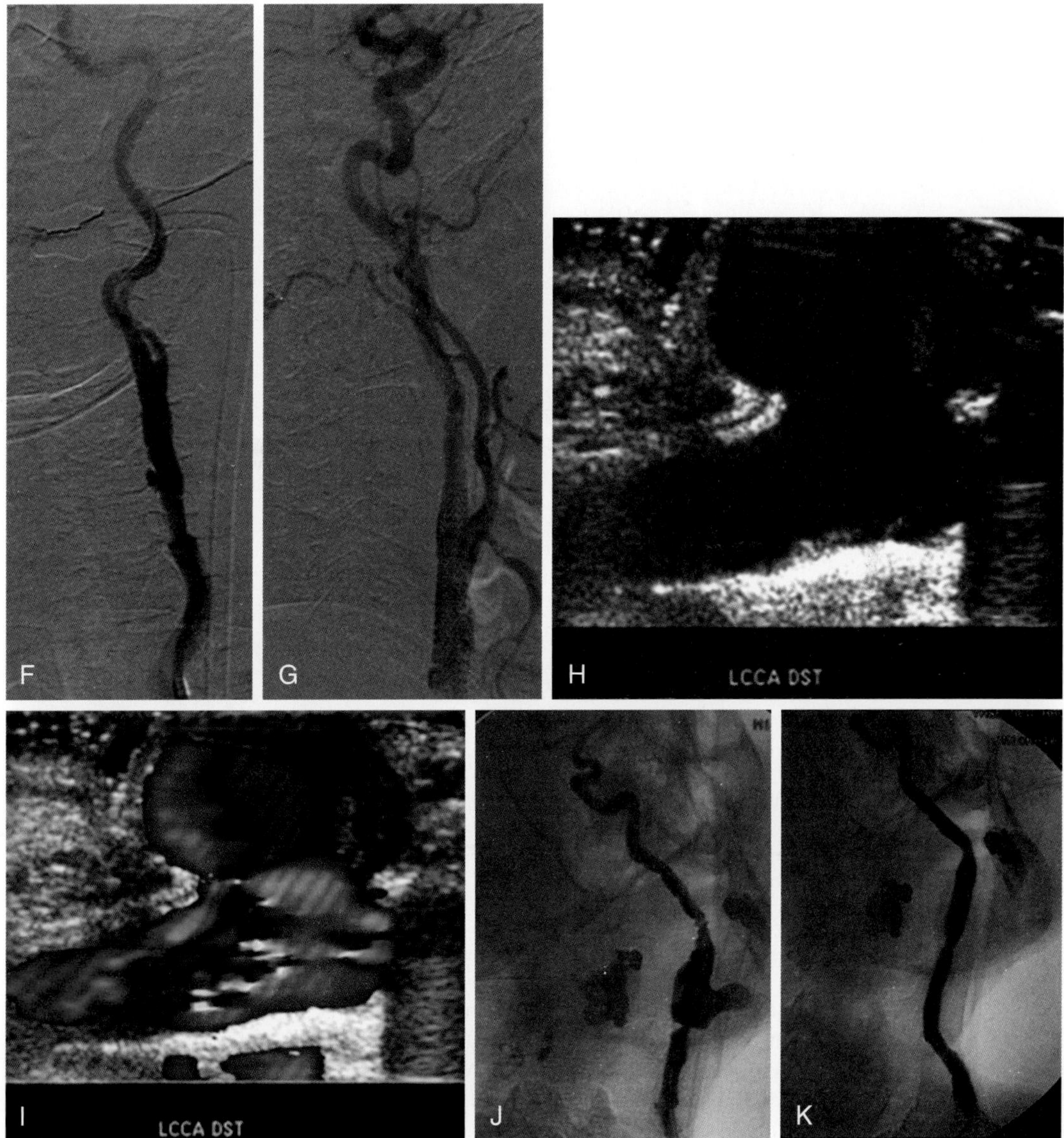

FIGURE 3.8 Cont'd

i. Furthermore, the transradial approach has certain anatomic advantages over the transfemoral approach.
ii. The radial is superficial and easily compressible without major susceptible surrounding structures, which significantly decrease potential postprocedure complications.[39] Despite these advantages, good patient selection, mastering techniques, and meticulous postprocedural care are critical to minimize postprocedural complications. A small radial artery less than 2 mm and dialysis fistula constitutes relative contraindications.[39]
iii. Bedside tests to evaluate the patency of the palmar arch have not been shown to predict ischemic complications or radial artery occlusion, and the Allen's maneuver or Barbeau test are no longer recommended prior to radial artery access.[43]

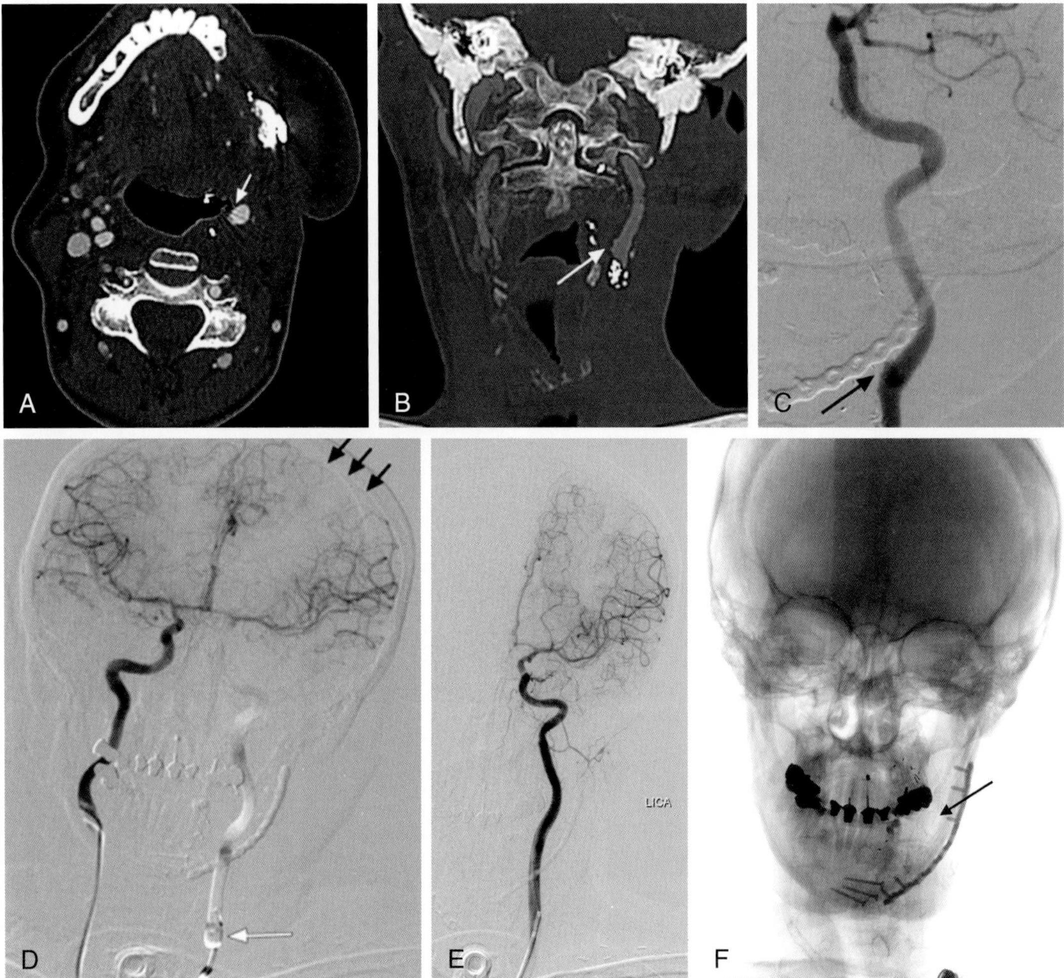

FIGURE 3.9: Carotid blowout (CBO). A and B, This 50-year-old woman with recurrent tonsillar cancer presented with massive oral bleeding, and CTA shows an irregular projection from the carotid directly adjacent to the pharynx (arrows), which was confirmed by DSA. C-F, The initial plan was to sacrifice the carotid, but a balloon occlusion tolerance test (white arrow in Panel D) shows reduced cerebral perfusion on the left (black arrows) and covered stents (arrow in panel F) were placed with preservation of the cerebral flow.

4. The **micropuncture technique** is outlined as follows.
   a. The wrist is placed in hyperextended anatomic position with a rolled towel or radial board used as support.
   b. After giving local anesthesia, the radial artery is punctured with a 21-gauge needle under ultrasound guidance.
   c. A 0.018-inch wire is advanced through the needle; the needle is then exchanged for a 5 French coaxial dilator, which is then exchanged over a 0.035-inch Bentson wire for a 4-7 Fr vascular sheath.
      i. Alternatively specialized radial artery sheaths are available that can be advanced directly over an 0.018-inch wire.

d. For patients undergoing evaluation of carotid stenosis, a pigtail catheter is advanced over a Bentson wire into the ascending aorta, and an aortogram is performed.
   i. Further catheter and guidewire selection depends on the side of the carotid stenosis and anatomic origin of the great vessels.

IX. Techniques for Carotid Artery Stenting

A. Angioplasty and Stenting

1. The early application of angioplasty and stenting for treatment of carotid stenosis was performed with bare metal stents analogous to stent placement in other peripheral arteries.

2. The significant incidence of stroke at the time of angioplasty and stenting led to the development of strategies for embolic protection. A series of trials were pivotal in the establishment of routine use of embolic protection devices (EPDs) in carotid angioplasty and stenting.

B. EVA-3S Trial

1. In 2011, there was a secondary analysis of CAS patients from the endarterectomy versus angioplasty in patients with symptomatic severe carotid stenosis (EVA-3S) trial (CAS vs CEA—France 2000-2005), which was stopped for futility.[44]
   a. In this study 262 patients fulfilled the inclusion criteria (1 was initially allocated to surgery, and in 13 patients stent insertion failed).
   b. 25 patients (9.5%) had a stroke or death during the first 30 days postprocedure.

2. Analysis revealed that the risk of stroke was higher in those patients with internal carotid artery/common carotid artery angulation of greater than or equal to 60% and lower in those patients protected with cerebral EPD.

3. Additional risk factors revealed in a systematic review of a total of 56 studies (34,398 patients) included increased internal carotid artery common carotid angulation, left-sided carotid angioplasty, and stenting, and target internal carotid stenosis was greater than 10 mm.
   a. Type III aortic arch, aortic arch calcification with or without ostial involvement, calcifications, ulcerations, or degree of stenosis did not demonstrate increase in stroke or death risk.
   b. There was no correlation found between the type of stent or the type of cerebral protection device in this systematic review.

4. The timing of procedural strokes in the EVA-3S analysis was informative. Among 17 strokes on day 0 (at the time of the procedure) 5 occurred during aortic arch navigation before common carotid cannulation, 3 during navigation across the stenosis, 1 during protection device placement, and 8 after dilatation and stent placement across the stenosis.

C. Statutory Quality Assurance (2009, 2014)

1. Review of a German nationwide statutory quality assurance database including all open surgical and endovascular procedures on the extracranial carotid artery revealed a total of 13,086 stenting procedures for asymptomatic carotid stenosis between 2009 and 2014.

2. The use of embolic protection was independently associated with decreased hospital risk for stroke or death.[45]

X. Embolic Protection Devices

A. Purpose of EPDs

1. Conceptually there are two primary types of EPDs that can be utilized to protect against cerebral embolization during carotid artery stenting, those that provide embolic protection from a position distal to the target stenosis, and those that provide protection from a position proximal to the target stenosis.

2. The ideal EPD would be easy to use, provide complete protection for all parts of the procedure, and should be applicable to all types of plaque.

3. The device should capture debris of all sizes, and there should be a plan for effective aspiration of debris prior to removal of the device.

B. Distal Embolic Protection

1. Distal embolic protection is performed using a filter device or distal balloon in the internal carotid artery.
   a. A balloon (or filter) placed in the distal internal carotid to provide embolic protection does isolate the brain from debris during the intervention, but placement requires that the target lesion be crossed prior to the establishment of protection.
   b. Following the predilatation, stent placement, and postdilatation, the proximal internal carotid artery is aspirated to remove any debris left behind prior to removal of the device.
   c. The use of the distal balloon requires collateral flow via an intact Circle of Willis and cannot be employed in the case of a contralateral internal carotid occlusion.
   d. This distal balloon method is rarely used with the availability of newer filters and the development of proximal protection device alternatives.

2. Distal embolic protection is most often performed using a filter device, which is basket-like in shape, with a distal straight (curveable) wire.
   a. The device is advanced in the closed position through the level of stenosis. The EPD is deployed and then the procedure takes place over the wire used as a monorail for predilatation, stent placement, and postdilatation after which an end-hole catheter can be advanced over the EPD wire for particulate aspiration.

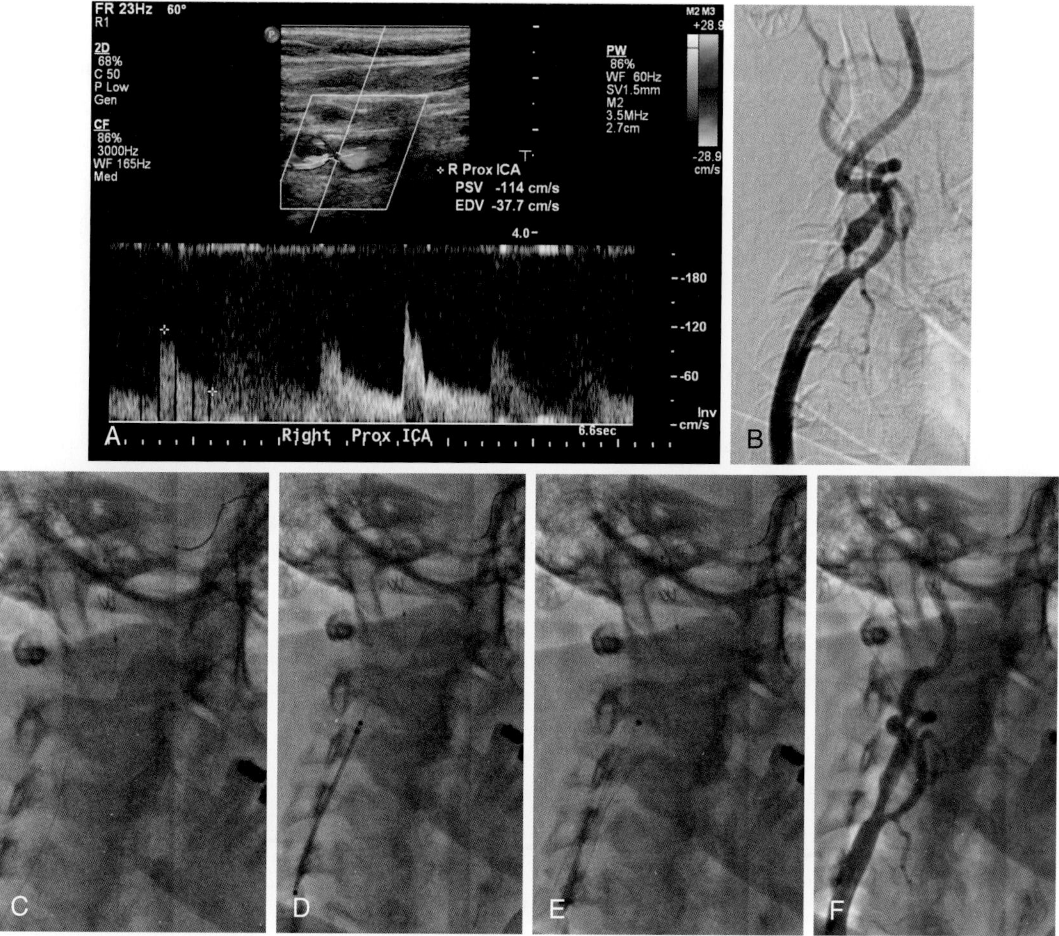

FIGURE 3.10: Filter embolic protection device (EPD). A, DUS demonstrates internal carotid artery stenosis with increased velocities. B, DSA confirms stenosis and favorable anatomy for distal protection. C, The EPD is deployed. D and E, The stent is advanced and deployed with the EPD in place. F, Final DSA post stent deployment.

b. Cerebral perfusion can be maintained throughout the procedure unlike balloon distal protection (Fig. 3.10).
c. Although most commonly used, distal EPD is not ideal because there is no protection while the lesion is crossed.
d. The landing zone in the distal cervical carotid must be straight to allow the device to deploy without causing dissection and to attain correct apposition of the device to the vessel wall. If the device is not well opposed, debris/particles less than 150 μm embolize past the device.
e. The filter may also become filled with debris and require aspiration before closing the device prior to removal postprocedure.
f. The device may become filled with debris requiring catheter aspiration prior to closing (Fig. 3.11; Table 3.2).

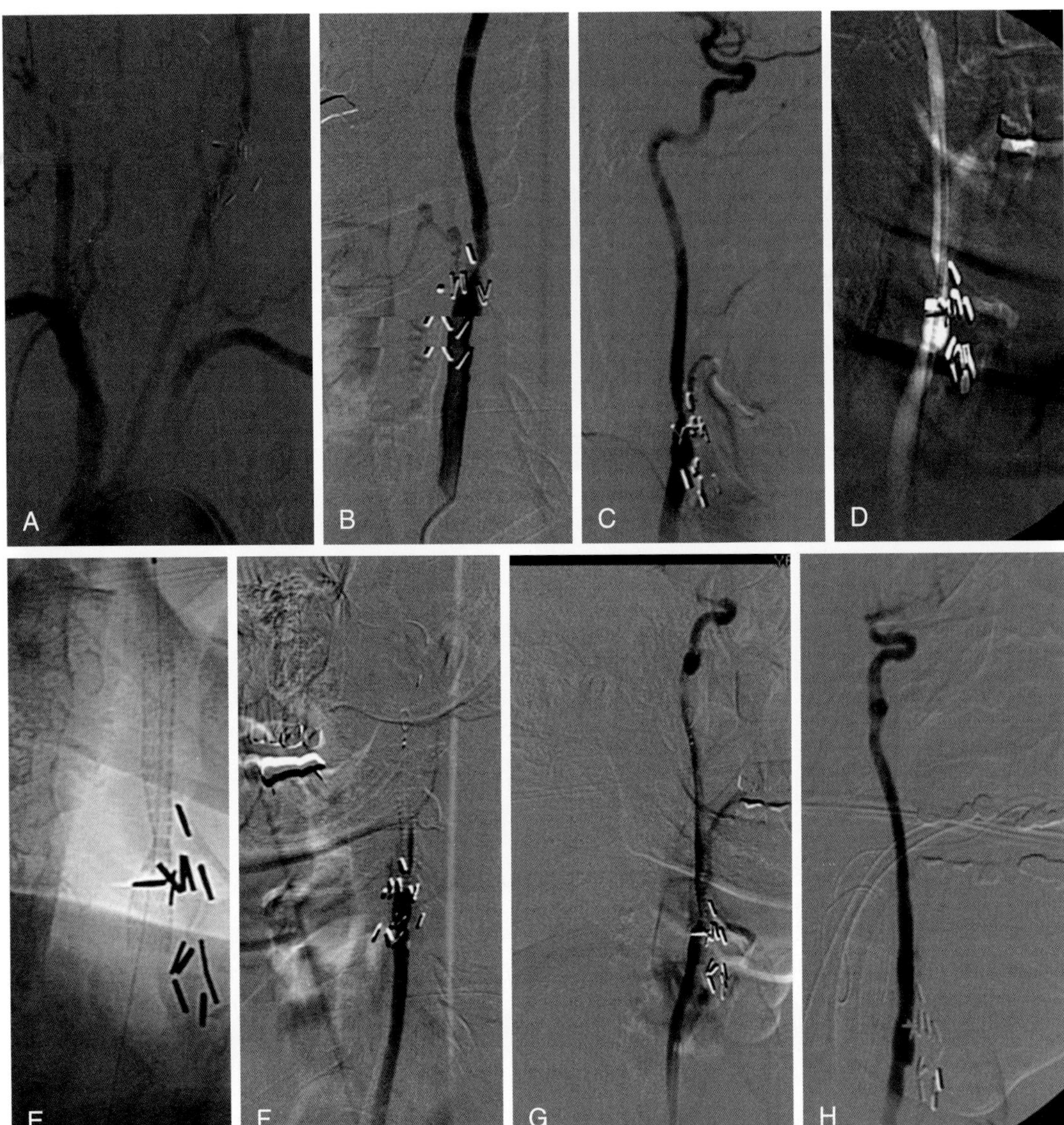

FIGURE 3.11: Filter embolic protection device (EPD) with filling and embolization post removal. A-C, Arch and LCCA DSA demonstrate a tight internal carotid artery stenosis with near occlusion of the ECA in a patient with tonsillar carcinoma post radiation and surgery. D and E, Transfemoral CAS with distal protection was uneventful until the poststent DSA showed no flow beyond the stent (F). The concern is that the filter was filled with debris. The export catheter was utilized to clear the basket and the flow was improved. H, I When the EPD was removed, it contained debris. H, I. Unfortunately, the carotid looked improved, but there was distal embolization of debris to the brain. J, Despite intracranial TPA, the patient had a large left hemispheric stroke.

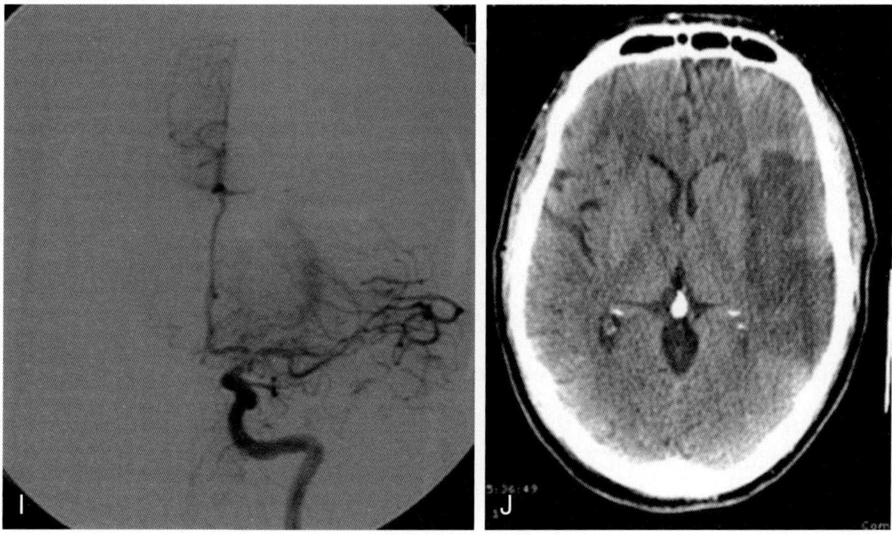

FIGURE 3.11 Cont'd

C. Proximal EPD

1. With a proximal EPD, protection is established first prior to crossing the target lesion or performing an intervention.
   a. It can also be used in a tortuous internal carotid artery because no distal landing zone is required.
2. With proximal protection, there is occlusion of the external carotid and the common carotid artery with flow reversal.
3. Use of this type of EPD requires a patent external carotid artery on the side of the target internal carotid stenosis.[46]
   a. The aortic arch and common carotid configuration must also accommodate the 9 French guiding catheter (6 French working channel).

TABLE 3.2. Steps for Percutaneous Transfemoral Carotid Angioplasty and Stenting Using Distal Embolic Protection Device
Vascular access via femoral artery
Placement of 6F 80-90 cm sheath into the common carotid artery using diagnostic catheter coaxially versus exchange
Target lesion angioplasty using monorail system (5 mm balloon)
Following removal of the balloon, the stent is advanced into ideal position using roadmap and bony landmarks
Post stent deployment, the lesion is postdilated
The filter device is retrieved using a retrieval catheter
Post stent deployment, the lesion is postdilated at the discretion of the operator
Postprocedural angiogram should include both the neck and the cerebral vasculature
Vascular closure using manual pressure with or without mechanical closure device

b. As with the distal internal carotid balloon, this proximal EPD also requires collateral flow via an intact Circle of Willis and *may* not be an option in the case of a contralateral internal carotid occlusion.
c. The common carotid balloon is inflated first and subsequently the external carotid balloon is inflated with the combination suspending flow in the internal carotid artery during the performance of the interventions.
d. Debris is removed via catheter aspiration.
e. Following aspiration, the external carotid balloon is deflated first followed by the common carotid balloon deflation (Fig. 3.12; Table 3.3).

D. Transcarotid Carotid Artery Revascularization

1. A recent variation to the concept of proximal protection is a hybrid open and endovascular technique whereby access to the common carotid is achieved by a cutdown just above the clavicle.
2. Femoral vein access is also achieved with a venous return sheath and dilator, which serves to create a conduit between the common carotid artery and the femoral vein.
3. This conduit is established in order that flow reversal can be employed during carotid angioplasty and stenting without the need for percutaneous distal or proximal EPD devices.
   i. This has been studied with a proprietary device, the Silk Road Enroute Transcarotid Neuroprotection System.[47]

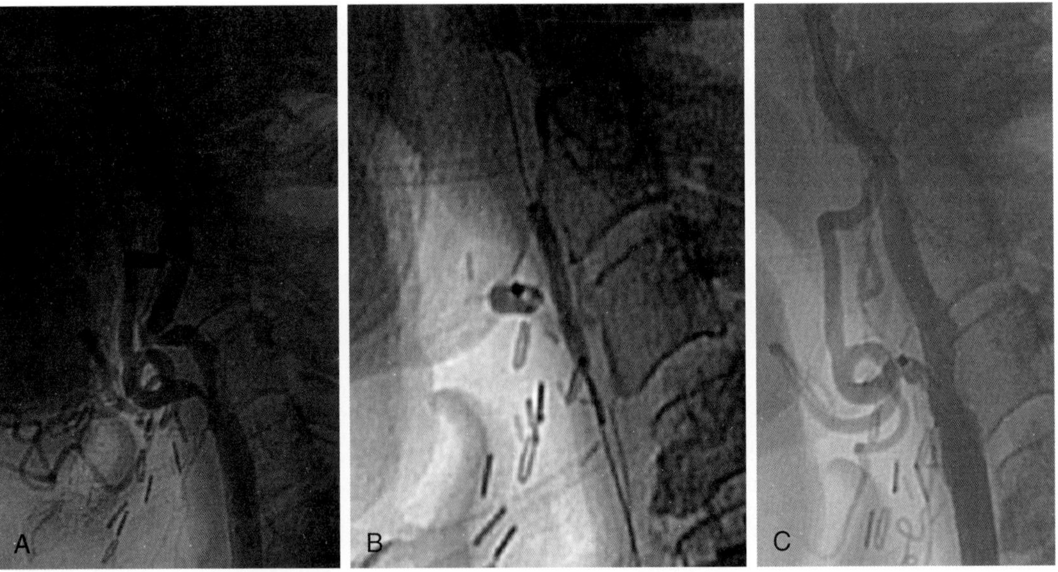

FIGURE 3.12: Proximal embolic protection device (EPD)-Mo.Ma (Medtronic). A, Carotid stenosis involves the bulb, and both the internal and external carotid origins and the kink in the internal carotid above the stenosis would pose challenges to placement of a distal protection device. B, The balloon is placed in the external carotid artery and the stent and angioplasty balloons are placed under flow reversal. C, Final stent placement DSA with balloon deflated. Case courtesy of Dr. Carlos Mena.

TABLE 3.3. Steps for Percutaneous Transfemoral Carotid Angioplasty and Stenting Using Mo.Ma (Medtronic) Device
Vascular access via femoral artery
Placement of 6F 80-90 cm sheath into the common carotid artery using diagnostic catheter coaxially versus exchange
For proximal EPD use: The distal balloon is place into the external carotid artery and the more proximal balloon is placed into the common carotid artery
The balloons are inflated and the lesion is crossed with the wire to be used as a monorail
Target lesion angioplasty using monorail system (5 mm balloon)
Following removal of the angioplasty balloon, the stent is advanced into ideal position using roadmap and bony landmarks
Post stent deployment, the lesion is postdilated
The balloons are deflated: external carotid first followed by the common carotid balloon
Postprocedural angiogram should include both the neck and the cerebral vasculature
Vascular closure using manual pressure with or without mechanical closure device

ii. In the Safety and Efficacy Study for Reverse Flow Used During Carotid Artery Stenting Procedure (ROADSTER) multicenter trial, the device was found to be safe with an overall risk of stroke, risk or myocardial infarction of 3.5% with a 99% technical success rate (Fig. 3.13; Table 3.4).

E. Considerations

1. By considering these three options available for cerebral EPDs and the clinical trial data, EPD use is mandatory for reimbursement by Medicare and it is used in 95% of all CAS cases.[48,49]

2. Stabile et al studied proximal versus distal protection devices and found fewer embolic complications in those cases where proximal protection devices were employed.[50]

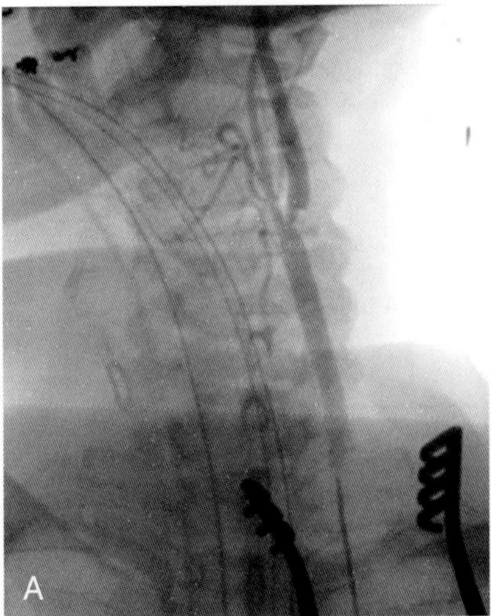

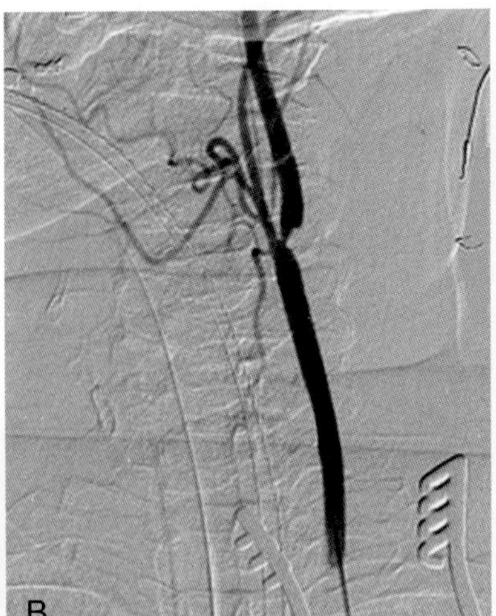

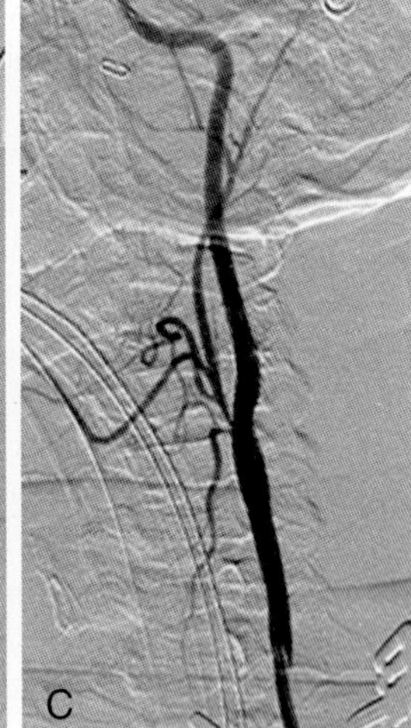

FIGURE 3.13: Transcarotid Carotid Artery Revascularization (TCAR). A, Unsubtracted DSA demonstrates internal carotid stenosis and the vascular access route just above the clavicle on the left. B and C, Subtracted DSA images before and after successful stent placement.

TABLE 3.4. Steps for Transcarotid Carotid Artery Revascularization for Carotid Angioplasty and Stenting
Vascular access via carotid artery cutdown just above the clavicle
Placement of 6F short sheath into the common carotid artery
Establishment of femoral vein access for conduit for cerebral protection
Target lesion angioplasty using monorail system (5 mm balloon)
Following removal of the angioplasty balloon, the stent is advanced into ideal position using roadmap and bony landmarks
Post stent deployment, the lesion is postdilated
Antegrade flow is reestablished
Postprocedural angiogram should include both the neck and the cerebral vasculature
Vascular closure

XI. Summary

Disease involving the extracranial and cervical carotid and vertebral arteries is most commonly related to atherosclerotic disease but may occur because of trauma, radiation exposure, collagen vascular disease, or extrinsic compression. Regardless of the cause, stenosis, occlusion, and atherosclerotic plaque involving the carotid and vertebral arteries are risk factors for ischemic stroke. There have been considerable advances over the last three decades with regard to optimal medical therapy for the prevention of stroke. Interventions such as CEA and CAS are safe methods of revascularization in symptomatic and asymptomatic patients, and vascular providers must consider the patient's disease process, medical comorbidities, and operative risk when planning the best method of revascularization.

References

1. Grant EG, Benson CB, Moneta GL, et al. Carotid artery stenosis: grayscale and Doppler ultrasound diagnosis–Society of Radiologists in Ultrasound consensus conference. *Ultrasound Q.* 2003;19(4):190-198.
2. Wintermark M, Arora S, Tong E, et al. Carotid plaque computed tomography imaging in stroke and nonstroke patients. *Ann Neurol.* 2008;64(2):149-157.
3. Silvennoinen HM, Ikonen S, Soinne L, Railo M, Valanne L. CT angiographic analysis of carotid artery stenosis: comparison of manual assessment, semiautomatic vessel analysis, and digital subtraction angiography. *AJNR Am J Neuroradiol.* 2007;28(1):97-103.
4. Menon BK, d'Esterre CD, Qazi EM, et al. Multiphase CT angiography: a new tool for the imaging triage of patients with acute ischemic stroke. *Radiology.* 2015;275(2):510-520.
5. Roberts HC, Dillon WP, Smith WS. Dynamic CT perfusion to assess the effect of carotid revascularization in chronic cerebral ischemia. *AJNR Am J Neuroradiol.* 2000;21(2):421-425.
6. Alvarez-Linera J, Benito-Leon J, Escribano J, Campollo J, Gesto R. Prospective evaluation of carotid artery stenosis: elliptic centric contrast-enhanced MR angiography and spiral CT angiography compared with digital subtraction angiography. *AJNR Am J Neuroradiol.* 2003;24(5):1012-1019.
7. Larose E, Kinlay S, Selwyn AP, et al. Improved characterization of atherosclerotic plaques by gadolinium contrast during intravascular magnetic resonance imaging of human arteries. *Atherosclerosis.* 2008;196(2):919-925.
8. Wasserman BA, Smith WI, Trout HH III, Cannon RO III, Balaban RS, Arai AE. Carotid artery atherosclerosis: in vivo morphologic characterization with gadolinium-enhanced double-oblique MR imaging initial results. *Radiology.* 2002;223(2):566-573.

9. Randoux B, Marro B, Koskas F, et al. Carotid artery stenosis: prospective comparison of CT, three-dimensional gadolinium-enhanced MR, and conventional angiography. *Radiology*. 2001;220(1):179-185.
10. Natsis KI, Tsitouridis IA, Didagelos MV, Fillipidis AA, Vlasis KG, Tsikaras PD. Anatomical variations in the branches of the human aortic arch in 633 angiographies: clinical significance and literature review. *Surg Radiol Anat*. 2009;31(5):319-323.
11. Brott TG, Hobson RW II, Howard G, et al. Stenting versus endarterectomy for treatment of carotid-artery stenosis. *N Engl J Med*. 2010;363(1):11-23.
12. Ferguson GG, Eliasziw M, Barr HW, et al. The North American Symptomatic Carotid Endarterectomy Trial: surgical results in 1415 patients. *Stroke*. 1999;30(9):1751-1758.
13. Bartlett ES, Walters TD, Symons SP, Fox AJ. Quantification of carotid stenosis on CT angiography. *AJNR Am J Neuroradiol*. 2006;27(1):13-19.
14. Spence JD, Song H, Cheng G. Appropriate management of asymptomatic carotid stenosis. *Stroke Vasc Neurol*. 2016;1(2):64-71.
15. Spence JD. Management of patients with an asymptomatic carotid stenosis–medical management, endovascular treatment, or carotid endarterectomy? *Curr Neurol Neurosci Rep*. 2016;16(1):3.
16. Wong KS, Chen C, Fu J, et al. Clopidogrel plus aspirin versus aspirin alone for reducing embolisation in patients with acute symptomatic cerebral or carotid artery stenosis (CLAIR study): a randomised, open-label, blinded-endpoint trial. *Lancet Neurol*. 2010;9(5):489-497.
17. Warlow CP. Symptomatic patients: the European Carotid Surgery Trial (ECST). *J Mal Vasc*. 1993;18(3):198-201.
18. Mayberg MR, Wilson SE, Yatsu F, et al. Carotid endarterectomy and prevention of cerebral ischemia in symptomatic carotid stenosis. Veterans Affairs Cooperative Studies Program 309 Trialist Group. *JAMA*. 1991;266(23):3289-3294.
19. Gurm HS, Yadav JS, Fayad P, et al. Long-term results of carotid stenting versus endarterectomy in high-risk patients. *N Engl J Med*. 2008;358(15):1572-1579.
20. Markus HS, King A, Shipley M, et al. Asymptomatic embolisation for prediction of stroke in the Asymptomatic Carotid Emboli Study (ACES): a prospective observational study. *Lancet Neurol*. 2010;9(7):663-671.
21. Rothwell PM. ACST: which subgroups will benefit most from carotid endarterectomy? *Lancet*. 2004;364(9440):1122-1123; author reply 1125-1126.
22. Rothwell PM, Goldstein LB. Carotid endarterectomy for asymptomatic carotid stenosis: asymptomatic carotid surgery trial. *Stroke*. 2004;35(10):2425-2427.
23. Halliday A, Harrison M, Hayter E, et al. 10-year stroke prevention after successful carotid endarterectomy for asymptomatic stenosis (ACST-1): a multicentre randomised trial. *Lancet*. 2010;376(9746):1074-1084.
24. Spence JD, Coates V, Li H, et al. Effects of intensive medical therapy on microemboli and cardiovascular risk in asymptomatic carotid stenosis. *Arch Neurol*. 2010;67(2):180-186.
25. Levy EI, Mocco J, Samuelson RM, Ecker RD, Jahromi BS, Hopkins LN. Optimal treatment of carotid artery disease. *J Am Coll Cardiol*. 2008;51(10):979-985.
26. Howard VJ, Meschia JF, Lal BK, et al. Carotid revascularization and medical management for asymptomatic carotid stenosis: protocol of the CREST-2 clinical trials. *Int J Stroke*. 2017;12(7):770-778.
27. Biller J, Feinberg WM, Castaldo JE, et al. Guidelines for carotid endarterectomy: a statement for healthcare professionals from a Special Writing Group of the Stroke Council, American Heart Association. *Circulation*. 1998;97(5):501-509.
28. Randomised trial of endarterectomy for recently symptomatic carotid stenosis: final results of the MRC European Carotid Surgery Trial (ECST). *Lancet*. 1998;351(9113):1379-1387.
29. Lal BK, Beach KW, Roubin GS, et al. Restenosis after carotid artery stenting and endarterectomy: a secondary analysis of CREST, a randomised controlled trial. *Lancet Neurol*. 2012;11(9):755-763.
30. Chimowitz MI, Lynn MJ, Turan TN, et al. Design of the stenting and aggressive medical management for preventing recurrent stroke in intracranial stenosis trial. *J Stroke Cerebrovasc Dis*. 2011;20(4):357-368.

31. Chimowitz MI, Lynn MJ, Howlett-Smith H, et al. Comparison of warfarin and aspirin for symptomatic intracranial arterial stenosis. *N Engl J Med.* 2005;352(13):1305-1316.
32. Compter A, van der Worp HB, Schonewille WJ, et al. Stenting versus medical treatment in patients with symptomatic vertebral artery stenosis: a randomised open-label phase 2 trial. *Lancet Neurol.* 2015;14(6):606-614.
33. Meschia JF, Bushnell C, Boden-Albala B, et al. Guidelines for the primary prevention of stroke: a statement for healthcare professionals from the American Heart Association/American Stroke Association. *Stroke.* 2014;45(12):3754-3832.
34. Kernan WN, Ovbiagele B, Black HR, et al. Guidelines for the prevention of stroke in patients with stroke and transient ischemic attack: a guideline for healthcare professionals from the American Heart Association/American Stroke Association. *Stroke.* 2014;45(7):2160-2236.
35. Mettinger KL, Ericson K. Fibromuscular dysplasia and the brain. I. Observations on angiographic, clinical and genetic characteristics. *Stroke.* 1982;13(1):46-52.
36. Engelter ST, Grond-Ginsbach C, Metso TM, et al. Cervical artery dissection: trauma and other potential mechanical trigger events. *Neurology.* 2013;80(21):1950-1957.
37. Seldinger SI. Catheter replacement of the needle in percutaneous arteriography. A new technique. *Acta Radiol Suppl (Stockholm).* 2008;434:47-52.
38. Campeau L. Percutaneous radial artery approach for coronary angiography. *Cathet Cardiovasc Diagn.* 1989;16(1):3-7.
39. Fischman AM, Swinburne NC, Patel RS. A technical guide describing the use of transradial access technique for endovascular interventions. *Tech Vasc Interv Radiol.* 2015;18(2):58-65.
40. Feldman DN, Swaminathan RV, Kaltenbach LA, et al. Adoption of radial access and comparison of outcomes to femoral access in percutaneous coronary intervention: an updated report from the national cardiovascular data registry (2007-2012). *Circulation.* 2013;127(23):2295-2306.
41. Ruzsa Z, Nemes B, Pinter L, et al. A randomised comparison of transradial and transfemoral approach for carotid artery stenting: RADCAR (RADial access for CARotid artery stenting) study. *EuroIntervention.* 2014;10(3):381-391.
42. Ferrante G, Rao SV, Juni P, et al. Radial versus femoral access for coronary interventions across the entire spectrum of patients with coronary artery disease: a meta-analysis of randomized trials. *JACC Cardiovasc Interv.* 2016;9(14):1419-1434.
43. Mason PJ, Shah B, Tamis-Holland JE, et al. An update on radial artery access and best practices for transradial coronary angiography and intervention in acute coronary syndrome: a scientific statement from the American Heart Association. *Circ Cardiovasc Interv.* 2018;11(9):e000035.
44. Mas JL, Trinquart L, Leys D, et al. Endarterectomy versus angioplasty in patients with symptomatic severe carotid stenosis (EVA-3S) trial: results up to 4 years from a randomised, multicentre trial. *Lancet Neurol.* 2008;7(10):885-892.
45. Knappich C, Kuehnl A, Tsantilas P, et al. The Use of embolic protection devices is associated with a lower stroke and death rate after carotid stenting. *JACC Cardiovasc Interv.* 2017;10(12):1257-1265.
46. Kassavin DS, Clair DG. An update on the role of proximal occlusion devices in carotid artery stenting. *J Vasc Surg.* 2017;65(1):271-275.
47. Kwolek CJ, Jaff MR, Leal JI, et al. Results of the ROADSTER multicenter trial of transcarotid stenting with dynamic flow reversal. *J Vasc Surg.* 2015;62(5):1227-1234.
48. Giri J. Letter by Giri regarding article, "comparative effectiveness of carotid revascularization therapies: evidence from a national hospital discharge database". *Stroke.* 2015;46(2):e41.
49. Giri J, Parikh SA, Kennedy KF, et al. Proximal versus distal embolic protection for carotid artery stenting: a national cardiovascular data registry analysis. *JACC Cardiovasc Interv.* 2015;8(4):609-615.
50. Stabile E, Biamino G, Sorropago G, Rubino P. Proximal endovascular occlusion for carotid artery stenting. *J Cardiovasc Surg (Torino).* 2013;54(1):41-45.

CHAPTER 4

Subclavian Artery Stenosis/ Interventions

Atul Singla, MD, Imaad Razzaque, MD, and Chiranjiv S. Virk, MD

Key Points

- Subclavian stenosis is four times more common in the left subclavian in comparison to the right.
- Symptoms of subclavian stenosis include upper limb claudication, vertebrobasilar steal, and, in case of mammary artery graft to coronary arteries, symptoms of coronary ischemia and cardiomyopathy.
- Endovascular revascularization is undertaken by femoral, brachial, or radial access.
- Balloon expandable stents with intravascular ultrasound (IVUS) guidance is recommended for proximal lesions.
- 5 year patency rates of subclavian stent placement have been showed to be greater than 80% in different series.

I. Introduction

Subclavian artery stenosis is uncommon but is associated with significant morbidity and mortality.[1,2] It is usually focal, and the left side is four times more commonly affected than right in the majority of lesions.[3–5] It is most frequently due to atherosclerosis but may also be caused by fibromuscular dysplasia, Takayasu arteritis, thoracic outlet compression, radiation induced, or trauma.

Anatomically, the left subclavian artery originates as the most distal branch of the aortic arch whereas right subclavian artery is a branch of brachiocephalic artery. The subclavian artery gives rise to the vertebral artery, the internal mammary artery, and the thyrocervical trunk, before terminating as the axillary artery (Fig. 4.1).

II. Subclavian Artery Lesions

A. **Asymptomatic** Patients with isolated subclavian artery lesions are often asymptomatic because of the presence of a rich collateral supply.

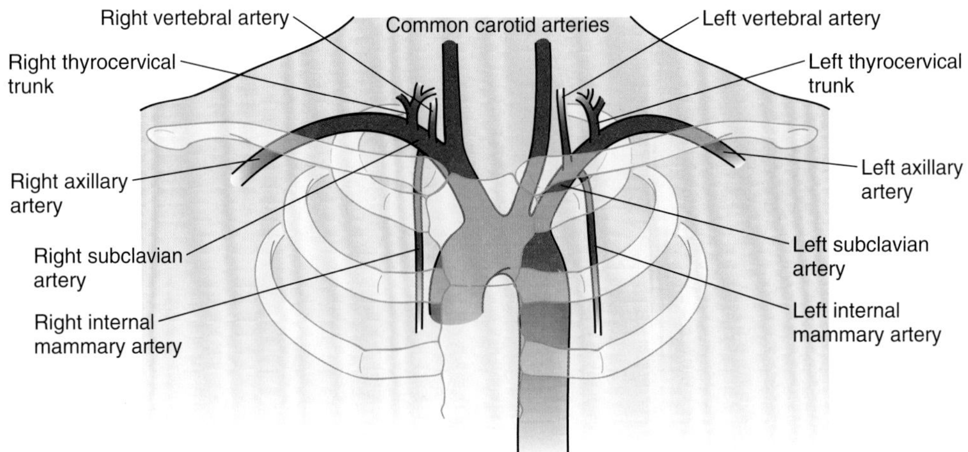

FIGURE 4.1: Anatomy of subclavian artery.

B. Symptomatic

1. Upper limb ischemia/arm claudication and fatigue.
2. **Subclavian steal syndrome:** Owing to severe proximal obstruction, blood flow reverses along the vertebral artery to supply the respective arm (vertebral-subclavian steal) resulting in disorientation, loss of balance, dizziness, diplopia, nystagmus, tinnitus, or hearing loss, consistent with vertebrobasilar insufficiency.
3. **Coronary steal phenomenon:** Severe proximal stenosis can also cause reversal of flow in the coronary artery bypass graft (either left or right internal mammillary artery) to supply the arm leading to angina, myocardial infarction, and ischemic cardiomyopathy if the degree of steal is significant (Fig. 4.2).

III. Evaluation

A. Clinical evaluation of suspected significant subclavian artery stenosis should begin with measuring blood pressure of both arms. A difference >15 mm Hg suggests significant stenosis.[6,7] This may not hold true in the presence of bilateral disease, which, fortunately, is an infrequent finding.

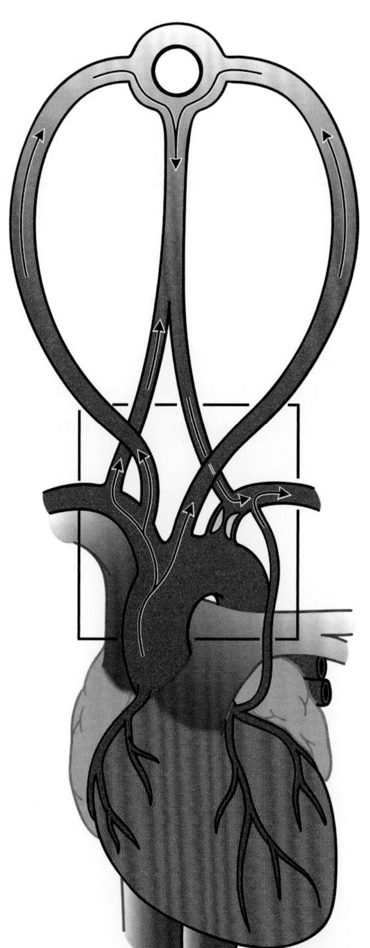

FIGURE 4.2: Subclavian artery stenosis depicting reversal of flow across left vertebral artery depicting steal physiology.

B. Decreased amplitude of the pulse, atrophic changes with the skin and/or nails of the affected arm, and auscultation of a bruit in the supraclavicular fossa suggest subclavian artery stenosis.

C. Noninvasive imaging such as duplex ultrasound with color flow can provide anatomical and functional assessment of a significant subclavian stenotic lesion. Findings such as waveform dampening, monophasic waveform, flow reversal, color aliasing suggestive of turbulent flow, or increased velocities at the suspected site of stenosis are suggestive of significant obstruction.

D. Other noninvasive imaging modalities include magnetic resonance angiogram (MRA) and computer tomographic angiography (CTA), the latter providing excellent resolution of the lesion as well as surrounding structures, helpful in planning endovascular treatment.

IV. Angiography

A. **Invasive Digital Subtraction Angiography** Invasive digital subtraction angiography remains the gold standard imaging modality for assessing significant subclavian artery stenosis. **Technique:** For diagnostic angiography most commonly, common femoral artery access is utilized. Ipsilateral brachial or radial can be accessed if necessary (eg, aortoiliac occlusions). Introducer sheaths between 4 Fr and 6 Fr sheath can be used.

B. **Arch Aortography** Arch aortography is performed utilizing nonangled pigtail catheter positioned in the ascending aorta in left anterior oblique (LAO) 30-45° projection (Fig. 4.3). Usually power injection with 15-20 mL/s for a total of 30-40 mL contrast can be used depending on renal function of the patient. We commonly dilute contrast with 50% contrast and 50% heparinized saline to reduce the total contrast volume.

C. **Subclavian or Innominate Angiography**

1. Selective subclavian or innominate angiography can be performed using one of the several catheters available (Judkins right (JR) 4, angled glide, multipurpose, vertebral, Simmons, Vitek, IM etc. [Fig. 4.4]). We commonly use the JR4 catheter. The catheter is advanced over a 0.035″ glidewire advanced to the distal subclavian artery to obtain a selective angiogram. Care should be taken when engaging or

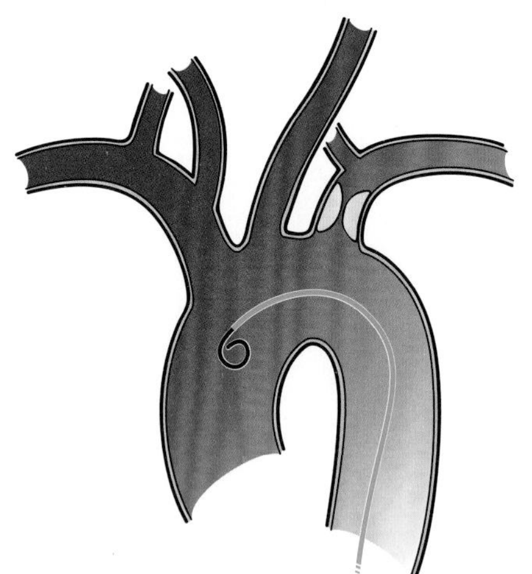

FIGURE 4.3: Arch Aortography performed utilizing non-angled pigtail catheter.

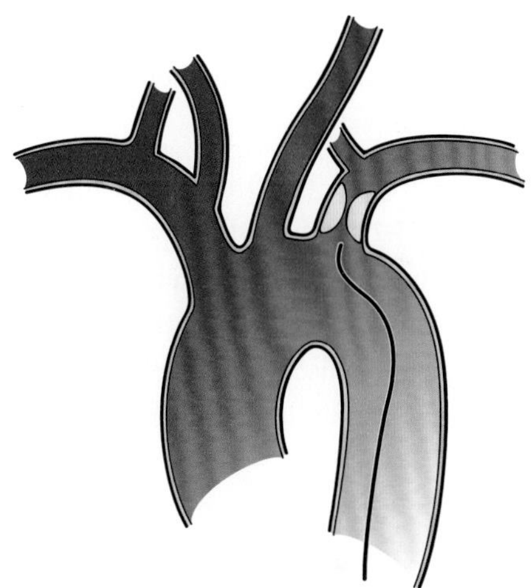

FIGURE 4.4: Selective subclavian angiography.

manipulating catheters to avoid dislodgement of aortic atheroma to minimize the risk of stroke. In cases when thoracic outlet syndrome is suspected, angiograms are repeated with the arm abducted and internally rotated.

2. Anteroposterior (AP) and ipsilateral oblique projections are utilized to assess the origin of the artery and its correlation with the vertebral and internal mammary artery.
3. Once significant stenosis is suspected angiographically, a pullback pressure gradient is measured with a 4 Fr or 5 Fr catheter. Ideally the gradient is measured by recording simultaneous pressure readings proximal and distal to the stenosis using two different pressure manifolds. A gradient of 20-30 mm Hg is considered significant.

V. Treatment

A. Patients with asymptomatic stenosis (either identified incidentally or by imaging) have increased risk of morbidity/mortality and benefit from medical therapy including aspirin, beta blockade, angiotensin-converting enzyme inhibitor, and statin.[5]

B. Indications for revascularization include arm ischemia, vertebral-subclavian steal syndrome, coronary-subclavian steal syndrome, and planned coronary bypass surgery using the ipsilateral internal mammary artery.[8]

C. Revascularization can be achieved surgically (axillary-axillary bypass, carotid-subclavian bypass, and transposition of the subclavian artery) or percutaneously. In current era, endovascular treatment with stenting has become the preferred option with an acceptable rate of restenosis.

VI. Intervention

A. Dosage and Procedures

1. All patients should receive full-dose aspirin and loading dose of Plavix 24-48 hours before intervention. 70-80 units per kilogram of unfractionated heparin is administered with additional heparin boluses provided to maintain an activated clotting time

range of 250-300 seconds. Other antithrombotic regimens (Bivalirudin and GPIIb/IIIa inhibitors) can be extrapolated from coronary angioplasty literature, but there are no data to validate their use in subclavian angioplasty.

2. On average, the subclavian artery diameter ranges from 7 to 10 mm in diameter. The brachiocephalic artery diameters on average are 8-11 mm in diameter. For this reason, a 7-8 Fr guide catheter or 6 Fr 90 cm guiding sheath (Cook shuttle sheath, Bloomington IN) is reasonable to use to allow for balloon and stent catheters to be delivered at the site of the lesion. For nonocclusive stenotic disease and simplicity, the preferred strategy is femoral approach (unless there is abdominal aortic disease that hinders advancing equipment).

   Initially, a smaller size diagnostic catheter (usually 5 Fr JR4 or multipurpose) is telescoped through the sheath and used to engage the ostium of the left subclavian artery or brachiocephalic artery. A support wire, either 0.014″ or 0.018″, is used to cross the lesion (Fig. 4.5). We commonly use soft 0.014″ work horse wires such as Asahi Prowater (Abbott Vascular) or Runthrough (Terumo). Next, the diagnostic catheter is advanced across the lesion. Once across the lesion, the 0.014″ or 0.018″ wire is exchanged for a soft-tipped 0.035″ Wholey or Rosen wire for better support before balloon angioplasty and stenting. The diagnostic catheter is removed, and balloon angioplasty is performed, typically with the balloon diameter undersized to the vessel (5-6 mm diameter balloon with a length that ranges from 20-40 mm). It is imperative not to compromise the ostium/origin of the vertebral or the internal mammary artery. Similarly, care must be taken to identify the origin of common carotid artery when performing right subclavian and/or brachiocephalic artery intervention. We routinely perform IVUS at this point before stent deployment for sizing and optimal vessel preparation.

3. It is common to proceed with stenting after balloon angioplasty, as angioplasty if performed alone is associated with recoil, abrupt closure, dissection, and suboptimal lumen gain.[9,10] For proximal subclavian lesions, balloon expandable stents are utilized for their radial strength and precise deployment. For the mid and distal vessel, angioplasty alone is preferred, as stenting is highly prone to fracture between clavicle and first rib causing thoracic outlet syndrome physiology. Self-expendable stents have reportedly a higher tendency to develop stent compression and higher restenosis rate.

4. It is imperative to cover the ostium of subclavian or brachiocephalic artery by having proximal 2-3 mm of the stent hang out in the aortic arch. Precise stent placement requires good wire support and imaging in multiple orthogonal views before deployment (for left subclavian artery, LAO projection is preferred; for right subclavian artery RAO projection is preferred).

5. To avoid geographic miss of the ostium during stent deployment, an additional step maybe used by advancing the guide catheter or the long sheath across the lesion. The stent is advanced over the wire within the guide catheter and positioned across the lesion. The guide catheter is withdrawn, "unsheathing" the stent in proper position. It is imperative not to oversize the stent owing to risk of dissection and potential catastrophic intrathoracic hemorrhage. Repeat angiogram is warranted to ensure no complications occurred. IVUS is optional post stent deployment.

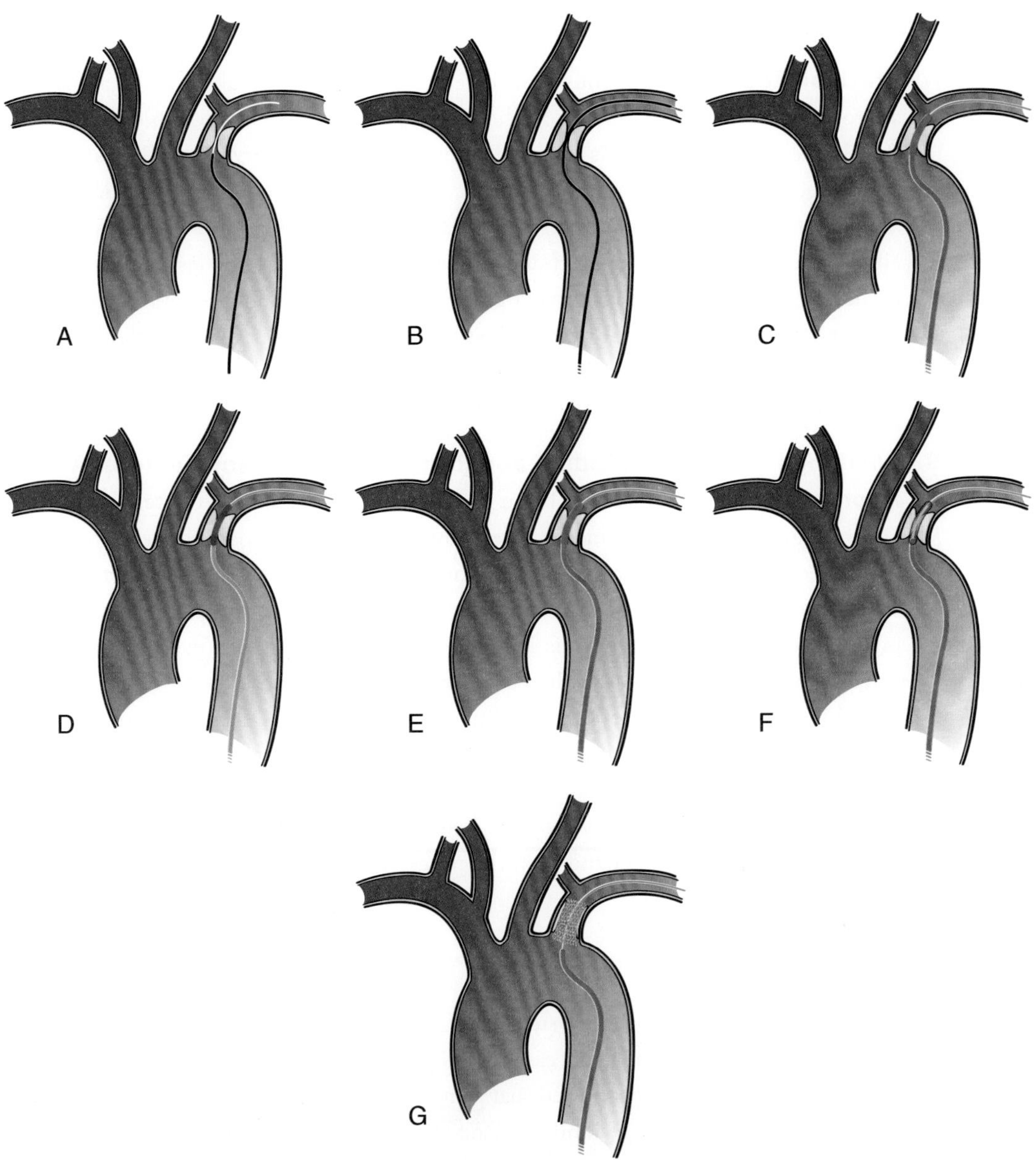

FIGURE 4.5: A, A 0.014″ workhorse wire across the lesion into the axillary artery. B, JR4 catheter or angled glide catheter is advanced over the wire across the lesion and through this catheter the wire is exchanged out for a stiffer wire eg, rosen or stiff glide wire. C, 6 Fr 90 cm shuttle sheath advanced over the catheter beyond the lesion. D, Predilatation balloon catheter at the lesion site, followed by withdrawing the sheath below the lesion (unsheathing the catheter). E, After performing balloon dilatation, sheath is advanced over the deflating balloon across the lesion. F, Stent is positioned at the lesion site and sheath withdrawn with 1-2 mm of stent hanging out in the aortic arch (unsheathing the stent). G, Stent deployment.

B. **Follow-Up** Post stenting patients are followed at 1-, 6-, and 12-month intervals and yearly thereafter. Our protocol is to perform history and physical examination, with bilateral arm blood pressure measurements at each visit. If restenosis is suspected, color duplex ultrasound is performed.

VII. Subclavian Total Occlusions

A. **Brachial Approach** For flush occluded subclavian arterial lesions, a brachial approach is the preferred method. The technique varies from the femoral approach. A 6-French shuttle sheath is inserted into the brachial artery carefully, as the brachial subclavian arterial junction is prone to dissection. Delivery of the sheath over an amplatz wire may reduce the rate of dissection. A 0.035″ glidewire supported by either a diagnostic catheter or glide catheter is used to cross the lesion. Once across the lesion, the technique to intervene is the same as outlined in the femoral approach. Precise position of the stent over the ostium is challenging, as it is difficult to visualize the ostium when injecting from the arm and one may have to rely on the bony landmarks/calcification.

B. **Combined Antegrade (Radial) and Retrograde (Common Femoral Access) Approach** Other option is to obtain dual access using combined antegrade (radial) and retrograde (common femoral access) approach. Initial imaging is performed by dual injection using a 6 Fr glidesheath for radial access with a JR4 catheter and an aortogram performed by pigtail catheter via transfemoral approach. Once imaging is obtained, a 0.035″ glidewire is inserted to the distal cap within the JR4 catheter or glide catheter. A support catheter is used to help cross the lesion. Once the wire is within the ascending aorta, repeat imaging should be performed to confirm location. Glidewire from radial access is snared out of the femoral sheath, establishing radial to femoral rail. After establishing the radial to femoral wire, tension is applied at each end by grasping the wire with hemostats. Femoral sheath is then advanced across the subclavian lesion and then the procedure is completed through the femoral access as described earlier.

VIII. Outcomes

A. Balloon angioplasty followed by stent placement in the subclavian artery has a 5 year proven patency of 82% based on a case series by Wang.[11] Another study by Huttl et al. on brachiocephalic angioplasty showed that primary and secondary patency at 10 years were 98% and 93%, respectively.[12] Similarly, Paukovits demonstrated a primary patency rate of 98% at 2 years and 70% at 8 years in 77 innominate artery angioplasties, thus suggesting that brachiocephalic stenting should be considered as first-line therapy given the overall high technical success rate and very low rates of procedure complications (2.6% distal embolization, including transient ischemic attacks only).[13] Restenosis occurs in about 10% of patients who undergo stenting.[14]

B. Surgical intervention maybe required for more complex tubular lesions. Various techniques have been described such as carotid-subclavian bypass, carotid transposition, or axillo-axillary bypass surgeries, which have all maintained a patency rate of 70% at 5 years, with higher patency rates in common carotid bypass (80%) versus lower patency rates in axillo-axillary bypass (46%).[15] Of note, patients who have symptomatic carotid stenosis should have the carotid stenosis intervened on before intervening for subclavian stenosis.

C. Patients with high surgical risk and unfavorable anatomy for percutaneous interventions should be treated medically with antiplatelet therapy and primary prevention for other cardiovascular diseases.

References

1. Hennerici M, Rautenberg W, Mohr S. Stroke risk from symptomless extracranial arterial disease. *Lancet.* 1982;2(8309):1180-1183.
2. Moran KT, Zide RS, Persson AV, Jewell ER. Natural history of subclavian steal syndrome. *Am Surg.* 1988;54(11):643-644.
3. Rodriguez-Lopez JA, Werner A, Martinez R, Torruella LJ, Ray LI, Diethrich EB. Stenting for atherosclerotic occlusive disease of the subclavian artery. *Ann Vasc Surg.* 1999;13(3):254-260.
4. Schillinger M, Haumer M, Schillinger S, Mlekusch W, Ahmadi R, Minar E. Outcome of conservative versus interventional treatment of subclavian artery stenosis. *J Endovasc Ther.* 2002;9(2):139-146.
5. Ochoa VM, Yeghiazarians Y. Subclavian artery stenosis: a review for the vascular medicine practitioner. *Vasc Med.* 2011;16(1):29-34.
6. Osborn LA, Vernon SM, Reynolds B, Timm TC, Allen K. Screening for subclavian artery stenosis in patients who are candidates for coronary bypass surgery. *Catheter Cardiovasc Interv.* 2002;56(2):162-165.
7. Lobato EB, Kern KB, Bauder-Heit J, Hughes L, Sulek CA. Incidence of coronary-subclavian steal syndrome in patients undergoing noncardiac surgery. *J Cardiothorac Vasc Anesth.* 2001;15(6):689-692.
8. Patel SN, White CJ, Collins TJ, et al. Catheter-based treatment of the subclavian and innominate arteries. *Catheter Cardiovasc Interv.* 2008;71(7):963-968.
9. Bachman DM, Kim RM. Transluminal dilatation for subclavian steal syndrome. *AJR Am J Roentgenol.* 1980;135(5):995-996.
10. Zeitler E, Richter EI, Roth FJ, Schoop W. Results of percutaneous transluminal angioplasty. *Radiology.* 1983;146(1):57-60.
11. Wang KQ, Wang ZG, Yang BZ, et al. Long-term results of endovascular therapy for proximal subclavian arterial obstructive lesions. *Chin Med J (Engl).* 2010;123(1):45-50.
12. Huttl K, Nemes B, Simonffy A, Entz L, Berczi V. Angioplasty of the innominate artery in 89 patients: experience over 19 years. *Cardiovasc Intervent Radiol.* 2002;25(2):109-14.
13. Paukovits TM, Lukacs L, Berczi V, Hirschberg K, Nemes B, Huttl K. Percutaneous endovascular treatment of innominate artery lesions: a single-centre experience on 77 lesions. *Eur J Vasc Endovasc Surg.* 2010;40(1):35-43.
14. Filippo F, Francesco M, Francesco R, et al. Percutaneous angioplasty and stenting of left subclavian artery lesions for the treatment of patients with concomitant vertebral and coronary subclavian steal syndrome. *Cardiovasc Intervent Radiol.* 2006;29(3):348-353.
15. Salam TA, Lumsden AB, Smith RB. Subclavian artery revascularization: a decade of experience with extra-thoracic bypass procedures. *J Surg Res.* 1994;56(5):387-392.

CHAPTER **5A**

Coarctation of the Aorta

Chandni Patel, MD, Kurt Bjorkman, MD, and Jeremy D. Asnes, MD

Key Points

- Coarctation of the aorta may be first identified in adolescence or adulthood with hypertension often being the first presenting sign.
- Intervention for coarctation should be approached cautiously and methodically.
- For native coarctation, current recommendations suggest a multidisciplinary approach incorporating input from surgeons, cardiologists, and interventionalists with adult congenital heart disease expertise to determine surgical versus catheter-based intervention.
- For recurrent discrete coarctation, guidelines favor percutaneous catheter intervention over surgery.
- Stent angioplasty has been shown to have superior outcomes and lower complication rates as compared with both balloon angioplasty and surgery.
- Covered stents should be available during interventional procedures in the event of serious aortic wall injury.
- Given the risk of aortic wall injury with catheter-based intervention for coarctation, routine follow-up with either CT angiography or MR angiography should be performed.

I. Introduction

A. **Coarctation** of the aorta describes a wide variation of anatomic narrowing of the aorta, most commonly occurring as a discrete lesion in the proximal thoracic aorta opposite the insertion site of the ductus arteriosis.[1] However, even when discrete, coarctation is considered to be part of a generalized arteriopathy.[2] It is one of the more common congenital lesions, accounting for 5%-10% of all congenital heart disease. Genetic influences on coarctation have long been suspected with a well-documented male predominance of disease with an incidence ratio of 1.7:1.[3] This genetic link is further evidenced by coarctation appearing in 35% of patients with Turner syndrome (45X). NOTCH1 and MCTP2 have recently been recognized as possible loci for disease.[4,5]

B. Permutations of this disease exist not only in location but also in length, severity, coexisting conditions, time of presentation, and complications.[1] Rarely, coarctation involves the ascending or abdominal aorta.[6] Although most often diagnosed in infancy or childhood, aortic coarctation may first be identified in adolescence or adulthood. Furthermore, with increasing survival and patient longevity, significant rates of residual coarctation, as well as recurrence postintervention, are seen well into adulthood.[7-10]

C. Hypertension of the aorta and its branches proximal to the obstructed aortic segment is the most obvious consequence of this disease. However, coarctation-associated hypertension is only one component of a complex arteriopathic disease. Moreover, although it is tempting to consider treatment of coarctation as a simple procedure directed at relief of aortic obstruction and hypertension, the care of the patient with aortic coarctation requires a life-long, often multidisciplinary approach that should include experts in adult congenital heart disease.

II. Coexisting Disease

A. Occurrence

1. Coarctation most commonly occurs in conjunction with other congenital heart lesions including aortic arch hypoplasia, ventricular septal defects (VSDs), patent ductus arteriosus, transposition of the great arteries, atrioventricular canal defects, and left-sided obstructive lesions including abnormalities of the mitral valve and the subaortic region.[11]

2. Bicuspid aortic valve is seen in more than 50% of affected patients.[12] In a series of 500 patients with coarctation undergoing MRI assessment, only 14% had isolated coarctation.[13]

B. Anomalies

a. Coarctation is also associated with extracardiac vascular anomalies including important variations in brachiocephalic artery anatomy, a robust collateral arterial circulation, and intracranial aneurysms.[1,11,14]
b. Arterial collaterals may arise from the internal thoracic and subclavian arteries, thyrocervical trunks, and vertebral and anterior spinal arteries and provide blood supply to the descending aorta, bypassing the obstruction caused by the coarctation itself.[15] The aortic wall itself is abnormal and predisposed to dissection and rupture.[16]

III. Natural History

A. The natural history of uncorrected coarctation of the aorta was described by Campbell in 1970 after reviewing the records of 465 patients who had survived the first year of life.

1. Of these, there was a mean age of death at 34 years, and 75% of patients died by age 46 years, with the most common causes of death including congestive heart failure (26%), aortic rupture (21%), endocarditis (18%), and intracranial hemorrhage (12%).[3]

B. Life expectancy is significantly improved with intervention, but still notably reduced from nonaffected populations with survival rates of 72% at 30 years after operation in those operated on at median age of 16 years, and 81% survival at 50 years after surgery in those operated on before the age of 5 years.[17,18]

C. In patients who have had corrective intervention, the most common causes of late death are coronary artery disease, sudden cardiac death, heart failure, cerebrovascular accidents, and ruptured aortic aneurysm.[17] Thus, intervention is essential to prevent significant morbidity and mortality.

IV. Presentation and Examination Findings

A. Presentation

1. The most common presenting sign of disease in the patient with aortic coarctation is systolic hypertension, and perhaps the most easily identified finding is a differential between the upper extremity and lower extremity systolic blood pressure.[19]
   a. Patients presenting with coarctation-associated hypertension fall into one of the three categories: those with "native" coarctation for which no prior intervention has been undertaken; those with residual or recurrent obstruction at or adjacent to a site of prior catheter or surgical intervention, so called recurrent coarctation; and those with well-repaired coarctation, no residual aortic arch obstruction, and persistent hypertension (Fig. 5A.1).
   b. Regardless of which category they are in, patients are often asymptomatic. Rarely, they may present with headache, epistaxis, claudication, aortic dissection, or heart failure.[16,20] We will discuss the management of those patients with native, residual, and recurrent obstruction in this chapter.
2. Not discussed in this chapter is the far more uncommon presentation of a patient with complications of aortic aneurysm related to a prior coarctation repair.

B. Examination Findings

1. Aside from hypertension, notable physical examination findings may include diminished and delayed femoral pulses as compared with the radial pulse (*pulsus parvus et tardus*) as well as a cardiac murmur.
2. A systolic ejection murmur from the coarctation may be heard in the left upper sternal border, at the base of the heart, and in the back. In addition, continuous murmurs may be heard over the anterior chest wall and back in patients with a robust collateral arterial system.
3. Associated lesions such as aortic valve stenosis, VSDs, or mitral stenosis will produce their own distinct murmurs as well.[1]
4. Surgery for coarctation may be performed from a left or right lateral thoracotomy, or from a median sternotomy (most often in the setting of concomitant cardiac disease or arch hypoplasia). Surgical scars will help guide an understanding of the approach taken in patients without a well-known history.

V. Evaluation

A. Testing and Imaging

1. Blood pressure assessment in all four extremities
2. Full physical examination including identification of scars related to prior surgery
3. Echocardiogram to assess associated congenital cardiac disease and/or surgical repairs and myocardial function
4. Thoracic CTA (CT angiography) or MRA (MR angiography) for detailed assessment of the entire thoracic aorta and its branches

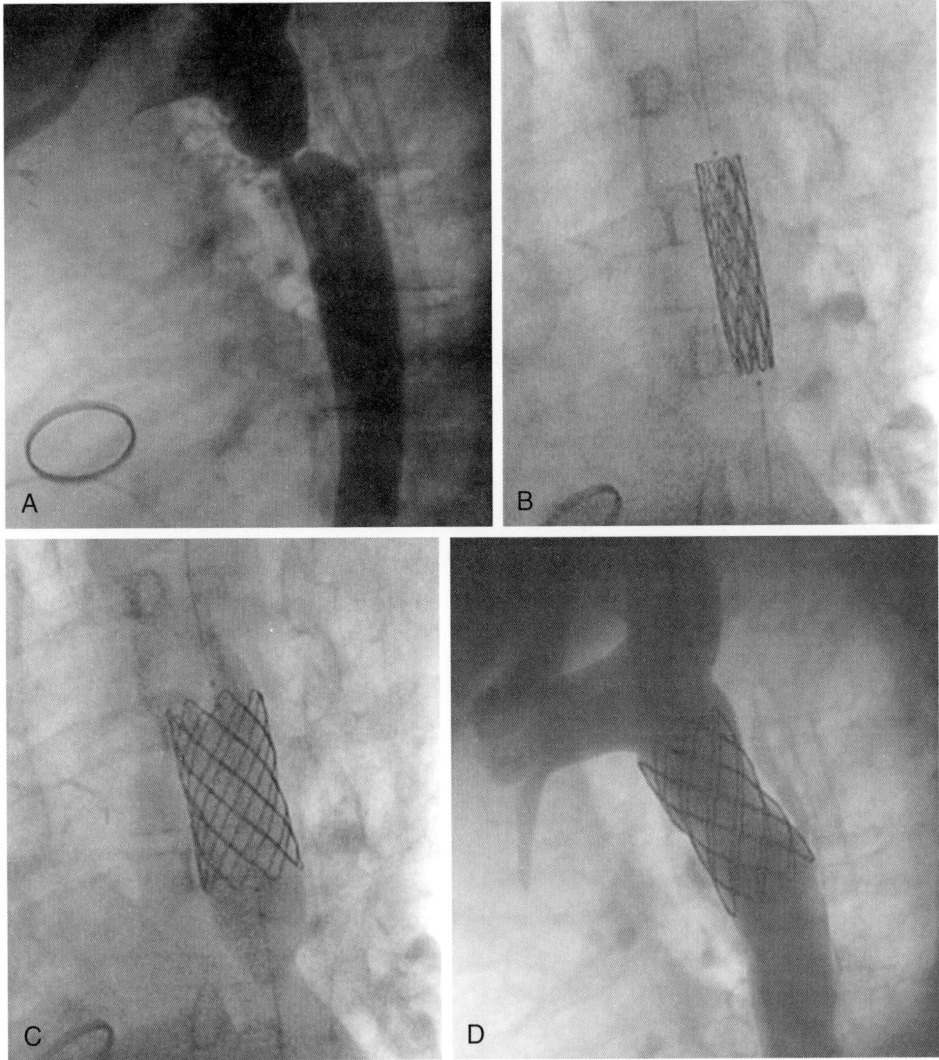

FIGURE 5A.1: A, Native coarctation in a 40-year-old man who had previously undergone ascending aorta and aortic valve replacement (narrowest diameter 4.5 mm). B, 4.5-cm-long Cheatham Platinum Covered Stent premounted on 22 mm balloon-in-balloon catheter; deployment with inner balloon inflated. C, Outer balloon inflated at 3 atm. D, Final angiogram following covered stent angioplasty.

5. Imaging of the intracranial vasculature (CTA or MRA) is recommended to exclude coexisting aneurysms, which can be seen in up to 10% of patients with coarctation[16,21]

6. In the older adult or others at risk for peripheral vascular disease, consideration should be given to assessment of the femoral and iliac arteries (CTA or MRA)

B. Anatomic Considerations

1. Notably, 3%-4% of patients with coarctation will have an aberrant right subclavian artery arising from the descending aorta distal to the obstruction, complicating the assessment of a blood pressure differential.

2. Furthermore, in patients with a robust arterial collateral circulation, the blood pressure differential may be reduced, masking the severity of the aortic obstruction.

3. In addition, surgical approaches to coarctation may include sacrifice of the left subclavian artery as a component of the repair (subclavian flap technique).
   a. In these patients, the blood pressure in the left arm is unreliable.
   b. Owing to a combination of anatomic variation and/or surgical repair, there is no reliable, noninvasive means of assessing the systolic blood pressure proximal to a segment of narrowed aorta.

VI. Indications for Treatment

American and European guidelines for the treatment of adult patients with congenital heart disease include specific recommendations regarding the treatment of aortic coarctation.[2,16] A summary of indications for intervention can be found in Table 5A.1.

VII. Goals of Therapy

A. The primary goal of any interventional therapy for aortic coarctation is to normalize the luminal diameter of the narrowed segment of the aorta and thereby eliminate the pressure gradient across the coarctation. In most but not all patients, this will lead to improvement in hypertension and a decrease in the need for antihypertensive medication.

B. Determining the appropriate or "normal" target diameter of the aorta in a patient with coarctation requires assessment of that individual's aortic dimensions from the transverse arch to the distal thoracic aorta at the level of the diaphragm. There is often aneurysmal dilation of the ascending aorta, particularly when a bicuspid aortic valve is present. There may also be associated transverse arch hypoplasia, which in and of itself can lead to hypertension in the proximal arch and ascending aorta even after successful treatment of a discrete coarctation. Typically, there is aneurysmal dilation of the aorta just distal to the coarctation, but the dimensions of aorta at the level of the diaphragm are preserved. Thus, the diameter of the aorta at the diaphragm is often used as a therapeutic target.

C. Garcier et al. reported aortic lumen dimensions measured by MRI in 66 healthy adults with a mean age of 44.5 years (range 19.3-82.4 y).[22] The mean diameter from the distal aortic arch to the midthoracic aorta ranged from 25 mm (range 16.4-35 mm) at the distal arch to 22.7 mm (range 13.8-32 mm) at the level of the left ventricle.[22] Because of the coexisting aortopathy, these dimensions may not apply to individuals with aortic coarctation. However, when considering therapy in a young patient with growth potential, they must be kept in mind.

TABLE 5A.1. Indications for Intervention in Patients With Aortic Coarctation
• Peak-to-peak coarctation gradient ≥20 mm Hg • Peak-to-peak coarctation gradient <20 mm Hg in the presence of anatomic imaging evidence of significant coarctation with radiological evidence of significant collateral flow • Pathologic blood pressure response to exercise • ≥ 50% luminal narrowing relative to the aortic lumen at the level of the diaphragm (independent of blood pressure gradient)

VIII. Treatment Options

A. Measures of Success

1. The successful treatment of aortic coarctation must be measured across multiple domains. In the hypertensive patient with native or recurrent coarctation, the overarching goal is reduction of systolic blood pressure.
   a. However, it is well known that resting and exercise hypertension is common in this population, even in the absence of persistent aortic obstruction.
   b. Furthermore, hypertension can be partially mitigated with pharmacologic therapies in some patients with aortic obstruction.
   c. Thus, measures of therapeutic success may include not only angiographic improvement in aortic lumen size but also reduction in gradient, reduction in blood pressure at rest and/or with exercise, reduction in symptoms (when present), and reduction in antihypertensive medication requirements.

2. Measures of procedural success include not only therapeutic success but also the absence of significant procedure-related morbidity and mortality including aortic wall injury and aneurysm formation.

B. Surgery

1. Surgical repair of aortic coarctation may be accomplished through several different approaches including coarctectomy with direct end-to-end anastomosis or extended end-to-end anastomosis, interposition graft placement, bypass graft placement, and subclavian flap or patch aortoplasty. In patients with recurrent coarctation, understanding the initial surgical approach is critical to understanding the cause of recurrent obstruction and how to best manage it.

2. Current guidelines recommend surgical intervention for long-segment recoarctation and coarctation in the setting of aortic arch hypoplasia.[16]
   a. Furthermore, these guidelines recommend that surgery be performed by surgeons with expertise in congenital heart surgery.
   b. With regard to discrete native coarctation, guidelines do not specify a preference for surgery or transcatheter approach, but rather recommend a multidisciplinary approach incorporating input from surgeons, cardiologists, and interventionalists with adult congenital heart disease expertise.
   c. For recurrent discrete coarctation, guidelines favor percutaneous catheter intervention over surgery.

C. Intervention Recommendations Surgery carries up to a 10% reintervention risk for older children and adults[23]and in one study spanning several decades was associated with a perioperative mortality of 4.5%.[17] Thus, there has been a shift recently toward percutaneous approaches (balloon angioplasty or stent placement) for primary intervention in adults with uncomplicated native coarctation.[16,23,24] In patients with recoarctation, the general consensus favors, with rare exception, the transcatheter approach regardless of the age. In particular, stent angioplasty has come into favor as the intervention of choice in adults with native or recurrent coarctation because of its superior outcomes and lower complication rates as compared with both balloon angioplasty and surgery.[25] We describe in the sections that follow the available percutaneous options for treatment of coarctation of the aorta.

IX. Percutaneous Treatment Options

A. Balloon Angioplasty

1. Balloon angioplasty can result in hemodynamic and angiographic improvements in both native and recurrent coarctation. Animal studies have demonstrated that successful balloon angioplasty for aortic coarctation results in tears of the aortic intima.[26] Achieving a successful tear generally requires expansion of the stenotic lesion by two to three times its initial diameter.

2. The gradient relief achieved with balloon angioplasty is less predictable, and the risk of undesirable aortic wall injury is higher than with stent angioplasty or surgery. This is likely related to the overdistension needed to achieve a therapeutic result.

3. Some studies have shown the risk of postangioplasty aortic aneurysm formation to be as high as 35%.[27,28] Rates of recoarctation following balloon angioplasty have been reported to range anywhere from 8% to 32%.[27,29,30] In a prospective, multi-institutional, observational study, balloon angioplasty was found to be inferior to stent angioplasty for the treatment of native aortic coarctation. In this study, gradient reduction with balloon angioplasty alone was less than that seen with stent angioplasty or surgery. Furthermore, the rate of aortic wall injury and aneurysm formation was significantly higher with balloon angioplasty compared with stent angioplasty. Compared with its use in native coarctation, balloon angioplasty results in better gradient reduction and less aortic wall injury when used for the treatment of recurrent coarctation.

4. In our practice, balloon angioplasty is generally reserved for the treatment of recurrent coarctation in infants and young children whose vasculature is too small to allow placement of a stent capable of reaching anticipated adult aortic dimensions. See Table 5A.2 for equipment.

B. Technique and Procedural Considerations for Balloon Angioplasty

1. **Key Points** Excellent and detailed discussion of the techniques and materials required for coarctation balloon angioplasty can be found in Dr Charles Mullins' textbook *Cardiac Catheterization in Congenital Heart Disease.*[31] The following key points should be considered:
   a. We recommend that all patients undergo preprocedural imaging—either CTA or MRA.
   b. We recommend the use of general anesthesia, as aortic wall interventions are painful and inadvertent patient movement can result in significant complications.
   c. Type and cross-matched blood should be available in the room during the procedure.

TABLE 5A.2.	Balloon Angioplasty Equipment: Description and Uses

Catheters	• Soft-tipped, atraumatic end-hole catheters
	  • Helpful for crossing the coarctation and delivering guidewires
	• Multimarker pigtail angiographic catheters
	  • Helpful for calibration and length assessment
	• Multi-Track angiographic catheter (NuMED, Inc., Hopkinton, NY)
	  • Allows for hemodynamic and angiographic assessment without need to remove the guidewire

Balloons	• Noncompliant angioplasty balloons with short shoulders are preferred • Precise inflation pressure/balloon diameter relationships are needed for safe angioplasty
Guidewires	• Exchange length guidewires with enhanced stiffness such as Rosen Wires or Amplatz Extra-Stiff wires
Sheaths	• Sheaths must be able to accommodate the angioplasty balloons being used and provide good hemostasis at aortic pressure when a wire and catheter (such as the Multi-Track catheter) are across the hemostatic valve • Large diameter (12-14 French), long (75-90 cm) sheaths should be available, should emergent covered stent placement be necessary
Large-diameter covered stents	• In the event of a serious aortic wall injury such as a large dissection, acute aneurysm formation, or aortic wall rupture, covered stents—balloon expandable or self-expanding—of sufficient diameter for use in the aorta should be immediately available, and the operator should be comfortable with their use. Given the spectrum of aortic coarctation, this necessitates an inventory of various sizes and lengths • In our practice, we rely on the Mounted CP Covered Stent (NuMED, Inc., Hopkinton, NY). These can be delivered through a 12 or 14 French sheath and most can be expanded to 30 mm. These stents exhibit significant foreshortening, and thus careful review of the stent length at the intended implant diameter is necessary

d. A careful hemodynamic assessment should be performed prior to intervention. In cases where the indication for intervention will depend on the invasive hemodynamic assessment, one may want to perform a baseline assessment prior to induction of general anesthesia. If the presence of a significant obstruction is confirmed, the patient can then be induced prior to intervention.

e. Detailed, multiplane angiography should be performed prior to any intervention.
   i. In our practice, we routinely use rotational angiography to assess the aortic arch and coarctation and determine the optimal gantry angle for intervention.
   ii. Utilize an angiographic catheter with calibration markers to allow for accurate measurements; the width of a catheter does not provide a sufficiently accurate reference.

2. **Balloon Dilation**

a. Usually performed with a single dilation balloon in a retrograde fashion.

b. Select a balloon that is 2.5-3 times larger than the narrowest coarctation diameter but not larger than diameter of the smallest adjacent "normal" aortic lumen. Balloons >3 times the narrowest diameter increase the risk for vessel disruption, whereas those larger than the adjacent normal vessel increase the risk of injury to the normal aortic wall.

c. The length of the balloon should be long enough to cover the area of coarctation completely, without extending too far in either direction, thus avoiding injury to the normal aortic wall.

d. The distal end of the wire is usually fixed in the right or left subclavian artery. If these locations are inadequate, the wire can be fixed in the aortic root; however, this position offers less stability. Under no circumstances should the wire be positioned in a carotid or vertebral artery. The balloon should be meticulously prepped prior to insertion so that it is free of air—ie, "negative prep". This will avoid inadvertent air embolization in the event of a balloon rupture.

e. The balloon should be centered across the stenosis, and care should be taken to be sure the proximal shoulder does not extend into a small caliber vessel—ie, the subclavian artery.
f. A pressure manometer should be used, and inflation pressures should not exceed the balloon burst pressure or 4-6 atm—whichever is less.
g. Balloon inflation should be stopped if an adequate waist does not appear or the balloon becomes displaced.
h. Leaving the guidewire in place, postdilation angiography should be repeated to assess for improvement in the coarctation and to evaluate for aortic wall complications including dissection, aneurysm formation, and rupture.
i. To avoid vessel dissection or perforation, the dilated segment should only be recrossed over the previously placed guidewire.

3. **Prograde Catheter** The use of a prograde catheter is reserved for special cases.
   a. A prograde catheter from a radial or brachial arterial access site can be used to assist in balloon positioning; to monitor pressures before, during, and after the dilation; and for angiography.
      i. **Advantages:** Allows for these measurements and angiography prior to obtaining arterial access. Postprocedure, allows for angiography without requiring any manipulation of wires/catheters across a freshly dilated coarctation.
   b. A prograde catheter can also be used from a venous access site via a transseptal approach.

C. Complications From Balloon Angioplasty

1. Complications related to transcatheter balloon angioplasty of aortic coarctation can be classified into 3 categories: (1) **technical**, (2) **aortic**, and (3) **peripheral vascular**.[24]
   a. Technical complications include issues with the equipment or procedural technique and include balloon rupture, balloon displacement, and guidewire injury.
   b. Aortic wall injury is common and includes intimal tears, aortic dissection, and aneurysm formation.
      i. In the CCISC study, there was a 10% incidence of acute aortic wall injury and an incidence of 21.4% in short-term follow-up (3-18 mo postprocedure).[25]
      ii. Acutely, all cases of aortic wall injury were related to dissection, whereas in the short-term follow-up group, the majority of cases were due to aneurysm formation.
      iii. In intermediate follow-up (18-60 mo postprocedure), the incidence of aortic wall injury increases to 43.8%, most of which are due to aneurysm formation.[25]
      iv. This speaks to the importance of pre- and postintervention angiography and interval follow-up. As discussed previously, it is critical to maintain an inventory of appropriately sized covered stents for use in emergency situations such as acute aneurysm formation or rupture.

c. Peripheral vascular complications are similar to those seen in any cardiac catheterization with arterial access and include cerebral vascular accidents, peripheral emboli, and injury to access vessels.

2. Access site complications are of particular concern, as these procedures often require the use of large-size arterial sheaths.
   a. Adequacy of femoral and iliac vessel size should be assessed prior to the introduction of large-diameter sheaths.
   b. In our experience, arteriotomy closure techniques such as "preclosure" of the access site with the PerClose ProGlide (Abbott Vascular, Santa Clara, CA) can help reduce postprocedural bleeding and hematoma formation in appropriate-size patients.

D. Stent Angioplasty

1. **Studies and Evaulations:** Balloon-expandable stent angioplasty for both native and recurrent aortic coarctation has been extensively evaluated over the past decade. In some studies, stent angioplasty has been shown to be superior to balloon angioplasty and surgery for the treatment of native aortic coarctation.[25,29]
   a. Additionally, the rates of aneurysm formation and other aortic wall complications following stent angioplasty of recurrent coarctation are less than those associated with balloon angioplasty alone.
   b. A prospective, multi-institutional registry study of 302 patients (median age 15 y, range 2-63 y) undergoing stent angioplasty for coarctation (55% native) found no procedural mortality. Procedural adverse events were seen in 5% including acute and intermediate aortic wall complications in 1% and 2%, respectively.[32]

2. **Preferences:** In our practice, we favor stent angioplasty for both native and recurrent aortic coarctation in adolescent and adult patients. A variety of stents are available with achievable diameters sufficient for use in the treatment of aortic coarctation. However, only the Cheatham Platinum (CP) Stent and the Covered CP Stent (NuMED, Hopkinton, NY) carry a specific indication for use in native and recurrent aortic coarctation. In our practice, we use a variety of balloon-expandable stents. The use of self-expanding nitinol stents and stent grafts for the treatment of native and recurrent coarctation has been described; however, available data regarding their use and outcomes are limited to small case series.[33] Thus, this chapter will focus on balloon-expandable stents.

3. **Stent Selection:** Stent selection depends upon several factors: the diameter required to avoid residual obstruction; the necessary radial strength to maintain stent and lumen integrity; the anatomy of the landing zone (straight or curvilinear); the need to cross or jail brachiocephalic vessels; and the need for a covered stent. It should be noted that only the CP stent and Covered CP stent are available premounted on a delivery balloon catheter. Currently, all other stents must be hand-crimped onto an appropriately sized balloon.
   a. The Palmaz XL 10 series of stents (J&J) are closed-cell stents laser-cut from a very rigid stainless-steel tube and are capable of expanding to 28 mm in diameter. They are available in 30, 40, and 50 mm, lengths, but at aortic diameters (16-28 mm),

there is marked foreshortening. Thus, it is important to have a foreshortening chart available so that an appropriate stent length is selected. These stents have high radial strength but are inflexible and unmalleable, thus they are ideal for discrete coarctations in straight segments of the aorta. They will not conform to curvilinear anatomies and may cause severe distortion or vessel injury when used in such an environment. Finally, the closed-cell design limits the ability to open cells beyond a few millimeters in situations where a brachiocephalic vessel is intentionally or unintentionally jailed. The Palmaz Genesis family of stents are available in 3 size ranges—medium, large, and XD—"extra-diameter."

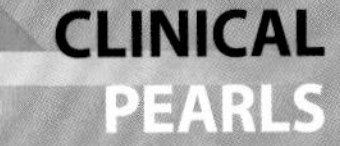

- Large diameter covered stents such as the Covered CP stent should be immediately available in case of aortic wall injury.
- Stent selection is multifactorial: the anatomy of the landing zone, diameter required to relieve the obstruction, radial strength of the stent, the need to jail head and neck vessels and the need for a covered stent are all important considerations.

These stents can only reach 18 mm in diameter, limiting their use to patients with overall smaller aortic dimensions. The Genesis XD is available in lengths from 19 to 59 mm. Like the Palmaz XL stents, the Genesis XD stents are laser-cut from stainless steel, have good radial strength (although less than that of the XL stents), and have a closed-cell design. This stent introduced an "S"-shaped "sigma hinge," allowing the stent to flex around curves, and reduced the degree of shortening upon full stent expansion. Thus, in patients with a relatively small aorta, the Genesis XD is a good choice for use in curvilinear anatomies. The closed-cell design of the Palmaz Genesis series may limit the ability to open the cells in situations where brachiocephalic vessels are crossed. However, with currently available ultra-high-pressure balloons, the stent struts can usually be fractured when necessary, although this may negatively affect stent integrity. As mentioned, these stents have less radial strength than the Palmaz XL stents and, in our experience, are at increased risk for fracture over time.

b. The ev3 IntraStent LD Max was approved for use in 2002. These stents have unique characteristics including an open-cell design that reduces stent foreshortening and allows for expansion of cells up to 12 mm. With staged or sequential expansion, these stents can be expanded to 24-26 mm with minimal foreshortening. However, when expanded to full diameter with a single balloon inflation, they will foreshorten. Thus, they should only be deployed using a balloon-in-balloon (BIB) catheter (NuMED, Hopkinton, NY) as discussed later. They are available in lengths of 16, 26, and 36 mm. The open-cell design affords a great deal of flexibility making this stent quite amenable to placement in curvilinear anatomies. Their radial strength is less than that of the Genesis XD stents. Also, the open-cell design results in less metallic coverage and thus less support of the aortic wall. We reserve use of this stent to narrowing within the curvature of the aortic arch and in situations where we anticipate jailing a brachiocephalic vessel.

c. The NuMED CP stent is the only stent specifically approved for use in aortic coarctation. The CP stent was designed to have rounded edges to reduce aortic wall injury. The zig-zag pattern of the stent creates a closed-cell configuration with some added flexibility. In 2007, the Coarctation of the Aorta Stent Trial (COAST) was initiated to assess the safety and efficacy of the CP stent when used in adults and children with native or recurrent coarctation.[34] In long-term follow-up, these stents have generally been believed to be safe and effective. Stent fracture has been common in follow-up, but clinically insignificant. The reintervention rate was 13% and generally due to aortic wall injury or for planned stent dilation.[34] This stent has large cells and is quite malleable making it a good choice for curvilinear anatomies. It is available both premounted (on a BIB catheter) and unmounted. It is available in lengths from 16 to 45 mm and in diameters from 12 to 30 mm. As with the Palmaz XL stents, the CP stents foreshorten significantly with expansion, and thus it is crucial to refer to a foreshortening chart to accurately predict the final stent length at the intended implant diameter.

d. The Covered Cheatham Platinum stent (CCPS) is a bare-metal CP stent covered along almost its entire length with an expandable sleeve of ePTFE (expanded polytethrafluoroethylene; Fig. 5A.1). The fabric surrounding the stent is thought to provide several advantages over bare-metal stents: (1) additional structural support, (2) a protective barrier at the site of stent placement, (3) a reduction in shear stress.[27] One limitation of this stent is the need for larger sheath sizes. Moreover, the stent must be carefully positioned to avoid unintended obstruction of brachiocephalic vessels. The ePTFE does not extend all the way to the edge of the stent; this must be considered when attempting to cover a specific anatomic location. The COAST II trial demonstrated the ability of the CCPS to treat and/or prevent aortic wall injuries related to coarctation.[23] Long-term follow-up is ongoing. These stents (or a large diameter, covered, self-expanding stent or endograft) can provide life-saving coverage of potentially catastrophic aortic wall injuries and thus should be immediately available when performing balloon or bare-metal stent angioplasty. In patients with resistant lesions, ie, coarctations that will not resolve at < 5-6 atm with either balloon or bare-metal stent angioplasty, we recommend implanting a CCPS that extends well past the lesion prior to higher-pressure expansion. In older patients, especially those with visible calcium within the aortic wall, we implant a CCPS primarily because of the known risks of aortic wall injury in this population.[20,35]

4. **Equipment:** Much of the equipment needed for balloon angioplasty should also be available for stent angioplasty procedures, including, soft-tipped end-hole catheters, stiff guidewires, Multi-Track angiographic catheters, calibrated pigtail catheters, large-diameter long sheaths, and large-diameter covered stents.

5. **Specific Balloons:** We almost exclusively use the BIB catheter (NuMED, Hopkinton, NY) for stent implantation in adolescent and adult patients.
   a. This BIB catheter is specifically designed for stent placement and consists of two "nested", independently inflatable balloons on a single catheter shaft. It is available with outer balloon diameters of 8-30 mm. The inner balloon is ½ the diameter and 10 mm shorter than the outer balloon.
   b. When manually mounting a stent, the stent is centered and crimped on the outer balloon. The premounted CP stent and CCPS come mounted on these balloons. Once at the target lesion, the inner balloon is inflated, expanding the center portion of the stent prior to the proximal and distal ends. This prevents "dog-boning," where the shoulders of the balloon and hence the ends of the stent expand first, and reduces the risk of the stent "milking" during expansion. Furthermore, with the stent fixed at ½ its intended diameter, angiography and reposition can be performed prior to inflation of the outer balloon. The ability to perform staged expansion allows the ev3 Mega LD stents to be implanted with minimal foreshortening.
   c. Postimplant dilation is occasionally required after placement of a covered stent in a resistant stenosis. Our inventory includes Z-Med II balloons (NuMED Inc., Hopkinton, NY) and VIDA balloons (BARD, Tempe AZ) for this purpose. The VIDA balloons are low profile and are often used for late postdilation months after initial implant, thus limiting the need for large sheaths.
6. **Wires**
   a. Most operators use a long, stiff wire with a soft tip such as a Rosen wire or the Amplatz Super-Stiff wire
   b. All BIB catheters track over 0.035 inch wires
7. **Sheaths**
   a. All hand-mounted catheters require delivery through a long sheath. Most popular: straight Cook RB-Mullins sheaths.
   b. To accommodate the added stent material, a sheath 2-3 French sizes larger than required for the angioplasty balloon should be chosen.
8. **Large-Diameter Covered Stents**
   a. In the event of a serious aortic wall injury such as a large dissection, acute aneurysm formation, or aortic wall rupture, covered stents—balloon-expandable or self-expanding—of sufficient diameter for use in the aorta should be immediately available, and the operator should be comfortable with their use. Given the spectrum of aortic coarctation, this necessitates an inventory of various sizes and lengths.
   b. In our practice, we rely on the Mounted CP Covered Stent (NuMED, Inc., Hopkinton, NY). These can be delivered through a 12 or 14 French sheath and most can be expanded to 30 mm. These stents exhibit significant foreshortening, and thus careful review of the stent length at the intended implant diameter is necessary.

E. Technique and Procedural Considerations for Stent Angioplasty

1. **Key Points:** Excellent and detailed discussion of the techniques and materials required for coarcation stent angioplasty can be found in Dr Charles Mullins' textbook *Cardiac Catheterization in Congenital Heart Disease*[36] and in *Coarctation of the aorta: Stenting in children and adults*, an excellent review by Drs Golden and Hellenbrand.[24] The following key points should be considered:
   a. General anesthesia should be used, as stent angioplasty is painful and patient movement can result in a myriad of complications.
   b. Cross-matched blood should be immediately available.
   c. As described earlier for balloon angioplasty, careful measurement of the gradient across the coarctation and detailed, multiplane angiography should be completed prior to the intervention.
   d. Use of a calibrated angiographic catheter is essential. Detailed measurements of the coarctation, proximal and distal aortic diameters, the length of the lesion, and the distance to the brachiocephalic vessels should be made. This will dictate balloon and stent size selection.
   e. Similar to balloon angioplasty, a stiff wire should be anchored deep in a subclavian artery:
      i. For lesions in the transverse arch, wire positioning in the right subclavian artery can help keep the balloon and stent straight.
      ii. For lesions in the proximal descending aorta, wire placement in the left subclavian artery is ideal.
   f. In tortuous and or highly stenotic lesions, it may be helpful to cross the lesion from a radial or brachial artery approach and then snare and externalize a guidewire from the descending aorta to allow retrograde passage of catheters.
   g. Some operators choose to test the compliance of the coarctation lesion prior to intervention:
      i. Use a balloon that is at least 2 mm smaller in diameter than the intended stent.
      ii. Inflate balloon to low pressure (ie, not more than 2-3 atm). If there is a significant waist remaining on the balloon, one may choose to implant the stent at a smaller diameter and postpone complete expansion of the stent until a second catheterization 6 or more months later. This allows time for the stent and surrounding tissue to mature and may decrease the risk of aortic wall complications.
      iii. Predilation of the coarctation with the intent to disrupt the intima should not be performed prior to stent placement. This has been shown to increase the risk of aortic wall complications.

2. **Stent Selection (Table 5A.3)**
   a. One must be cognizant of the maximum diameter of the stent being selected. The Genesis XD stent can only reach 18 mm in diameter and thus should only be used in fully grown patients with relatively small aortic caliber.

TABLE 5A.3. Available Stents for Stenting of Coarctation of the Aorta (CoA)

Stent-Alone	Available Lengths (mm)	Maximum Diameter (mm)	Cell Design	Coarctation Application
Palmaz XL	30, 40, 50	28	Closed/fixed	Discrete CoA in straight segments of the aorta
Max LD	16, 26, 36	26	Open/dilatable 12 mm	Transverse arch; lesions with risk of impinging on head vessels; curvilinear segments
Mega LD	16, 26, 36	18	Open/dilatable 12 mm	Transverse arch; lesions with risk of impinging on head vessels; curvilinear segments
Genesis XD	19, 25, 29, 39, 59	18	Closed/dilatable	Smaller aortas; curvilinear segments
Cheatham Platinum[a]	16, 22, 28, 34, 39, 45	24	Closed/dilatable	Curvilinear segments
Covered Cheatham Platinum[a]	16, 22, 28, 34, 39, 45	24	Closed/covered	Lesions with high risk of aortic wall injury

[a]Available unmounted or premounted on a balloon-in-balloon delivery catheter.

b. The anatomic landscape—curvilinear segment versus straight aortic segment—may necessitate a more flexible stent.

c. The need to cross or jail brachiocephalic branches may warrant use of an open-cell stent so that the covering cell can be dilated.

d. Some operators choose to implant a covered stent in most if not all patients. Certainly, in older adults and those with calcification at or adjacent to the coarctation, a covered stent should be used primarily, as there is a higher risk for aortic wall disruption in these patients.

e. In patients with noncompliant lesions—ie, those requiring > 4-5 atm of pressure to open—a covered stent should be used. This holds true for patients undergoing a staged expansion with a bare-metal stent. If, at the time of the second procedure, the lesion is still resistant, a covered stent should be placed inside the original bare-metal stent (extending beyond both ends of the bare-metal stent to avoid endoleak) prior to using higher pressure to expand the lesion.

3. **Balloon Selection**

   a. The diameter of the aorta either at the transverse arch or at the diaphragm is typically used as an ultimate target diameter. The aortic segment just distal to the coarctation is typically aneurysmal, and one should not attempt to match this diameter.

   b. A balloon that is equal to or just slightly shorter than the selected stent length should be used.

   c. The NuMED BIB balloon is ideal for coarctation stent implant. The outer balloon length should match the selected stent length.

4. **Hand-crimping:** The stent will need to be hand-crimped onto the balloon.

   a. The following techniques can be used to prevent the stent from slipping off the balloon during advancement through the delivery sheath:

i. After hand-crimping the stent, a length of umbilical tape can be looped around the stent/balloon at its center and pulled tight to help tighten the stent down. This can be repeated a few millimeters from each end of the stent as well. One should avoid the ends of the stent, as this technique can cause the sharp ends of the stent to puncture the balloon.
ii. The balloon can be inflated to 0.5 atm prior to or immediately after introduction into the delivery sheath. For the NuMED BIB balloon, the outer balloon should be inflated.

b. Hand-crimped stents should always be delivered to their target vessel through a long sheath. The sheath size should be 1-2 French sizes larger than that needed for the balloon catheter alone.

5. It is crucial to position the shoulder of the balloon proximal to the origin of whichever subclavian is used to anchor the guidewire. Failure to do so will cause the balloon to "milk" out of the subclavian artery during inflation and will result in failure to deploy stent in the desired location.

6. In our practice, if the stenosis does not resolve at ≤ 5 atm of pressure, we will bring the patient back at a second setting 6-12 months later for further expansion. This provides time for the tissue to heal and mature, and often the lesion will become more compliant.

7. **Compliance:** When treating highly compliant lesions or lesions with only a mild amount of stenosis, rapid right ventricular pacing can be used to decrease cardiac output and aortic pulse pressure, thereby improving balloon stability during implant. This is generally not necessary in tight stenoses.
   a. Pace at 180-200 bpm with the goal of decreasing the pulse pressure by 10 mm Hg and decreasing the systolic BP to <100 mm Hg.
   b. Pacing should be terminated **after** the delivery balloon is deflated to avoid a sudden change in output that could force a partially inflated balloon through the stent and dislodge it.

8. When using a NuMED BIB balloon for stent delivery, an angiogram can be performed either through the delivery sheath or through an antegrade catheter to confirm the position of the stent prior to full expansion.

9. After the balloon catheter is removed, angiography can be performed using a Multi-Track catheter or a cut pigtail catheter over a wire.
   a. Assess for stent position, size, and any vascular complications
   b. Repeat a pullback to obtain a poststent gradient

10. Have inventory of large-diameter stents covered with polytetrafluoroethylene (PFTE) for use in emergency situations (see stent discussion in the previous section).

11. **Prograde Catheter:** The use of a prograde catheter is reserved for special cases.

a. A prograde catheter from a radial or brachial arterial access site can be used to assist in balloon positioning; to monitor pressures before, during, and after the dilation; and for angiography.
   i. **Advantages:** Allows for these measurements and angiography prior to obtaining arterial access. Postprocedure, allows for angiography without requiring any manipulation of wires/catheters across a freshly dilated coarctation.
b. A prograde catheter can also be used from a venous access site via a transseptal approach.

F. Complications From Stent Angioplasty

1. Similar to balloon angioplasty, complications of transcatheter stenting of aortic coarctation can be classified into 3 categories: (1) **technical**, (2) **aortic**, and (3) **peripheral vascular**.
   a. Technical complications include issues with the equipment or procedural technique and include stent migration, stent fracture, balloon rupture, and overlap of brachiocephalic vessels. Stent migration can occur because of an improperly sized balloon or balloon rupture.
      i. In the CCISC study, 4.8% of cases involved stent migration with 64% of these cases occurring with the use of oversized balloons.[25] Stent fracture was rare and occurred in 6 out of 588 patients in the same study. Balloon rupture occurred in 2.2% of patients in the CCISC study, primarily with the use of older Palmaz 8-series stents. Balloon rupture can result in other complications including aortic wall injury, embolization of balloon fragments, and stent migration. Although unintentional overlap or jailing of the brachiocephalic vessels may be viewed as a complication, it is not uncommon to intentionally jail such vessels—the left subclavian artery in particular. When this occurs with a bare-metal stent, there is typically preserved flow into the vessel. If an appropriate stent is chosen, the cell overlying the vessel origin can be dilated to reduce metallic coverage. The CCISC study followed 61 such cases (bare-metal stents) with no evidence of hemodynamic issues or embolic events.
      ii. However, when using a covered stent, several factors must be considered: (1) did the vessel have normal antegrade flow initially; (2) is there sufficient collateral flow—either through dilated collaterals or through the Circle of Willis—to avoid compromising cerebral blood flow; (3) is there sufficient collateral flow to avoid subclavian steal. Consultation with a vascular surgeon is recommended. In some cases, a surgical carotid-subclavian bypass prior to stent implantation may be warranted.[37]
   b. Aortic wall injuries may include intimal tears, aortic dissection, and aneurysm formation. Stent angioplasty is generally believed to result in less aortic wall injury than balloon angioplasty alone. This is likely because stent angioplasty does not require overdistension of the tissue beyond the intended diameter, and the stent provides support for the aortic wall itself.

i. The CCISC reported 1.3% instance of angiographic evidence of intimal tears with two cases requiring further intervention, one at the time of the procedure and one 10 months later.[25]

ii. Aortic dissection is a rare, but potentially fatal complication. This speaks to the importance of pre- and postintervention angiography and the importance of maintaining an inventory of covered stents, should such a complication arise. About 1.5% of cases in the CCISC study had aortic dissection with 3 requiring emergent surgery.

iii. Similarly, aortic aneurysms are a rare but potentially dangerous complication occurring in about of 13 cases of 160, followed up longitudinally in the CCISC study.[25] They can present late and therefore, we recommend follow-up imaging (MRI or CT or angiography) 6 months after stent placement.

c. Peripheral vascular complications are similar to those seen with any cardiac catheterization with arterial access and include cerebral vascular accidents, peripheral emboli, and injury to access vessels. In our experience, arteriotomy closure techniques such as "preclosure" of the access site with the PerClose ProGlide (Abbott Vascular, Santa Clara, CA) can help reduce postprocedural bleeding and hematoma formation in appropriate-size patients.

X. Follow-up

Balloon angioplasty and stent angioplasty for aortic coarctation are associated with low long-term risks for evolving aortic wall injury including dissection and aneurysm formation. Thus routine imaging of the aorta with either CTA or MRA is warranted. We recommend imaging be obtained 3-6 months after intervention or sooner if there is particular concern. Subsequent to that, follow-up imaging is generally recommended every 5 years.

References

1. Beekman III RH. *Coarctation of the aorta.* In: *Moss and Adams' Heart Disease in Infants, Children, and Adolescents.* 7th ed. Philadelphia, PA: Lippincott Williams & Wilkins; 2008.
2. Erbel R, Aboyans V, Boileau C, et al. 2014 ESC guidelines on the diagnosis and treatment of aortic diseases. *Eur Heart J.* 2014;35(41):2873-2926. doi:10.1093/eurheartj/ehu281.
3. Campbell M. Natural history of coarctation of the aorta. *Br Hear J.* 1970;32(5):633-640.
4. McBride KL, Riley MF, Zender GA, et al. NOTCH1 mutations in individuals with left ventricular outflow tract malformations reduce ligand-induced signaling. *Hum Mol Genet.* 2008;17(18):2886-2893. doi:10.1093/hmg/ddn187.
5. Lalani SR, Ware SM, Wang X, et al. MCTP2 is a dosage-sensitive gene required for cardiac outflow tract development. *Hum Mol Genet.* 2013;22(21):4339-4348. doi:10.1093/hmg/ddt283.
6. Parent JJ, Bendaly EA, Hurwitz RA. Abdominal coarctation and associated comorbidities in children. *Congenit Hear Dis.* 2014;9(1):69-74. doi:10.1111/chd.12082.
7. Avila P, Mercier LA, Dore A, et al. Adult congenital heart disease: a growing epidemic. *Can J Cardiol.* 2014;30(12 suppl):S410-S419. doi:10.1016/j.cjca.2014.07.749.
8. Kappetein AP, Zwinderman AH, Bogers AJ, Rohmer J, Huysmans HA. More than thirty-five years of coarctation repair. An unexpected high relapse rate. *J Thorac Cardiovasc Surg.* 1994;107(1):87-95.
9. Patel Y, Jilani MI, Cho K. Coarctation of the aorta presenting in a 79-year-old male. *Thorac Cardiovasc Surg.* 1998;46(3):158-160. doi:10.1055/s-2007-1010216.

10. Alegria JR, Burkhart HM, Connolly HM. Coarctation of the aorta presenting as systemic hypertension in a young adult. *Nat Clin Pr Cardiovasc Med.* 2008;5(8):484-488. doi:10.1038/ncpcardio1258.
11. Becker AE, Becker MJ, Edwards JE. Anomalies associated with coarctation of aorta: particular reference to infancy. *Circulation.* 1970;41(6):1067-1075.
12. Niwa K, Perloff JK, Bhuta SM, et al. Structural abnormalities of great arterial walls in congenital heart disease: light and electron microscopic analyses. *Circulation.* 2001;103(3):393-400. https://www.ncbi.nlm.nih.gov/pubmed/11157691.
13. Teo LLS, Cannell T, Babu-Narayan SV, Hughes M, Mohiaddin RH. Prevalence of associated cardiovascular abnormalities in 500 patients with aortic coarctation referred for cardiovascular magnetic resonance imaging to a tertiary center. *Pediatr Cardiol.* 2011;32(8):1120-1127. doi:10.1007/s00246-011-9981-0.
14. Schievink WI, Raissi SS, Maya MM, Velebir A. Screening for intracranial aneurysms in patients with bicuspid aortic valve. *Neurology.* 2010;74(18):1430-1433. doi:10.1212/WNL.0b013e3181dc1acf.
15. Leschka S, Alkadhi H, Wildermuth S. Images in cardiology. Collateral circulation in aortic coarctation shown by 64 channel multislice computed tomography angiography. *Heart.* 2005;91(11):1422. doi:10.1136/hrt.2004.054346.
16. Warnes CA, Williams RG, Bashore TM, et al. ACC/AHA 2008 guidelines for the management of adults with congenital heart disease: a report of the American College of Cardiology/American Heart Association task force on practice guidelines (writing committee to develop guidelines on the management of adults with congenital heart disease). *Circulation.* 2008;118(23):e714-e833. doi:10.1161/CIRCULATIONAHA.108.190690.
17. Cohen M, Fuster V, Steele PM, Driscoll D, McGoon DC. Coarctation of the aorta. Long-term follow-up and prediction of outcome after surgical correction. *Circulation.* 1989;80(4):840-845. https://www.ncbi.nlm.nih.gov/pubmed/2791247.
18. Toro-Salazar OH, Steinberger J, Thomas W, Rocchini AP, Carpenter B, Moller JH. Long-term follow-up of patients after coarctation of the aorta repair. *Am J Cardiol.* 2002;89(5):541-547.
19. Strafford MA, Griffiths SP, Gersony WM. Coarctation of the aorta: a study in delayed detection. *Pediatrics.* 1982;69(2):159-163.
20. Cardoso G, Abecasis M, Anjos R, et al. Aortic coarctation repair in the adult. *J Card Surg.* 2014;29(4):512-518. doi:10.1111/jocs.12367.
21. Perloff JK. The variant associations of aortic isthmic coarctation. *Am J Cardiol.* 2010;106(7):1038-1041. doi:10.1016/j.amjcard.2010.04.046.
22. Garcier JM, Petitcolin V, Filaire M, et al. Normal diameter of the thoracic aorta in adults: a magnetic resonance imaging study. *Surg Radiol Anat.* 2003;25(3-4):322-329. doi:10.1007/s00276-003-0140-z.
23. Taggart NW, Minahan M, Cabalka AK, Cetta F, Usmani K, Ringel RE. Immediate outcomes of covered stent placement for treatment or prevention of aortic wall injury associated with coarctation of the aorta (COAST II). *JACC Cardiovasc Interv.* 2016;9(5):484-493. doi:10.1016/j.jcin.2015.11.038.
24. Golden AB, Hellenbrand WE. Coarctation of the aorta: stenting in children and adults. *Catheter Cardiovasc Interv.* 2007;69(2):289-299. doi:10.1002/ccd.21009.
25. Forbes TJ, Kim DW, Du W, et al. Comparison of surgical, stent, and balloon angioplasty treatment of native coarctation of the aorta: an observational study by the CCISC (Congenital Cardiovascular Interventional Study Consortium). *J Am Coll Cardiol.* 2011;58(25):2664-2674. doi:10.1016/j.jacc.2011.08.053.
26. Lock JE, Bass JL, Amplatz K, Fuhrman BP, Castaneda-Zuniga W. Balloon dilation angioplasty of aortic coarctations in infants and children. *Circulation.* 1983;68(1):109-116. doi:10.1161/01.CIR.68.1.109.
27. Torok RD. Coarctation of the aorta: management from infancy to adulthood. *World J Cardiol.* 2015;7(11):765. doi:10.4330/wjc.v7.i11.765.
28. Cowley CG, Orsmond GS, Feola P, McQuillan L, Shaddy RE. Long-term, randomized comparison of balloon angioplasty and surgery for native coarctation of the aorta in childhood. *Circulation.* 2005;111(25):3453-3456. doi:10.1161/CIRCULATIONAHA.104.510198.
29. Harris KC, Du W, Cowley CG, Forbes TJ, Kim DW. A prospective observational multicenter study of balloon angioplasty for the treatment of native and recurrent coarctation of the aorta. *Catheter Cardiovasc Interv.* 2014;83(7):1116-1123. doi:10.1002/ccd.25284.

30. Fawzy ME, Fathala A, Osman A, et al. Twenty-two years of follow-up results of balloon angioplasty for discreet native coarctation of the aorta in adolescents and adults. *Am Heart J.* 2008;156(5):910-917. doi:10.1016/j.ahj.2008.06.037.
31. Mullins CE. *Dilation of coarctation of the aorta- native and re/residual coarctation.* In: *Cardiac Catheterization in Congenital Heart Disease.* 1st ed.: Blackwell Publishing; 2006:454-471.
32. Holzer R, Qureshi S, Ghasemi A, et al. Stenting of aortic coarctation: Acute, intermediate, and long-term results of a prospective multi-institutional registry-Congenital cardiovascular interventional study consortium (CCISC). *Catheter Cardiovasc Interv.* 2010;76(4):553-563. doi:10.1002/ccd.22587.
33. Kische S, D'Ancona G, Stoeckicht Y, Ortak J, Elsässer A, Ince H. Percutaneous treatment of adult isthmic aortic coarctation acute and long-term clinical and imaging outcome with a self-expandable uncovered nitinol stent. *Circ Cardiovasc Interv.* 2015;8(1):1-10. doi:10.1161/CIRCINTERVENTIONS.114.001799.
34. Meadows J, Minahan M, McElhinney DB, McEnaney K, Ringel R. Intermediate outcomes in the prospective, multicenter coarctation of the aorta stent trial (COAST). *Circulation.* 2015;131(19):1656-1664. doi:10.1161/CIRCULATIONAHA.114.013937.
35. Oliver JM, Gallego P, Gonzalez A, Aroca A, Bret M, Mesa JM. Risk factors for aortic complications in adults with coarctation of the aorta. *J Am Coll Cardiol.* 2004;44(8):1641-1647. doi:10.1016/j.jacc.2004.07.037.
36. Mullins CE. *Coarctation of the aorta and miscellaneous arterial stents.* In: *Cardiac Catheterization in Congenital Heart Disease.* Blackwell Publishing; 2006:642-660.
37. Shennib H, Rodriguez-Lopez J, Ramaiah V, et al. Endovascular management of adult coarctation and its complications: intermediate results in a cohort of 22 patients. *Eur J Cardio-thoracic Surg.* 2010;37(2):322-327. doi:10.1016/j.ejcts.2009.04.071.

CHAPTER 5B

Endovascular Management of the Ascending Aorta and the Aortic Arch

Camilo A. Velasquez, MD, Young Erben, MD, Mohammad A. Zafar, MD, Chandni Patel, MD, Ayman Saeyeldin, MD, Anton A. Gryaznov, MD, PhD, Bulat Ziganshin, MD, PhD, and John A. Elefteriades, MD, PhD (hon)

Key Points

- Thoracic aortic aneurysms are usually asymptomatic and not easily detectable until an acute and often catastrophic complication occurs.
- Diameters greater than 6 cm increase the risk of death and complication threatening to produce death. Recently, evidence has shown hinge points at 5.25 cm and 5.75 cm, suggesting a leftward shift in the aortic diameter at which intervention should be recommended.
- The imaging modalities used for diagnosing pathology of the ascending aorta are computed tomography, magnetic resonance imaging, and echocardiography.
- Type A acute aortic dissection is a surgical emergency requiring immediate consultation and intervention.
- Open surgical intervention with the replacement of the ascending aorta or the aortic arch with a graft is the gold standard for the treatment of thoracic aortic pathology.
- High-risk patients who are unable to undergo open surgical repair may fairly be managed with medical therapy with adequate outcomes.
- Endovascular management of aortic pathology is an alternative for high-risk patients in whom the open approach is prohibited.
- There are no specific approved devices for the endovascular management of the ascending aorta and the aortic arch.

I. Introduction

A. Thoracic aortic diseases are virulent, often capable of leading to death of the patient.[1,2] Generally, the thoracic aorta is a silent organ that only becomes symptomatic when a catastrophic event such as death or a major complication that threatens to produce death occurs.[1] According to data from the Centers for Disease Control and Prevention, from the years 1999 to 2015, aortic aneurysm was the 19th leading cause of death in all ages and the 16th cause of death in patients older than 65 years.[3] Approximately, 10,000 aortic deaths per year have been reported, with a decrease in incidence from 15,807 deaths in 1999 to 9988 deaths by 2015.[1,3]

B. The aorta itself is considered an active organ with mechanical properties and an intrinsic and complex biology. Diseases of the aorta are categorized based on location: aortic root, ascending aorta, aortic arch, and descending aorta. The diseases affecting the aorta are separated in two distinct entities at the level of the ligamentum arteriosum: above the ligament (ascending aorta and aortic arch), the disease is nonarteriosclerotic in nature, whereas below the ligament (descending aorta and abdominal aorta), arteriosclerosis is abundant.[1]

C. **Thoracic endovascular aortic repair (TEVAR)** has been shown to reduce perioperative mortality and morbidity with a sustained benefit during follow-up. However, recent studies of endovascular approaches to aneurysms in the abdominal and thoracic aorta show a seriously disturbing tendency to endoleak by 5 years.[4-6] In recent years, TEVAR has become an accepted treatment for patients with suitable anatomy in the descending thoracic aorta.[7,8]

  a. However, an endovascular approach for repair of the ascending aorta and aortic arch pathology is troublesome. Anatomic and physiologic challenges are formidable for the adequate deployment of endovascular systems. Fundamental problems abound. Proximal graft fixation close to both the aortic valve and the coronary ostia is difficult and dangerous. Distal landing zones may impinge on the innominate artery. These are examples of the complexity of endovascular techniques applied in the "high-rent" region proximal to the ligamentum arteriosum.[1] Additionally, the hemodynamic forces experienced in the ascending aorta can be an obstacle for accurate graft deployment.

D. There are no current societal guidelines for endovascular management of ascending aortic aneurysm. In fact, several case reports constitute the bulk of the current literature.[9] Therefore, this chapter aims to provide the reader with the current state of the art in the emerging endovascular treatment of the ascending aorta and the aortic arch. The pathologies amenable to intervention will be discussed, and the current devices and techniques available for the ascending and arch segments will be described.

II. Aortic Pathology for the Endovascular Treatment of the Ascending Aorta

A. Current Management and Treatments

In recent years, interest in the management of aortic diseases with endovascular devices has seen an expansion beyond the treatment of the abdominal aorta to an increased attention to more proximal segments of the thoracic aorta. The ascending aorta and the aortic arch became the ultimate frontiers for utilization of endovascular techniques.[8,10] Additionally, with the increased safety of open aortic surgery,[11,12] the endovascular approach has been reserved for patients who pose a prohibitive risk for an open procedure, or as a last resort in emergent conditions in which an open surgical approach is not feasible and sole medical management can be expected to lead to decreased survival.[10] Endovascular management of the ascending aorta and aortic arch can be applied in high-risk patients with the following conditions: type A aortic dissection, aortic pseudoaneurysm, penetrating aortic ulcer (PAU), intramural hematoma (IMH), ascending aortic aneurysm, and ascending aortic rupture.[8,10]

B. Thoracic Aortic Dissection

1. Comorbidities that are associated with an increase in the wall stress (hypertension, weightlifting, coarctation, cocaine use) or aortic media abnormalities (Marfan disease, Loeys-Dietz, Ehlers-Danlos, bicuspid aortic valve, familial aortic aneurysm, steroid treatment) can predispose to the development of aortic dissection (Table 5B.1).[13]

TABLE 5B.1. Risk Factors Associated With the Development of Aortic Dissection[13]
Conditions Associated With Increased Aortic Wall Stress
• Uncontrolled hypertension
• Pheochromocytoma
• Cocaine and other stimulants
• Weightlifting and Valsalva maneuvers
• Trauma
• Deceleration or torsional injury
• Coarctation of the aorta
Conditions Associated With Aortic Media Abnormalities
Genetic
• Marfan syndrome
• Ehlers-Danlos syndrome, vascular form (type IV)
• Bicuspid aortic valve
• Turner syndrome
• Loeys-Dietz syndrome
• Familial thoracic aortic aneurysm and dissection syndrome
Inflammatory Vasculitis
• Takayasu arteritis
• Giant cell arteritis
• Bechet arteritis
Others
• Pregnancy
• Polycystic kidney disease
• Chronic corticosteroid and immunosuppression agent administration
• Infections involving the aortic wall

2. Depending on the severity and degree of dissection, multiple organ systems can be affected, including cardiovascular, pulmonary, renal, neurologic, gastrointestinal, and peripheral vascular (Table 5B.2).[14]
3. Overall, type A dissections are treated emergently with operative repair. This is in contrast to patients with type B dissections, who are initially treated conservatively with anti-impulse therapy, with surgery being reserved for patients with complications.[15,16] The indications for surgical, endovascular, and medical therapy are as follows (Table 5B.3):
   a. Acute type A aortic dissections pose substantial risk of aortic rupture, aortic regurgitation with heart failure, stroke, cardiac tamponade, and visceral ischemia.
   b. In the IRAD registry, patients with type A aortic dissection who were medically managed had a mortality rate of 58% compared with 26% in those who underwent surgery.[17]

TABLE 5B.2. Complication by Organ System in Patients With Aortic Dissection[14]

Cardiovascular
Cardiac arrest
Syncope
Aortic regurgitation
Congestive heart failure
Coronary ischemia
Myocardial infarction
Cardiac tamponade
Pericarditis

Pulmonary
Pleural effusion
Hemothorax
Hemoptysis (aortotracheal or bronchial fistula)

Renal
Acute renal failure
Renovascular hypertension
Renal ischemia or infarction

Neurologic
Stroke
Transient ischemic attack
Paraparesis or paraplegia
Encephalopathy
Coma
Spinal cord syndrome
Ischemic neuropathy

Gastrointestinal
Mesenteric ischemia or infarction
Pancreatitis
Hemorrhage (aortoenteric fistula)

Peripheral vascular
Upper or lower extremity ischemia

Systemic
Fever

TABLE 5B.3. Indications for Surgical Intervention in Patients With Aortic Dissection[2,13]

Surgical Therapy

- Acute type A dissection
- Retrograde dissection into the ascending aorta

Endovascular and/or Surgical Therapy

- Endovascular therapy in acute type A dissection for patients with prohibitive risk for surgical therapy
- Acute type B dissection complicated by
  - Visceral ischemia
  - Limb ischemia
  - Rupture or impending rupture
  - Aneurysmal dilatation
  - Refractory pain

Medical Therapy

- Uncomplicated type B aortic dissection
- Uncomplicated isolated arch dissection

c. The goal of repair is to excise/obliterate the proximal entry tear, prevent pericardial rupture, prevent or treat coronary ostial dissection, correct aortic valve regurgitation, restore flow into the true lumen, correct malperfusion, and, if possible, obliterate the distal false channel.[14]

4. If the aortic valve is unable to be repaired, aortic valve replacement is often required. Therefore, the emergent treatment of type A dissection consists in the replacement of the ascending aorta, often together with replacement of the aortic valve and the dissected aortic arch.[1] In patients in whom open repair is not feasible, endovascular techniques have been applied. These involve placement of an endograft in the ascending aorta and the aortic arch. However, such applications are investigational in nature and often carried out on a compassionate use basis.

C. Thoracic Aortic Aneurysm

1. Thoracic aortic aneurysms (TAAs) are defined as enlargements of the aorta greater than 1.5 times its normal size.[1] We often use a diameter greater than 4 cm as the definition for TAA. True aneurysms involve the three layers of the aortic wall without losing continuity; however, inherent weakness of the aortic wall predisposes to diameter expansion and rupture.[13,14,18] On the other hand, false aneurysms, or pseudoaneurysms, occur when there is a loss of continuity in the aortic wall itself, with bleeding that is contained by the adventitia or the surrounding perivascular tissues. Pseudoaneurysms generally pose an increased risk of rupture compared with true aneurysms.[14]

2. The pathophysiology of aortic dilatation is generally attributed to cystic medial degeneration and inflammatory changes within the aortic wall. In cystic medial degeneration, there is a disruption and loss of elastic fibers with increased deposition of proteoglycans in the medial layers. During inflammatory changes, there is a shift toward excessive degradation of the extracellular matrix, overriding its synthesis, thus adversely affecting the delicate homeostasis that normally exists between the vascular smooth muscle cells and the extracellular proteins in the medial layer of the aorta.[1,19,20] The activity of the proteolytic enzymes such as matrix metalloproteinases (MMPs) plays a major pathophysiologic role in aortic aneurysm formation. MMPs, especially the MMP-2 and MMP-9 subtypes, degrade the elastin, fibrillin, and collagen in the medial layer of the aortic wall. Normally, MMPs are regulated by the presence of tissue inhibitors of metalloproteinases (TIMPs), but in aneurysmal patients, the balance between MMPs and TIMPs is shifted toward an increase in proteolysis, correlating with the observed degradation and thinning seen in the aortic wall.[1,21] Additionally, inflammatory conditions such as Takayasu arteritis, rheumatoid arthritis, and giant cell arteritis, among others, can lead to the development of TAAs, further exemplifying the inflammatory role in aneurysm formation.[1]

3. **Anatomical Categorization of Ascending Thoracic Aortic Aneurysms:** TAAs can be categorized in three general classes according to the pattern of aortic root involvement (see Fig. 5B.1).[1]

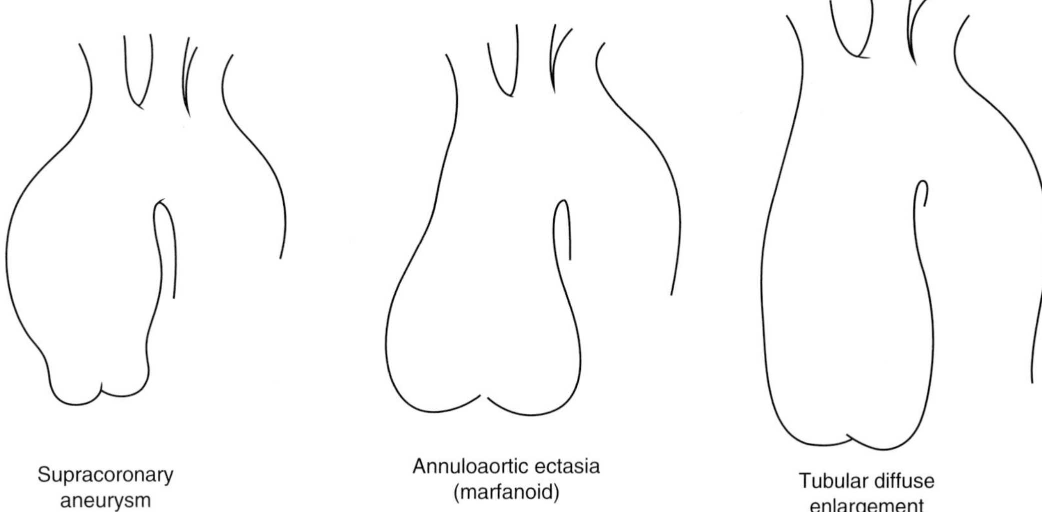

FIGURE 5B.1: Three common patterns of ascending aortic aneurysm disease: supracoronary, annulo-aortic ectasia, and tubular (see text for discussion). Reproduced with permission from Elefteriades JA. Thoracic aortic aneurysm: reading the enemy's playbook. *Curr Probl Cardiol.* 2008;33(5):203-277.

a. **Supracoronary aneurysm:** The aortic annulus and the short segment of aorta between the annulus and the coronary orifices are of normal size, with supracoronary dilatation of the ascending aorta.
b. **Marfanoid aneurysm:** Also termed annuloaortic ectasia, this type of aneurysm involves a dilatation of the aortic annulus and the proximal portion of the aorta.
c. **Tubular aneurysm:** In this category, the aortic annulus and the proximal aorta are somewhat but not markedly dilated, with a uniform caliber throughout the ascending aorta conferring a "tubular" appearance.
   i. On rare occasions, one may also see a saccular aneurysm, which protrudes like a sack from the aortic lumen, involving only a small portion of the aortic wall length and circumference.
   ii. These patterns of anatomic enlargement are important because surgical therapy is predicated on the precise pattern of enlargement.

4. **Long-term Complications of Thoracic Aortic Aneurysms**
   a. Growth of TAAs predisposes the patient in the long term to suffer aortic dissection or rupture.

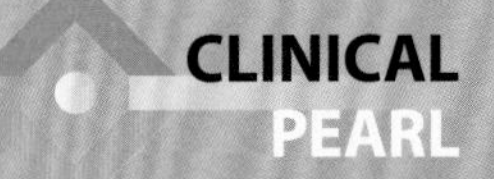

In the ascending aorta, rupture rarely occurs without aortic dissection.

i. Work done to unveil the natural history of ascending aortic aneurysms has revealed diameter "hinge points" at which risk of rupture and dissection increases dramatically.[1]

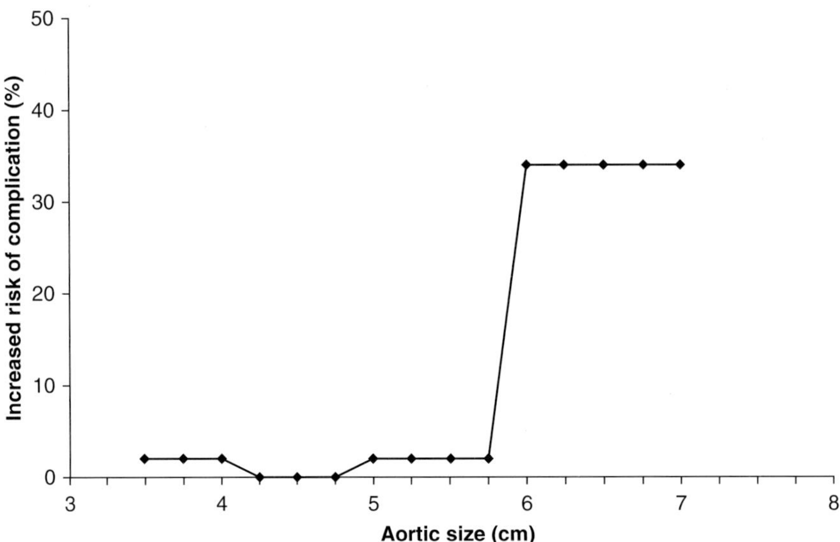

FIGURE 5B.2: Note the "hinge point" at 6 cm diameter, at which the natural risk of an ascending aneurysm increases dramatically. Reproduced with permission from Elefteriades JA. Natural history of thoracic aortic aneurysms: indications for surgery, and surgical versus nonsurgical risks. *Ann Thorac Surg.* 2002;74(5): S1877-S1880; discussion S1892-S1898.

ii. Traditionally, in the case of ascending aortic aneurysms, the hinge point has been 6 cm, where 31% of the patients will have suffered a dissection or rupture by the time the aneurysm reaches this point[1,22-24] (see Fig. 5B.2).

iii. Current data, more granular as the number of studied patients has grown, have shown hinge points at 5.75 cm and again at 5.25 cm suggesting that criteria for intervention should be moved leftward to smaller sizes.[25]

b. Clinical features of an acute aortic event (rupture or dissection) depend on the location of the pathology. Generally, ascending aortic dissections produce tearing, severe, substernal pain. Generally, descending aortic aneurysms produce severe interscapular pain, which often radiates and progresses caudally down the body.

5. Criteria for Surgical Intervention

a. The generally accepted criterion for intervention in patients with chronic ascending thoracic aneurysms is a diameter of the ascending aorta greater than 5.5 cm. For institutions with large experience, which can deliver operation at low risk, 5.0 cm is an accepted criterion. However, a critical point for emphasis is that dimensional criteria apply for *asymptomatic* aneurysms only.

b. Symptomatic aneurysms require operation regardless of size, as pain in an aneurysm portends rupture. It is said that rapid growth of the thoracic aorta, at or above 0.5 cm/y, requires operation. In matter of fact, such rapid growth is extremely rare in the thoracic aorta.

c. Putative growth at this rate is usually due to measurement error (oblique measurements or comparison on noncorresponding aortic segments). Furthermore, connective tissue diseases and familial TAAs may require a more aggressive surgical approach, because dissections can occur at quite small sizes.

d. We often operate even before 5 cm for patients with Marfan syndrome, Loeys-Dietz, Ehlers-Danlos, and other inherited aortopathies (see Fig. 5B.3).[26] In Turner syndrome, where dissection can occur suddenly at small sizes, surgery can be considered when the ascending aorta reaches 3.5 cm or greater[1,13] (Table 5B.4).

6. **Surgical Procedures**
   a. Surgical treatment for ascending aortic aneurysms usually involves resection and grafting +/– aortic valve replacement. Generally, surgery of the ascending aorta requires arresting of the heart during the aortic reconstruction and institution of artificial blood circulation via the use of cardiopulmonary bypass. One of the biggest challenges in the surgical approach to ascending aortic aneurysms is intervention on the aortic arch. When the aortic arch is intervened upon, blood flow to the head vessels generally must be interrupted (requiring methods for cerebral protection, such as deep hypothermic circulatory arrest [DHCA]) or substituted artificially. Currently, three methods for cerebral protection are used independently or concurrently: DHCA, antegrade cerebral perfusion (ACP),

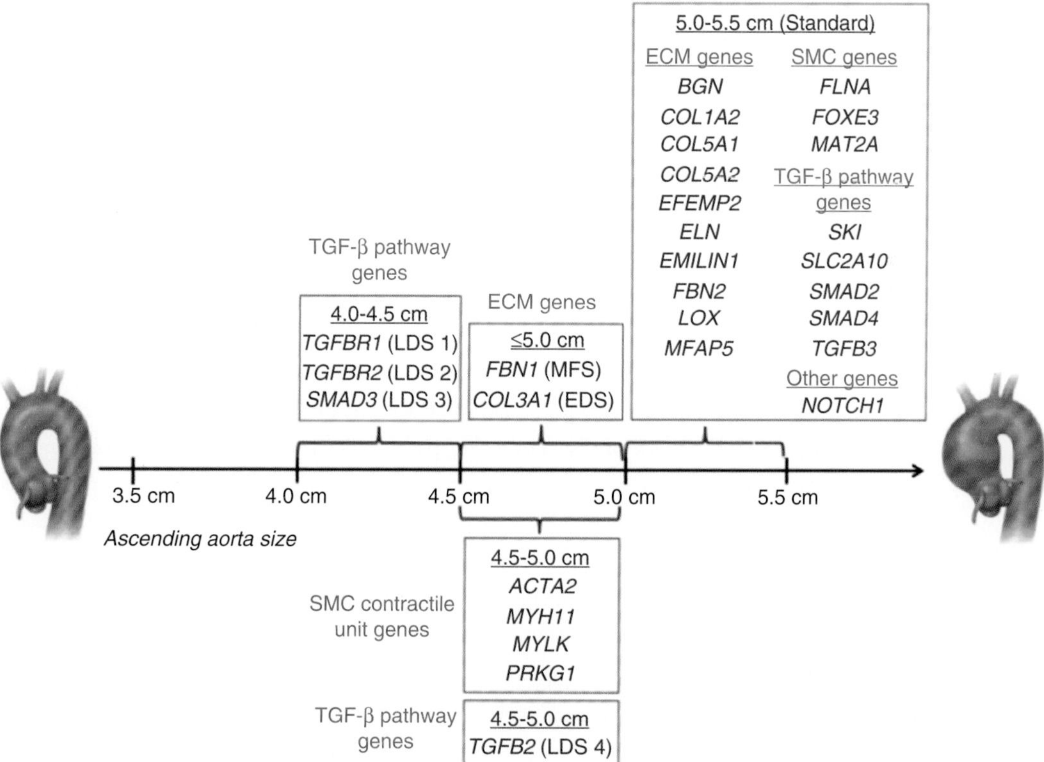

FIGURE 5B.3: Simplified schematic illustration of ascending aorta dimensions for prophylactic surgical intervention divided by gene category: ECM genes, SMC contractile unit and metabolism genes, and TGF-β signaling pathway genes. ECM, extracellular matrix; LDS, Loeys-Dietz syndrome; MFS, Marfan syndrome; SMC, smooth muscle cell; EDS, Ehlers-Danlos syndrome. Reproduced with permission from Brownstein AJ, Ziganshin BA, Kuivaniemi H, Body SC, Bale AE, Elefteriades JA. Genes associated with thoracic aortic aneurysm and dissection: an update and clinical implications. *Aorta (Stamford).* 2017;5(1):11-20.

TABLE 5B.4. Indications for Surgery According to Ascending Aortic Diameter

	Ascending aortic diameter at which surgery is recommended
TAA (no other coexisting conditions)	5.5 cm
BAV, Marfan, familial TAA	5 cm
Loeys-Dietz	4.4-4.6 cm by CT or MRI; 4.2 cm by TEE
Turner syndrome	>3.5 cm

and retrograde cerebral perfusion (RCP). Furthermore, three approaches for the aortic arch replacement are generally applied according to anatomic indications.[14]

i. **Proximal hemiarch resection:** In this procedure, the arch vessels are left intact while just the undersurface of the aortic arch is replaced. This suffices for many ascending aneurysms that taper gradually as they reach the arch zone.
ii. **Complete arch resection:** In these procedures, the entire aortic arch is replaced. Cerebral blood flow is reconstituted either by reattaching an "island" of aortic wall carrying the great vessels (Carrel patch) or by grafts to the head vessels themselves.
iii. **Elephant trunk procedure:** This procedure is used if the aneurysm extends into the descending aorta, requiring a two-stage approach. During the first stage one accomplishes placement of an "elephant trunk" sewn to the end of the aortic arch with the distal end of the graft hanging freely in the descending aorta. During the second stage, about 4 weeks later, the descending aneurysm is resected and the distal end of the elephant trunk is attached to the normal aorta below.

b. Currently, open surgery of the ascending aorta and aortic arch has proven to be exceptionally safe, with a mortality of 2.1% at 30 days; including a 1.5% mortality for elective cases and a 6.3% mortality for emergent cases.[12] Therefore, open surgical repair is the current standard of treatment for patients with ascending aortic pathology. Furthermore, several other pathologies such as aortic pseudoaneurysm, PAU, IMH, and a rupture of the ascending aorta can be effectively approached with an open surgical repair, thus eliminating their inherent risk of catastrophic events. Endovascular repair is reported in the literature less frequently for these pathologies than for aortic dissection; however, the focal localization of these lesions in the aorta makes them amenable to the placement of an endograft.[8,10]

7. **Aortic Pseudoaneurysm:** A true aneurysm, as previously described, is a weakening of the three layers of the aortic wall. However, a pseudoaneurysm is a loss of continuity with blood accumulation that is contained by the adventitia of the aorta or surrounding scar tissue. This can be seen at surgical anastomotic sites, such as proximal and distal graft anastomoses and coronary reimplantation sites. Pseudoaneurysms also develop after complex aortic valve surgery with root enlarging procedures or in settings of endocarditis and tissue destruction. Because of pressurized flow into the sac, pseudoaneurysms pose an increased risk of rupture into the mediastinum and pleural spaces that is very often fatal.[27]

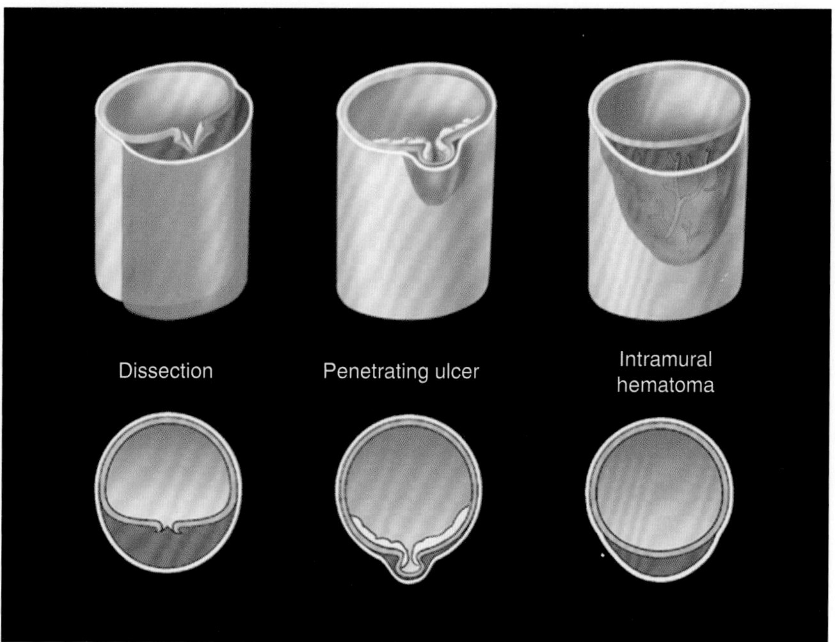

FIGURE 5B.4: Variant forms of aortic dissection: typical aortic dissection, penetrating aortic ulcer, and intramural hematoma (IMH). Note the concentric nature of the hematoma in IMH. Reproduced with permission from Elefteriades JA. Thoracic aortic aneurysm: reading the enemy's playbook. *Curr Probl Cardiol.* 2008;33(5):203-277.

8. **Penetrating Aortic Ulcer:** PAU is characterized by a region of the aorta with atherosclerotic changes and an ulcer-like projection appearance (see Fig. 5B.4). The intima is transgressed and the lesion progresses through the aortic wall; also, it may or may not be associated with an overlying thrombus. PAU can be an entry point for the development of dissection and may be associated with the development of a hematoma within the media that leads to dissection or even rupture.[28,29]

9. **Intramural Hematoma:** IMH is a variant of aortic dissection (see Fig. 5B.4); there is an involvement of the medial layer of the aortic wall in the absence of an intimal tear; however, it can be associated with the presence of microtears and the development of a hematoma. IMH is hypothesized to occur after the spontaneous rupture of the vasa-vasorum or disruption of the media induced by a PAU. IMH has a thinner outer media that increases the risk of rupture in comparison with patients with aortic dissection.[28,30]

III. Endovascular Management of the Ascending Aorta and Aortic Arch

A. Implementation of Techniques

The successful implementation of endovascular techniques in the abdominal aorta has rendered the open procedure as a second-line of treatment in patients with abdominal aortic diseases. Endovascular repair instead, became the gold standard for the management of acute and elective abdominal aortic conditions. Therefore, enthusiasm expanded to the thoracic aortic segments for the management of conditions such as aneurysms, dissections, and PAUs with the intention of reducing complications such as early death, paraplegia, renal insufficiency, and cardiac events associated with the open surgical repair.[8] The proximal aortic segments are the ultimate frontier for endovascular techniques. However, the closer endovascular therapy gets to the aortic valve, the more complex and dangerous it becomes. Anatomical and physiological complexities complicate the adequate deployment and application of endovascular devices. Additionally, there is a lack of ascending aorta–specific devices that are necessary to fit the anatomy and hemodynamic forces that are experienced in the proximal portion of the aorta.[8]

B. Anatomic and Hemodynamic Challenges

1. The anatomy of the ascending aorta and the aortic arch poses a challenge for the implementation of endovascular techniques. The proximity of the aortic valve and coronary ostia below the sinotubular junction can lead to aortic insufficiency or myocardial infarction following stent deployment in so proximal a position. Also, the presence of the head vessels (innominate artery, left common carotid artery, and left subclavian artery) places the patient at risk of cerebrovascular accident if there is a deployment or migration beyond the point of origin of the innominate artery.[8] Thus, the effective area of intervention for the ascending aorta is limited to the zone above the sinotubular junction to the origin of the innominate artery, generally representing a length of 5-7 cm.[31] An additional parameter that affects the proper use of endovascular techniques is the larger diameter of the ascending aorta, on average 1 cm larger than the descending aorta; this limits the range of stents that can be borrowed from those commonly employed during TEVAR.[8,10,32] Furthermore, because of the short segment of the ascending aorta, achieving the generally recommended 20 mm landing zone can be challenging; hence, some reports recommend paring the landing zone to a new lower minimum of 10 mm to avoid obstructing the coronary ostia or the aortic valve, proximally, and the innominate artery distally.[8,33]

2. The hemodynamic forces and the pronounced diameter changes during the cardiac cycle in the ascending aorta can hinder the precise deployment of stents. The higher systolic flow in comparison with the descending aorta can lead to migration of the stent while being deployed, a phenomenon known as "windsock."[34]Consequently, the use of special technical maneuvers may be necessary; these include rapid ventricular pacing to 180 bpm, adenosine injection for transient cardiac arrest, vena cava occlusion, or medications such as nitrates—all applied to decrease afterload, blood pressure, and cardiac output during endograft placement.[8,10,33] The greatest changes in diameters during the cardiac cycle reach 5 mm just distal to the coronary arteries, representing a mean change of 17%, and also 5 mm noted proximal to the innominate artery, a change of 14 %. To plan optimally, ECG-gated computed tomographic angiography (CTA) can specifically evaluate the pulsatility of the ascending aorta for better sizing.[7]

C. Indications and Patient Selection

1. Patients with advanced age or multiple medical comorbidities and those who are otherwise unfit to undergo surgery often have poor outcomes with exclusive medical management for advanced ascending aortic pathology. For instance, patients with type A aortic dissection have an in-hospital mortality approaching 60% when treated medically.[33] In fact, an overall of 28% of patients with ascending aortic pathology are deemed to be unsuitable for an open surgical procedure.[33] When a patient is deemed inoperable, the endovascular approach takes its relevance. Promising results of endovascular stenting in case series and case reports support use of this approach for focal lesions located in the area above the sinotubular junction but below the origin of the innominate artery.[8,10] The minimally invasive endovascular approach has been used for acute and chronic type A aortic dissections (48%), aortic pseudoaneurysms (27.7%), ascending aortic aneurysm (5.1%), PAU (4.2%), IMH (2.5%), and rupture of the ascending aorta (2.5%).[8,10] Despite the use of the endovascular technique almost exclusively in high-risk patients, high technical success (96%) and low conversion rates to open surgery (0.7%) have been reported.[35]
2. The anatomical likelihood of suitability of an endovascular approach for the ascending aorta in patients with type A aortic dissection is based on several specific anatomic variables: absence of aortic valvular pathology (aortic regurgitation), adequate aortic length for sealing zones, favorable location of coronary ostia (to avoid occlusion). More specifically, the following prerequisites are suggested to choose a subset of patients most likely to benefit from an endovascular approach:
   a. Presence of proximal and distal landing zones with a length >10 mm,
   b. No difference in diameters (<10%) between proximal and distal landing zones,
   c. True aortic lumen diameter ≤ 38 mm,
   d. Total aortic diameter >16 mm and <46 mm,
   e. Absence of coronary artery bypass originating from the ascending aorta,
   f. Absence of calcification or thrombotic material in ascending or neighboring aortic zones,
   g. Intimal tear >10 mm above the sinotubular junction,
   h. Intimal tear > 5 mm below the innominate artery,
   i. Absence of grade 3 or 4 aortic regurgitation, and
   j. Diameter of the common and external iliac arteries >7 mm.[7,34]
3. Endovascular repair of the ascending aorta is contraindicated in the presence of severe aortic valve regurgitation, if the type A aortic dissection involves the aortic root proper, and (in the mind of most authorities) patients with connective tissue disease (Marfan's, Loeys-Dietz, Ehlers-Danlos). However, in patients with connective tissue pathologies, endovascular therapy can be utilized as a bridge until a definitive open surgical approach can be done, deferring the acuteness of the process to a more subacute and controlled situation.[7]

D. Devices for the Ascending Aorta

1. **Devices:** The appeal of endovascular therapy for the ascending aorta is tempered by the lack of specific aortic devices. Endografts applied for the ascending aorta usually correspond to designs intended for treatment of descending thoracic aortic (TEVAR) and abdominal aortic pathologies.[31] However, some investigational devices have been designed specifically for the ascending aorta, including the Zenith Ascend (Cook Medical, Bjaeverskov, Denmark) and the Valiant PS-IDE device (Medtronic, Minneapolis, MN).
   a. **Zenith Ascend Device (Cook Medical, Bjaeverskov, Denmark):** The Zenith Ascend stent is an investigational device tailored to the ascending aorta for the treatment of type A aortic dissection and aneurysmal disease. It has first been used in Europe, with a few cases reported in the United States under compassionate use through an investigational device exemption protocol.[34] The Ascend device provides a lower profile, with polyester fabric and nitinol stents, with a shorter and flexible tip intended to decrease ventricular and valve trauma. Additional support and fabric apposition are achieved with proximal and distal bare-metal fixation stents, which decrease the risk of compromising the coronary or innominate arteries.[32,34] Ascend is recommended for use in patients with the following anatomic criteria: minimum 10 mm landing zones distal to the origin of the coronary arteries and proximal to the origin of the innominate artery, and an aortic diameter no greater than 40 mm and no less than 24 mm.[34,36]
   b. **Valiant PS-IDE (Medtronic, Minneapolis, MN):** The Valiant PS-IDE endograft is a modification of the Valiant Thoracic stent graft used in TEVAR. It has been modified to treat ascending aortic pathologies, adjusting the original configuration to fit the shorter segment and the wider diameter of the ascending aorta. It was used in a prospective study to determine the feasibility of successful implantation. Two configurations were proposed: a proximal FreeFlo taper with a distal closed-web and a proximal closed-web design with bare springs distally. The delivery system was identical to the Valiant Captiva, with a nontip capture device used for the proximal closed-web design and a tip capture system for the FreeFlo configuration. It was configured to be used in patients with at least 10 mm of landing zones proximally and distally to the diseased area, an ascending aortic diameter between 28 mm and 44 mm, and high-risk surgical candidates with an American Society of Anesthesiology (ASA) score of 4.[32]
2. Table 5B.5 lays out the different endografts (both ascending specific and borrowed from TEVAR) that have been applied to the endovascular management of the ascending aorta.[8,10]

E. Deployment of Endografts

1. When a patient is deemed high risk for open surgery and an endovascular approach is considered, not only the anatomic and hemodynamic profiles may pose a challenge for endograft deployment but also anatomic variables affecting vascular access to the ascending aorta. Normally, with experience acquired in transcatheter aortic valve

TABLE 5B.5. Different Types of Stents Used for the Endovascular Treatment of the Ascending Aorta[a],[8,10]

Device/Stent Graft
Zenith TX2 Pro-Form endograft (Cook Medical, Bloomington, IN)
Thoracic TAG (Gore Medical, Flagstaff, AZ)
Talent thoracic stent graft (Medtronic, Minneapolis, MN)
Valiant stent graft (Medtronic, Minneapolis, MN)[a]
Zenith ascending dissection device (Cook Medical, Bjaeverskov, Denmark)[a]
Seal thoracic stent graft (S&G Biotech)
Najuta thoracic stent graft system (Kawasumi)
Custom-made grafts
Excluder abdominal cuff (Gore Medical, Flagstaff, AZ)
Endurant aortic cuff (Medtronic, Minneapolis, MN)
Relay NBS thoracic stent graft (Bolton Medical, Sunrise, FL)
Zenith aortic cuff extender (Cook Medical, Bloomington, IN)

[a]Stents Specifically Designed for the Ascending Aorta
BAV, bicuspid aortic valve aneurysm; TAA, thoracic aortic aneurysm; TEE, transesophageal echocardiography.

replacement (TAVR), the transfemoral approach is chosen, provided that there is adequate diameter of the iliofemoral vessels to accommodate the delivery sheaths.[7] However, the long distance to the sinotubular junction, compared with the relatively short length required for abdominal and the thoracic devices, poses a technical challenge. Also, long and rigid nosecones present a risk of ventricular perforation and aortic valve leaflet damage. Therefore, alternative access approaches that allow a more straight and direct route to the ascending aorta have been utilized. Delivery has been accomplished through the right and left carotid artery, right and left axillary artery, right and left subclavian artery, and iliac artery. Transseptal and transapical approaches have also been described in the literature.[32]

2. The transapical approach tries to solve the aforementioned problems, eliminating the need for long and stiff nosecones, and thus minimizing risk of associated complications. With the shorter distance from the LV apex to the ascending aorta, operator control during deployment is improved. When combined with maneuvers to decrease the cardiac output transiently, the apical approach leads to a more precise landing of the device. Additionally, with a more controlled technique for deployment of the graft, a better coaxial placement can be achieved to reduce the development of type I endoleaks. One of the advantages of this technique is the certainty of deployment in the true lumen in patients with type A dissection achieved by accessing the ascending aorta through a nondissected plane (via the left ventricle).[32]

F. Perioperative Imaging and Testing

1. For the successful deployment of an endovascular device in the ascending aorta, especially thorough preoperative planning is required. First, preoperative imaging with gated contrast enhanced computed tomography (CT) or noncontrast time-of-flight

magnetic resonance imaging (MRI) provides an understanding of the aortic anatomy. Essential information includes aortic size and the presence of atherosclerotic plaques and PAUs. Furthermore, precise imaging permits evaluation of the proximal and distal landing zones, size and angulation of access vessels, and the presence and location of vital side branches. Additionally, for interventions that cover aortic branches, fusion images integrating preoperative CTA or MRA with intraoperative fluoroscopy provide precise intraoperative roadmaps for the surgeon.[7]

2. Transesophageal echocardiography (TEE) also plays a critical role. In the preoperative stage, TEE allows for better visualization of aortic valve function. Intraoperatively, TEE guides the ideal selection of the transapical access site and confirms the position of the guidewire in the true lumen. Furthermore, TEE helps to detect any complication after stent deployment, such as iatrogenic aortic valve regurgitation and regional wall motion abnormalities due to obstruction of the coronary ostia.[7]
3. Intraoperatively, neurologic monitoring can be used to confirm the integrity of blood flow through the supra-aortic arch vessels and adequate cerebral perfusion. For instance, transcutaneous near-infrared spectroscopy and transcranial cerebral oximetry can provide real-time information about cerebral perfusion and oxygenation. Additionally, transcranial Doppler of intracranial vessels can detect changes in blood flow and microemboli, which can inform the surgical team of partial or total occlusion of the arch vessels, compromising cerebral blood flow, or distal embolization.[7]
4. Finally, for direct visualization of the endolumninal surface, intravascular ultrasound (IVUS) is a valuable resource, allowing measurement of the luminal diameter and precise determination of the position of branch vessels. Also, IVUS permits the localization of plaques or thrombi and enhances selection and achievement of landing zones. In type A aortic dissection, IVUS can be used reliably to identify the true lumen (differentiating from the false). IVUS also can confirm appropriate graft deployment and rule out any endoleaks.[7]

G. Complications

Most of the complications seen with endovascular management of the ascending aorta are novel even to the specialist; however, most of them are expected because of the anatomic singularities of this segment of aorta. The most common complications reported in the literature are as follows. Perforation of the left ventricle and/or formation of a left ventricular aneurysm may be seen when a rigid delivery system that must pass through the aortic valve is used. In the same setting, damage to the aortic leaflets is also plausible. Injury and dissection of the aortic root and occlusion of the coronary arteries with ensuing myocardial infarction can be encountered when the device is positioned close to the sinotubular junction, because of the exertion of strong radial forces to enhance proximal fixation in the ascending aorta.[32,37] Neurologic complications, such as ischemic stroke, can occur secondary to aortic arch branch vessel occlusion. Furthermore, particulate and/or air embolism may be seen following excessive wire and catheter manipulation in a diseased, atherosclerotic aortic arch. Also described are deployment failure, development of endoleaks, stent migration, need for reintervention, and conversion to open surgery.[8]

IV. Endovascular Therapy of the Aortic Arch

A. Challenges

The aortic arch together with the ascending aorta is among the most challenging areas for endovascular therapy. The curvature of the aortic arch, the high blood flow in the area, and the presence of vital branches that supply the upper body (including the brain) make any approach to this segment prone to devastating complications.[38]

B. Approaches and Misconceptions

1. Normally, conventional open surgical treatment for arch pathology involves a sternotomy incision, cardiopulmonary bypass, and a circulatory arrest with deep hypothermia with or without ACP or RCP. Despite persistent misconceptions to the contrary, surgical advances have rendered elective aortic arch surgery remarkably safe; reported postoperative mortality and permanent neurologic deficit are 2.9% and 2.2%, respectively.[12]
2. Recent advances in endovascular materials and techniques permit the application of endovascular and combined endovascular/open (hybrid) approaches for management of the aortic arch, with the goal of reducing complications of open and staged procedures.[38]
3. Despite endovascular advances in the management of the aortic arch, the risks of paraplegia, endoleak, stroke, and retrograde type A dissection remain. Embolism to the cerebral circulation, especially for patients with highly atheromatous aortic arches, is reported in up to 15% of patients following hybrid arch repair and accounts for the majority of strokes. Paraplegia, due to spinal cord hypoperfusion, manifests with rates about 6 %. The paraplegia risk increases with the length of aortic coverage; and previous infrarenal aortic surgery also increases the risk.[39] Retrograde dissection is an extremely serious complication encountered in patients treated for type B aortic dissection. Retrograde dissection seems to be more common when the stent grafts are oversized more than 10%. Rates of retrograde dissection from 2% to 6.5% following hybrid arch repair have been described. Type Ia endoleak is seen in 6% of aortic arch interventions, with reintervention rates of 18% at 1 year, 21% at 2 years, and 36% at 5 years.[39]

C. Aortic Arch Landing Zones

1. For placement of an endograft in the aortic arch, the stents require a minimum of 15 mm of a landing zone proximally and distally. However, when the aortic arch is highly angulated, the landing zone required increases to 20 mm.
2. Additionally, ideal sealing zone parameters for the aortic arch include a diameter of the aorta smaller than 40 mm, a length of disease-free aorta greater than 20 mm, and an angulation less than 60°.[39] Ishimaru and colleagues[40] established five aortic arch zones that are used as landing landmarks for the endovascular deployment of stents.
   a. **Zone 0** is the area proximal to the innominate artery involving its origin and the ascending aorta.
   b. **Zone 1** involves the origin of the common carotid artery.
   c. **Zone 2** involves the origin of the subclavian artery.

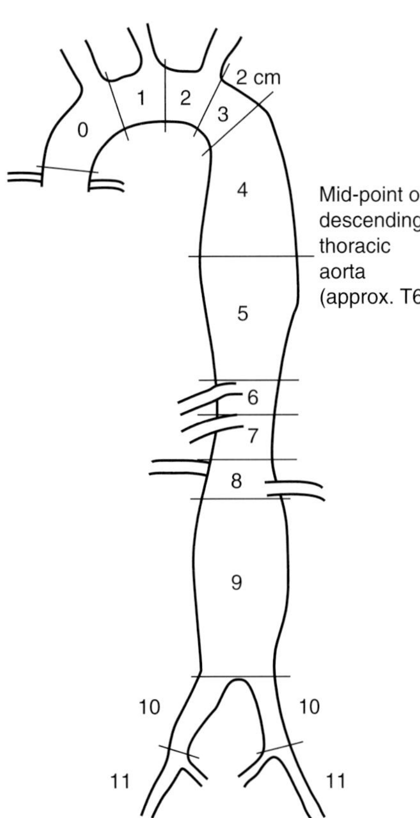

FIGURE 5B.5: Schematic representation of the aortic zones for proper landing of endovascular stents. Reprinted with permission from Fillinger MF, Greenberg RK, McKinsey JF, Chaikof EL; Society for Vascular Surgery Ad Hoc Committee on TRS. Reporting standards for thoracic endovascular aortic repair (TEVAR). *J Vasc Surg*. 2010;52:1022-1033, 1033.e1015.

d. **Zone 3** is between the left subclavian artery and 2 cm distal to it.
e. **Zone 4** includes the remainder of the thoracic aorta more than 2 cm distal to the left subclavian artery (Fig. 5B.5).[39,41]

V. Total Endovascular Technique for the Aortic Arch

When approaching the aortic arch, diverse techniques from hybrid to fully endovascular methods can be used. The total endovascular approach includes the parallel stent technique, use of endovascular branched endografts, and in situ fenestration.[38]

A. The Parallel Stent Technique

1. Also called snorkel or chimney technique, the parallel stent technique is used to maintain blood flow in the vital branches within the sealing zones of the endovascular stent without the need for fenestrated or branched grafts. In this technique, a covered stent is deployed into vital arch branches parallel to the main aortic graft.

2. The aortic stent is prolonged beyond the origin of the aortic branches, and the parallel graft works as a functional arm of the stent graft. The primary difficulty with the chimney technique is the development of type Ia endoleaks due to the insufficient apposition of the main body of the stent to the aortic wall. The "gutters" around the parallel graft encourage endoleak flow.

3. The parallel graft technique has been reported to have an operative success of 99%, a perioperative mortality of 4.5%, and a stroke rate of 4%. The high rate of stroke is due to emboli from manipulation of the aortic branches.[39,42,43]

4. Nevertheless, the snorkel or chimney graft technique is an option for emergent or urgent cases in patients who are not surgical candidates, or as a bailout procedure in unplanned coverage of the aortic branches.[39]

B. Branched Endografts

1. Branched endografts are indicated when there is an insufficient area for proximal sealing distal to the left subclavian artery (zone 3 and zone 4); therefore, proximal coverage involving the vital aortic arch branches is required (zone 0 to zone 3). Branched endografts maintain the benefits of an endovascular technique while avoiding malperfusion to the aortic branches.[44] Branched endografts have been available outside the United States under individual manufacturer-sponsored custom programs for many years. However, in the United States branched endografts have been employed in a few selected sites under a FDA investigational device exemption, mostly as investigational devices.[44]

2. Several branched endografts are currently under investigation (Table 5B.6).
   a. **Cook Arch Branch device (Cook Medical, Bloomington, IN):** This is a two-branch endograft designed for deployment into zone 0. It is made of a low-profile woven polyester material and a combination of nitinol and stainless steel, with two integral branches corresponding to the innominate artery and the left common carotid artery.[44]
   b. **Bolton Arch Branch device (Bolton Medical, Sunrise, FL):** The device is offered under "custom-made" orders outside the United States. It is based on the Relay NBS platform and made of polyester fabric and nitinol stents without a proximal bare-spring segment. Branches are internal and are referred as tunnels: these are oriented so that the anterior one can be optimally joined to the left carotid and the posterior one to the innominate artery.[44]
   c. **Medtronic Arch Branch device (Medtronic, Santa Rosa, CA):** This device, referred to as Mona-LSA, is a single-branch device used for zone 2 deployments. It is based on the Valiant thoracic endograft platform and is made of polyester and nitinol material. In principle, the device can be used for more proximal

TABLE 5B.6. Current Endovascular Aortic Arch stent Grafts[39]

Manufacturer	Scallop	Fenestration	Branch	Proximal Landing Zone
Bolton Medical	Yes	Yes	Yes. Single or double	0
Cook Zenith	Yes	Yes	Yes. Single or double	0
Gore TAG	No	No	Yes. Single	0
Medtronic	No	No	Yes. Single	2
Kawasumi	No	Yes	No	0

arch zones as long as indispensable covered vessels can be revascularized. The geometry is a modified fenestration with an inverted funnel appearance that allows the external segment to engage the origin of the subclavian artery or any alternate arch vessel and the bridging stent to flare with the widened mouth of the fenestration.[44]

d. **W.L. Gore Arch Branch device (W.L. Gore Medical, Flagstaff, AZ):** This device, referred to as GORE TAG thoracic branch endoprosthesis, is a single-branch arch device, based on the cTAG platform and made of expanded polytethrafluoroethylene (ePTFE) covering a nitinol frame. It was designed for deployment in zone 0 and zone 2; however, more proximal arch zones would require surgical revascularization of indispensable arch branches.[44]

C. In Situ Fenestration

1. This technique was first described in 2004 by McWilliams and colleagues.[45] This technique is reserved for zone 1 and zone 2 without the use of extracorporeal perfusion to maintain cerebral circulation due to only temporary coverage of the supra-aortic branches.[38]

2. The basic principle is to allow blood flow to the vital arch branches by fenestrating a thoracic endograft after deployment.[45]

3. Initial efforts involved a stiff guidewire followed by a needle and a cutting balloon angioplasty. It was found later that this technique causes tears in the expanded ePTFE stent graft. Therefore, laser or radiofrequency puncture has been invoked to create a retrograde in situ fenestration during TEVAR, followed by balloon angioplasty and deployment of a covered stent.[38]

4. In addition to the fenestration technique, the following fenestrated graft, developed by Kawasumi Laboratories Najuta, has been described:
   a. **The Najuta endograft system (Kawasumi Laboratories Najuta, Tokyo, Japan):** It is a fenestrated graft without branches that was constructed with longitudinally connected Z stents covered with ePTFE.[39]

D. Physician-Modified Stent Grafts

1. Custom-made branched and fenestrated endografts can be useful during elective cases but are not easily applicable during urgent and emergent cases, because of the prolonged manufacturing delay. Therefore, physicians have opted to modify infrarenal and thoracic devices "on the back table" by adding branches and fenestrations.

2. Devices are usually created with reinforced fenestrations or branches constructed from portions of self-expanding stent grafts. Such creative efforts make these homemade devices an option for patients in need of urgent operation. However, long-term outcomes are not known, placing a great responsibility on the physician, especially if the urgent case is not done under a formal investigation device exemption (IDE) study within the United States.[46]

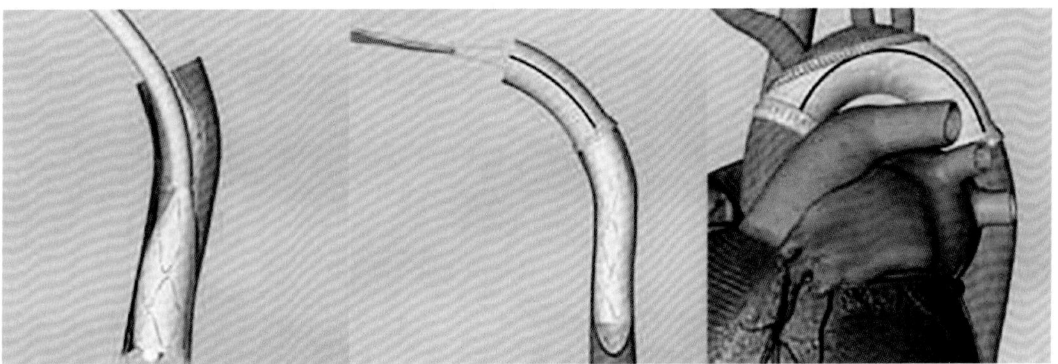

FIGURE 5B.6: Deployment of E-vita open plus and reconstruction of the aortic arch. © JOTEC GmbH, a full owned subsidiary of CryoLife Inc.

VI. Hybrid Procedure Approach for the Aortic Arch

A. In an attempt to reduce the risks associated with an open procedure, but at the same time to avoid the limitations of an endovascular approach, hybrid techniques are described. There are two types of hybrid interventions: first, an open aortic arch repair with distal extension using the stent graft or frozen elephant trunk procedure, and second, an extra-anatomic bypass involving the supra-aortic branches combined with a thoracic stent placement to allow for a proximal extension of the landing zones or debranching procedure (Fig. 5B.6).

B. Frozen Elephant Trunk Procedure

1. The elephant trunk procedure was first described by Borst and colleagues[47] in 1983 to treat extensive aneurysmal disease of the entire thoracic aorta. In this procedure, a free elephant graft is left dandling in the descending aorta for later utilization in the replacement of the descending aorta during a second stage. Kato and colleagues[48] reported the first experience with a modification of the two-staged elephant trunk procedure. It consisted in the open surgical approach of the aortic arch with a deployment of an endovascular stent to treat the descending aorta. The original technique has been modified from a free distal anastomosis to a hand-sewn proximal end of the frozen elephant trunk to avoid migration. This technique allows for the management of extensive aortic aneurysmal disease with an open repair of the aortic arch and an antegrade deployment of the thoracic endograft. Additionally, it is used in the management of type A aortic dissections to reduce aneurysmal degeneration of the descending aorta.[38]
2. There are two prefabricated grafts available outside the United States.
    a. **The E-Vita Open and the E-Vita Plus (JOTEC, Hechingen, Germany):** These devices have the longest registry dating back to 2005. They have demonstrated rates of in-hospital mortality of 16% for aortic dissection and 13% for nondissections; postoperative stroke and spinal cord injury have been found to be 8% and 4%, respectively. With these devices, a landing zone lower than T10 has been identified as a risk factor for paraplegia (Fig. 5B.7).[38]

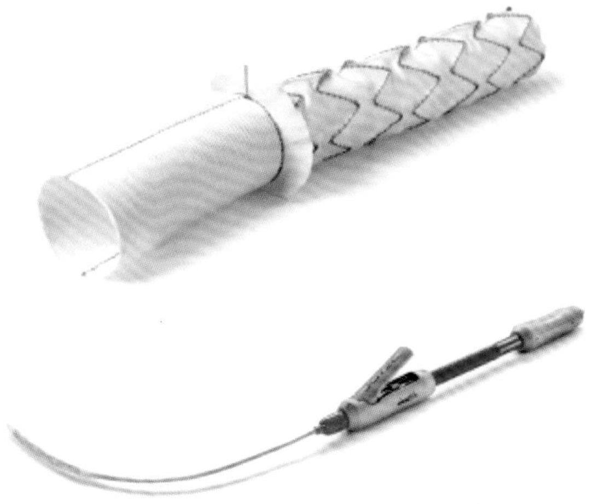

FIGURE 5B.7: The E-vita open plus hybrid prosthesis and its delivery system. © JOTEC GmbH, a full owned subsidiary of CryoLife Inc.

b. **Thoraflex™ Hybrid Plexus and Thoraflex™ Hybrid Ante-Flo. Terumo Aortic (Inchinnan, United Kingdom):** This device has a four-branch (Plexus) configuration as well as a straight version (Ante-Flo) that permit the implantation of the aortic arches individually or as a carrel patch, respectively. It has reported rates of 7% for perioperative mortality and 7% for spinal injury. The Thoraflex™ Hybrid devices is currently under investigation in the United States for aortic dissection, aneurysm and rupture (Fig. 5B.8).[38,49]

C. Surgical Debranching Procedure

1. An extra-anatomical bypass from the ascending aorta to the supra-aortic branches using a median sternotomy was first described in the late 1990s. In 2000, the first extra-anatomical bypass from the left common carotid to left subclavian associated with a TEVAR was described for treatment of an acute type B aortic dissection. Debranching procedures may be performed with or without sternotomy. Options vary based on the location of the pathologic process along the aortic arch zones.[38]

2. These debranching procedures may be performed in a staged fashion or at the same operation together with TEVAR.[39] Careful consideration is essential for patients with diseases affecting zone 0.[38]
   a. **Zone 0 surgical debranching:** Zone 0 deployment of endografts is used when the aortic pathology covers the ascending aorta and the proximal aortic arch. A bypass from the ascending aorta can be used to circumvent the origins of the aortic arch branches that are covered with the thoracic stent. If the origin of the innominate artery is compromised, an extra-anatomic bypass form the ascending aorta to the innominate artery is done. In case of needed revascularization for the left common carotid, an extra-anatomic bypass for the left common carotid artery is constructed using the bypass of the innominate artery as an inflow. In case of coverage of the left subclavian artery, a bypass can be anastomosed to the left common carotid artery graft. If the left subclavian artery is difficult to access,

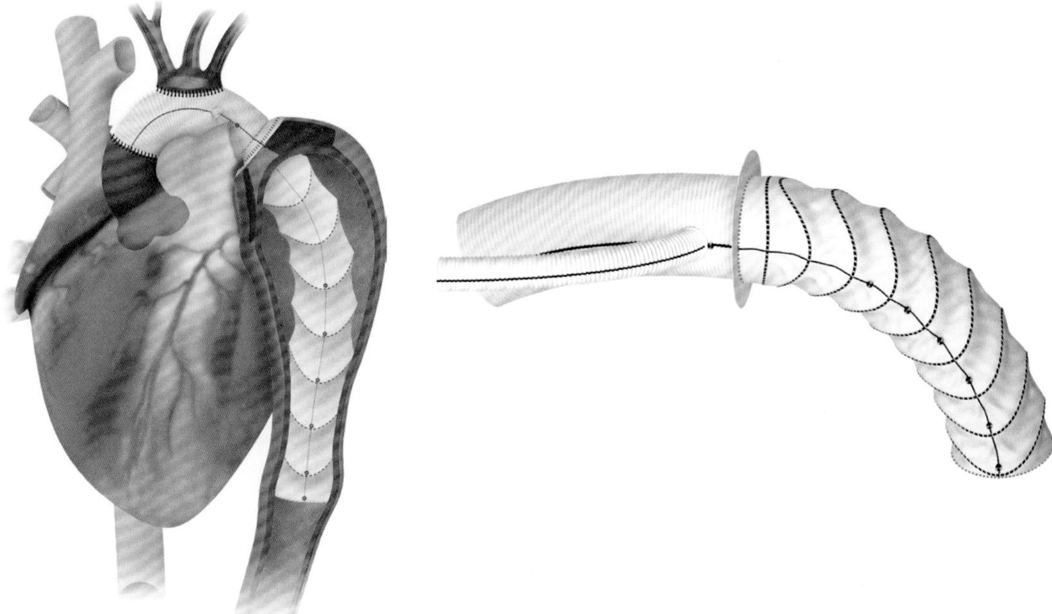

FIGURE 5B.8: The Thoraflex™ hybrid prosthesis and its delivery system. © 2019 Terumo Aortic.

it can be later revascularized with subclavian transposition or left subclavian to carotid artery bypass. Postoperative mortality has been reported to be 0%-8% and stroke rate to be 0%-17%.[38]

b. **Zone 1 surgical debranching:** Zone 1 debranching is indicated for patients with distal aortic arch pathology that has a proximal landing zone greater than 2 cm from the innominate artery. First, an extrathoracic left carotid to right carotid bypass is performed using an 8 mm Dacron graft; this can be performed via the anterior subplatysmal plane or the retroesophageal route, the latter providing the shortest and the most secure route because of the deep position of the graft in the neck. Also, some surgeons prefer the transposition technique avoiding the use of prosthetic material; however, that procedure must be done using a sternotomy or hemisternotomy. In this case, at the time of bypass the proximal left carotid artery is ligated to prevent type II endoleak, and the proximal left subclavian is also ligated as needed. Finally, TEVAR is performed. Postoperative mortality has been reported to be 0%-11% and stroke rate to be 11%.[38]

c. **Zone 2 surgical debranching:** Zone 2 TEVAR requires preoperative surgical revascularization of the left subclavian artery to avoid ischemic complications. Subclavian revascularization is especially important in specific circumstances. These are listed here, with the potential complication of nonrevascularization indicated in parentheses: when there is a patent left internal mammary graft (immediate myocardial infarction), functional left upper extremity arteriovenous fistula (fistula closure), planned long segmental coverage (>20 cm) of the descending aorta (paraplegia), absent or atretic right vertebral artery (posterior fossa stroke), prior infrarenal aortic operation (paraplegia), hypogastric artery occlusion (various), and the presence of aneurysms where upcoming intervention involving the aortic arch is anticipated (paraplegia). Usually, a zone 2 debranching procedure is used for treatment of type B aortic dissection and proximal descending aortic aneurysms. Postoperative mortality has been reported to be 0%-3.4% and stroke rate 3% to be 8.7%.[38]

VII. Summary

Endovascular management of aortic pathology has emerged as a near gold standard for the treatment of the abdominal aorta. The good results from these abdominal interventions have generated enthusiasm for expanding the technology into more proximal aortic segments. The descending aorta has been the more proximal aortic segment in which most of the interest has been placed. However, the ascending aorta and the aortic arch have been approached as well—perhaps the ultimate frontiers for implementation of the endovascular treatment.

Despite the interest in handling more proximal segments endovascularly, many difficulties arise. The ascending aorta is a high-stake zone due to the proximal location of the aortic valve and coronary ostia and the distal presence of the head vessels. Any misplacement of a thoracic stent can result in devastating consequences such as myocardial infarction or stroke. Finally, the hemodynamic forces experienced in these segments increase the difficulty for adequate deployment, requiring techniques that decrease the blood pressure and the cardiac output.

Moreover, the aortic arch requires meticulous surgical planning to best decide the approach that will limit the risk of stroke due to instrumentation of the head vessels.

The lack of specific devices for the ascending aorta and the investigational nature of aortic arch devices make endovascular management of these segments a new and developing area; such interventions are largely limited to high-risk patients in whom conventional open surgery is not possible or safe. Thus, endovascular techniques provide an alternative to sole medical management (in nonsurgical patients), which would be expected to result in high mortality and morbidity.

It must be remembered that open surgical techniques have achieved previously unimaginable levels of effectiveness and safety. An experienced open surgical opinion should be invoked before pursuit of exciting but complex endovascular therapies with unproven large-scale, long-term results.

CLINICAL PEARLS

- Aortic aneurysm is a silent disease requiring close monitoring because the first clinical manifestation can be a life-threatening complication.
- Aortic dissection requires a high index of suspicion, especially in patients with abrupt onset of chest or back pain.
- The open surgical approach for the management of the ascending aorta and the aortic arch is the gold standard for treatment of thoracic aortic pathology, with dramatic improvements in safety compared with earlier eras.
- Endovascular management of the ascending aorta and the aortic arch is largely reserved for high-risk surgical patients in whom conventional approaches are prohibited.

Recommended Reading

1. Hiratzka LF, Bakris GL, Beckman JA, et al. ACCF/AHA/AATS/ACR/ASA/SCA/SCAI/SIR/STS/SVM guidelines for the diagnosis and management of patients with thoracic aortic disease: executive summary. *Circulation.* 2010;121:1544-1579.
2. Braverman AC. Diseases of the aorta. In: Braunwald E, Mann DL, Zipes DP, Libby P, Bonow R, eds. *Braunwald's Heart Disease a Textbook of Cardiovascular Medicine.* Saunders Elsevier; 2014.
3. Elefteriades JA, Farkas EA. Thoracic aortic aneurysm clinically pertinent controversies and uncertainties. *J Am Coll Cardiol.* 2010;55(9):841-857. doi:10.1016/j.jacc.2009.08.08.
4. Elefteriades JA. Thoracic aortic aneurysm: reading the enemy's playbook. *Curr Probl Cardiol.* 2008;33:203-277.
5. Muetterties CE, Menon R, Wheatley GH III. A systematic review of primary endovascular repair of the ascending aorta. *J Vasc Surg.* 2018;67(1):332-342.
6. Tanaka A, Estrera A. Endovascular treatment options for the aortic arch. *Cardiol Clin.* 2017;35(3):357-366.

References

1. Ziganshin BA, Elefteriades JA. Thoracic aortic disease. In: Stergiopoulos K, Brown DL, eds. *Evidence-Based Cardiology Consult.* London: Springer London; 2014:331-353.
2. Erbel R, Aboyans V, Boileau C, et al. 2014 ESC guidelines on the diagnosis and treatment of aortic diseases: document covering acute and chronic aortic diseases of the thoracic and abdominal aorta of the adult. The task force for the diagnosis and treatment of aortic diseases of the European Society of Cardiology (ESC). *Eur Heart J.* 2014;35(41):2873-2926.
3. Prevention CfDaC. *WISQARS Leading Causes of Death Reports, 1999-2015.* [cited 2017 November]; Available at: http://webappa.cdc.gov/sasweb/ncipc/leadcaus10.html.
4. Patel R, Powell JT, Sweeting MJ, Epstein DM, Barrett JK, Greenhalgh RM. The UK EndoVascular Aneurysm Repair (EVAR) randomised controlled trials: long-term follow-up and cost-effectiveness analysis. *Health Technol Assess.* 2018;22(5):1-132.
5. Le TB, Park KM, Jeon YS, Hong KC, Cho SG. Evaluation of delayed endoleak compared with early endoleak after endovascular aneurysm repair. *J Vasc Interv Radiol.* 2018;29(2):203-209.
6. Lal BK, Zhou W, Li Z, et al. Predictors and outcomes of endoleaks in the veterans affairs Open Versus Endovascular Repair (OVER) trial of abdominal aortic aneurysms. *J Vasc Surg.* 2015;62(6):1394-1404.
7. Shah A, Khoynezhad A. Thoracic endovascular repair for acute type A aortic dissection: operative technique. *Ann Cardiothorac Surg.* 2016;5(4):389-396.
8. Muetterties CE, Menon R, Wheatley GH III. A systematic review of primary endovascular repair of the ascending aorta. *J Vasc Surg.* 2018;67(1):332-342.
9. Gandet T, Alric P, Bommart S, Canaud L. Endovascular aortic repair of a chronic ascending and arch aortic aneurysm. *J Thorac Cardiovasc Surg.* 2017.
10. Baikoussis NG, Antonopoulos CN, Papakonstantinou NA, Argiriou M, Geroulakos G. Endovascular stent grafting for ascending aorta diseases. *J Vasc Surg.* 2017;66(5):1587-1601.
11. Achneck HE, Rizzo JA, Tranquilli M, Elefteriades JA. Safety of thoracic aortic surgery in the present era. *Ann Thorac Surg.* 2007;84(4):1180-1185; discussion 1185.
12. Bin Mahmood SU, Velasquez CA, Zafar MA, et al. Current safety of ascending aortic surgery. Abstracts of the American Association of Thoracic Surgery Aortic Symposium, New York. 2018.
13. Hiratzka LF, Bakris GL, Beckman JA, et al. 2010 ACCF/AHA/AATS/ACR/ASA/SCA/SCAI/SIR/STS/SVM guidelines for the diagnosis and management of patients with thoracic aortic disease: a report of the American College of Cardiology Foundation/American Heart Association Task Force on Practice Guidelines, American Association for Thoracic Surgery, American College of Radiology, American Stroke Association, Society of Cardiovascular Anesthesiologists, Society for Cardiovascular Angiography and Interventions, Society of Interventional Radiology, Society of Thoracic Surgeons, and Society for Vascular Medicine. *Circulation.* 2010;121(13):e266-e369.

14. Braverman AC. Diseases of the aorta. In: Braunwald E, Mann DL, Zipes DP, Libby P, Bonow R, eds. *Braunwald's Heart Disease a Textbook of Cardiovascular Medicine*. Saunders Elsevier; 2014.
15. Peterson MD, Diethrich EB, Rudakewich G. *Acute Aortic Dissection. Aortic Diseases: Clinical Diagnostic Imaging Atlas*. Philadeplphia: PA: Saunders Elsevier; 2009. 55-112.
16. Nienaber CA, Eagle KA. Aortic dissection: new frontiers in diagnosis and management: Part I: from etiology to diagnostic strategies. *Circulation*. 2003;108(5):628-635.
17. Hagan PG, Nienaber CA, Isselbacher EM, et al. The International Registry of Acute Aortic Dissection (IRAD): new insights into an old disease. *JAMA*. 2000;283(7):897-903.
18. Botta D, Elefteriades JA, Koullias G, et al. *Acute Aortic Disease*. CRC Press; 2007.
19. Sinha I, Bethi S, Cronin P, et al. A biologic basis for asymmetric growth in descending thoracic aortic aneurysms: a role for matrix metalloproteinase 9 and 2. *J Vasc Surg*. 2006;43(2):342-348.
20. Koullias GJ, Ravichandran P, Korkolis DP, Rimm DL, Elefteriades JA. Increased tissue microarray matrix metalloproteinase expression favors proteolysis in thoracic aortic aneurysms and dissections. *Ann Thorac Surg*. 2004;78(6):2106-2110; discussion 2110-2111.
21. Elefteriades JA. Thoracic aortic aneurysm: reading the enemy's playbook. *Yale J Biol Med*. 2008;81(4):175-186.
22. Elefteriades JA. Natural history of thoracic aortic aneurysms: indications for surgery, and surgical versus nonsurgical risks. *Ann Thorac Surg*. 2002;74(5):S1877-S1880; discussion S1892-S1898.
23. Coady MA, Rizzo JA, Goldstein LJ, Elefteriades JA. Natural history, pathogenesis, and etiology of thoracic aortic aneurysms and dissections. *Cardiol Clin*. 1999;17(4):615-635; vii.
24. Coady MA, Rizzo JA, Hammond GL, et al. What is the appropriate size criterion for resection of thoracic aortic aneurysms? *J Thorac Cardiovasc Surg*. 1997;113(3):476-491; discussion 489-491.
25. Zafar MA, Li Y, Rizzo JA, et al. Height alone (rather than body surface area) suffices for risk estimation in ascending aortic aneurysm. *J Thorac Cardiovasc Surg*. 2017. In Press.
26. Brownstein AJ, Ziganshin BA, Kuivaniemi H, Body SC, Bale AE, Elefteriades JA. Genes associated with thoracic aortic aneurysm and dissection: an update and clinical implications. *Aorta (Stamford)*. 2017;5(1):11-20.
27. Otto CM. Diseases of the great arteries. In: Otto CM, ed. *Textbook of Clinical Echocardiography*. 6th ed. Philadelphia, PA: Elsevier; 2018. 446-472.
28. *Overview of Acute Aortic Dissection and Other Acute Aortic Syndromes [database on the Internet]*. 2018.
29. Elefteriades JA. Thoracic aortic aneurysm: reading the enemy's playbook. *Curr Probl Cardiol*. 2008;33(5):203-277.
30. Velasquez CA, Bin Mahmood SU, Zafar MA, et al. Precipitous resolution of type-A intramural hematoma with medical management in a patient with metastatic stage 4 renal cell carcinoma. *Int J Angiol*. 2017;26(4):267-270.
31. Shults CC, Chen EP, Thourani VH, Leshnower BG. Transapical thoracic endovascular aortic repair as a bridge to open repair of an infected ascending aortic pseudoaneurysm. *Ann Thorac Surg*. 2015;100(5):1883-1886.
32. Khoynezhad A, Donayre CE, Walot I, Koopmann MC, Kopchok GE, White RA. Feasibility of endovascular repair of ascending aortic pathologies as part of an FDA-approved physician-sponsored investigational device exemption. *J Vasc Surg*. 2016;63(6):1483-1495.
33. Kumpati GS, Gray R, Patel A, Bull DA. Endovascular repair of acute ascending aortic disruption via the right axillary artery. *Ann Thorac Surg*. 2014;97(2):700-703.
34. Oderich GS, Pochettino A, Mendes BC, Roeder B, Pulido J, Gloviczki P. Endovascular repair of saccular ascending aortic aneurysm after orthotopic heart transplantation using an investigational zenith ascend stent-graft. *J Endovasc Ther*. 2015;22(4):650-654.
35. Horton JD, Kolbel T, Haulon S, et al. Endovascular repair of type A aortic dissection: current experience and technical considerations. *Semin Thorac Cardiovasc Surg*. 2016;28(2):312-317.
36. Tsilimparis N, Debus ES, Oderich GS, et al. International experience with endovascular therapy of the ascending aorta with a dedicated endograft. *J Vasc Surg*. 2016;63(6):1476-1482.
37. Yang ZH, Xia LM, Wei L, Wang CS. Complications after endovascular repair of Stanford type A (ascending) aortic dissection. *Eur J Cardiothorac Surg*. 2012;42(5):894-896.

38. Tanaka A, Estrera A. Endovascular treatment options for the aortic arch. *Cardiol Clin*. 2017;35(3):357-366.
39. Rudarakanchana N, Jenkins MP. Hybrid and total endovascular repair of the aortic arch. *Br J Surg*. 2018;105(4):315-327.
40. Mitchell RS, Ishimaru S, Ehrlich MP, et al. First International Summit on Thoracic Aortic Endografting: roundtable on thoracic aortic dissection as an indication for endografting. *J Endovasc Ther*. 2002;9(suppl 2):II98-II105.
41. Fillinger MF, Greenberg RK, McKinsey JF, Chaikof EL, Society for Vascular Surgery Ad Hoc Committee on TRS. Reporting standards for thoracic endovascular aortic repair (TEVAR). *J Vasc Surg*. 2010;52(4):1022-1033, 1033 e15.
42. Moulakakis KG, Mylonas SN, Dalainas I, et al. The chimney-graft technique for preserving supra-aortic branches: a review. *Ann Cardiothorac Surg*. 2013;2(3):339-346.
43. Lachat M, Frauenfelder T, Mayer D, et al. Complete endovascular renal and visceral artery revascularization and exclusion of a ruptured type IV thoracoabdominal aortic aneurysm. *J Endovasc Ther*. 2010;17(2):216-220.
44. Anthony Lee W. Status of branched grafts for thoracic aortic arch endovascular repair. *Semin Vasc Surg*. 2016;29(1-2):84-89.
45. Glorion M, Coscas R, McWilliams RG, Javerliat I, Goeau-Brissonniere O, Coggia M. A Comprehensive review of in situ fenestration of aortic endografts. *Eur J Vasc Endovasc Surg*. 2016;52(6):787-800.
46. Mastracci TM, Greenberg RK. Thoracic and thoracoabdominal aneurysms: branched and fenestrated endograft treatment. In: Cronenwett JL, Johnston W, eds. Rutherford's Vascular Surgery. 8th ed. Elsevier; 2014:2149-2168.
47. Borst HG, Walterbusch G, Schaps D. Extensive aortic replacement using "elephant trunk" prosthesis. *Thorac Cardiovasc Surg*. 1983;31(1):37-40.
48. Kato M, Ohnishi K, Kaneko M, et al. New graft-implanting method for thoracic aortic aneurysm or dissection with a stented graft. *Circulation*. 1996;94(9 suppl):II188-II193.
49. Ma WG, Zheng J, Sun LZ, Elefteriades JA. Open stented grafts for frozen elephant trunk technique: technical aspects and current outcomes. *Aorta (Stamford)*. 2015;3(4):122 135.

CHAPTER 6

Endovascular Repair of the Descending Aorta

Ayman Saeyeldin, MD, Young Erben, MD, Mohammad A. Zafar, MD, Afsha Aurshina, MBBS, Camilo A. Velasquez, MD, Wei-Guo Ma, MD, Chandni Patel, MD, Jeremy D. Asnes, MD, Bulat Ziganshin, MD, PhD, John A. Elefteriades, MD, PhD (hon), and Bauer E. Sumpio, MD, PhD

Key Points

- TEVAR is a safe and effective method for treatment of various pathologies affecting the descending thoracic aorta.
- Various devices are currently FDA approved for TEVAR, with growing evidence supporting their safety and efficacy.
- Careful preoperative planning is indispensable in order to choose the correct stent type and minimize complications.
- Revascularization and debranching procedures (hybrid repair) should be considered on an individualized basis.
- Endovascular treatment has less perioperative morbidity and mortality than open repair; however, long-term results regarding the durability and reliability of these devices are scarce.

I. Introduction

Since the preliminary reports on thoracic endovascular aortic repair (TEVAR) in 1994,[1] major advancements have been achieved in the stent materials, sizes, conformability, graft tapering, techniques of deployment, and the applications of this life-saving method of treatment. TEVAR has successfully reoriented the current treatment guidelines of descending thoracic aortic aneurysms (DTAs) as TEVAR permits the introduction of a stent graft into the descending or thoracoabdominal aorta through a minimally invasive incision. Although TEVAR was initially introduced for the treatment of degenerative aneurysmal aortic diseases in nonsurgical candidates, TEVAR is now considered a valid treatment option for an array of other aortic pathologies, with the advantages of lower morbidity, avoidance of a thoracotomy incision, and the elimination of the need for partial or total circulatory support. This chapter discusses the endovascular repair of aortic pathologies afflicting the descending thoracic aorta.

II. Anatomic Background

The descending aorta is the longest segment of the thoracic aorta, beginning at the isthmus between the origin of the left subclavian artery and the ligamentum arteriosum and coursing anterior to the vertebral column, giving off paired thoracic arteries (T1-T12), and then traversing the aortic hiatus in the diaphragm into the abdomen to continue as the abdominal aorta. The abdominal aorta extends retroperitoneally to its bifurcation into the common iliac arteries at the level of the fourth lumbar vertebra.

A. **Landing Zones** For the purpose of describing the extent of endovascular coverage, the thoracic aorta is divided into landing zones,[2] which determine the location of the stent and define the need for a concomitant debranching procedure (Fig. 6.1):

- Zone 0: Proximal to the takeoff of the innominate artery
- Zone 1: Distal to the innominate artery, but proximal to the origin of the left common carotid artery

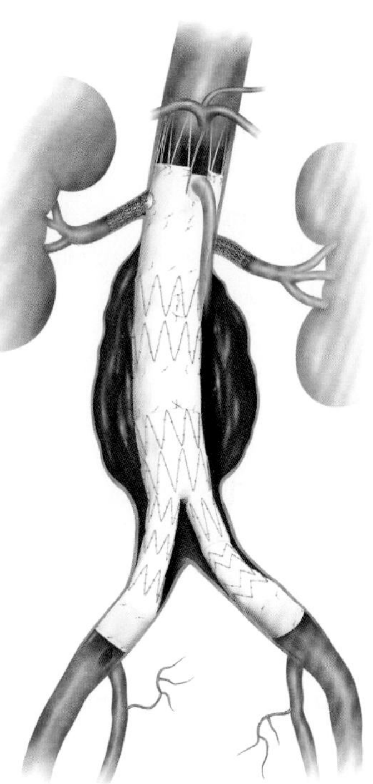

FIGURE 6.1: Zones of attachment. Reprinted with permission from Fillinger MF, Greenberg RK, McKinsey JF, Chaikof EL. Society for Vascular Surgery Ad Hoc Committee on TRS. Reporting standards for thoracic endovascular aortic repair (TEVAR). *J Vasc Surg*. 2010 52:1022-1033, 1033. e1015.

- Zone 2: Distal to the origin of the left common carotid artery, but proximal to the left subclavian artery
- Zone 3: ≤2 cm from the left subclavian artery without covering it
- Zone 4: >2 cm distal to the left subclavian, but within the proximal half of the descending aorta (T6)
- Zone 5: Starts in the distal half of the descending thoracic aorta, but proximal to the celiac artery
- Zone 6: Coeliac origin to the top of the superior mesenteric artery
- Zone 7: Superior mesenteric artery origin, suprarenal aorta
- Zone 8: Covers at least one renal artery
- Zone 9: Infrarenal
- Zone 10: Common iliac
- Zone 11: External iliac

B. **Spinal Perfusion** The spinal cord is supplied by branches of the vertebral artery: one anterior spinal artery (supplying the anterior two-thirds of the spinal cord) and two posterior spinal arteries (supplying the posterior one-third), which anastomose distally at the conus medullaris. The thoracic aorta is dependent on radicular contributions to the anterior spinal artery via the artery of Adamkiewicz, which can be found between T9 and T12 in 75% of individuals, and other segmental (intercostal) arteries.[3]

III. Indications for TEVAR

TEVAR was initially introduced for the treatment of thoracic aortic aneurysms in patients who could not tolerate open repair. Keystone trials led to approval by the United States Food and Drug Administration (FDA) in 2005.[4] Since then, TEVAR has been a treatment modality for other aortic pathologies, such as aortic dissection, blunt traumatic aortic injury, and penetrating aortic ulcers.[5,6] TEVAR has also expanded its reach beyond the original nonsurgical patients to patients who would also be suitable for open surgery.

A. Thoracic Aortic Aneurysms

1. Patients with large DTAs are at risk of dire complications such as rupture or dissection. The risk of complications increases as the diameter of the descending aorta enlarges, with a "hinge point" at 7 cm.[7,8] However, by the time the aorta reaches this size, 43% of patients suffer a devastating complication.[9] Survival can be improved with preemptive open surgical repair of the aorta, before these critical diameters are reached.[10,11] Although there is a paucity of data comparing endovascular repair to medical management, it is plausible to assume that outcomes would be better with endovascular repair (rather than purely medical management) in patients with indications for open surgical intervention.

2. The current recommendations for TEVAR in patients with degenerative aneurysms of the descending thoracic aorta include aortic size exceeding 5.5 cm, saccular aneurysms, or postoperative pseudoaneurysms (class: Ib).[10] TEVAR aims to exclude the aortic aneurysm from the circulation by implanting a membrane-covered stent-graft across the lesion, in order to prevent further enlargement and eventual aortic rupture. In DTAs, it is recommended that stent-graft exceed the reference aortic diameter at the landing zone by at least 10%-15% (to produce a "seal").

B. Thoracic Aortic Dissection

1. Repair of descending aortic dissection (DescAD) (type B in Stanford classification, or type III in DeBakey classification) is indicated in patients with complications, which typically occur within the first 2 weeks of diagnosis, affecting approximately 25% of patients.[10–13] The suitable complications include the following:
   a. End-organ malperfusion
   b. Refractory pain in spite of optimized medical treatment (OMT)
   c. Rapid expansion if the false lumen (which may be appreciated over the first several months following an acute presentation)
   d. Impending or frank rupture
   e. Aneurysmal dilation in a chronic DescAD meeting criteria for repair

2. TEVAR aims to stabilize the dissected aorta to prevent late complications by inducing favorable aortic remodeling. Obliteration of the intimal tear by implantation of a stent-graft helps redirect blood flow into the true lumen (TL), thus improving distal perfusion.[14] At least 1 or 2 cm of dissected aorta must be covered to provide stent fixation. Thrombosis of the false lumen (FL) is also promoted by stent grafting, which induces the beneficial process of aortic remodeling.

3. For uncomplicated DescAD, reports from the International Registry of Acute Aortic Dissection (IRAD) show no benefit of TEVAR over medical therapy.[15] For complicated acute DescAD, TEVAR is the treatment of choice.[16]

4. The INvestigation of STEnt grafts in patients with type B Aortic Dissection (INSTEAD trial),[17] which compared TEVAR + OMT with OMT alone in patients with uncomplicated type B AD, has shown no significant difference in the 2-year all-cause mortality, with 88.0% survival at 2 years in the TEVAR group, versus 95.6% in the OMT group. Five-year follow-up (the INSTEAD-XL trial) was conducted via a special (controversial) statistical analysis method (Landmark analysis).[18] Analysis showed that all-cause mortality in the TEVAR + OMT group versus OMT-alone group was 11.1% versus 19.3% (P = 0.13), aortic deaths were 6.9% versus 19.3% (P = 0.04), and progression of the pathology occurred in 27% versus 46.1% (P = 0.04), respectively.

5. The INSTEAD-XL trial was designed to evaluate patients with more chronic dissections (56 days in the stent-graft group vs 75 days in the medical management group). The controversy arose in that the Landmark method does not include periprocedural early mortality in the analysis. Detractors point out that the choice of Landmark analysis may have produced better apparent outcomes than would have been seen with standard analytic methods.

C. **Other Pathologies** TEVAR can also be utilized in patients with blunt thoracic aortic injuries due to high-speed deceleration, with significantly lower perioperative morbidity and mortality compared with open repair.[19] Other lesions in the spectrum of aortic dissection (e.g., intramural hematoma/penetrating aortic ulcer) can also be managed with an endovascular technique, so as to exclude the aortic lesion, or to cover the intimal tear in any coexistent dissection. Endovascular techniques can also be utilized in cases of aortoesophageal fistula as a temporizing measure to prevent exsanguination and allow for fluid resuscitation.[20]

IV. Endograft Structure

Endovascular grafts are usually inserted via a transfemoral approach. Upon deployment, the endograft self-expands to exclude the native diseased aorta from the circulation and comes in contact with the aortic wall proximally and distally in a tight-seal fashion (Fig. 6.2). Significant variations in graft design exist. However, all stents are composed of a delivery system, main device, and device extensions.[21]

A. **Delivery System** The size of the delivery sheath depends on the diameter of the endograft that needs to be deployed to provide appropriate fixation. Delivery is usually accomplished via a femoral approach by direct surgical cutdown. If the diameter of the femoral or iliac artery is too small to withstand the delivery system, access can be obtained by direct puncture of the iliac artery or the aorta via a retroperitoneal incision, or by suturing a synthetic conduit onto the iliac artery.

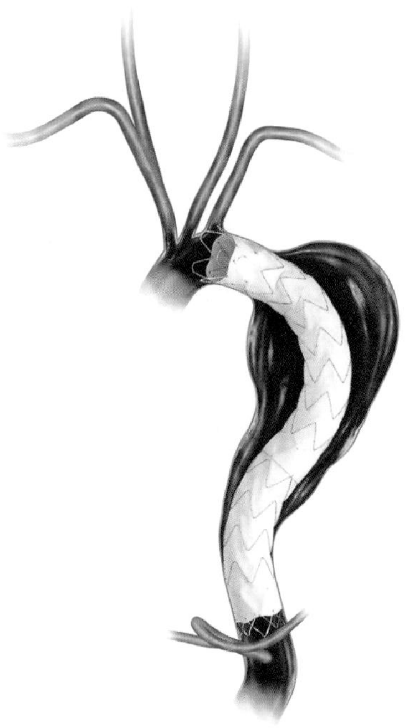

FIGURE 6.2: The Zenith Alpha thoracic stent graft. Thoracic endovascular grafts require proximal and distal seal zones of least 2 cm. Permission for use granted by Cook Medical, Bloomington, Indiana.

B. **Main Device** The endograft can be straight or tapered and may or may not have a longitudinal support. The graft self-expands, but subsequent ballooning is an option. Fixation systems may include barbs or uncovered proximal stents.

C. **Extensions** These are utilized during deployment if adequate positioning of the endograft is not obtained, or if postdeployment aortography reveals endoleaks. Proximal or distal extension devices can provide a complete seal.

V. Available Endografts for TEVAR

Multiple devices are currently FDA approved for thoracic endovascular repair from different manufacturers (Table 6.1). These devices include the Gore TAG and CTAG (W.L. Gore & Associates, Newark, DE), Zenith TX2 and Zenith Alpha (Cook Medical, Bloomington, IN), Valiant (Medtronic Vascular, Santa Rosa, CA), and the Relay (Bolton Medical, Sunrise, FL).

A. TAG and CTAG

1. The TAG device (W.L. Gore & Associates) is a flexible tube-shaped stent-graft, lined with polytetrafluorethylene (ePTFE) “Teflon” and covered with an additional layer of Teflon and fluorinated ethylene propylene (FEP), to further reduce friction and the occurrence of endoleaks (Fig. 6.3). It is supported through its entire length with a nitinol exoskeleton. The proximal end of the graft consists of exposed stent apices, whereas the distal end remains in line with the graft material. Radiopaque bands are present at each end to facilitate placement under fluoroscopy. These flared endings are intended to improve sealing and attachment of the graft to the aortic wall.[22]

TABLE 6.1. Summary of Thoracic Device Characteristics

Device	TAG	CTAG	Zenith TX2	Zenith Alpha	Valiant	Relay
Manufacturer	W.L. Gore & Associates	W.L. Gore & Associates	Cook Medical	Cook Medical	Medtronic Vascular	Bolton Medical
Device structure	Tube-shaped stent-graft lined with ePTFE/FEP, and supported by a nitinol exoskeleton	Similar design to the TAG, but more conformable	Dacron graft sewn to a stainless steel stent	Similar to TX2	Self-expanding tube with nitinol scaffolding sewn to the outside of the graft material. Lacks a longitudinal support bar, for more flexibility	Self-expanding nitinol stent, sutured to a polyester fabric graft. Longitudinal support achieved via a nitinol wire
Proximal and distal ends	Flared exposed stent apices	Similar to the TAG device	External barbs proximally and distally. Extension BMS is available	Similar to TX2	Proximal end is bare stent with eight shorter bare stents. Distal stent graft with a closed web configuration	Two versions, the Relay with proximal bare stent, and the Relay-NBS, without bare stent. One distal configuration is available
Diameter (mm)	26-45	21-45	28-42	18-34	24-46	22-46
Length (cm)	10-20	10-20	12-21.6	10.5-16	Up to 22.7	10-25
Delivery system	20-24 F sheath	Sheathless delivery system	20-22 F delivery sheath	16-20 F sheath	Xcelerant delivery system	20-26 F delivery sheath

BMS, bare metal stent; ePTFE, polytetrafluorethylene; FEP, fluorinated ethylene propylene.

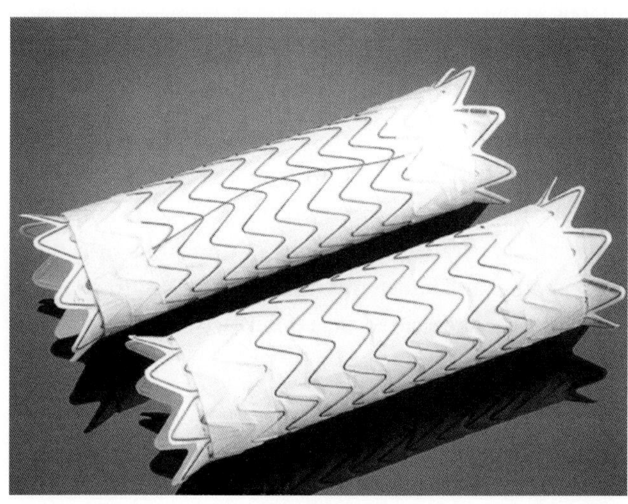

FIGURE 6.3: Original (top) and redesigned (bottom) GORE TAG devices. Reprinted with permission from Makaroun MS, Dillavou ED, Kee ST, et al. Endovascular treatment of thoracic aortic aneurysms: results of the phase II multicenter trial of the GORE TAG thoracic endoprosthesis. *J Vasc Surg*. 2005;41:1-9.

2. A next-generation device, the Conformable TAG (CTAG) shares a similar design but offers more conformability to accommodate more acute angles, often found in the aortic arch. This is achieved through modification of the material and the attachment of the exoskeleton to the graft.
3. TAG device is available in diameters from 26 to 45 mm in 10, 15, and 20 cm lengths. The delivery sheath ranges from 20 to 24 French in diameter depending on the

device size. CTAG offers a wider range of diameters (21-45 mm),[23] with a sheathless delivery system. The endoprosthesis is constrained inside a deployment sleeve and mounted onto the leading end of the delivery catheter. Pulling the deployment knob, which is attached to the deployment line system, unlaces the sleeve and allows the self-expanding endoprosthesis to deploy. This allows the CTAG to conform to smaller and more tapered aortas and to provide a solution for nonaneurysmal aortic pathologies such as blunt aortic injury.[22]

4. The safety and efficacy of the TAG endograft have been demonstrated. Although the initial results with the TAG device were disappointing, and the trial was stopped owing to complications,[24] further modifications of the device have proven to be efficacious. In a multicenter study comparing endovascular DTA repair using the TAG device with open repair, aorta-specific survival was significantly better in the endovascular group at 5 years (96% vs 88%, $P = 0.24$), and major adverse events were reduced at 30 days (21% vs 71%, $P < 0.001$) and at 1 year (42% vs 77%. $P < 0.001$).[4,25]
5. The Aortic Dissection Stent-graft OR Best Medical Treatment (ADSORB) trial, comparing outcomes of OMT only versus OMT and the Gore TAG device, in patients with uncomplicated type B dissection, demonstrated the safety of the device.[26] The false lumen (FL) decreased in size in the OMT + TAG group ($P < 0.001$), whereas in the OMT group it increased. The true lumen (TL) increased in the OMT + TAG ($P < 0.001$), whereas in the OMT group it remained unchanged. The overall transverse diameter was the same at the beginning and after 1 year in the OMT group (42.1 mm), but in the OMT + TAG group it decreased (38.8 mm; $P = 0.062$). Remodeling with thrombosis of the FL, and reduction of its diameter is induced by the stent graft; however long-term results are still needed.
6. Criticism to the ADSORB study concerned the definition of FL thrombosis, which was not the same in the OMT plus TEVAR and OMT only groups. For patients treated with OMT plus TEVAR, the FL was considered thrombosed as long as no flow was visualized in the false lumen parallel to the endograft, excluding the distal 2 cm, whereas in the OMT group, the false lumen was only considered thrombosed if there was no flow in any segment of the thoracic aorta, a difference that would appear substantially to favor the TEVAR group.[27]
7. The safety and efficacy of the CTAG device was evaluated in a nonrandomized study with 51 patients suffering from blunt aortic injury,[28] with no operative mortality and no major device events. Thirty-day mortality, unrelated to device, was 7.8%.

B. Zenith TX2 and Zenith Alpha

1. Zenith TX2 endograft (Cook Medical) and Zenith Alpha (new generation, low profile stents[29]) are two-piece systems, proximal and distal. They are constructed of full-thickness woven polyester fabric (i.e., Dacron), sewn to self-expanding special stainless steel stents, with braided polyester and monofilament polypropylene suture.

The graft body stents and the distal sealing stent are made from superelastic electropolished nitinol wire[30] (Fig. 6.2). Active fixation at the proximal and distal ends is achieved via external barbs for each component. An extension bare metal stent is available, which can be used to distally fixate the graft over the origins of the visceral arteries. A modification of the TX2 device (Pro-form) is intended to improve conformability and apposition of the graft in the aortic arch during proximal descending thoracic aortic deployments, in order to minimize the risk of graft folding and collapse.[31]

2. Proximal and distal Zenith TX2 device components are available in diameters ranging from 28 to 42 mm, and the components range in length from 12 to 21.6 cm. Delivery sheath is a 20 or 22 French.[29] Zenith Alpha is available in diameters from 18 to 34 mm, with component lengths from 10.5 to 16 cm.[29] The devices are delivered through a 16-20 French sheath depending on the diameter of the device. Both devices are self-expanding; however, subsequent ballooning is an option when needed.

3. The safety and efficacy of the Zenith TX2 endograft were evaluated in a multicenter study of 230 patients with DTAs, who were treated with TEVAR (n = 160) or open repair (n = 70).[30] Perioperative morbidity was significantly lower for endovascular repair (composite index 1.3 vs 2.9, $P < 0.01$). Endovascular repair was also associated with fewer cardiovascular and pulmonary adverse events; however, incidence of neurologic events was not significantly different. At 12 months, aneurysm growth was identified in 7.1%, endoleak in 3.9%, and migration (>10 mm) in 2.8% of the endovascular patients.

4. The Zenith TX2 dissection system shares a similar design, and its efficacy was evaluated in the STABLE trial, in 40 patients with complicated DescAD, defined by branch vessel malperfusion, impending rupture, aortic diameter ≥40 mm, rapid aortic expansion, and persistent pain or hypertension despite maximum medical therapy.[32] Seven combinations of stent grafts and dissection stents were used, and all devices were successfully deployed and patent. One-year survival rate was 90%. Morbidity occurring within 30 days included stroke (7.5%), transient ischemic attack (2.5%), paraplegia (2.5%), retrograde dissection (5%), and renal failure (12.5%). Favorable aortic remodeling was observed during the course of follow-up, indicated by an increase in the TL size, and a concomitant decrease in the FL size along the dissected aorta, with completely thrombosed thoracic FL observed in 31% of patients at 12 months.

C. Valiant Thoracic Stent-Graft System

1. The Valiant endograft (Medtronic Vascular) is a modified version of the earlier Talent endograft system (withdrawn by manufacturer). It is composed of a self-expanding tube. The nitinol scaffolding of the stent graft is composed of a series of serpentine five-peaked springs stacked in a tubular configuration. The scaffolding in this device

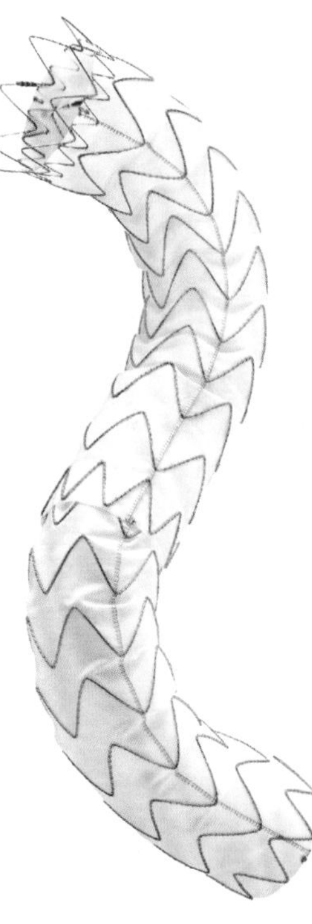

FIGURE 6.4: The Valiant thoracic stant graft. Reprinted with permission from Fairman RM, Tuchek JM, Lee WA, et al. Pivotal results for the medtronic valiant thoracic stent graft system in the VALOR II trial. *J Vasc Surg.* 2012;56:1222-1231.e1221.

is sewn to the outside of the graft material (not the inside, as with the Talent device) (Fig. 6.4). Valiant device lacks the longitudinal support bar of the earlier device, which gives more flexibility. The device has a modified proximal bare stent with eight shorter bare stents proximally. A distal stent graft component has a closed web configuration at the proximal end (no bare spring) and a closed web or an eight-peak bare-spring configuration at the distal stent end.[33]

2. The graft is available in straight or tapered versions, with diameters ranging from 24 to 46 mm, and lengths up to 22.7 cm. It is compressed and preloaded into the Xcelerant delivery system (Medtronic Vascular), which consists of a single-use disposable catheter with an integrated handle.[33]
3. Valiant endograft efficacy was evaluated in a retrospective study with 180 patients,[34] treating various descending aortic pathologies (66 patients with thoracic aneurysms, 22 with thoracoabdominal aneurysms, 19 with an acute aortic syndrome, 52 with aneurysmal degeneration of a chronic dissection, and 21 patients with traumatic aortic transection). Overall 30-day mortality for the series was 7.2%, with a stroke rate of 3.8% and a paraplegia rate of 3.3%. Mortality rates differed according to the indication, with the highest rate for thoracoabdominal aneurysms (27.3%) and lowest for acute traumatic rupture (0%).
4. The VALOR II trial (Evaluation of the Clinical Performance of the Valiant Thoracic Stent Graft System in the Treatment of Descending Thoracic Aneurysms of

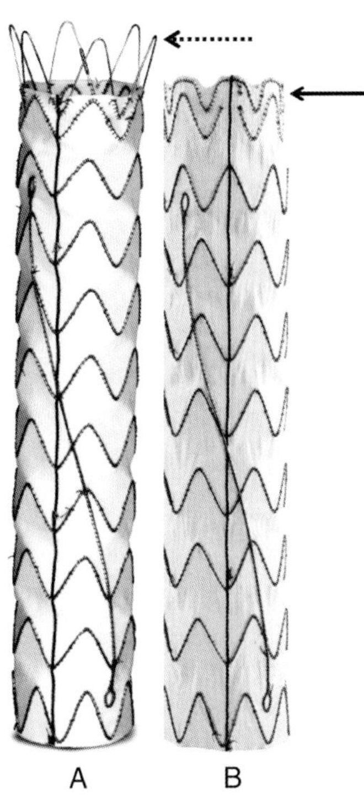

FIGURE 6.5: In the Relay stent-graft, the curved nitinol wire starts below the second row of proximal covered stents and ends close to the distal stent, allowing for sufficient column strength while at the same time providing flexibility and torque response. A, Relay has an alignment zone (dotted arrow) to provide optimal alignment with aortic anatomy and allow proximal capture of the stent-graft for accurate placement. B, In Relay-NBS, the proximal end is covered with polyester vascular graft fabric (solid arrow) to optimize apposition of the proximal end of the graft to the lumen wall while minimizing trauma to the intima and risk of fabric infolding. Reprinted with permission from Zipfel B, Czerny M, Funovics M, et al. Endovascular treatment of patients with types A and B thoracic aortic dissection using Relay thoracic stent-grafts: results from the RESTORE Patient Registry. *J Endovasc Ther.* 2011;18:131-143.

Degenerative Etiology in Subjects Who Are Candidates for Endovascular Repair) has led to the approval of the Captivia Delivery System (Medtronic vascular) in the United States.[33,35] A cohort of 160 patients with degenerative DTAs and thoracoabdominal aneurysms were followed up for 5 years. Technical success rate was 96.3%, and the 30-day mortality was 3.1%. 38.1% of patients had ≥1 major adverse event at 30 days, while 48.7% of patients had ≥1 major adverse event at 12 months.

5. Five-year survival was 64%, with 5% aneurysm-related mortality. Secondary intervention occurred in 6.8% of patients.

D. Relay

1. The Relay thoracic stent-graft system (Bolton Medical) is composed of a self-expanding nitinol stent, sutured to a polyester fabric graft, with a curved longitudinal nitinol wire for the purpose of providing longitudinal strength (Fig. 6.5). Two different proximal standard configurations are available, the RELAY, with the proximal bare stent, and a non-bare-stent model (RELAY-NBS). Only one distal configuration is present.[36]
2. It is available in straight and tapered configurations, with diameters ranging from 22 to 46 mm, and lengths from 10 to 25 cm. The delivery sheath ranges from 20 to 26 French, depending on the diameter of the device.
3. The European experience with Relay was demonstrated in the RESTORE registry, with a success rate of 97.3%.[37] A cohort of 150 patients were prospectively

accrued, in whom thoracic aortic aneurysms was treated in 64.7%, and DescAD in 19.3%. Paraplegia rate was 3.3%, recovered paraparesis 3.3%, and stroke only 0.6%. Reinterventions were necessary in 8.7% of the cases. The 30-day mortality rate was 10%. Reintervention rate during 2-year follow-up was 8.9%, owing to two stent graft migrations, three proximal type I endoleak, four type III endoleak, and five distal type I endoleaks. No open conversion was needed during follow-up.

4. The use of Relay system in DescAD was evaluated in another study of the RESTORE registry,[38] in which the majority of patients had type B AD (84%). The technical success rate was 95%. Thirty-day mortality was 8%, and the type I endoleak rate was 7%. The 2-year survival rate was 82% in the overall population, and 84% in patients with type B AD.

5. Bolton Medical's next generation device, the (Relay Pro), is currently being developed, offering diameters as small as 19 French, in both stented and NBS configurations.

   The pivotal trials providing evidence regarding the thoracic devices have been summarized (Tables 6.2 and 6.3).

VI. Investigational Devices

These devices are currently being investigated but have not yet been approved in the United States. These include the LeMaitre TAArget device, the JOTEC E-Vita stent-graft system, and the Streamliner Multilayer Flow Modulator.

A. TAArget

1. The TAArget thoracic stent-graft (previously labeled EndoFit, LeMaitre Vascular) is composed of a nitinol skeleton of Z-shaped stents that are encapsulated between two thin sheets of expanded ePTFE. The Z-shaped stents aim at providing longitudinal support without a support bar. The device can be straight or tapered, and the proximal end is available with and without external fixation with a bare metal stent, allowing for different configurations of the device.[39]

2. The graft is available in diameters from 30 to 42 mm, with lengths from 7 to 22 cm. The graft is deployed through a 22 or 24 French sheath depending on the diameter of the device.[40]

3. In a study with 41 patients with various descending aortic pathologies, who were managed using the TAArget device, the graft was successfully deployed in all 41 patients. In-hospital mortality was 7.3%, and three patients developed endoleaks, with only one patient requiring intervention. One patient suffered from spinal cord ischemia. Two-year mortality was 17%, with 11% aneurysm-related mortality.[39]

4. Another study with 46 aneurysm patients and 41 with DescAD, managed using the TAArget device,[40] showed 100% deployment success rate. In-hospital mortality was 9.2%, and neurological complications occurred in 9.3% of patients, including five strokes (two fatal) and three cases of paraplegia. Five patients had immediate

TABLE 6.2. Summary of Evidence About Various Thoracic Devices in Aortic Dissection

Study	Year	Device	Aim	Number of Patients	Type of Dissection	Success	Results	Mortality	Complications	Comments
INSTEAD trial[17]	2009	Talent graft	Compare TEVAR + OMT to OMT alone in uncomplicated type B AD	140	Uncomplicated chronic type B AD	Access obtained in 70/72 cases randomized to TEVAR + OMT (97.2%)	Aortic remodeling occurred in 91.3% with TEVAR vs 19.4% in OMT group ($P < 0.01$)	No difference in 2-y all-cause mortality	Paraplegia: 3 cases in TEVAR vs 1 in OMT group	
INSTEAD-XL trial[18]	2013	Talent graft	Long-term follow-up of the INSTEAD trial	140	Uncomplicated chronic type B AD	Access obtained in 97.2% of cases	Landmark analysis suggested a benefit of TEVAR for all end points (mortality and progression) between 2 and 5 y	• All-cause mortality was lower in TEVAR group: 11.1% vs 19.3% ($P = 0.13$) • Aorta-specific mortality was lower in TEVAR group (6.9% vs 19.3%; $P = 0.04$) at 5 y		Landmark method does not include periprocedural early mortality in the analysis
ADSORB trial[26]	2014	Gore TAG	Compare OMT + TAG device to OMT alone in uncomplicated type B AD	61	Uncomplicated acute type B	Access obtained in 100% of cases	• Incomplete FL thrombosis: 43% in TAG group vs 97% in OMT group • FL decreased and TL increased in TAG group and increased in the OMT group (P < 00.1)	• No mortality within 30 d • One death in the TAG + OMT group during follow-up due to cardiac arrest, but no autopsy was performed		

(Continued)

TABLE 6.2. Summary of Evidence About Various Thoracic Devices in Aortic Dissection—Continued

Study	Year	Device	Aim	Number of Patients	Type of Dissection	Success	Results	Mortality	Complications	Comments
STABLE trial[32]	2012	Proximal Zenith TX2 and distal BMS	Evaluate the composite TX2 device in complicated type B AD	40	Complicated acute type B AD	Technical success: 100%	Complete FL thrombosis: 31% at 1 y	1-y survival: 90%	30-d morbidities: • Stroke: 7.5% • TIA: 2.5% • Paraplegia: 2.5% • Renal failure: 12.5%	Complications defined by branch vessel malperfusion, impending rupture, aortic diameter ≥40 mm, rapid aortic expansion, and persistent pain or hypertension despite maximum medical therapy
RESTORE trial[37]	2008	Relay	Evaluate the efficacy of the Relay graft in DTA and DescAD	150	Acute uncomplicated type B AD	Technical success: 97.3%	Aneurysm was the most common pathology treated (64.7%) followed by dissections (19.3%)	30-d mortality was 10%	• Paraplegia: 3.3% • Recovered paraparesis: 3.3% • Stroke: 0.6% • Reintervention at 2 y: 8.9%	
Zipfel et al[38]	2011	Relay	To evaluate the safety and performance of Relay stent-grafts in patients with acute or chronic aortic dissections	91	Acute and chronic uncomplicated type A and type B AD	Technical success: 95% (97% in acute, 95% in chronic, and 93% in type B dissections)	Relay stent graft showed favorable outcomes in treatment of thoracic aortic dissections	• 30-d mortality was 8% (13% in acute and 5% in chronic dissections); all deaths occurred in patients with type B dissections • 2-y survival: • Overall: 82% • Type B AD: 84%	• Paraplegia, paraparesis, and stroke occurred in 4, 1, and 2 patients, respectively; 2 cases of paraplegia occurred in patients with acute type B dissections • Type I endoleak: 7% (7% in acute and 8% in chronic dissections); all occurred in patients with type B dissections	

AD, aortic dissection; ADSORB, acute dissection stent graft or best medical treatment; BMS, bare metal stent; DTA, descending thoracic aneurysm; FL, false lumen; INSTEAD, investigation of stent graft in aortic dissection; OMT, optimized medical treatment; RESTORE, European experience in the RELAY endovascular registry for thoracic disease STABLE, study of thoracic aortic type B dissection using endoluminal repair; TEVAR, thoracic endovascular aortic repair; TL, true lumen.

TABLE 6.3. Summary of Evidence About Various Thoracic Devices in Descending Thoracic Aneurysms

Study	Year	Device Used	Aim of Study	No. of Patients	Results
Cho et al[25]	2006	Gore TAG	Compare endovascular repair of DTAs using the TAG device, to open repair	142	• Technical success: 98% (139/142) • Operative mortality: 2.1% in TAG group vs 11.7% in surgical group • MAE at 1 y: (42% vs 77%) • Aneurysm-related survival at 5 y: (98% vs 88%)
Farber et al[135]	2012	CTAG	To evaluate CTAG device in BAT	51	• Technical success: 100% • 30-d mortality: 7.8% • MAE: 35.3%
Matsumura et al[30]	2008	Zenith TX2	Compare the TX2 device to open repair	230	• Perioperative morbidity was lower for TX2 device (composite index 1.3 vs 2.9) • Neurologic complications were not significantly different • Aneurysms growth at 12 mo in the TX2 group was 7.1%

Thompson et al[34]	2007	Valiant endograft	Evaluate the efficacy of Valiant endograft in multiple descending aortic pathologies	180	• 30-d mortality: 7.2%
					• Stroke: 3.8%
					• Paraplegia: 3.3%
					• Mortality rate differed with indication:
					  • Thoracoabdominal aneurysm: 27.3%
					  • BAT: 0%

VALOR II trial[33]	2012	Valiant endograft	Evaluation of the Valiant graft in degenerative DTAs	160	• Technical success: 96.3%
					• 30-d mortality: 3.1%
					• MAE: 38.1%:
					  • Paraplegia: 0.6%
					  • Paraparesis: 1.9%
					  • Stroke: 2.5%
					• 1-y aneurysm-related mortality: 4%
					• Graft migration: 2.0%
					• Endoleaks:13%

VALOR II long-term trial[35]	2017	Valiant endograft	Long-term outcomes of the VALOR II trial	160	• 5-y survival: 64% • Aneurysm-related death at 5 y: 5% • Secondary intervention: 6.8% • Average aortic diameter decreased in 48%

BAT, blunt aortic trauma; DTA, descending thoracic aneurysm; MAE, major adverse events; VALOR, evaluation of the clinical performance of the Valiant thoracic stent graft system in the treatment of descending thoracic aneurysms of degenerative etiology in subjects who are candidates for endovascular repair.

proximal type I endoleak. Mortality rate over a follow-up period of 5.2 months was 11.4% but was not felt to be aneurysm or stent-graft related.

5. The DEDICATED registry has been established and aims at evaluating the use and efficacy of the TAArget stent graft for the treatment of acute and chronic aortic type B AD.[41]

B. E-Vita

1. The E-Vita stent graft system (CryoLife JOTEC, Kennesaw, GA) has been on the European market since May 2004. It is composed of a low porosity woven polyester graft with nitinol springs support structure, sutured to inner side of the graft in a tip-to-tip fashion. The device has no longitudinal support, making it very flexible. It is available in 24-44 mm diameters, and in 12, 15, 17, and 23 cm in length.[42] Multiple graft configurations are available for this device.

2. Safety and efficacy of the E-Vita device were evaluated in a review of 126 patients with multiple descending aortic pathologies. Graft was successfully deployed in 77% of patients. Overall perioperative mortality within 30 days was 12.3%. Stroke occurred in 2.8% of cases, and transient spinal cord dysfunction was observed in two cases.[42]

C. Streamliner Multilayer Flow Modulator

1. The Streamliner Multilayer Flow Modulator (SMFM; Cardiatis) is a self-expanding stent, composed of cobalt alloy wires that are interconnected in five layers.[43] It is designed to allow blood flow through the stent to maintain patency of branch vessels, which may be an alternative the hybrid technique, especially when applied in the aortic arch (Fig. 6.6). The SMFM was approved in Europe in 2010.

2. Evidence regarding the SMFM is limited.[44–46] In a nonrandomized trial (STRATO), 23 high-risk surgical patients with Crawford type II or III thoracoabdominal aneurysms were managed with the SMFM device.[47] Stable aneurysm thrombosis was achieved in 15 out of 20 patients at 1 year. The rate of branch patency was 96% at 1 year, 100% at 2 years, and 97% at 3 years. Nine patients had endoleaks requiring 11 interventions.

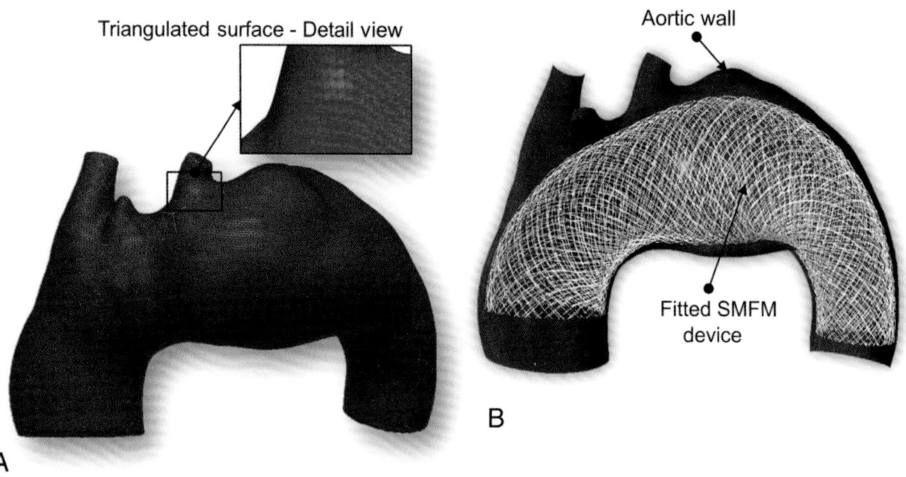

FIGURE 6.6: Computational fluid dynamics workflow from medical data to blood flow simulation setup. A, Aortic Arch three-dimensional geometry represented by a volume enclosed in a triangulated surface. B, SMFM (Cardiatis, Isnes, Brussels, Belgium) device; spatial representation as fitted through a diseased aortic arch. Reprinted with permission from Stefanov F, Morris L, Elhelali A, et al. Insights from complex aortic surgery with a Streamliner device for aortic arch repair (STAR). *J Thorac Cardiovasc Surg.* 2016;152:1309-1318. e1305.

VII. Preprocedural Planning

A. Imaging

1. Precise imaging of the entire aorta and its branches is essential before planning an endovascular repair. Computed tomograpic angiography (CTA) with three-dimensional reformatting of the chest, abdomen, and pelvis is the method of choice. Assessment of the external and endoluminal diameter of the aorta is vital to appropriately choose the diameter and length of the endograft and the location of the landing zones. Furthermore, assessment of the burden of calcification, angulation, and tortuosity of the aorta is required to plan the perfect deployment technique[48,49] and to assess the likelihood of endoleaks.[50] CTA also helps to identify the important side branches and diameters of the iliac arteries to better choose the delivery device. Generally, an 8 mm external iliac artery—which has approximately 24 French outer diameters—should accommodate a 22 French sheath.[51]

2. Magnetic resonance angiography (MRA) can also be used; however, it does not demonstrate vessel wall calcification, which has implications for vascular access.

B. Landing Zones

1. Tight seal of the graft to the aortic wall is required to exclude blood flow from a thoracic aneurysm sac. The endograft must provide an adequate seal proximally—at the aneurysm neck—and distally, which are called the "landing zones." A minimum seal zone of 2 cm is recommended in the thoracic aorta to prevent migration and endoleak.

2. Proximally, the landing above the neck of the aneurysm may involve the aortic arch. When device deployment involves the arch, the proximal end of the graft must closely appose to the inner curve of the arch in order to avoid migration or device collapse.[52,53] Further, deployment in the arch can jeopardize the blood flow to the branch vessels, namely the left subclavian, left common carotid, and the brachiocephalic trunk. Earlier generation stents faced the problem of not being able to conform to the arch anatomy, leading to "bird beaking" (Fig. 6.7), and increasing the risk of graft failure. Current devices are characterized by improved flexibility and design at proximal graft that permit better conformation to the aortic arch. Careful planning is essential to assess the need for "debranching procedures," which involve "moving" the branch vessels to a more proximal location to preserve blood flow after stent deployment (hybrid approaches).[54]

3. Distal seal zone must also be at least 2 cm in length, which in some cases might necessitate covering of the celiac trunk. Visceral arteries bypass procedures might be required to preserve the blood flow to the gut.[55]

C. Choosing the Correct Graft As mentioned, CTA should be utilized to assess the diameter of the aorta before planning endovascular repair, in order to choose the correct size and length of the graft. Larger native thoracic aortas require larger diameter

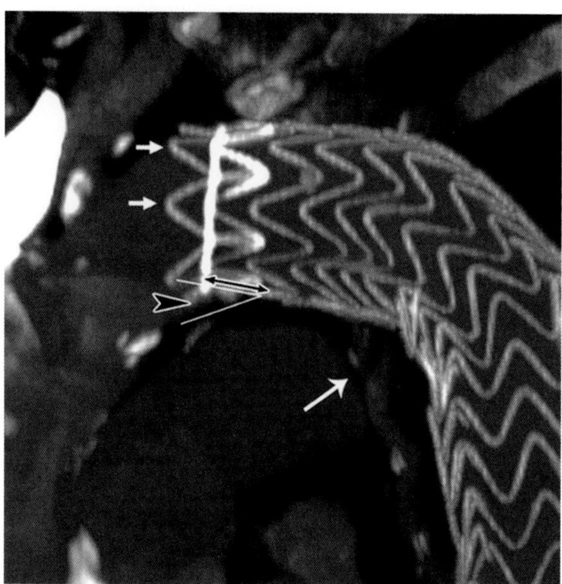

FIGURE 6.7: Image obtained in an 84-year-old woman who underwent TEVAR for an atherosclerotic aortic aneurysm show bird-beak configuration resulting in type Ia endoleak. Thin-slab maximum intensity projection shows bird-beak configuration (arrowhead)—imperfect apposition at proximal end of stent-graft to lesser curve of aortic arch—resulting in wedge-shaped gap between undersurface of the stent-graft and aortic wall. Length (two-headed arrow) and angle of the bird-beak were measured with three-dimensional workstation functions. Scalloped flares (small arrows) at the proximal end of the device were excluded from measurement of bird-beak length. Leakage of contrast medium is observed flowing continuously from the bird-beak into the aneurysmal sac, signifying type Ia endoleak (big arrow). Reprinted with permission from Ueda T, Fleischmann D, Dake MD, Rubin GD, Sze DY. Incomplete endograft apposition to the aortic arch: bird-beak configuration increases risk of endoleak formation after thoracic endovascular aortic repair. *Radiology*. 2010;255:645-652.

stent-grafts. Nonaneurysmal thoracic aortic pathologies (e.g., blunt aortic injures) require smaller stent-grafts. Commercial devices are available in diameters from 21 to 45 mm, which can accommodate various types of aortic pathologies. Fifteen to twenty percent oversizing is recommended for thoracic aortic endograft; however, excessive oversizing may lead to dreaded retrograde aortic dissection.[56] It is important to note that the aortic diameter decreases dramatically in patients with traumatic aortic injury with hemodynamic instability due to hypotension. This decrease in aortic diameter could lead to inaccurate aortic measurements and undersizing of the endograft.[57]

D. **Debranching Procedures** The need for debranching procedures for important branch vessels should be determined preoperatively by studying the proximal and distal landing zones.[55]

1. **Arch Vessel Bypass**
   a. Arch vessel bypass needs to be considered when the proximal landing zones involve any of the aortic arch vessels. Not infrequently, one or more of the arch branches may need to be covered for an adequate seal to be obtained. For the subclavian artery, a meta-analysis of 1161 patients has shown that left subclavian

artery revascularization did not significantly reduce the risk of strokes, spinal cord injury, or mortality.[58] In another review, symptoms of upper extremity ischemia requiring subsequent revascularization occurred in only 4% of patients.[59]

b. Preemptive revascularization should be performed in patients with a dominant left vertebral artery, hypoplastic right vertebral artery, or incomplete circle of Willis, as interruption in circulation would lead to an increased risk of stroke and paraplegia.[60,61] Planned revascularization can also be considered in patients with patent left inferior mammary artery-coronary bypass or functioning left upper extremity dialysis arteriovenous access.[62] Carotid-subclavian bypass or subclavian-carotid transposition procedures can restore the left subclavian flow. The optimal procedure should be based on duplex ultrasonography of the vertebral and carotid arteries. However, both procedures have not produced a benefit in terms of neurological outcomes and mortality.[63]

c. If the proximal landing zone is anticipated to cover the left common carotid artery or the brachiocephalic trunk, open, antegrade bypass from the ascending aorta or carotid transposition can be performed. Alternatively, extra-anatomic bypass (e.g., carotid-carotid bypass) can be performed to avoid sternotomy.[64,65]

d. Timing of debranching procedure can be in the same setting, or few days before the endovascular procedure.

2. **Visceral Bypass**

a. Celiac artery coverage may frequently be indicated in order to gain adequate distal sealing of the graft to avoid type Ib endoleak. Celiac coverage can pose a risk for mesenteric ischemia. However, successful cases of covering the celiac artery have been reported in patients with a documented patent pancreaticoduodenal system, with a low incidence of mesenteric ischemia.[66,67] In a recent literature review, covering the celiac artery, without deliberate accompanying ceiliac embolization, resulted in only three type II endoleaks in 72 patients, which required treatment by coil embolization.[68]

b. Landing distal to the superior mesenteric artery or the renal vessels requires special measures, either by open surgical bypass, use of special fenestrated grafts,[69] use of branched grafts,[70] or revascularization using snorkel or chimney stents[71,72] (Fig. 6.8). Debranching procedures can also provide blood flow via alternative vessels to allow coverage of the visceral segment of the aorta.[73] Debranching procedures can be performed in the same setting or several days before repair.

E. **Other Approaches** For juxtarenal aortic aneurysms, fenestrated endovascular aneurysm repair (FEVAR) continues to evolve to avoid the need for debranching procedures.[74,75] The Zenith Fenestrated Endovascular Graft (Cook Medical) is the primarily studied device. The use of accessory stents, such as the chimney/snorkel technique,[76,77] or in situ fenestration of the graft using a needle or laser has also been described, especially in association with emergency surgery to avoid debranching procedures.[78] Branched grafts are being investigated for thoracic or thoracoabdominal aneurysms,[79] but the rate of repair-related mortality may be higher than conventional grafts.

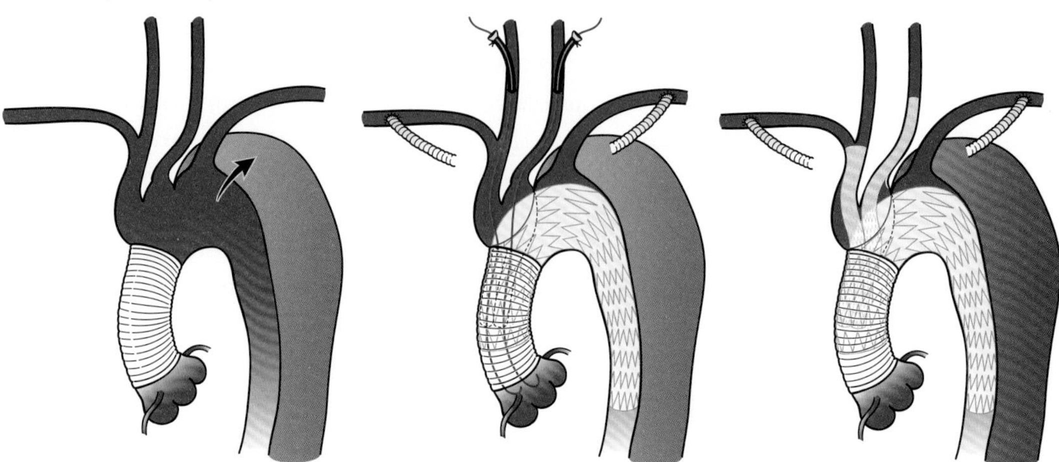

FIGURE 6.8: TEVAR with dual branch device for residual aortic dissection after graft replacement of ascending aorta for type A aortic dissection. TEVAR, thoracic endovascular aortic repair. Reprinted with permission from Kuratani T. Best surgical option for arch extension of type B dissection: the endovascular approach. *Ann Cardiothorac Surg*. 2014;3:292-299.

VIII. Preoperative Preparation

A. **Antibiotics** Practice guidelines recommend antibiotic prophylaxis with Cefazolin within 30 minutes of the skin incision[80] (vancomycin or clindamycin may be used in case of penicillin allergy). Antibiotics should be discontinued within 24 hours given the lack of proven benefit beyond that time.

B. Renal Injury

1. Ten to fifteen percent of patients following TEVAR can suffer acute kidney injury (AKI), most of whom are type B DescAD patients, typically treated only after organ malperfusion has occurred.[81] Risk factors for renal injury are poor preoperative kidney function, aneurysms of the renal arteries, and need for blood transfusion.[82]

2. Contrast-induced nephropathy from use of contrast during CTA can be avoided with appropriate hydration before endovascular repair, and by adequate preoperative planning of landing zones to achieve a tight seal without the use of large amounts of contrast.

C. Cerebrospinal Fluid Drainage

1. Spinal cord perfusion pressure equals the mean arterial pressure minus the cerebrospinal fluid pressure. Spinal drainage aims at decreasing the pressure in the subarachnoid space around the spinal cord, thereby increasing the spinal cord perfusion pressure, and decreasing the incidence of spinal cord ischemia during or after endovascular stenting of thoracic aorta. This is achieved via insertion of a drain at the level of the L3-L4 disc in the subarachnoid space.[83]

2. Data from the European Collaborators on Stent/Graft Techniques for Aortic Aneurysm Repair (EUROSTAR) registry highlighted the importance of collateral circulation for the spinal cord perfusion during endovascular repair.[84] A spinal drain is indicated when extensive coverage of the thoracic aorta is required, when there are multiple internal iliac artery occlusions, or when there is a prior history of open or endovascular repair.[85–87] In a study with 72 patients, the risk of spinal cord ischemia was 12.5% in patients with prior abdominal aortic aneurysm repair, versus 1.7% in patients without prior repair.[85] Another retrospective cohort study of endovascular repair of Crawford Type II thoracoabdominal aneurysms showed that staged repair was associated with lower risk of spinal cord ischemia, compared with single staged repair (11.1% vs 37.5%).[88] A promising spinal cooling catheter has been developed, which drains cerebrospinal fluid (CSF) as well as producing localized spinal cord hypotension. Clinical application of this catheter is expected soon.[89]

IX. Technique of Placement

Endovascular repair of thoracic aorta is performed under general anesthesia, which allows respiratory control and more precise imaging. In the EUROSTAR registry, technical success was achieved in 87% of aneurysm patients and 89% of DescAD patients.[90]

A. Access Vessels

1. Large-bore sheaths need to be introduced through the femoral artery, typically by femoral cutdown. Unlike abdominal aortic repair, percutaneous access is usually difficult because of larger devices; however, trials using the "Preclose technique" for TEVAR have been successful.[91] It is likely that in the future, percutaneous access will be implemented for thoracic aneurysms as well.[92]

2. In 3.8%-9.4% of patients, femoral cutdown is not suitable and other access sites are required.[93] Tortuous, calcific, or narrow iliac arteries may not be suitable to pass such large devices, so access can be obtained through an iliac conduit, direct exposure of the common iliac artery, direct delivery through the abdominal aorta, or by balloon angioplasty of the iliac arteries before procedures. In challenging access situations, antegrade access through the ascending aorta has been described for descending thoracic endografts.[94]

B. Deployment

1. Wire access is gained into the ascending aorta and exchanged for a stiff wire to allow tracking of the device. Positioning the graft is typically achieved under fluoroscopy, along with other techniques such as transesophageal echocardiography (TTE) and intravascular ultrasound.[95] After vascular access has been obtained, lowering blood pressure is needed only transiently at the moment of deployment. Blood pressure is lowered, pharmacologically or by rapid pacing, down to the 60s, in order to prevent the graft from moving distally owing to pressure (i.e., wind-sock effect).

2. When the proximal landing zone involves the arch, a 30-60° left anterior oblique (LAO) projection is used to precisely splay out the arch vessels. For the distal landing zone near the celiac trunk, a lateral projection is used. Once the device is deployed in position, the stent-graft is expanded and can be ballooned at the proximal and distal landing zones to stabilize in place.

C. **Evaluating for Endoleaks** Aortography is typically performed after deployment to ensure correct positioning of the graft, patency of branch vessels, aneurysmal sac occlusion, and to check for the presence of an endoleak, which is the persistence of flow in the aneurysm sac after repair. Removal of the sheath and repair of the arteriotomy is then performed.

D. **Postoperative Imaging** It is recommended to obtain a CTA within 1 month of the procedure, at 6 months and then annually to evaluate for endograft integrity and location, for persistence of the aneurysm sac, and for late complications and endoleaks[96]

X. Complications

A. Perioperative Mortality and Morbidity

1. With the advancement of TEVAR devices and techniques, perioperative mortality rates in some studies are lower than in open repair. In a multicenter study for descending thoracic aneurysms in low-risk patients, perioperative mortality rates were 2.1% for endovascular repair versus 11.7% in patients undergoing open repair ($P < 0.001$).[97] According to the National Surgical Quality Improvement Program (NSQIP) database, the operative indications for TEVAR procedure were not found to be a predictor of poor patient outcome. However, patients presenting with emergency conditions, such as rupture or aortic dissection, had higher rates of 30-day mortality (22.6% vs 6.2%),[98] as well as higher late mortality rates.[99]

2. In the NSQIP database, perioperative morbidity associated with TEVAR was found to be 9%,[30] with the cumulative major morbidity scores significantly lower than the open group at 30 days (1.3 ± 3.0 vs 2.9 ± 3.6, respectively, $P<.01$). No difference in survival between males and females was noted.[100–103]

B. Endoleaks

1. Endoleak is a term that describes the presence of persistent flow of blood into the aneurysm sac after endograft placement, which poses a risk for aneurysm expansion and rupture. Endoleak is usually recognized upon aortography after deployment of the endograft, or at postprocedure CT scan. However, endoleak can appear up to 5 years after repair.[104] Long-term follow-up of patients who underwent endovascular repair for abdominal aortic aneurysms showed high rates of endoleak development, reaching approximately 30%, with an average follow-up of 6 years.[105] This suggests that TEVAR may recapitulate the high endoleak rate when many late cases become available for analysis.

2. Classification of endoleaks is based on the source of the leak[106] (Table 6.4), which helps determine the appropriate management plan. Type II endoleak is the most prevalent type and is due to patent aortic branches, especially intercostal and lumbar arteries.[107] Continued aneurysm sac expansion without a demonstrable endoleak on any imaging modality is referred to as endoleak of undefined origin, also called type V endoleak or endotension.[108]

3. The rate of endoleaks with TEVAR has been noted to be somewhere between 3.9%[30] and 15.6% in another review.[109]

4. It is noted that complex fenestrated, branched, and chimney endografts introduce the potential for additional modes of failure in terms of component separation and endoleaks. Treatment of endoleaks associated with these devices remains challenging.[110]

C. Spinal Cord Ischemia

1. TEVAR carries a real risk of spinal cord ischemia and paraplegia, comparable to rates reported after open surgical repair. The rates of spinal cord injury and paraplegia after open thoracoabdominal aortic repair in contemporary series range from 3% to 12%,[111–118] and from 5% to 10% in endovascular and hybrid procedures.[90,115,119–122] In a retrospective cohort of 724 patients who were treated with either TEVAR (n = 352) or open repair (372), for thoracic or thoracoabdominal aneurysms, the rates of spinal cord injuries were not significantly different (4.3% in the endovascular group vs 7.5% in the open group).

2. The extent of coverage of the aorta is the major risk factor for spinal cord ischemia.[111]

3. Patients with prior endovascular repair also tend to have an increased risk, as well as those with preoperative renal insufficiency.[123] In the European Registry of Endovascular Aortic Repair Complications (EuREC), simultaneous closure of at least two vascular territories supplying the spinal cord was found to increase the risk of spinal cord injury, along with long perioperative hypotension.[124]

TABLE 6.4. Classification of Endoleaks

Type of Endoleak	Description
Type I	
Ia	Inadequate seal at the proximal end
Ib	Inadequate seal at the distal end
Ic	Inadequate seal at iliac occluder
Type II	Sac filling via an aortic branch vessel
IIa	Single vessel
IIb	Two vessels or more
Type III	Leak through a defect in graft fabric
IIIa	Junctional separation of the modular component
IIIb	Holes involving the endograft
Type IV	Leak through porous graft material
Type V	Continued aneurysm sac expansion without a demonstrable endoleak on any imaging modality

D. **Stroke** In situations where the aneurysm sac extends to the arch, proximal landing zones can come in proximity to the carotid and vertebral arteries, leading to embolic strokes and cerebrovascular complications. Prior strokes, along with the presence of heavy atheromatous burden in the aortic arch, are strong risk factors for development of such events.[125] Posterior circulation strokes can result from emboli reaching the circle of Willis from the vertebral and subclavian arteries (subclavian stump syndrome).[126]

In one study with 1002 patients, stroke occurred in 4.8% of patients undergoing TEVAR, in whom, prior revascularization of the subclavian artery seemed to protect against posterior circulation strokes.[127] Another study has found the risk of stroke to be 6.25%, with higher rates of complications in patients presenting with emergent conditions.[128]

E. Ischemia

1. **Extremity ischemia.** Although infrequent, coverage of the left subclavian artery can lead to ischemic complications, in patients requiring proximal landing in the arch. Planned revascularization of the subclavian artery before TEVAR should be considered in at-risk patients; this can decrease the ischemic complications, albeit increasing the intraoperative morbidity.[60]

2. **Visceral ischemia.** Coverage of celiac trunk or the superior mesenteric artery can lead to visceral ischemia in patients with thoracoabdominal aneurysms involving these vital structures. Careful planning of debranching procedures or the use of other intraoperative techniques should be carried out before TEVAR.

   Renal ischemia and acute kidney injury (AKI) can also occur, with risk factors being preoperative decreased GFR, extent of thoracoabdominal repair, and postoperative transfusion.[82]

F. **Access Complications** Owing to the large devices, vascular complications at the access sites are not infrequent. Calcific, small tortuous vessels are at higher risk. When iliac rupture occurs, balloon occlusion can be used for temporary vascular control until the artery can be repaired.

G. **Postimplantation Syndrome** Endothelial activation by the endograft can lead to a systemic inflammatory response, characterized by fever, leukocytosis, and elevation of inflammatory markers, with the response being more apparent in acute aortic pathologies.[129,130]

XI. Late Complications

A. Survival and Outcomes

1. Medicare database information from 2005 to 2010 of more than 1100 patients who underwent TEVAR has revealed the median survival to be 57.6 months.[131] The early and late incidence of death varied significantly by aortic disease. Patients with aortic

rupture, acute aortic dissection, and aortic trauma had the highest early incidence of death, whereas late survival was highest in patients with acute aortic dissection, aortic trauma, and isolated thoracic aortic aneurysm, particularly those not requiring subclavian artery coverage.

2. Combined experience from the EUROSTAR and United Kingdom Thoracic Endograft registries has shown the 1-year mortality among patients treated for aortic aneurysm and aortic dissection to be 20% and 10%, respectively. It is important to mention that most of these patients had multiple comorbidities and were not surgical candidates.

3. Questions about the durability and integrity of these endografts are yet to be answered and continued use of registries should provide data from long-term follow-up.

B. **Migration of the Graft** Caudal migration of the graft can happen, especially with oversizing, tortuous aortas, and inability to obtain appropriate tight seals at the landing zones. In one study, the rate of migration (>10 mm) was 2.8%.[30] Device enfolding or collapse can also occur, leading to occlusion manifestations.[132]

C. **Secondary Intervention**

1. Secondary intervention is usually required after endoleaks, device migration, or organ ischemia, with multiple reports on the incidence of these important complications. In a study with 680 patients who were treated with TEVAR from 2000 to 2012, reintervention was needed in 73 patients (11.7%), with a median interval of 210 days. Endograft failures included endoleak in 45, proximal aortic events (retrograde type A or aneurysmal degeneration) in 11, distal aortic events (dissection or aneurysmal degeneration) in 15, endograft infection in 3, and others in 6.[133]

2. In another review of 585 patients, the need for secondary intervention was 12% with a median follow-up of 5.6 months.[134]

XII. Conclusion

Endovascular repair of the descending thoracic aorta has witnessed major advancements in the techniques, graft design, and applicability to various aortic pathologies. Careful planning before the procedure is indispensable in order to correctly address the pathology and to avoid complications. Technique of deployment depends on the device type and the pathology addressed. TEVAR has the advantage of absence of thoracotomy incision and aortic cross-clamping. Nonetheless, TEVAR carries real risks of morbidity and mortality. Long-term evidence about the reliability and durability of these devices remains unelucidated, as registries continue to build follow-up on the patients treated. A multidisciplinary approach is required in management of patients, to choose the best method of management, either with TEVAR or with open repair. Open repair is quite safe at experience centers and offers a nearly "bullet proof" permanence vis-a-vis the treated aortic segment.

References

1. Dake MD, Miller DC, Semba CP, Mitchell RS, Walker PJ, Liddell RP. Transluminal placement of endovascular stent-grafts for the treatment of descending thoracic aortic aneurysms. *N Engl J Med.* 1994;331:1729-1734.
2. Fillinger MF, Greenberg RK, McKinsey JF, Chaikof EL; Society for Vascular Surgery Ad Hoc Committee on TRS. Reporting standards for thoracic endovascular aortic repair (TEVAR). *J Vasc Surg.* 2010;52:1022-1033, 1033. e1015.
3. Biglioli P, Roberto M, Cannata A, et al. Upper and lower spinal cord blood supply: the continuity of the anterior spinal artery and the relevance of the lumbar arteries. *J Thorac Cardiovasc Surg.* 2004;127:1188-1192.
4. Makaroun MS, Dillavou ED, Kee ST, et al. Endovascular treatment of thoracic aortic aneurysms: results of the phase II multicenter trial of the GORE TAG thoracic endoprosthesis. *J Vasc Surg.* 2005;41:1-9.
5. Grabenwoger M, Alfonso F, Bachet J, et al. Thoracic Endovascular Aortic Repair (TEVAR) for the treatment of aortic diseases: a position statement from the European Association for Cardio-Thoracic Surgery (EACTS) and the European Society of Cardiology (ESC), in collaboration with the European Association of Percutaneous Cardiovascular Interventions (EAPCI). *Eur J Cardiothorac Surg.* 2012;42:17-24.
6. Coady MA, Ikonomidis JS, Cheung AT, et al. Surgical management of descending thoracic aortic disease: open and endovascular approaches: a scientific statement from the American Heart Association. *Circulation.* 2010;121:2780-2804.
7. Coady MA, Rizzo JA, Hammond GL, et al. What is the appropriate size criterion for resection of thoracic aortic aneurysms? *J Thoracic Cardiovasc Surg.* 1997;113:476-491; discussion 489–491.
8. Davies RR, Goldstein LJ, Coady MA, et al. Yearly rupture or dissection rates for thoracic aortic aneurysms: simple prediction based on size. *Ann Thorac Surg.* 2002;73:17-28.
9. Elefteriades JA. Natural history of thoracic aortic aneurysms: indications for surgery, and surgical versus nonsurgical risks. *Ann Thorac Surg.* 2002;74:S1877-S1880; discussion S1892–1878.
10. Hiratzka LF, Bakris GL, Beckman JA, et al. 2010 ACCF/AHA/AATS/ACR/ASA/SCA/SCAI/SIR/STS/SVM Guidelines for the Diagnosis and Management of Patients With Thoracic Aortic Disease. A Report of the American College of Cardiology Foundation/American Heart Association Task Force on Practice Guidelines, American Association for Thoracic Surgery, American College of Radiology, American Stroke Association, Society of Cardiovascular Anesthesiologists, Society for Cardiovascular Angiography and Interventions, Society of Interventional Radiology, Society of Thoracic Surgeons, and Society for Vascular Medicine. *Circulation.* 2010;121:e266-e369.
11. Erbel R, Aboyans V, Boileau C, et al. 2014 ESC Guidelines on the diagnosis and treatment of aortic diseases: document covering acute and chronic aortic diseases of the thoracic and abdominal aorta of the adult. The Task Force for the Diagnosis and Treatment of Aortic Diseases of the European Society of Cardiology (ESC). *Eur Heart J.* 2014;35:2873-2926.
12. Patterson B, De Bruin JL, Brownrigg JR, et al. Current endovascular management of acute type B aortic dissection—whom should we treat and when? *J Cardiovasc Surg.* 2014;55:491-496.
13. Fattori R, Tsai TT, Myrmel T, et al. Complicated acute type B dissection: is surgery still the best option?: a report from the International Registry of Acute Aortic Dissection. *JACC Cardiovasc Interv.* 2008;1:395-402.
14. Duebener LF, Lorenzen P, Richardt G, et al. Emergency endovascular stent-grafting for life-threatening acute type B aortic dissections. *Ann Thorac Surg.* 2004;78:1261-1266; discussion 1266–1267.
15. Fattori R, Montgomery D, Lovato L, et al. Survival after endovascular therapy in patients with type B aortic dissection: a report from the International Registry of Acute Aortic Dissection (IRAD). *JACC Cardiovasc Interv.* 2013;6:876-882.
16. Grabenwöger M, Alfonso F, Bachet J, et al. Thoracic Endovascular Aortic Repair (TEVAR) for the treatment of aortic diseases: a position statement from the European Association for Cardio-Thoracic Surgery (EACTS) and the European Society of Cardiology (ESC), in collaboration with the European Association of Percutaneous Cardiovascular Interventions (EAPCI). *Eur Heart J.* 2012;33:1558-1563.

17. Nienaber CA, Rousseau H, Eggebrecht H, et al. Randomized comparison of strategies for type B aortic dissection: the INvestigation of STEnt Grafts in Aortic Dissection (INSTEAD) trial. *Circulation.* 2009;120:2519-2528.
18. Nienaber CA, Kische S, Rousseau H, et al. Endovascular repair of type B aortic dissection: long-term results of the randomized investigation of stent grafts in aortic dissection trial. *Circ Cardiovasc Interv.* 2013;6:407-416.
19. Demetriades D, Velmahos GC, Scalea TM, et al. Operative repair or endovascular stent graft in blunt traumatic thoracic aortic injuries: results of an American Association for the Surgery of Trauma Multicenter Study. *J Trauma.* 2008;64:561-570; discussion 570–561.
20. Canaud L, Ozdemir BA, Bee WW, Bahia S, Holt P, Thompson M. Thoracic endovascular aortic repair in management of aortoesophageal fistulas. *J Vasc Surg.* 2014;59:248-254.
21. Kiguchi M, Chaer RA. Endovascular repair of thoracic aortic pathology. *Expert Rev Med Devices.* 2011;8:515-525.
22. Jordan WD Jr, Rovin J, Moainie S, et al. Results of a prospective multicenter trial of CTAG thoracic endograft. *J Vasc Surg.* 2015;61:589-595.
23. https://www.goremedical.com/products/ctag---specifications. Vol. 2018.
24. Melissano G, Tshomba Y, Civilini E, Chiesa R. Disappointing results with a new commercially available thoracic endograft. *J Vasc Surg.* 2004;39:124-130.
25. Cho JS, Haider SE, Makaroun MS. Endovascular therapy of thoracic aneurysms: Gore TAG trial results. *Semin Vasc Surg.* 2006;19:18-24.
26. Brunkwall J, Kasprzak P, Verhoeven E, et al. Endovascular repair of acute uncomplicated aortic type B dissection promotes aortic remodelling: 1 year results of the ADSORB trial. *Eur J Vasc Endovasc Surg.* 2014;48:285-291.
27. 27Voute MT, Bastos Goncalves F, Verhagen HJ. Commentary on 'ADSORB: a study on the efficacy of endovascular grafting in uncomplicated acute dissection of the descending aorta'. *Eur J Vasc Endovasc Surg.* 2012;44:37.
28. Farber MA, Giglia J, Starnes B, et al. TEVAR using the redesigned TAG Device (CTAG) for traumatic aortic transection: a nonrandomized multicenter trial. *J Vasc Surg.* 2012;55:622.
29. Melissano G, Tshomba Y, Rinaldi E, Chiesa R. Initial clinical experience with a new low-profile thoracic endograft. *J Vasc Surg.* 2015;62:336-342.
30. Matsumura JS, Cambria RP, Dake MD, et al. International controlled clinical trial of thoracic endovascular aneurysm repair with the Zenith TX2 endovascular graft: 1-year results. *J Vasc Surg.* 2008;47:247-257; discussion 257.
31. Lee WA, Martin TD, Hess PJ Jr, Beaver TM, Klodell CT. First United States experience of the TX2 Pro-Form thoracic delivery system. *J Vasc Surg.* 2010;52:1459-1463.
32. Lombardi JV, Cambria RP, Nienaber CA, et al. Prospective multicenter clinical trial (STABLE) on the endovascular treatment of complicated type B aortic dissection using a composite device design. *J Vasc Surg.* 2012;55:629-640. e622.
33. Fairman RM, Tuchek JM, Lee WA, et al. Pivotal results for the Medtronic Valiant Thoracic Stent Graft System in the VALOR II trial. *J Vasc Surg.* 2012;56:1222-1231. e1221.
34. Thompson M, Ivaz S, Cheshire N, et al. Early results of endovascular treatment of the thoracic aorta using the Valiant endograft. *Cardiovasc Intervent Radiol.* 2007;30:1130-1138.
35. Conrad MF, Tuchek J, Freezor R, Bavaria J, White R, Fairman R. Results of the VALOR II trial of the Medtronic Valiant Thoracic Stent Graft. *J Vasc Surg.* 2017;66:335-342.
36. Riambau V, Zipfel B, Coppi G, et al. Final operative and midterm results of the European experience in the RELAY Endovascular Registry for Thoracic Disease (RESTORE) study. *J Vasc Surg.* 2011;53:565-573.
37. Riambau V; RESTORE collaborators. European experience with relay: a new stent graft and delivery system for thoracic and arch lesions. *J Cardiovasc Surg.* 2008;49:407-415.
38. Zipfel B, Czerny M, Funovics M, et al. Endovascular treatment of patients with types A and B thoracic aortic dissection using Relay thoracic stent-grafts: results from the RESTORE Patient Registry. *J Endovasc Ther.* 2011;18:131-143.

39. Inglese L, Mollichelli N, Medda M, et al. Endovascular repair of thoracic aortic disease with the EndoFit stent-graft: short and midterm results from a single center. *J Endovasc Ther.* 2008;15:54-61.
40. Qu L, Raithel D. Two-year single-center experience with thoracic endovascular aortic repair using the EndoFit thoracic stent-graft. *J Endovasc Ther.* 2008;15:530-538.
41. Bergeron P, Inglese L, Gay J; Dedicated Registry Collaborators. Setting up of a multicentric European registry dealing with type B dissections in chronic and acute phases with thoracic EndoFit devices. *J Cardiovasc Surg.* 2007;48:689-695.
42. Zipfel B, Buz S, Hammerschmidt R, Krabatsch T, Duesterhoeft V, Hetzer R. Early clinical experience with the E-vita thoracic stent-graft system: a single center study. *J Cardiovasc Surg.* 2008;49:417-428.
43. Stefanov F, Morris L, Elhelali A, et al. Insights from complex aortic surgery with a Streamliner device for aortic arch repair (STAR). *J Thorac Cardiovasc Surg.* 2016;152:1309-1318. e1305.
44. Sultan S, Hynes N, Sultan M; Collaborators MFM. When not to implant the multilayer flow modulator: lessons learned from application outside the indications for use in patients with thoracoabdominal pathologies. *J Endovasc Ther.* 2014;21:96-112.
45. Vaislic CD, Fabiani JN, Chocron S, et al. One-year outcomes following repair of thoracoabdominal aneurysms with the multilayer flow modulator: report from the STRATO trial. *J Endovasc Ther.* 2014;21:85-95.
46. Hynes N, Sultan S, Elhelali A, et al. Systematic review and patient-level meta-analysis of the streamliner multilayer flow modulator in the management of complex thoracoabdominal aortic pathology. *J Endovasc Ther.* 2016;23:501-512.
47. Vaislic CD, Fabiani JN, Chocron S, et al. Three-year outcomes with the multilayer flow modulator for repair of thoracoabdominal aneurysms: a follow-up report from the STRATO trial. *J Endovasc Ther.* 2016;23:762-772.
48. Kaladji A, Spear R, Hertault A, Sobocinski J, Maurel B, Haulon S. Centerline is not as accurate as outer curvature length to estimate thoracic endograft length. *Eur J Vasc Endovasc Surg.* 2013;46:82-86.
49. Muller-Eschner M, Rengier F, Partovi S, et al. Accuracy and variability of semiautomatic centerline analysis versus manual aortic measurement techniques for TEVAR. *Eur J Vasc Endovasc Surg.* 2013;45:241-247.
50. Nakatamari H, Ueda T, Ishioka F, et al. Discriminant analysis of native thoracic aortic curvature: risk prediction for endoleak formation after thoracic endovascular aortic repair. *J Vasc Interv Radiol.* 2011;22:974-979. e972.
51. Gasper WJ, Reilly LM, Rapp JH, et al. Assessing the anatomic applicability of the multibranched endovascular repair of thoracoabdominal aortic aneurysm technique. *J Vasc Surg.* 2013;57:1553-1558; discussion 1558.
52. Kasirajan K, Dake MD, Lumsden A, Bavaria J, Makaroun MS. Incidence and outcomes after infolding or collapse of thoracic stent grafts. *J Vasc Surg.* 2012;55:652-658; discussion 658.
53. Jonker FH, Schlosser FJ, Geirsson A, Sumpio BE, Moll FL, Muhs BE. Endograft collapse after thoracic endovascular aortic repair. *J Endovasc Ther.* 2010;17:725-734.
54. Smith TA, Gatens S, Andres M, Modrall JG, Clagett GP, Arko FR. Hybrid repair of thoracoabdominal aortic aneurysms involving the visceral vessels: comparative analysis between number of vessels reconstructed, conduit, and gender. *Ann Vasc Surg.* 2011;25:64-70.
55. Greenberg RK, Lytle B. Endovascular repair of thoracoabdominal aneurysms. *Circulation.* 2008;117:2288-2296.
56. Canaud L, Ozdemir BA, Patterson BO, Holt PJ, Loftus IM, Thompson MM. Retrograde aortic dissection after thoracic endovascular aortic repair. *Ann Surg.* 2014;260:389-395.
57. Jonker FH, Verhagen HJ, Mojibian H, Davis KA, Moll FL, Muhs BE. Aortic endograft sizing in trauma patients with hemodynamic instability. *J Vasc Surg.* 2010;52:39-44.
58. Hajibandeh S, Hajibandeh S, Antoniou SA, Torella F, Antoniou GA. Meta-analysis of left subclavian artery coverage with and without revascularization in thoracic endovascular aortic repair. *J Endovasc Ther.* 2016;23:634-641.
59. Dunning J, Martin JE, Shennib H, Cheng DC. Is it safe to cover the left subclavian artery when placing an endovascular stent in the descending thoracic aorta? *Interact Cardiovasc Thorac Surg.* 2008;7:690-697.

60. Rehman SM, Vecht JA, Perera R, et al. How to manage the left subclavian artery during endovascular stenting of the thoracic aorta. *Eur J Cardiothorac Surg.* 2011;39:507-518.
61. Waterford SD, Chou D, Bombien R, Uzun I, Shah A, Khoynezhad A. Left subclavian arterial coverage and stroke during thoracic aortic endografting: a systematic review. *Ann Thorac Surg.* 2016;101:381-389.
62. Dexter D, Maldonado TS. Left subclavian artery coverage during TEVAR: is revascularization necessary? *J Cardiovasc Surg.* 2012;53:135-141.
63. Madenci AL, Ozaki CK, Belkin M, McPhee JT. Carotid-subclavian bypass and subclavian-carotid transposition in the thoracic endovascular aortic repair era. *J Vasc Surg.* 2013;57:1275-1282. e1272.
64. Szeto WY, Bavaria JE, Bowen FW, Woo EY, Fairman RM, Pochettino A. The hybrid total arch repair: brachiocephalic bypass and concomitant endovascular aortic arch stent graft placement. *J Card Surg.* 2007;22:97-102; discussion 103–104.
65. Bergeron P, Mangialardi N, Costa P, et al. Great vessel management for endovascular exclusion of aortic arch aneurysms and dissections. *Eur J Vasc Endovasc Surg.* 2006;32:38-45.
66. Vaddineni SK, Taylor SM, Patterson MA, Jordan WD Jr. Outcome after celiac artery coverage during endovascular thoracic aortic aneurysm repair: preliminary results. *J Vasc Surg.* 2007;45:467-471.
67. Leon LR Jr, Mills JL Sr, Jordan W, et al. The risks of celiac artery coverage during endoluminal repair of thoracic and thoracoabdominal aortic aneurysms. *Vasc Endovascular Surg.* 2009;43:51-60.
68. Jim J, Caputo FJ, Sanchez LA. Intentional coverage of the celiac artery during thoracic endovascular aortic repair. *J Vasc Surg.* 2013;58:270-275.
69. Yuri K, Yokoi Y, Yamaguchi A, Hori D, Adachi K, Adachi H. Usefulness of fenestrated stent grafts for thoracic aortic aneurysms. *Eur J Cardiothorac Surg.* 2013;44:760-767.
70. Shahverdyan R, Gawenda M, Brunkwall J. Triple-barrel graft as a novel strategy to preserve supra-aortic branches in arch-TEVAR procedures: clinical study and systematic review. *Eur J Vasc Endovasc Surg.* 2013;45:28-35.
71. Riesenman PJ, Reeves JG, Kasirajan K. Endovascular management of a ruptured thoracoabdominal aneurysm-damage control with superior mesenteric artery snorkel and thoracic stent-graft exclusion. *Ann Vasc Surg.* 2011;25:555. e555–559.
72. Pecoraro F, Pfammatter T, Mayer D, et al. Multiple periscope and chimney grafts to treat ruptured thoracoabdominal and pararenal aortic aneurysms. *J Endovasc Ther.* 2011;18:642-649.
73. Bockler D, Kotelis D, Geisbusch P, et al. Hybrid procedures for thoracoabdominal aortic aneurysms and chronic aortic dissections—a single center experience in 28 patients. *J Vasc Surg.* 2008;47:724-732.
74. Greenberg RK, Sternbergh WC III, Makaroun M, et al. Intermediate results of a United States multicenter trial of fenestrated endograft repair for juxtarenal abdominal aortic aneurysms. *J Vasc Surg.* 2009;50:730–737. e731.
75. Tambyraja AL, Fishwick NG, Bown MJ, Nasim A, McCarthy MJ, Sayers RD. Fenestrated aortic endografts for juxtarenal aortic aneurysm: medium term outcomes. *Eur J Vasc Endovasc Surg.* 2011;42:54-58.
76. Xue Y, Sun L, Zheng J, et al. The chimney technique for preserving the left subclavian artery in thoracic endovascular aortic repair. *Eur J Cardiothorac Surg.* 2015;47:623-629.
77. Zhu Y, Guo W, Liu X, Jia X, Xiong J, Wang L. The single-centre experience of the supra-arch chimney technique in endovascular repair of type B aortic dissections. *Eur J Vasc Endovasc Surg.* 2013;45:633-638.
78. Redlinger RE Jr, Ahanchi SS, Panneton JM. In situ laser fenestration during emergent thoracic endovascular aortic repair is an effective method for left subclavian artery revascularization. *J Vasc Surg.* 2013;58:1171-1177.
79. Wang ZG, Li C. Single-branch endograft for treating stanford type B aortic dissections with entry tears in proximity to the left subclavian artery. *J Endovasc Ther.* 2005;12:588-593.
80. Bratzler DW, Dellinger EP, Olsen KM, et al. Clinical practice guidelines for antimicrobial prophylaxis in surgery. *Am J Health Syst Pharm.* 2013;70:195-283.
81. Pisimisis GT, Khoynezhad A, Bashir K, Kruse MJ, Donayre CE, White RA. Incidence and risk factors of renal dysfunction after thoracic endovascular aortic repair. *J Thorac Cardiovasc Surg.* 2010;140:S161-S167.

82. Piffaretti G, Mariscalco G, Bonardelli S, et al. Predictors and outcomes of acute kidney injury after thoracic aortic endograft repair. *J Vasc Surg*. 2012;56:1527-1534.
83. Cheung AT, Weiss SJ, McGarvey ML, et al. Interventions for reversing delayed-onset postoperative paraplegia after thoracic aortic reconstruction. *Ann Thorac Surg*. 2002;74:413-419; discussion 420–411.
84. Buth J, Harris PL, Hobo R, et al. Neurologic complications associated with endovascular repair of thoracic aortic pathology: Incidence and risk factors. a study from the European Collaborators on Stent/Graft Techniques for Aortic Aneurysm Repair (EUROSTAR) registry. *J Vasc Surg*. 2007;46:1103-1110; discussion 1110–1101.
85. Schlosser FJ, Verhagen HJ, Lin PH, et al. TEVAR following prior abdominal aortic aneurysm surgery: increased risk of neurological deficit. *J Vasc Surg*. 2009;49:308-314; discussion 314.
86. Ullery BW, Quatromoni J, Jackson BM, et al. Impact of intercostal artery occlusion on spinal cord ischemia following thoracic endovascular aortic repair. *Vasc Endovascular Surg*. 2011;45:519-523.
87. Amabile P, Grisoli D, Giorgi R, Bartoli JM, Piquet P. Incidence and determinants of spinal cord ischaemia in stent-graft repair of the thoracic aorta. *Eur J Vasc Endovasc Surg*. 2008;35:455-461.
88. O'Callaghan A, Mastracci TM, Eagleton MJ. Staged endovascular repair of thoracoabdominal aortic aneurysms limits incidence and severity of spinal cord ischemia. *J Vasc Surg*. 2015;61:347-354. e341.
89. Moomiaie RM, Ransden J, Stein J, et al. Cooling catheter for spinal cord preservation in thoracic aortic surgery. *J Cardiovasc Surg*. 2007;48:103-108.
90. Leurs LJ, Bell R, Degrieck Y, et al. Endovascular treatment of thoracic aortic diseases: combined experience from the EUROSTAR and United Kingdom Thoracic Endograft registries. *J Vasc Surg*. 2004;40:670-679; discussion 679–680.
91. Lee WA, Brown MP, Nelson PR, Huber TS. Total percutaneous access for endovascular aortic aneurysm repair ("Preclose" technique). *J Vasc Surg*. 2007;45:1095-1101.
92. Skagius E, Bosnjak M, Bjorck M, Steuer J, Nyman R, Wanhainen A. Percutaneous closure of large femoral artery access with Prostar XL in thoracic endovascular aortic repair. *Eur J Vasc Endovasc Surg*. 2013;46:558-563.
93. Stone DH, Brewster DC, Kwolek CJ, et al. Stent-graft versus open-surgical repair of the thoracic aorta: mid-term results. *J Vasc Surg*. 2006;44:1188-1197.
94. Bhutia SG, Wales L, Jackson R, Kindawi A, Wyatt MG, Clarke MJ. Descending thoracic endovascular aneurysm repair: antegrade approach via ascending aortic conduit. *Eur J Vasc Endovasc Surg*. 2011;41:38-40.
95. Qu L, Raithel D. Techniques for precise thoracic endograft placement. *J Vasc Surg*. 2009;49:1069-1072; discussion 1072.
96. Rylski B, Blanke P, Siepe M, et al. Results of high-risk endovascular procedures in patients with non-dissected thoracic aortic pathology: intermediate outcomes. *Eur J Cardiothorac Surg*. 2013;44:156-162.
97. Bavaria JE, Appoo JJ, Makaroun MS, et al. Endovascular stent grafting versus open surgical repair of descending thoracic aortic aneurysms in low-risk patients: a multicenter comparative trial. *J Thorac Cardiovasc Surg*. 2007;133:369-377.
98. Ehlert BA, Durham CA, Parker FM, Bogey WM, Powell CS, Stoner MC. Impact of operative indication and surgical complexity on outcomes after thoracic endovascular aortic repair at National Surgical Quality Improvement Program Centers. *J Vasc Surg*. 2011;54:1629-1636.
99. Chung J, Corriere MA, Veeraswamy RK, et al. Risk factors for late mortality after endovascular repair of the thoracic aorta. *J Vasc Surg*. 2010;52:549-554; discussion 555.
100. Etezadi V, Schiro B, Pena CS, Kovacs M, Benenati JF, Katzen BT. Endovascular treatment of descending thoracic aortic disease: single-center, 15-year experience. *J Vasc Interv Radiol*. 2012;23:468-475.
101. Arnaoutakis GJ, Schneider EB, Arnaoutakis DJ, et al. Influence of gender on outcomes after thoracic endovascular aneurysm repair. *J Vasc Surg*. 2014;59:45-51.
102. Jackson BM, Woo EY, Bavaria JE, Fairman RM. Gender analysis of the pivotal results of the Medtronic Talent Thoracic Stent Graft System (VALOR) trial. *J Vasc Surg*. 2011;54:358-363, 363.e351.
103. Czerny M, Hoebartner M, Sodeck G, et al. The influence of gender on mortality in patients after thoracic endovascular aortic repair. *Eur J Cardiothorac Surg*. 2011;40:e1-e5.

104. Makaroun MS, Dillavou ED, Wheatley GH, Cambria RP, Gore TAG Investigators. Five-year results of endovascular treatment with the Gore TAG device compared with open repair of thoracic aortic aneurysms. *J Vasc Surg.* 2008;47:912-918.
105. Lal BK, Zhou W, Li Z, et al. Predictors and outcomes of endoleaks in the veterans affairs Open Versus Endovascular Repair (OVER) trial of abdominal aortic aneurysms. *J Vasc Surg.* 2015;62:1394-1404.
106. Chaikof EL, Blankensteijn JD, Harris PL, et al. Reporting standards for endovascular aortic aneurysm repair. *J Vasc Surg.* 2002;35:1048-1060.
107. Abularrage CJ, Crawford RS, Conrad MF, et al. Preoperative variables predict persistent type 2 endoleak after endovascular aneurysm repair. *J Vasc Surg.* 2010;52:19-24.
108. Veith FJ, Baum RA, Ohki T, et al. Nature and significance of endoleaks and endotension: summary of opinions expressed at an international conference. *J Vasc Surg.* 2002;35:1029-1035.
109. Preventza O, Wheatley GH III, Ramaiah VG, et al. Management of endoleaks associated with endovascular treatment of descending thoracic aortic diseases. *J Vasc Surg.* 2008;48:69-73.
110. Mastracci TM, Greenberg RK, Eagleton MJ, Hernandez AV. Durability of branches in branched and fenestrated endografts. *J Vasc Surg.* 2013;57:926-933; discussion 933.
111. Zoli S, Roder F, Etz CD, et al. Predicting the risk of paraplegia after thoracic and thoracoabdominal aneurysm repair. *Ann Thorac Surg.* 2010;90:1237-1244; discussion 1245.
112. Coselli JS, LeMaire SA, Preventza O, et al. Outcomes of 3309 thoracoabdominal aortic aneurysm repairs. *J Thorac Cardiovasc Surg.* 2016;151:1323-1337.
113. Estrera AL, Sandhu HK, Charlton-Ouw KM, et al. A quarter century of organ protection in open thoracoabdominal repair. *Ann Surg.* 2015;262:660-668.
114. Fehrenbacher JW, Siderys H, Terry C, Kuhn J, Corvera JS. Early and late results of descending thoracic and thoracoabdominal aortic aneurysm open repair with deep hypothermia and circulatory arrest. *J Thorac Cardiovasc Surg.* 2010;140:S154-S160; discussion S185–S190.
115. Conrad MF, Ye JY, Chung TK, Davison JK, Cambria RP. Spinal cord complications after thoracic aortic surgery: long-term survival and functional status varies with deficit severity. *J Vasc Surg.* 2008;48:47-53.
116. Greenberg RK, Lu Q, Roselli EE, et al. Contemporary analysis of descending thoracic and thoracoabdominal aneurysm repair: a comparison of endovascular and open techniques. *Circulation.* 2008;118:808-817.
117. Kulik A, Castner CF, Kouchoukos NT. Outcomes after thoracoabdominal aortic aneurysm repair with hypothermic circulatory arrest. *J Thorac Cardiovasc Surg.* 2011;141:953-960.
118. Lima B, Nowicki ER, Blackstone EH, et al. Spinal cord protective strategies during descending and thoracoabdominal aortic aneurysm repair in the modern era: the role of intrathecal papaverine. *J Thorac Cardiovasc Surg.* 2012;143:945-952. e941.
119. Drinkwater SL, Goebells A, Haydar A, et al. The incidence of spinal cord ischaemia following thoracic and thoracoabdominal aortic endovascular intervention. *Eur J Vasc Endovasc Surg.* 2010;40:729-735.
120. Guillou M, Bianchini A, Sobocinski J, et al. Endovascular treatment of thoracoabdominal aortic aneurysms. *J Vasc Surg.* 2012;56:65-73.
121. Martin DJ, Martin TD, Hess PJ, Daniels MJ, Feezor RJ, Lee WA. Spinal cord ischemia after TEVAR in patients with abdominal aortic aneurysms. *J Vasc Surg.* 2009;49:302-306; discussion 306–307.
122. Ferrer C, Cao P, De Rango P, et al. A propensity-matched comparison for endovascular and open repair of thoracoabdominal aortic aneurysms. *J Vasc Surg.* 2016;63:1201-1207.
123. Ullery BW, Cheung AT, Fairman RM, et al. Risk factors, outcomes, and clinical manifestations of spinal cord ischemia following thoracic endovascular aortic repair. *J Vasc Surg.* 2011;54:677-684.
124. Czerny M, Eggebrecht H, Sodeck G, et al. Mechanisms of symptomatic spinal cord ischemia after TEVAR: insights from the European Registry of Endovascular Aortic Repair Complications (EuREC). *J Endovasc Ther.* 2012;19:37-43.
125. Gutsche JT, Cheung AT, McGarvey ML, et al. Risk factors for perioperative stroke after thoracic endovascular aortic repair. *Ann Thorac Surg.* 2007;84:1195-1200; discussion 1200.

126. Patel R, Muthu C, Goh KH. Subclavian stump syndrome causing a posterior circulation stroke after thoracic endovascular aneurysm repair (TEVAR) with adjunctive carotid to subclavian bypass and endovascular embolization of the left subclavian artery. *Ann Vasc Surg.* 2014;28:1318. e1313–1316.
127. Patterson BO, Holt PJ, Nienaber C, Fairman RM, Heijmen RH, Thompson MM. Management of the left subclavian artery and neurologic complications after thoracic endovascular aortic repair. *J Vasc Surg.* 2014;60:1491-1497. e1491.
128. Knowles M, Murphy EH, Dimaio JM, et al. The effects of operative indication and urgency of intervention on patient outcomes after thoracic aortic endografting. *J Vasc Surg.* 2011;53:926-934.
129. Gabriel EA, Locali RF, Romano CC, Duarte AJ, Palma JH, Buffolo E. Analysis of the inflammatory response in endovascular treatment of aortic aneurysms. *Eur J Cardiothorac Surg.* 2007;31:406-412.
130. Eggebrecht H, Mehta RH, Metozounve H, et al. Clinical implications of systemic inflammatory response syndrome following thoracic aortic stent-graft placement. *J Endovasc Ther.* 2008;15:135-143.
131. Schaffer JM, Lingala B, Miller DC, Woo YJ, Mitchell RS, Dake MD. Midterm survival after thoracic endovascular aortic repair in more than 10,000 medicare patients. *J Thorac Cardiovasc Surg.* 2015;149:808-820; discussion 820–803.
132. Shukla AJ, Jeyabalan G, Cho JS. Late collapse of a thoracic endoprosthesis. *J Vasc Surg.* 2011;53:798-801.
133. Szeto WY, Desai ND, Moeller P, et al. Reintervention for endograft failures after thoracic endovascular aortic repair. *J Thorac Cardiovasc Surg.* 2013;145:S165-S170.
134. Scali ST, Beck AW, Butler K, et al. Pathology-specific secondary aortic interventions after thoracic endovascular aortic repair. *J Vasc Surg.* 2014;59:599-607.
135. Farber MA, Giglia JS, Starnes BW, et al. Evaluation of the redesigned conformable GORE TAG thoracic endoprosthesis for traumatic aortic transection. *J Vasc Surg.* 2013;58:651-658.

CHAPTER 7

Pulmonary Artery Stenosis

M. Abigail Simmons, MD and
Jeremy D. Asnes, MD

Key Points

- Pulmonary artery stenosis may be due to congenital or acquired disease.
- Pulmonary artery stenosis should be considered as part of the differential diagnosis for any adult undergoing evaluation of pulmonary hypertension.
- Indications to intervene on pulmonary artery stenosis include: 1) right ventricular systolic pressure greater than 2/3 systemic pressure, 2) Significant stenosis in the setting of right ventricular dysfunction, 3) pulmonary artery stenosis with a marked perfusion inequality or deficit, 4) regional pulmonary artery hypertension in unaffected lung segment, and 5) pulmonary artery narrowing/distortion in patients with cavopulmonary anastomoses.
- Interventional techniques to address pulmonary artery stenosis include simple balloon angioplasty, cutting balloon angioplasty, and stent angioplasty.

I. Introduction

A. Obstructions or stenoses with the pulmonary arterial tree result from a diverse group of intrinsic and extrinsic factors.

B. Pulmonary artery stenoses may involve the main pulmonary artery, the left and right branch pulmonary arteries, and the lobar, segmental, and subsegmental branches of the more distal pulmonary arterial tree. Obstruction may be isolated to a single vessel or may occur at multiple sites and multiple levels.[1] Management strategies for pulmonary artery stenosis include balloon angioplasty, cutting balloon angioplasty, and stent angioplasty. Patient-specific strategies depend on etiology, lesion characteristics, and patient characteristics.

II. Etiology of Pulmonary Artery Stenosis

A. Pulmonary artery stenosis can be broadly classified as either congenital or acquired (Table 7.1). In a study by Franch, 60% of congenital stenoses were found in conjunction with congenital heart disease while 40% were isolated. Isolated congenital stenosis is often found in association with genetic syndromes including Williams, Alagille, and Noonan syndrome (Fig. 7.1). In these settings, the stenoses tend to be diffuse, involving multiple segments at multiple levels of the pulmonary tree.

B. Pulmonary artery stenoses may be acquired as a result of congenital heart disease surgery, particularly if the surgery involves manipulation of the pulmonary arteries themselves. Patch material, suture lines, and distortion due to kinking or stretching of the pulmonary vessel may all contribute to postsurgical pulmonary artery stenosis (Figs. 7.2A–C and 7.3A).

Table 7.1. Etiologies of Pulmonary Artery Stenosis

Congenital Malformation of Pulmonary Arterial System
- Congenital heart disease associated
  - Tetralogy of Fallot, pulmonary atresia, pulmonary valvar stenosis
  - Main, branch, or lobar artery stenoses
- Isolated pulmonary artery stenosis
  - Main or branch pulmonary artery stenosis

Genetic Syndromes
- Williams syndrome:
  - Diffuse involvement: branch, lobar, segmental pulmonary arteries
- Alagille syndrome: Peripheral pulmonary artery stenosis

Postsurgical
- Distal to site of pulmonary artery patch or anastomosis
- Site of previous Blalock-Taussig shunt
- Site of patent ductus arteriosus ligation or device implantation
- Following removal of pulmonary artery band
- Following arterial switch operation

Idiopathic Pulmonary Artery Stenosis
- Takayasu arteritis: Main, branch, and lobar pulmonary artery stenosis
- Fibrosing mediastinitis: Main and branch pulmonary artery stenosis

External Compression
- Compression from tumor (ie bronchogenic carcinoma) or lymphadenopathy
- Compression from infiltrative or fibrotic lung disease (ie sarcoidosis)

C. Pulmonary artery stenosis presenting *de novo* in the adult is a rare but important condition and is usually an acquired pathology.[2,3] Etiologies include external compression from tumor or lymphadenopathy, fibrosing mediastinitis, systemic vasculitis (eg Takayasu arteritis or Behcet disease), thromboembolic disease, and sarcoidosis. (Table 7.1). These are often misdiagnosed as idiopathic pulmonary arterial hypertension or pulmonary hypertension due to chronic venous thromboembolism. In cases of late diagnosis, patients have often received inappropriate or incomplete therapeutic strategies with little clinical benefit.

III. Pathophysiology

Pulmonary artery stenosis results in varying degrees of ventilation/perfusion mismatch, pulmonary hypertension, vascular injury in unaffected segments, elevations of right heart pressure, right ventricular dysfunction, and limitations of cardiac output. In the presence of an intra-cardiac shunt (eg, patent foramen ovale, atrial septal defect, or ventricular septal defect) obstruction to pulmonary blood flow can result in cyanosis from shunting of deoxygenated blood to the systemic circulation due to increased resistance to pulmonary blood flow. Untreated, pulmonary artery stenosis can contribute to exercise limitation, diminished quality of life, and, in the case of congenital lesions and stenosis due to previous cardiac surgery, limited pulmonary vascular growth and post-operative mortality.[4,5]

IV. Interventional Strategies

A. **First Balloon Angioplasty and Advancements** Lock *et al*, were the first to perform balloon angioplasty of pulmonary arteries. Their seminal work with an experimental lamb model was quickly translated to the congenital cardiac catheterization laboratory.[6,7]

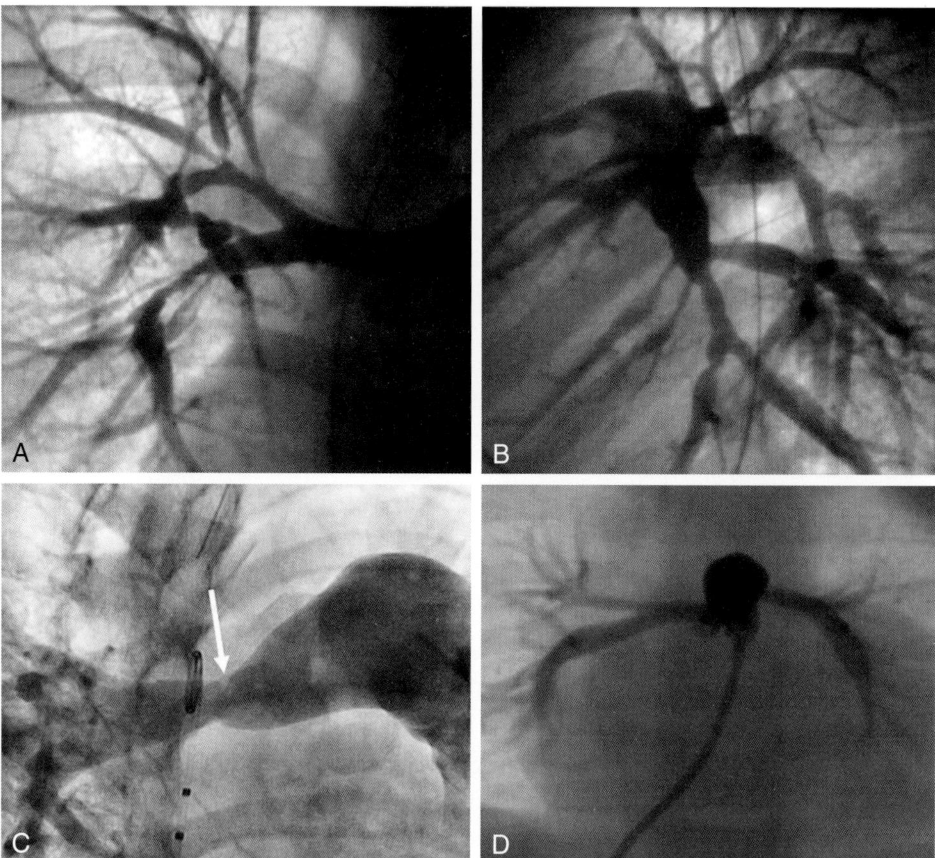

FIGURE 7.1: A and B, Anterior-posterior and lateral angiograms from a patient with Williams syndrome. There is diffuse disease with hypoplasia of the central pulmonary arteries and severe stenoses of almost all lobar and segmental branches. C, Severe discrete right pulmonary artery stenosis (white arrow) in a patient with Takayasu arteritis. D, Severe proximal pulmonary artery stenosis/hypoplasia in a patient with Alagille syndrome.

Rapid advancements in catheter, balloon, stent and guidewire technologies, as well as refinements in angioplasty techniques, broadened the scope of lesions that can be safely treated with transcatheter therapies. In the current era, simple balloon angioplasty, cutting balloon angioplasty, and stent angioplasty are the primary interventions for pulmonary arterial stenosis.

B. **Indications for Intervention** Generally agreed upon indications for intervention are[8,9]

1. Significant elevation in right ventricular systolic pressures (≥2/3 systemic)
2. Significant stenosis in the setting of right ventricular dysfunction
3. Pulmonary artery stenosis with a marked perfusion inequality or deficit
4. Regional pulmonary artery hypertension in unaffected lung segments (mean distal pressure >25 mm Hg)
5. Pulmonary artery narrowing/distortion in patients with cavopulmonary anastomoses

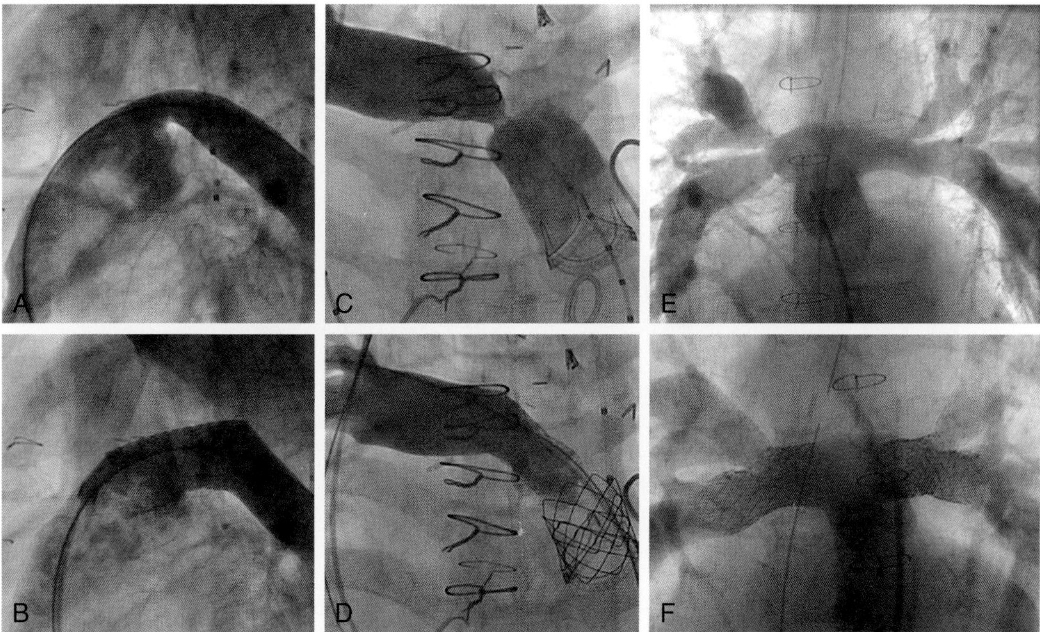

FIGURE 7.2: A and B, Stenosis due to folding of the proximal left pulmonary artery at the site of a surgical patch before (A) and after (B) stent placement. C and D, Severe right pulmonary artery stenosis related to surgical patch material before (C) and after (D) stent placement and transcatheter valve-in-valve pulmonary valve implant. D, Pulmonary artery angiogram in a patient with transposition of the great arteries following arterial switch operation. There are stenoses of the lobar branches related to surgical manipulation of the pulmonary vasculature (E) successfully treated with stent angioplasty (F).

V. Goals of Therapy and Measures of Success

The goals of intervention include reduction in right ventricle pressure, improved distribution of pulmonary blood flow, preservation and improved growth of distal pulmonary vasculature, pressure reduction in unobstructed lung segments, and improvement in exercise capacity. Therapeutic success is measured by angiographic and/or clinical/physiologic improvement.[10] Nuclear perfusion imaging helps assess regional pulmonary perfusion and the need for and success of an intervention.

VI. Standard Balloon Angioplasty

Successful balloon angioplasty tears the intima and media of the pulmonary arterial wall.[11,12]

A. Balloon Expansion

1. In general, balloons either expand uniformly with a discrete waist at the site of highest resistance, or nonuniformly without a discrete waist.
2. The latter is often associated with stenosis due to external compression, kinking, or stretching of the vessel.
3. These vessels typically exhibit significant recoil limiting therapeutic benefit of balloon angiogplasty.

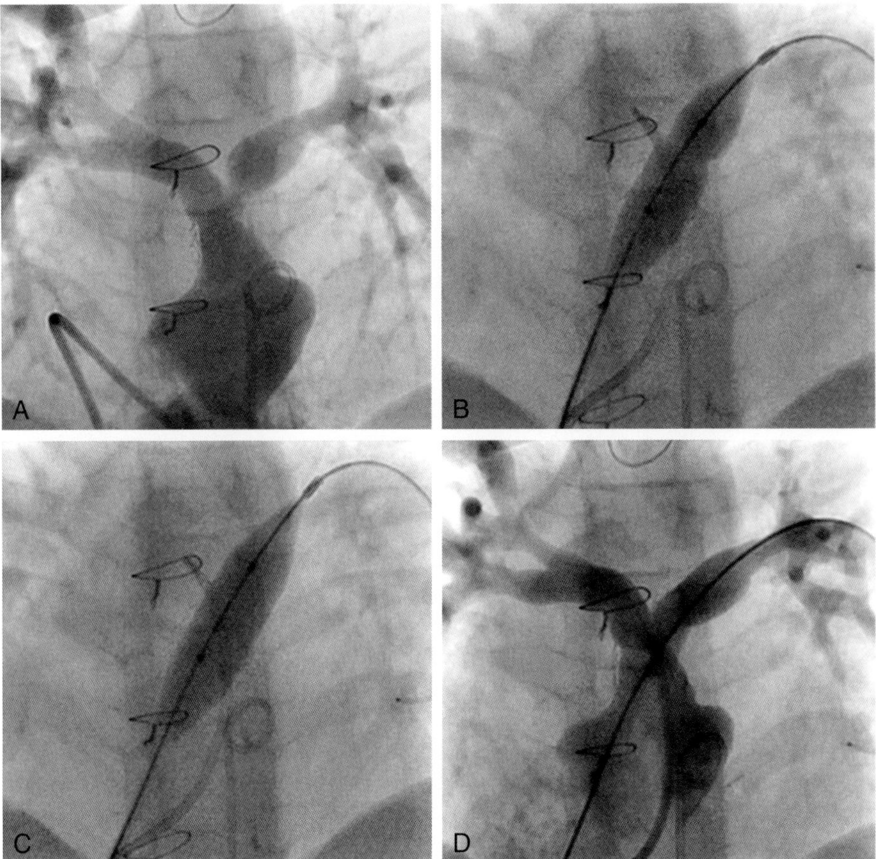

FIGURE 7.3: Balloon angioplasty of proximal left pulmonary artery stenosis related to surgical patch augmentation, before (A) and following (D) successful balloon angioplasty in a patient with tetralogy of Fallot. Note the discrete waist in the angioplasty balloon (B) that resolves with high-pressure inflation (C).

4. When a waist is present, successful angioplasty is dependent on its eradication.[13]
5. Angiography following successful balloon angioplasty often shows a non-obstructive intra-luminal filling defect indicative of an appropriate intimal and medial tear.

B. **Types of Balloon Angioplasty Catheters** A wide array of balloon angioplasty catheters is available for pulmonary artery balloon angioplasty. Balloon selection depends on both patient and target vessel characteristics with differences in guidewire size, shaft flexibility, balloon compliance, balloon and balloon shoulder length, and nominal/maximal inflation pressure impacting angioplasty catheter choice.

1. *Low-pressure balloon angioplasty.* Low-pressure balloon angioplasty (4-10 atm) using balloons 2-4 times larger than the target minimal lumen diameter has been successful in up to 60% of lesions.[13,14]
2. *High-pressure balloon angioplasty.* Success rates with high-pressure balloon angioplasty (10-22 atm) exceed those seen with low-pressure balloons. Furthermore, successful

high-pressure angioplasty is frequently achieved at lower balloon:minimal lumen ratios than those needed for low-pressure angioplasty.[15] Thus, with high-pressure angioplasty, a more conservative approach, starting with ratios of 2-3:1, with incremental increases in the absence of success may be preferable.

3. In recent studies, up to one-third of pulmonary artery stenoses remain resistant to high-pressure balloon angioplasty.[9] Resistance to angioplasty is more common in distal pulmonary arteries while proximal vessels exhibit higher rates of recoil. This is likely related to the variable mechanisms of stenosis at these sites. Restenosis rates of 10%-35% have been reported following simple balloon angioplasty.[9,16]

VII. Cutting Balloon Angioplasty

Cutting balloon angioplasty for pulmonary artery stenosis was first reported in 1999[17] and has since been reported in multiple series and studied in a randomized trial comparing cutting balloon angioplasty to high-pressure balloon angioplasty.[18] Cutting balloons improve the overall success rate for pulmonary artery angioplasty, particularly for lesions resistant to standard high-pressure balloon dilation. The microsurgical blades of the cutting balloon create precise longitudinal "incisions" along the length of the target lesion. The incisions are formed at lower pressures than those required to create an intimal/medial tear with a standard angioplasty balloon, and thus cutting balloons may reduce the risk of vessel rupture. Results are best in pulmonary artery stenoses that exhibit a discrete waist during standard angioplasty. Success in long-segment stenoses, diffusely hypoplastic pulmonary arteries, and pulmonary arteries exhibiting significant recoil is limited.[19]

Small diameter, 6-, 10-, and 15-mm long cutting balloons are available from 2.0 mm to 4.0 mm in diameter in 0.25 mm increments (Flextome, Boston Scientific). These are available as both over-the-wire and monorail systems. Importantly, these only accept a 0.014″ guidewire; thus guidewire exchange is frequently required when switching from a standard angioplasty balloon to a small diameter cutting balloon. Large diameter cutting balloons are limited to 2 cm lengths and are available from 5-8 mm in diameter in 1 mm increments. These balloons require a 0.018″ guidewire.

As with standard balloon angioplasty, cutting balloon size selection is dependent on the minimal lumen diameter of the target lesion and the diameter of the adjacent normal vessel. Successful dilation frequently requires balloon diameters 200%-400% of the minimal lumen diameter. However, the balloon should not be >1-2 mm larger than the adjacent normal vessel. Some operators recommend choosing cutting balloon diameters based on the diameter of the standard angioplasty balloon waist at 8-15 atm, selecting a balloon 0.5-1.0 mm larger than the waist.[10] Cutting balloon dilation can then be followed by angioplasty with a slightly larger standard balloon thus reducing the risk of injury to adjacent normal vasculature.

A. **Complications** Although balloon angioplasty is a relatively safe procedure, there are several complications which the interventionalist should be aware of and prepared to address. Reported complications of balloon angioplasty include: death, pulmonary edema, pneumothorax, hemoptysis, arrhythmia, hypotension, stroke, access site injury, cardiac arrest, target vessel aneurysm formation, occlusive intimal flaps, contained and uncontained transmural pulmonary artery tears.[10] Death is most commonly due to uncontained tears. Mortality rates of 1% to 9% were reported in early case series. However, refinement in technique and improvement in available technologies have reduced the risk of death.

Several factors increase the risk of vessel tears. Balloons exceeding twice the diameter of the proximal or distal "normal" vessel result in significant over-distension and increase the risk for vessel rupture and aneurysm formation, particularly in the smaller distal vessel. Proximal movement of the balloon during inflation may indicate oversizing, and continued forced dilation may result in vessel rupture. Risk is also increased in the setting of severe pulmonary hypertension.

In the case of vessel rupture, coil embolization and covered stent implant may be life saving.[20] Techniques to address an obstructing intimal flap include: covered or bare metal stent implantation.

Reperfusion injury due to the sudden increase in flow and pressure that accompanies a successful angioplasty can result in regional pulmonary edema in the segment subtended by the dilated vessel. This can require prolonged mechanical ventilation and diuretic therapy but typically resolves within 72 hours.[10,21] In the setting of significant ventilation perfusion mismatch, impaired gas exchange due to edema can be severe and even lethal. Increases in distal mean pressure to >20 mm Hg or >150% change in pressure are associated with development of edema.[21]

B. Procedural Considerations

1. General anesthesia allows for airway control/clearance in the setting of pulmonary edema or hemorrhage and improved patient comfort and positioning during long procedures
2. Cross-matched blood should be immediately available
3. Guidewires should be positioned in the largest distal branch possible to minimize distention of the distal vessel by the angioplasty balloon
4. Balloon deployment via a long sheath positioned just proximal to the angioplasty site allows for: rapid angiography between dilations; rapid assessment of pressure; rapid deployment of coils, occlusion devices, and stents if necessary; shielding of cutting balloon microtomes during passage through the heart; and enhanced stability of the balloon during inflation
5. Stenoses limiting flow to the largest segment of lung should be addressed first. If more distal stenoses are present, these should be addressed first to limit passage through previously dilated segments and to allow for timely recognition of reperfusion edema

VIII. Stent Angioplasty

While balloon angioplasty remains an important therapy for the treatment of pulmonary artery stenoses, long-term results are often unsatisfactory.[14] This is particularly true in stenoses related to external compression, kinking, or stretching of the pulmonary artery. Animal and clinical studies have shown that intravascular stents can maintain pulmonary artery patency and improve distal vasculature growth[22-26] (Fig. 7.2B,D, and E). Restenosis due to neointimal proliferation does occur in pulmonary artery stents and has been associated with overdilation, insufficient overlap between adjacent stents, and bifurcation stenosis stenting[25] (Fig. 7.4). While earlier reports demonstrated restenosis rates of 2%-3%,[24,27] a more recent report by Hallbergson et al showed restenosis in 24% of patients. Patients with tetralogy of

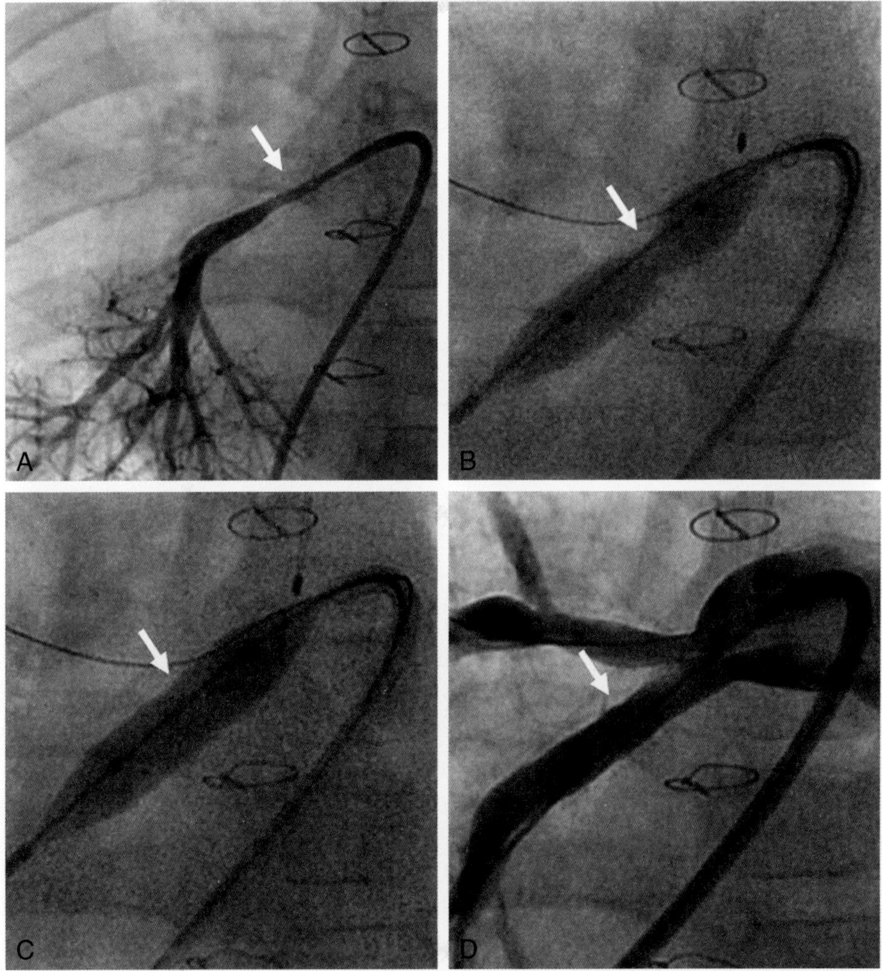

FIGURE 7.4: Balloon pulmonary angioplasty in a patient with Williams syndrome. A, Pulmonary angiogram demonstrating severe in-stent restenosis (arrow). B, Balloon angioplasty demonstrating a discrete waist (arrow) as the balloon expands. C, High pressure balloon angioplasty results in complete resolution of the waist (arrow). D, Post-angioplasty angiogram demonstrating no residual stenosis (arrow).

Fallot and major aortopulmonary collaterals appear to be at particular risk for restenosis and warrant close follow-up after stent placement.[28] Restenosis can most often be addressed with repeat angioplasty.[24,25,27]

A. Considerations and Circumstances for Stent Angioplasty[4,8,29]

1. Central branch pulmonary artery stenosis
2. Stenosis due to stretch or kinking
3. Stenosis that exhibits recoil following balloon angioplasty
4. Stenosis due to external compression
5. Early postoperative stenosis
6. Stenosis due to occlusive intimal flaps following balloon angioplasty
7. Long-segment stenosis

B. Additional Considerations Standard or cutting balloon angioplasty is frequently attempted as a first-line therapy in stenotic pulmonary arteries with stent placement reserved for those vessels that exhibit immediate failure due to significant recoil, occlusive dissection, or late restenosis after angioplasty. Primary stent angioplasty may be considered in long segment stenoses, stenoses due to external compression or "kinking," and bifurcation stenoses as these lesions typically do not respond to simple balloon angioplasty. Stent angioplasty in lesions resistant to balloon expansion can worsen obstruction due to intimal growth if the stenosis is not relieved. Stents places to treat stenoses in the distal vasculature may exhibit greater degrees of late stent stenosis.[30]

Early postoperative pulmonary artery stenoses following congenital heart surgery can significantly increase morbidity and mortality. Stent angioplasty of such stenoses has been shown to be more effective and safer than balloon angioplasty.[4] Although rare, primary stent angioplasty has also been effective in the relief of pulmonary artery obstruction caused by fibrosing mediastinitis and systemic arteritis involving the pulmonary arteries. Reintervention is frequently required due to recurrent obstruction; however, significant improvement in symptoms and survival is possible.[31-33]

IX. Stent Selection

There are no stents specifically designed or approved for use in the pulmonary arteries. Thus operators must repurpose systemic vascular and biliary stents (Table 7.2). Stent selection must take into account patient age and growth potential; the ultimate "adult" pulmonary vessel size must be considered. For example, a stent implanted in the proximal right pulmonary artery must ultimately be able to reach a diameter of at least 16-18 mm. Recent efforts to fracture pulmonary artery stents with ultrahigh-pressure balloons have shown promise. This technique allows for relief of obstruction caused by small but maximally dilated stents that would otherwise require surgical modification.[34,35]

Table 7.2. Available Stents for Pulmonary Artery Stenting

Unmounted Stents (hand crimping required)					
Stent	Available Lengths (mm)	Max Diameter (mm)	Cell Design	Pulmonary Artery Application	
Palmaz XL	30, 40, 50	28	Closed/fixed	Central pulmonary artery branches	
Max LD	16, 26, 36	26	Open/dilateable 12mm	Central pulmonary artery branches; Lobar branches	
Mega LD	16, 26, 36	18	Open/dilateable 12mm	Central pulmonary artery branches; Lobar branches	
Genesis XD	19, 25, 29, 59	18	Closed/dilateable	Central pulmonary artery branches; Lobar branches	
Premounted Stents					
Balloon	Available Diameters (mm)	Max Diameter (mm)	Available Lengths	Guidewire	Cell Design
Large Genesis					
OptaPro	5-10	10	19, 29, 39, 59, 79	0.035	Closed/dilateable
Medium Genesis					
OptaPro	4-8	8	12, 15, 18, 24	0.035	Closed/dilateable
Slalom	3-8	8	15, 18, 24, 39	0.018	Closed/dilateable
Palmaz Blue					
Aviator	4-7	7	15, 17, 20, 25	0.014	Closed/dilateable

Although attractive for their flexibility and low-profile delivery system requirements, use of self-expanding stents in the pulmonary arteries should be avoided. These stents exhibit exuberant neointimal proliferation, lack potential for over-dilation, and have been shown to migrate after implant.[36]

A. **Commonly Used Stents** The most commonly used stents for pulmonary artery stenoses are the Palmaz Genesis series, Palmaz XL series, and the IntraStent Max LD Biliary Stent (Table 7.2).

1. The Genesis stents are available in 3 size ranges—medium, large, and XD "extra-diameter." While the medium- and large-size Genesis stents are attractive because they come premounted on an angioplasty balloon, only the unmounted Genesis XD stents can reach diameters >12 mm. Medium Genesis stents can only reach 8-9 mm in diameter, and thus their use should be limited to segmental and subsegmental pulmonary artery branches. Despite their labeling, large Genesis stents can only reach 10-12 mm in diameter. Thus, although useful for lobar or smaller pulmonary artery branches, they should not routinely be used in proximal branch pulmonary arteries. Genesis XD stents can reach 18 mm in diameter and thus can be used in the central branch pulmonary arteries. However, these stents are only available unmounted and must be crimped by hand onto an angioplasty balloon for delivery. The closed-cell design of the Palmaz Genesis series may limit the ability to open the

cells in situations where a side branch is crossed. However, with currently available ultrahigh-pressure balloons, the stent struts can usually be fractured when necessary; this may negatively impact stent integrity.

2. The Palmaz XL series stents are capable of expanding to 28-30 mm in diameter. However, at these diameters, there is marked foreshortening. These stents have high radial strength but are inflexible, making delivery to the branch pulmonary arteries challenging. In current practice they are most often used for stenting in the main pulmonary artery and right ventricular outflow tract before transcatheter pulmonary valve implantation. Like the Genesis XD series, Palmaz XL stents are only available unmounted and must be hand-crimped onto an angioplasty balloon. They are closed-cell, and fracture of the struts can be difficult. Thus if a side-branch jailing is necessary in a central pulmonary artery, consideration should be given to use of the IntraStent Max LD stents (see below).
3. The IntraStent Max LD stents can achieve diameters up to 26 mm. These stents are significantly more flexible than the Palmaz XL stents but have less radial strength and are more prone to late fracture. They have an open-cell design allowing expansion of the cells to at least 12 mm. Their flexibility and open-cell design allow them to be placed within curvilinear vessels with less distortion than is seen with the closed-cell stents. Lobar, segmental, and subsegmental pulmonary artery stenoses can largely be managed with premounted stents. However, the proximal branch pulmonary arteries and main pulmonary artery require placement of stents capable of reaching diameters of at least 16-18 mm. None of the stents capable of reaching these diameters are currently available premounted. Rather, one must choose a balloon catheter of appropriate size and hand-crimp the stent onto the balloon. In our practice, we most often select a BIB balloon (B Braun) for stent delivery. This balloon-in-balloon catheter consists of two "nested," independently inflatable balloons on a single catheter shaft. It is available with outer balloon diameters of 8-30 mm. The inner balloon is ½ the diameter and 10 mm shorter than the outer balloon. The stent is centered and crimped on the outer balloon. Once at the target lesion, the inner balloon is inflated expanding the center of the stent before the proximal and distal ends. This prevents "dog-boning," where the shoulders of the balloon and hence the ends of the stent expand first. The risk of stent dislodgement is thus reduced. Furthermore, with the stent fixed at ½ its intended diameter, angiography and reposition can be performed before inflation of the outer balloon.
4. For implant of unmounted stents at diameters <8 mm, we use the OptaPro PTA Dilation Catheter (Cordis). While other lower profile balloons are available, we have found that it is difficult to securely hand-crimp a stent onto these very-low-profile balloons.

B. Technique Considerations

Excellent and detailed discussion of the techniques and materials required for pulmonary artery stent angioplasty can be found in Dr. Charles Mullins' textbook "Cardiac Catheterization in Congenital Heart Disease;" (Chapters 22 and 23).[37] The following key points should be considered:

1. Stent procedures should be performed in a biplane angiography–equipped laboratory.
2. General anesthesia should be used for these complex procedures.
3. Cross-matched blood should be immediately available.
4. Arterial access for blood pressure monitoring is recommended.
5. As a consequence of the manufacturing process, premounted medium and large Genesis stents are tightly adherent to their delivery balloon and can thus be safely delivered to the pulmonary arteries over a guidewire without the use of a long delivery sheath.[38] While this technique may be advantageous when implanting stents in infants or postoperative stenoses, in the majority of cases this practice is to be discouraged.
6. Hand-crimped stents should always be delivered to their target vessel through a long sheath. Manually crimped stents can snag and dislodge on Chiari network strands, tricuspid valve leaflets and chordae, outflow tract muscle bands, calcified patches, etc as they transit the right heart.
7. To accommodate the added stent material, a sheath 2-3 French sizes larger than required for the angioplasty balloon should be chosen.
8. Stiff wires, sheaths, and catheters can distort the target anatomy. Check-angiography should be performed through the side-arm of the long sheath or through an additional catheter positioned via a separate access site before balloon inflation. After confirming position, a controlled inflation should be performed. Rapid inflation limits the operator's ability to respond to changes in balloon position and can result in stent malposition.
9. The freshly implanted stent is not adherent to the vessel wall and is at risk for dislodgement; this is particularly true where the stent is not addressing a rigid stenosis (ie stenoses due to external compression or vessel stretch). Techniques to avoid dislodgement should be considered in such situations.[39]

c. **Complications** Complications associated with stent angioplasty include stent malposition, stent migration/dislodgement, occlusion/jailing of side branches, vessel rupture, dissection, compression of adjacent structures including bronchi and coronary arteries, pulmonary edema, and thrombosis.[25,40,41]

X. Therapeutic Algorithm

Therapeutic algorithms for pulmonary artery stenosis are complex and require consideration of etiology, location, patient age and growth potential, underlying cardiopulmonary physiology, and need for future surgery. Bergersen and Lock[10] provide an excellent review of catheter-based therapies for pulmonary artery stenosis. As a general framework the following algorithm can be followed as shown in Fig. 7.5.

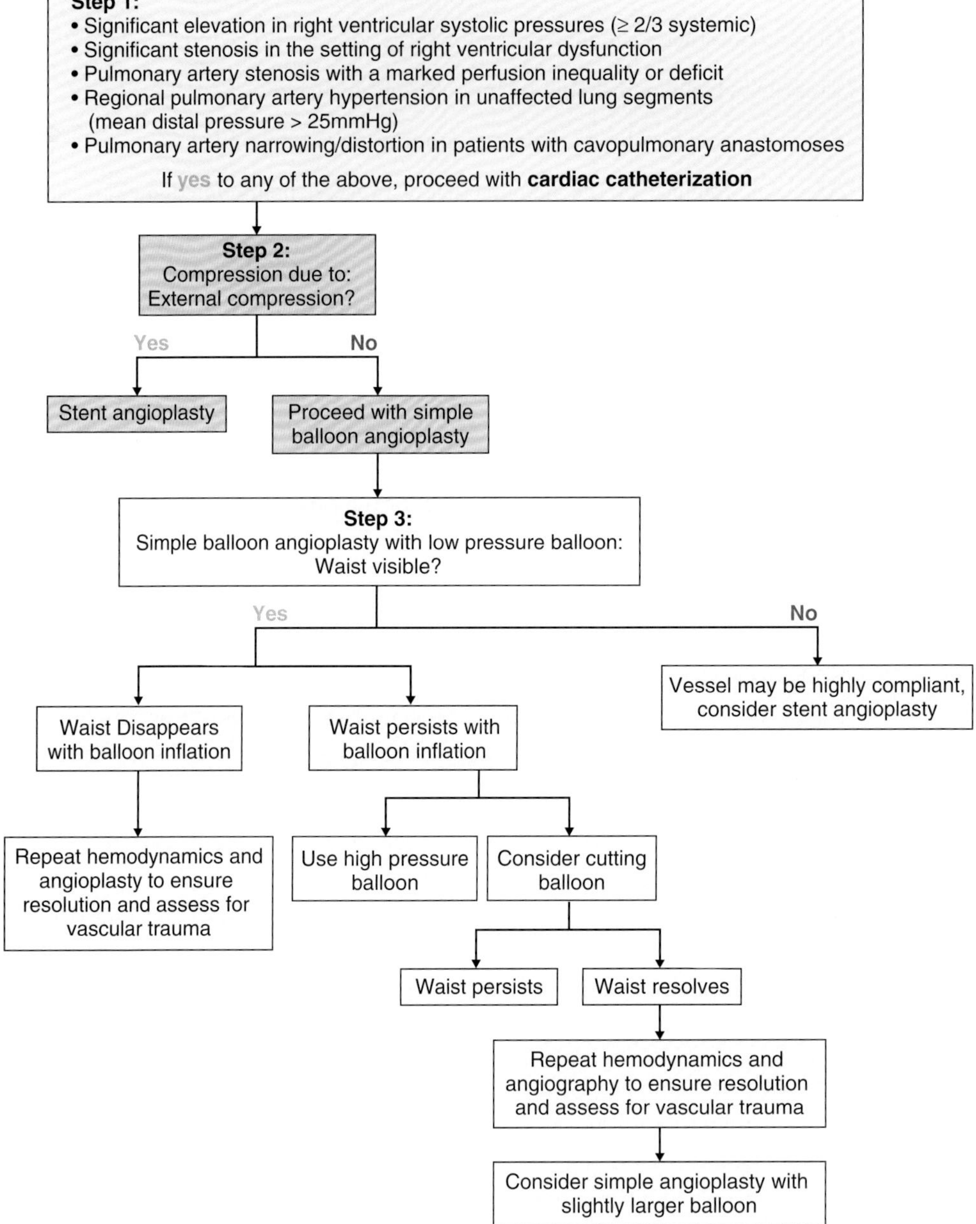

FIGURE 7.5: Therapeutic algorithm for the management of pulmonary artery stenosis.

References

1. Franch R, Gay BB. Congenital stenosis of the pulmonary artery branches: a classification, with postmortem findings in two cases. *Am J Med*. 1963;35:512-529.
2. Kreutzer J, Landzberg MJ, Preminger TJ, et al. Isolated peripheral pulmonary artery stenoses in the adult. *Circulation*. 1996;93(7):1417-1423.
3. Tonelli AR, Ahmed M, Hamed F, Prieto LR. Peripheral pulmonary artery stenosis as a cause of pulmonary hypertension in adults. *Pulm Circ*. 2015;5(1):204-210.

4. Rosales AM, Lock JE, Perry SB, Geggel RL. Interventional catheterization management of perioperative peripheral pulmonary stenosis: balloon angioplasty or endovascular stenting. *Catheter Cardiovasc Interv.* 2002;56(2):272-277.
5. Sutton NJ, Peng L, Lock JE, et al. Effect of pulmonary artery angioplasty on exercise function after repair of tetralogy of Fallot. *Am Heart J.* 2008;155(1):182-186.
6. Lock JE, Niemi T, Einzig S, Amplatz K, Burke B, Bass JL. Transvenous angioplasty of experimental branch pulmonary artery stenosis in newborn lambs. *Circulation.* 1981;64(5):886-893.
7. Rocchini AP, Kveselis D, Dick M, Crowley D, Snider AR, Rosenthal A. Use of balloon angioplasty to treat peripheral pulmonary stenosis. *Am J Cardiol.* 1984;54(8):1069-1073.
8. Bacha EA, Kreutzer J. Comprehensive management of branch pulmonary artery stenosis. *J Interv Cardiol.* 2001;14(3):367-376.
9. Bergersen L, Gauvreau K, Lock JE, Jenkins KJ. Recent results of pulmonary arterial angioplasty: the differences between proximal and distal lesions. *Cardiol Young.* 2005;15(06):597-604.
10. Bergersen L, Lock JE. What is the current option of first choice for treatment of pulmonary arterial stenosis?. *Cardiol Young.* 2006;16(4):329-338.
11. Edwards BS, Lucas R, Lock JE, Edwards JE. Morphologic changes in the pulmonary arteries after percutaneous balloon angioplasty for pulmonary arterial stenosis. *Circulation.* 1985;71(2):195-201.
12. Stock JH, Reller MD, Sharma S, Pavcnik D, Shiota T, Sahn DJ. Transballoon intravascular ultrasound imaging during balloon angioplasty in animal models with coarctation and branch pulmonary stenosis. *Circulation.* 1997;95(10):2354-2357.
13. Gentles TL, Lock JE, Perry SB. High pressure balloon angioplasty for branch pulmonary artery stenosis: early experience. *J Am Coll Cardiol.* 1993;22(3):867-872.
14. Rothman A, Perry SB, Keane JF, Lock JE. Early results and follow-up of balloon angioplasty for branch pulmonary artery stenoses. *J Am Coll Cardiol.* 1990;15(5):1109-1117.
15. Ettinger LM, Hijazi ZM, Geggel RL, Supran SE, Cao Q-L, Schmid CH. Peripheral pulmonary artery stenosis: acute and mid-term results of high pressure balloon angioplasty. *J Interv Cardiol.* 1998;11(4):337-344.
16. Bush DM, Hoffman TM, Del Rosario J, Eiriksson H, Rome JJ. Frequency of restenosis after balloon pulmonary arterioplasty and its causes. *Am J Cardiol.* 2000;86(11):1205-1209.
17. Schneider M, Zartner P, Magee A. Cutting balloon for treatment of severe peripheral pulmonary stenoses in a child. *Heart.* 1999;82(1):108.
18. Bergersen L, Gauvreau K, Justino H, et al. Randomized trial of cutting balloon compared with high-pressure angioplasty for the treatment of resistant pulmonary artery stenosis. *Circulation.* 2011;124(22):2388-2396.
19. Sugiyama H, Veldtman GR, Norgard G, Lee KJ, Chaturvedi R, Benson LN. Bladed balloon angioplasty for peripheral pulmonary artery stenosis. *Catheter Cardiovasc Interv.* 2004;62(1):71-77.
20. Baker CM, McGowan FX, Keane JF, Lock JE. Pulmonary artery trauma due to balloon dilation: recognition, avoidance and management. *J Am Coll Cardiol.* 2000;36(5):1684-1690.
21. Arnold LW, Keane JF, Kan JS, Fellows KE, Lock JE. Transient unilateral pulmonary edema after successful balloon dilation of peripheral pulmonary artery stenosis. *Am J Cardiol.* 1988;62(4):327-330.
22. Mullins CE, O'laughlin MP, Vick GW, et al. Implantation of balloon-expandable intravascular grafts by catheterization in pulmonary arteries and systemic veins. *Circulation.* 1988;77(1):188-199.
23. O'laughlin MP, Perry SB, Lock JE, Mullins CE. Use of endovascular stents in congenital heart disease. *Circulation.* 1991;83(6):1923-1939.
24. Ing FF, Grifka RG, Nihill MR, Mullins CE. Repeat dilation of intravascular stents in congenital heart defects. *Circulation.* 1995;92(4):893-897.
25. Krisnanda C, Menahem S, Lane GK. Intravascular stent implantation for the management of pulmonary artery stenosis. *Heart Lung Circ.* 2013;22(1):56-70.
26. Takao CM, El Said H, Connolly D, Hamzeh RK, Ing FF. Impact of stent implantation on pulmonary artery growth. *Catheter Cardiovasc Interv.* 2013;82(3):445-452.
27. McMahon CJ, El-Said HG, Grifka RG, Fraley JK, Nihill MR, Mullins CE. Redilation of endovascular stents in congenital heart disease: factors implicated in the development of restenosis and neointimal proliferation. *J Am Coll Cardiol.* 2001;38(2):521-526.

28. Hallbergson A, Lock JE, Marshall AC. Frequency and risk of in-stent stenosis following pulmonary artery stenting. *Am J Cardiol.* 2014;113(3):541-545.
29. Peters B, Ewert P, Berger F. The role of stents in the treatment of congenital heart disease: current status and future perspectives. *Ann Pediatr Cardiol.* 2009;2(1):3.
30. Vranicar M, Teitel DF, Moore P. Use of small stents for rehabilitation of hypoplastic pulmonary arteries in pulmonary atresia with ventricular septal defect. *Catheter Cardiovasc Interv.* 2002;55(1):78-82.
31. Furtado AD, Shivanna DN, Rao SPK, Bhat S, Suresh S, Peer SM. Pulmonary artery bypass for in-stent stenosis following angioplasty for isolated pulmonary takayasu arteritis. *J Card Surg.* 2012;27(3):365-367.
32. Albers EL, Pugh ME, Hill KD, Wang L, Loyd JE, Doyle TP. Percutaneous vascular stent implantation as treatment for central vascular obstruction due to fibrosing mediastinitis. *Circulation.* 2011;123(13):1391-1399.
33. Ferguson ME, Cabalka AK, Cetta F, Hagler DJ. Results of intravascular stent placement for fibrosing mediastinitis. *Congenit Heart Dis.* 2010;5(2):124-133.
34. Morray BH, McElhinney DB, Marshall AC, Porras D. Intentional fracture of maximally dilated balloon-expandable pulmonary artery stents using ultra-high-pressure balloon angioplasty: a preliminary analysis. *Catheter Cardiovasc Interv.* 2016;9(4).
35. Maglione J, Bergersen L, Lock JE, McElhinney DB. Ultra-high-pressure balloon angioplasty for treatment of resistant stenoses within or adjacent to previously implanted pulmonary arterial stents. *Circ Cardiovasc Interv.* 2009;2(1):52-58.
36. Cheung Y-f, Sanatani S, Leung MP, Human DG, Chau AK, Culham JG. Early and intermediate-term complications of self-expanding stents limit its potential application in children with congenital heart disease. *J Am Coll Cardiol.* 2000;35(4):1007-1015.
37. Mullins CE. *Cardiac Catheterization in Congenital Heart Disease: Pediatric and Adult*: John Wiley & Sons; 2008.
38. Pass RH, Hsu DT, Garabedian CP, Schiller MS, Jayakumar KA, Hellenbrand WE. Endovascular stent implantation in the pulmonary arteries of infants and children without the use of a long vascular sheath. *Catheter Cardiovasc Interv.* 2002;55(4):505-509.
39. Recto MR, Frank F, Grifka RG, Nihill MR, Mullins CE. A technique to prevent newly implanted stent displacement during subsequent catheter and sheath manipulation. *Catheter Cardiovasc Interv.* 2000;49(3):297-300.
40. Hamzeh RK, El-Said HG, Moore JW. Left main coronary artery compression from right pulmonary artery stenting. *Catheter Cardiov Interv.* 2009;73(2):197-202.
41. O'Byrne ML, Rome N, Santamaria RWL, et al. Intra-procedural bronchoscopy to prevent bronchial compression during pulmonary artery stent angioplasty. *Pediatr Cardiol.* 2016;37(3):433-441.

CHAPTER 8

Renovascular Disease

John F. Setaro, MD, FACC, FSCAI

Key Points

- Atherosclerotic disease underlies renal artery stenosis in 90% of cases.
- Guidelines recommend revascularization as a Class I indication for hemodynamically significant renovascular disease with recurrent unexplained heart failure or flash pulmonary edema.
- Invasive evaluation may include angiography with measurement of percentage stenosis as well as more physiologic measures such as resting ratio of distal artery to aortic pressure (Pd/Pa) <0.90, hyperemic fractional flow reserve value (Pd/Pa) <0.80, hyperemic mean gradient >20 mm Hg, hyperemic systolic gradient >20 mm Hg, or intravascular ultrasound (IVUS)–derived MLA <8.6 mm sq.
- Self-expanding stent placement by femoral access is the most common technique in treatment of renal artery stenosis.

I. Introduction

This chapter aims to survey disorders of the renal vessels, with an emphasis on diagnosis and treatment of arterial disease (medical, transcatheter, surgical), as well as to review novel catheter-based techniques (such as renal sympathetic denervation) designed to treat multi-drug-resistant hypertension and other circulatory conditions.

Renovascular disease, often termed renal artery stenosis, is typically of atherosclerotic origin and is a relatively frequent finding, particularly in the older population who may have concomitant atherosclerotic disease in other vascular distributions. Yet most structural renovascular disease that may be visible angiographically does not cause hypertension (renovascular hypertension) or renal ischemia as large angiographic series have demonstrated, with recent major trial evidence showing that optimized medical therapy rather than mechanical intervention may be appropriate in most cases. However, a subset of individuals who have resistant hypertension,[1] advancing renal dysfunction (especially with bilateral disease),[2] or flash pulmonary edema should be identified and treated by revascularization.[3]

II. Anatomic Considerations

In most cases, there is a single renal artery bilaterally (typically 5-7 mm diameter), with origins at the L1-L2 level of the aorta, each dividing into segmental, lobar, interlobar, arcuate, and interlobular branches.[4] In a minority of cases, anatomic variations may include dual renal arteries, accessory renal arteries, or early segmental branching renal arteries.[5] When the main renal artery is occluded, potential collateral sources (intercostal, lumbar, internal iliac, and adrenal arteries) may provide immediate viability but not long-term preservation of functioning renal mass.[4,6]

III. Pathophysiologic Factors and Natural History

A. **Systemic Hypertension Caused by Renovascular Disease** The mechanism of systemic hypertension caused by renovascular disease was first elucidated in 1934 through Goldblatt's experimental renal artery clamping models[7] and is founded upon reduced renal perfusion pressure leading to activation of the renin-angiotensin system with consequent release of serum renin and angiotensin II. Renin is released in response to diminished perfusion pressure at the juxtaglomerular apparatus of the afferent renal arterioles and in response to reduced sodium and chloride delivery to the macula densa segment of the ascending loop of Henle.[8] In turn, systemic vasoconstriction, sympathetic activation, and aldosterone-mediated depression of sodium excretion with consequent volume expansion will follow.

B. Pulmonary Congestion

1. These pathologic adaptations can promote sudden pulmonary congestion (flash pulmonary edema) and may exacerbate myocardial ischemia in vulnerable individuals. Locally, efferent arteriolar constriction governed by release of angiotensin II acts as a compensatory response favoring continued renal perfusion and explains why in the

setting of significant bilateral disease (or unilateral disease in a uninephric individual), there will be a rise in serum creatinine when antihypertensive pharmacologic inhibitors of the renin-angiotensin system are used. On the other hand, when unilateral disease is present, inhibitors of the renin-angiotensin system may be very useful in controlling hypertension (caused by activation of the renin-angiotensin system in renovascular hypertension), without a rise in serum creatinine, provided that the contralateral kidney is healthy and that functional renal mass is preserved.[9]

2. The abnormal vasoconstricted as well as volume-expanded pathophysiologic state of true renovascular hypertension highlights the importance of combined vasodilator and diuretic therapy for pharmacologic management.[8]

C. **Late Renal Ischemia and Dysfunction** It is interesting to consider that late renal ischemia and dysfunction may be founded upon several factors beyond simple reduced arterial blood flow, given that the kidney has relatively minimal oxygen requirements.[10,11] These extraischemic factors may encompass direct hypertensive injury to both ischemic and unaffected kidney, distal atheroembolic phenomena, and the generation of angiotensin II–based profibrotic mediators (transforming growth factor-beta [TGF-β], nuclear factor-kB, and platelet-derived growth factor [PDGF]).[4,12,13] Restoring renal artery blood flow alone through relief of stenosis may not be enough to reverse many of these late changes.[14]

D. **Atherosclerotic Renovascular Disease**

1. The progressive nature of atherosclerotic renovascular disease is underscored by several series that showed significant rates of progression of stenosis as well as occlusion by angiography or duplex ultrasound: progression in 44% of individuals and occlusion in 16% at 4 years,[15] progression in 11% of individuals at 2.6 years,[16] and progression in 35% of individuals at 3 years and 52% at 5 years (49% at 3 y if the baseline stenosis was >60%).[17]

2. Untreated severe disease with reduced renal blood flow may lead to the ischemic loss of functioning renal mass and has been linked to greater degree of stenosis and higher blood pressure.[18] In a second series, at 1 year there was at least a 1.0 cm reduction in kidney size in 13% of subjects with unilateral disease and in 43% of subjects who had bilateral disease.[19]

3. Overall, renovascular disease is a marker for poor long-term outcomes,[20] with far worse five-year survival in a recently surveyed community congestive heart failure cohort when compared with those subjects free of renovascular disease.[21]

IV. Clinical Presentations

A. **Literature** The medical literature supports a significant association between renovascular disease (typically defined as structural anatomic lesions greater than 50% stenosis diameter) and classical Framingham atherosclerotic risk factors (smoking, diabetes, hyperlipidemia, age), as well as aortic and peripheral vascular disease (38%)

and coronary artery disease (6.3%-23%), with a 7% prevalence of renovascular disease in the general older population.[3,4,22,23] A correlation has been noted between renovascular disease and two- to three-vessel coronary artery disease.[24] Longitudinal studies support the progressive nature of renovascular disease as noted above, especially when lesions are initially found to be severe, but it has been pointed out correctly that most of these retrospective as well as prospective series predate the inception of ideal medical therapies (aspirin, clopidogrel and other novel antiplatelet compounds, statins, modern antihyperglycemic agents, renin-angiotensin-aldosterone inhibitors) and lifestyle interventions (diet and weight control, exercise, sodium restriction, and smoking cessation).[4] This observation also sheds light on why optimized medical therapy has proved equally effective as revascularization in the most recent randomized prospective trials.[25] Presence and severity of renovascular disease is also associated with all-cause long-term mortality, likely reflecting the adverse implications of generalized systemic atherosclerotic vascular disease.[26]

B. **Population** The true prevalence of renovascular hypertension is less than 1% in the general population but may be much higher in states of resistant hypertension[27-29] or in the presence of other suggestive clinical features listed below (7.3% of 837 of such patients had at least a 70% stenosis of one or both renal arteries).[30,31] Clinical indicators of physiologically significant renovascular disease include (1) multidrug-resistant hypertension[1,32] or malignant hypertension (Grade III or IV Keith-Wagener retinal changes [hemorrhages and exudates, papilledema, respectively] have been associated) or the rapid acceleration of previously well-regulated hypertension,[33] (2) disparity in renal size or the presence of an atrophic (ischemic) kidney, (3) rise in serum creatinine following administration of inhibitors of the renin-angiotensin system (suggesting bilateral disease or unilateral disease in single kidney), or (4) sudden unexplained pulmonary edema or medically refractory angina pectoris. Onset of hypertension at a very young or a very old age may also provide a clue to significant renovascular disease (Table 8.1). The finding of a systolic and diastolic abdominal bruit radiating to the flank may be of contributory interest, yet as a physical sign lacks high sensitivity or specificity for the diagnosis of physiologically significant renovascular disease.

TABLE 8.1. Clinical Indicators Favoring a Search for Renovascular Hypertension
Onset of severe hypertension at extremes of age
Loss of regulation of previously well-controlled hypertension
Multidrug-resistant hypertension
Tobacco use
Atherosclerotic disease in multiple vascular distributions
Unexplained new renal impairment
Unexplained flash pulmonary edema
Refractory angina
Malignant hypertension, including retinal hemorrhages, exudates, and papilledema
Disparity in kidney size
Rise in serum creatinine after inception of renin-angiotensin system-inhibiting therapy

V. Atherosclerotic Renovascular Disease

A. It is estimated that atherosclerotic disease underlies renal artery stenosis in 90% of cases.[27] Nonatherosclerotic causes, the most frequent being fibromuscular dysplasia, are reviewed below. In most cases, the presence of structural atherosclerotic renovascular disease is not the cause of hypertension (renovascular hypertension) or ischemia of the kidney, and historically most catheter-based revascularizations that were performed without good evidence favoring true renovascular hypertension did not afford benefit.[34] In parallel with this observation, recent trial evidence, presented below, indicates that patients who have well controlled hypertension and normal renal function should be treated conservatively. Yet resistant hypertension, flash pulmonary edema, or progressive renal impairment with renal ischemia (especially in the context of bilateral disease), may require revascularization, thus improving clinical management and preventing the need for renal replacement therapy.[35,36]

B. Because there is considerable clinical overlap among states of (1) essential hypertension, (2) renovascular hypertension, (3) anatomic renal artery stenosis, (4) diabetic nephropathy, and (5) chronic renal impairment, methods of assessing the functional significance of anatomic renal artery disease will assume importance, as noted below.[37,38] Alternatively, although proteinuria is a feature in many forms of renal disease including ischemia, renal disease unrelated to stenosis may be reflected in an active urinary sediment (typically acellular in the setting of renal ischemia).[4,39] Additionally, elevated creatinine in the setting of unilateral stenotic disease suggests nonstenotic etiologies because a single remaining healthy contralateral kidney that is well perfused will maintain a normal creatinine value.[27] However, a rapid rise in serum creatinine may portend a better result postrevascularization, suggesting reversibility.[4,33] Of note, a group of investigators has reported a 24% prevalence of severe atherosclerotic renovascular disease in end-stage renal disease patients being considered for dialysis.[40]

VI. Nonatherosclerotic Renovascular Disease

A. Fibromuscular Dysplasia

1. The most common cause of nonatherosclerotic renovascular disease is fibromuscular dysplasia, often seen in younger women who are hypertensive yet otherwise free of classic atherosclerotic risk factors. One-third of cases of renal artery fibromuscular dysplasia are bilateral, and there is a familial component as well as a genetic association with polymorphisms of the renin-angiotensin system, specifically higher frequency of the angiotensin-converting enzyme (ACE) I allele.[41] It has been proposed that, because this allele is linked to lower circulating levels of angiotensin-converting enzyme and possibly lower tissue levels of angiotensin II (which regulates vascular smooth muscle growth and synthetic activity), the presence of the I allele may foster abnormal remodeling of the arterial media thus promoting fibromuscular dysplasia.[41]

2. Unlike the atherosclerotic lesion which classically involves the aorta and ostium and proximal renal artery, a fibromuscular dysplastic stenosis tends to show a beaded

appearance (reflecting the tissue webs or baffles that restrict blood flow), and resides in the distal two-thirds of the main renal artery or its principal branches[42] (Fig. 8.1).

3. As distinct from atherosclerotic renovascular disease, fibromuscular dysplasia rarely progresses to total occlusion or ischemic nephropathy. In addition to predilection for young females, fibromuscular dysplastic renovascular disease has been linked to tobacco consumption, alpha-1 antitrypsin deficiency, use of ergotamine or methysergide, pheochromocytoma, type IV Ehlers-Danlos syndrome, cystic medial necrosis, Alport syndrome, neurofibromatosis, and coarctation of the aorta.[43] This species of renovascular disease responds well to simple balloon angioplasty and exhibits durable results, without the need for intra-arterial stent placement[44] (Figs. 8.1–8.3).

B. **Other Rare Nonatherosclerotic Forms of Renovascular Disease** Other rare nonatherosclerotic forms of renovascular disease include vasculitis, neurocutaneous syndromes such as neurofibromatosis, Takayasu arteritis, aneurysms, congenital or posttraumatic arteriovenous fistulae, congenital bands, postradiation changes, spontaneous dissection, thromboembolization (typically cardiac in origin, from atrial fibrillation), atheroembolization, steal syndrome in the setting of celiac axis occlusion, or the vascular compressive effects of large renal cysts, pheochromocytoma, retroperitoneal fibrosis, or posttraumatic external scarring (Page kidney).[37,45] Regarding renal artery thromboembolization, there is scant experience reported in the literature describing catheter-based techniques for renal reperfusion, for instance local thrombolysis. Posttransplant renal vasculopathy, often appearing within 1 year of transplant, presents with renal impairment, hypertension, and circulatory congestion and is best managed with angioplasty and stenting.[46]

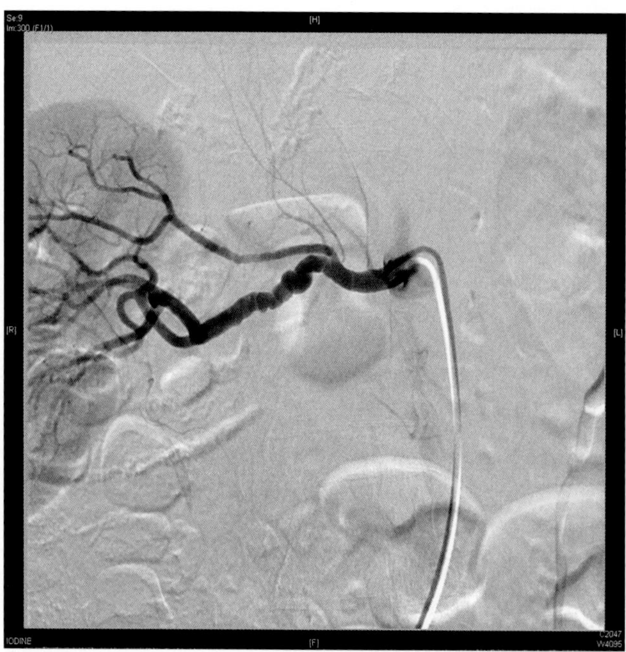

FIGURE 8.1: Renovascular disease: Fibromuscular dysplasia. Diagnostic angiography using a 5F internal mammary artery catheter to inject the right renal artery in a 67-year-old female patient who demonstrated three-drug-resistant hypertension. Procedure was conducted via the right common femoral artery. There is a slight inferior angulation to the origin of the right renal artery. Note the beaded appearance of the mid-vessel consistent with fibromuscular dysplasia. Courtesy of Jeptha P. Curtis MD.

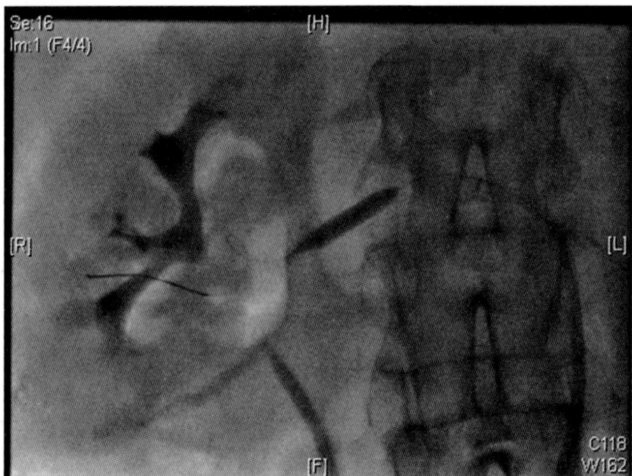

FIGURE 8.2: Renovascular disease: Fibromuscular dysplasia. Following administration of 7000-u unfractionated heparin, using a telescoping technique, a 7F renal double curve sheath guide was advanced over the 5F internal mammary artery catheter. Following the finding of a 15 mm Hg mean gradient across the stenotic region, angioplasty was performed using a 4.0 mm then a 5.0 mm balloon to a maximum pressure of 6 atm.

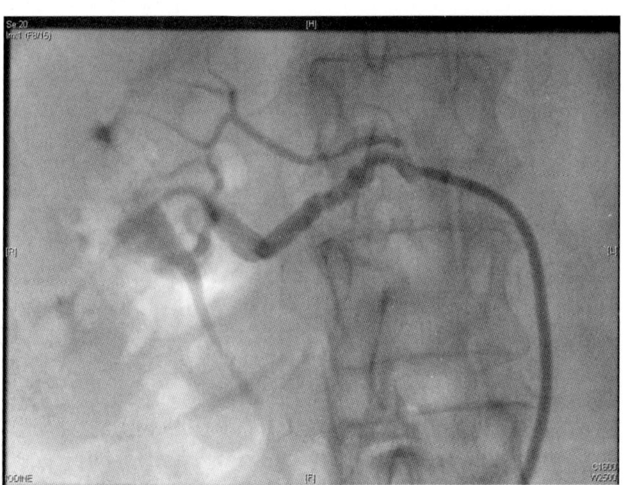

FIGURE 8.3: Renovascular disease: Fibromuscular dysplasia. Completion angiogram shows favorable result, revealing <20% residual stenosis. Subsequent clinical course is noteworthy for minimization of antihypertensive regimen and good preservation of renal function.

VII. Diagnostic Examinations

When clinical presentation is strongly suggestive of functionally significant renovascular disease, noninvasive assessment is indicated, with several methods each harboring advantages and disadvantages.

A. **Renal Duplex Ultrasound** Renal duplex ultrasound is useful when good acoustic windows are available in leaner individuals. When performed well technically and interpreted in a competent manner, this method can define kidney sizes, chart the progression of loss of renal mass, estimate the degree of echogenicity of the renal cortex, and illustrate the condition of the distal microvasculature. A physiologically significant stenosis may be reflected by a peak systolic velocity of >200 cm/s and a renal artery/aortic peak systolic velocity ratio of 3.5.[47] Renal resistive index (peak systolic velocity−end diastolic velocity/peak systolic velocity) can demonstrate the degree of microvascular resistance and may predict benefit of revascularization. However, threshold values have not yet been fully defined in the literature,[42] although 0.80 conventionally has been the upper limit of normal. Higher values suggest distal microvascular disease and have been linked with failure to improve clinically following main artery revascularization.[48]

B. **Captopril Renal Artery Scintigraphy** Captopril renal artery scintigraphy uses nuclear perfusion assessments before and after ACE inhibitor stimulation to determine whether arterial flow is dependent on efferent arteriolar vasoconstriction under the influence of angiotensin II, therefore confirming that functionally significant renovascular hypertension is present.[49] When comparing two kidneys, abnormal unilateral function may identify significant renovascular disease and predict improvement following revascularization.[50] However, while specificity is high, sensitivity may not be adequate, particularly in cases of bilateral disease (or unilateral disease in a single kidney) or low glomerular filtration rate. There is little role for previous methods such as intravenous pyelography or measurement of plasma renin activity. Early studies indicate a promising role for assays of brain natriuretic peptide (BNP, or B-type natriuretic peptide) in predicting blood pressure response postrevascularization.[51]

C. **Angiography**

1. **CT angiography** may provide useful images, but radiation burden and nephrotoxic radiocontrast exposure represent concerns. Moreover, this technique may fail to distinguish intraluminal stenosis from extravascular calcification.[42] Stenosis of >75% (or 50% with poststenotic dilatation) may be considered significant.
2. **MR angiography** is probably the most useful contemporary technique, requiring no radiation, although there is a false positive rate. A stenosis of >80% may be viewed as significant. However, its gadolinium contrast agent must be used with great caution when renal disease is present given the risk of development of nephrogenic systemic sclerosis. Questions also surround the significance of long-term deposition of gadolinium in bone and brain tissue.
3. **Invasive renal vein sampling** for renin measurement has suboptimal sensitivity and specificity, although lateralizing values predict treatment response.
4. **Percutaneous renal angiography** carries the risks of any invasive catheter-based procedure (bleeding, infection, embolization, vessel or kidney damage, radiation exposure, radiocontrast requirement), yet provides excellent images, is highly sensitive and specific for the depiction of vascular stenosis, permits immediate physiologic assessments, and allows balloon or stent revascularization in the same setting. Angiography is, however, relatively low risk and serves as the gold standard for visualization of the renal arteries.

   Femoral artery access is most commonly used, but upper extremity (radial or brachial artery) can be employed if the origin of the renal artery is angulated inferiorly[42] or if there is major infrarenal aortoiliac disease (Fig. 8.1). Nonselective abdominal aortography performed at the T12-L1 level uses a pigtail catheter with power injection using dilute radiocontrast and digital subtraction angiography.[47] The nonselective view elucidates the presence and number of renal arteries, as well as important aortic conditions such as protruding atherosclerotic plaque that could interfere with subsequent selective renal angiography.[42,47] With advanced renal impairment, carbon dioxide may act safely as a contrast medium.

5. In terms of angiographic views, selective renal artery angiography may require a slight degree of left anterior oblique angulation given the anterior origin of the right renal artery that is slightly superior to the orifice of the left renal artery, arising more posteriorly.[4] From the femoral approach, catheter selection may include internal mammary (Fig. 8.1), JR4, cobra, renal double curve, hockey stick, multipurpose, or SOS Omni.[42,47] Via upper extremity approaches, a 90-cm long 6F or 7F vascular sheath may prove useful, through which a 5F or 6F internal mammary artery, multipurpose, or JR4 catheter can be advanced to the orifice of the renal artery.

D. Discovery of Stenosis

1. If a stenosis is discovered, determination of physiologic or functional significance may be useful because there is a limited correlation between angiographic severity and functional significance, particularly in the case of fibromuscular dysplasia.[38] Simple measurement of translesional pressure gradient may be useful (Fig. 8.4) yet is not fully informative, however, because it does not consider other variables such as aortic pressure, catheter caliber, potential vasoconstricted condition of the downstream renal vasculature, and the ambient renal venous pressure (which could be elevated in many states, including congestive heart failure)[4] (Fig. 8.2). Translesional measurements can be accomplished by placing a 4F catheter distal to the stenosis, compared against a 6 or 7F guiding catheter, which would be located proximal to the stenosis. Because of its smaller size and therefore lesser propensity to increase artificially the measured gradient, a 0.014 pressure wire may be preferable here.[33] It has

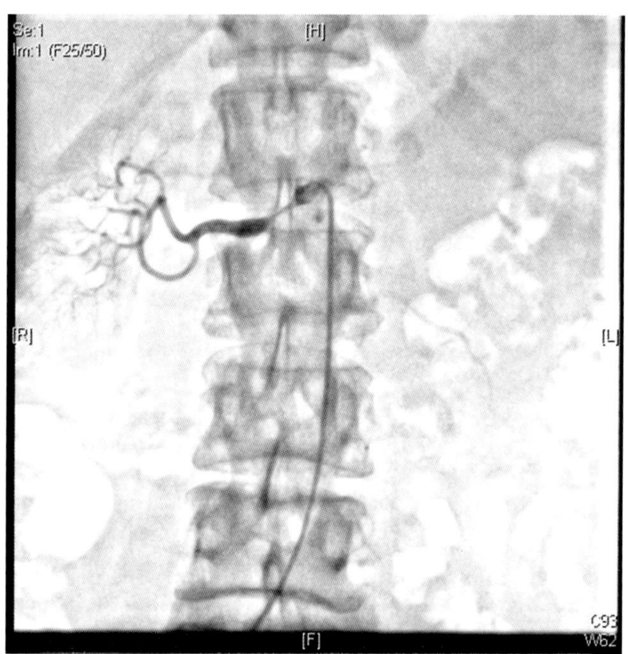

FIGURE 8.4: Renovascular disease. Atherosclerotic renal artery stenosis. Diagnostic angiography was performed via a telescoping 5 F internal mammary artery/7F renal double curve sheath guide in the case of a 65-year-old female who suffered with difficult to regulate angina, labile hypertension, and ultrasound-documented progressive loss of right renal mass. Procedure was conducted via the right common femoral artery, with discovery of a 90% right renal artery ostial stenosis. A 50% left renal artery stenosis was found to have a systolic gradient of <10 mm Hg, and was therefore selected for optimal medical therapy. Courtesy of Michael S. Remetz MD.

been suggested that a mean translesional gradient of 10 mm Hg or a peak-to-peak systolic gradient of 20 mm Hg should be considered significant for intervention.[33]

2. Stimulated hyperemic gradients and fractional flow reserve (using pressure wire) can pharmacologically eliminate distal vasoconstriction and, in a manner analogous to coronary lesion functional assessment, can provide a more accurate picture of lesion severity and may predict response to treatment. In most situations, the renal fractional flow reserve equals the ratio of the hyperemic pressure distal to the stenosis divided by the mean aortic pressure measured by pressure wire evaluation.[52] To stimulate the hyperemic response, papaverine (30-40 mg intra-arterial) has been recommended (and must be used with heparin-free saline to avoid an unwanted precipitate), and adenosine should not be used because of the possibility of paradoxical renal arteriolar vasoconstriction.[42] Other vasodilators such as dopamine (50 mcg/kg intra-arterial) and fenoldopam have been studied. IVUS for measurement of minimal luminal area (MLA) may be considered, and this technique may help to define severity of questionable lesions and to localize the true ostium if there is uncertainty.[33,53]

3. Recent recommendations favor the diagnosis of functionally significant renovascular disease (meriting revascularization) if one of the following criteria is present: (1) resting ratio of distal artery to aortic pressure (Pd/Pa) <0.90, (2) hyperemic fractional flow reserve value (Pd/Pa) <0.80, (3) hyperemic mean gradient >20 mm Hg, (4) hyperemic systolic gradient >20 mm Hg, or (5) IVUS-derived MLA <8.6 mm sq.[42]

4. It may be worth considering some limitations in physiologic measurements: because fractional flow reserve is dependent on the degree of hyperemic flow achieved pharmacologically, greater hyperemic flow creates higher pressure gradients and thus lower fractional flow reserve values (and vice versa).[38] Consequently, because of the lesser vasodilator reserve of the renal arterial bed (as opposed to the coronary circulation), the difference between baseline and stimulated hyperemic gradients is smaller than in the coronary circulation. It follows also that in the renal artery the differences between normal and abnormal fractional flow reserves are smaller and that the predictive value of resting gradients is nearly equal to that of pharmacologically provoked gradients.[38] Thus, investigative challenges remain in defining the optimal physiologic analytics for functional renovascular disease.

5. In addition to considering other causes for renal impairment or hypertension, kidney viability should be evaluated before revascularization is attempted. Useful parameters will include kidney size, recent decline in renal function, nuclear renal perfusion, and renal resistive index measurements.[4]

VIII. Renal Revascularization: Early Surgical Experience

Early surgical methods for treatment of renovascular hypertension encompassed nephrectomy of the pressor kidney and the use of venous conduits for aorto-renal artery bypass grafting, as well as extra-anatomic hepatorenal (right) or splenorenal (left) bypass grafting under selected clinical circumstances. More recently, because of the recognition of higher morbidity and mortality with surgery versus catheter-based methods, the latter have been preferred.

IX. Renal Revascularization: Balloon Angioplasty

Initially described by Gruntzig in 1978, percutaneous balloon angioplasty demonstrated reasonably durable results and became a widely used minimally invasive alternative to surgical renal artery bypass.[54] Although supplanted by endoluminal stenting in recent years, simple balloon angioplasty maintains an important role in the treatment of renovascular disease of fibromuscular dysplastic origin (Figs. 8.1–8.3).

X. Renal Revascularization: Endoluminal Stenting

Endoluminal stenting for renovascular disease has been shown to provide better procedural and long-term outcomes compared against simple balloon angioplasty in a prospective randomized trial.[42,55] Observational series have confirmed a very high technical success rate for renal artery stenting (3): overall mortality rate is low (0.8%), less than 8% risk of major complications (stroke, myocardial infarction, hemorrhage requiring transfusion, renal artery perforation, or urgent surgery), and less than 5% risk of eventual need for renal replacement therapy (dialysis or transplant).[4] With good technique, renal artery stent restenosis rates are less than 15%,[23] and the procedure can be accomplished safely and successfully even in the context of advanced renal impairment.[56] Renal duplex ultrasound represents a reasonable method of longitudinal poststent clinical noninvasive surveillance.

Before the procedure, aspirin and adequate prehydration to minimize contrast nephropathy are advisable. Most procedures are performed via the femoral approach, which accommodates larger (7F) catheters, although the upper extremity approaches (radial, brachial) may be linked to less frequent hemorrhage as well as allowing more favorable geometry for catheter seating considering the inferior angled origin of many renal arteries, as noted above.[42] Typically, 6-7F intravascular sheaths are used for renal artery stenting. For stenting, in addition to aspirin, clopidogrel 300-600 mg should be given orally (then 75 mg orally daily for 4 weeks [some authors recommend 6 weeks] following the stenting procedure), and intraprocedural anticoagulation may take the form of low-molecular-weight heparin, unfractionated heparin (goal activated clotting time 250), bivalirudin, or argatroban.

Balloon angioplasty alone may be performed via a 5F guiding system, but stent placement will usually require a 6F guiding catheter or a 5F guiding sheath. Although the guiding catheter offers better torquability (needed with the femoral approach), the smaller guiding sheath is useful from upper extremity access points where torquability is less important given the inferior angulation of renal artery origins.[4]

To access the renal artery origin from the common femoral artery approach in a safe and coaxial manner, two approaches have been well described[4]: the **no-touch** technique and the **direct method**.

A. **No-Touch Technique** The no-touch technique has been advocated whereby, using a guiding catheter or guiding sheath, a first guidewire is advanced superiorly (cephalad) in the aorta beyond the renal artery effectively holding the guiding system at a small yet safe distance away from the artery origin.[47] Then a second guidewire is passed into the renal artery to cross the stenosis. This wire will come to rest in a distal renal arterial branch.

The first guidewire is then withdrawn, permitting the guiding system to become seated safely and coaxially in the artery origin, minimizing the possibility of damage to the ostium.[33] If the proper seating of a guiding sheath is difficult, a smaller caliber diagnostic catheter can be telescoped through the guiding sheath (Fig. 8.1), followed by guidewire crossing of the stenosis, and then subsequent advancement of the guiding sheath over the combined wire and diagnostic catheter system.

B. **Direct Method** The **direct method** uses a small caliber (4-5F) diagnostic catheter that is telescoped through the guiding system to engage the renal artery origin, followed by the passing of a guidewire across the stenosis. Wire size is typically 0.014. To follow, the guiding system is then advanced over the small caliber catheter to engage the artery safely (Fig. 8.2). Both no-touch and direct engagement techniques serve to avoid guiding catheter trauma to the artery origin, frequently the site of plaque in atherosclerotic lesions.[4]

C. **Procedure Steps and Options**

1. The **next step in the procedure is balloon angioplasty** using a device size-matched to the artery, with the proximal end of the balloon located in the aorta to ensure complete coverage of an ostial lesion, if present, during balloon dilatation. Because balloon-expandable stents exhibit better radial strength, they are preferred to self-expanding stents. Stents are typically sized 5-7 mm, again with proximal end of the stent extending at least minimally out into the aorta to ensure unambiguous ostial coverage. At this point, the guiding system is withdrawn into the aorta to avoid stent deployment within the guiding system. The stent is then deployed. As the stent balloon deflates after deployment, the guiding system should be advanced so that the distal tip of the guiding system lies coaxially within the stent, thereby allowing a postdilatation balloon to pass into the newly placed stent uneventfully despite stent struts protruding into the aorta, while also facilitating the creation of a poststenting follow-up angiogram[4] (Figs. 8.4–8.6).

   Current stents approved for renal artery use include the Express SD (Boston Scientific), Formula (Cook), and RX Herculink Elite (Abbott Vascular)[33] (Figs. 8.5–8.6).

2. An **additional procedural option is that of distal embolic protection**, whereby atheroemboli can be collected using a netlike filter or balloon occlusion system deployed distally to prevent embolic migration into smaller arterial branches, thereby theoretically mitigating renal injury.[23] The general analogy would parallel the successful use of such devices for transcatheter carotid or coronary vein graft interventions. Proving benefit for routine renal artery use has been difficult, however, partly because of the lack of a biomarker such as troponin that measures end-organ injury or freedom thereof.[23] In one series evaluating patients with chronic kidney disease, although blood pressure and glomerular filtration rates improved overall, there was no difference in these measures between those receiving stenting with distal embolic protection and those receiving stenting alone.[56] Recovery of debris has been reported in most series where distal embolic

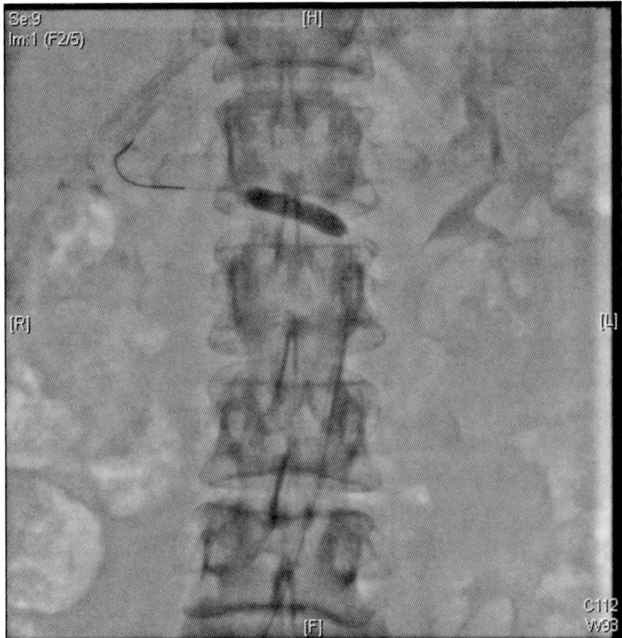

FIGURE 8.5: Renovascular disease. Atherosclerotic renal artery stenosis. The stenosis was crossed using a Hi-Torque Abbott Vascular Spartacore guide wire, followed by 5.0 mm balloon angioplasty predilatation with deployment of a 6 × 18 mm Abbott Vascular Herculink Elite stent.

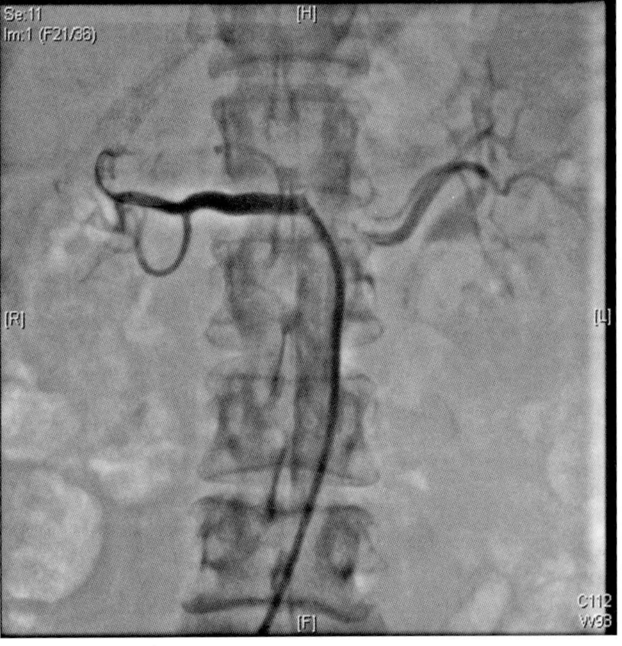

FIGURE 8.6: Renovascular disease. Atherosclerotic renal artery stenosis. Final angiographic view post–stent placement before wire removal shows excellent flow with no residual right renal artery stenosis. The subsequent clinical course has been remarkable for reduced frequency of angina, improved blood pressure control, and ultrasound-documented stabilization of kidney size.

protection was used consistently, irrespective of device used.[57,58] There are technical challenges, however, including the presence of early arterial branches, as well as the requirement that there be at least a 2-cm separation between the distal end of the stent and the resting location of the filter device.[4] At present, distal embolic protection is not used routinely in renal artery stenting.

XI. Medical Versus Transcatheter Management: Clinical Trial Evidence

Over the past decade, several prospective randomized trials have addressed the value of renal artery revascularization versus optimal medical therapy. Each of these trials has suffered from potential methodologic flaws. For example, EMMA and ASTRAL excluded many subjects who may have received benefit from stent revascularization.[59,60] However, a meta-analysis of all trials of renal revascularization versus medical therapy showed no overall benefit arising from revascularization on mortality, progression to end-stage renal impairment, major adverse cardiovascular events, or hypertension control.[61] Yet these trials, despite their limitations, mostly showed trends favoring modest improvements in blood pressure in the revascularization arms.[42] Below are details of the important trials.

A. **EMMA (Essai Multicentrique Medicaments vs Angioplastie) Study Group** The EMMA (Essai Multicentrique Medicaments vs Angioplastie) study group found no difference in ambulatory blood pressure between medically treated versus balloon angioplasty groups. Yet it was underpowered, had a high crossover rate from medical therapy to balloon angioplasty, had no stent option for suboptimal balloon results, enrolled mainly patients with moderate rather than severe stenotic disease, and did not include the most ill patients (advanced renal impairment, flash pulmonary edema, malignant hypertension).[59]

B. **Scottish and Newcastle Renal Artery Stenosis Collaborative Group** The Scottish and Newcastle Renal Artery Stenosis Collaborative Group showed that balloon revascularization tended to improve blood pressure in the bilateral disease arm (although not statistically significant) but not in the unilateral disease arm compared against medical therapy.[62]

C. **Dutch Renal Artery Stenosis Intervention Cooperative Study Trial (DRASTIC)** The Dutch Renal Artery Stenosis Intervention Cooperative Study trial (DRASTIC) compared balloon angioplasty against medical therapy, with no statistical difference in blood pressure control. However, nearly half of the medical patients crossed over to angioplasty, and angina and heart failure patients were excluded. Despite the statistically negative results, blood pressure control improved in most individuals in the balloon angioplasty cohort.[63]

D. **STAR Trial (Stent Placement in Patients With Atherosclerotic Renal Artery Stenosis and Impaired Renal Function)** The STAR Trial (Stent Placement in Patients with Atherosclerotic Renal Artery Stenosis and Impaired Renal Function) compared stenting to medical therapy in renovascular disease patients who showed renal impairment. Event rates were low overall, with many subjects manifesting moderate rather than severe disease. The result was not statistically significant. Three postprocedural mortalities in the stent arm is considered most unusual.[4,34]

E. **ASTRAL Trial (Angioplasty and Stenting for Renal Artery Lesions)** The ASTRAL Trial (Angioplasty and Stenting for Renal Artery Lesions) also examined subjects who had renal impairment and renovascular disease, the treatment arms being stenting versus medical therapy, with a negative result regarding the end point of changes in serum creatinine. There was a nonsignificant trend favoring stenting, however, and criticisms focused on the presence of only moderate disease in many subjects, as well as the inclusion of individuals who had considerably small kidney sizes.[4,64] In addition, there was an unexpectedly high number of periprocedural complications[38] in 31 of 359 patients (9%) who received revascularization (these events included pulmonary edema, myocardial infarction, renal embolizations, renal artery occlusions, renal artery perforations, femoral artery aneurysm, and cholesterol embolizations leading to peripheral gangrene and amputations).[64]

F. CORAL (Cardiovascular Outcomes in Renal Atherosclerotic Lesions)

1. CORAL (Cardiovascular Outcomes in Renal Atherosclerotic Lesions) was the largest stent versus optimized medical therapy trial. CORAL enrolled subjects who had either (1) unilateral or bilateral renovascular disease (angiographic stenosis >60% or peak Doppler velocity of >300 cm/s or >80% stenosis by MR angiography/CT angiography or >70% if other evidence of renal ischemia was present) or (2) hypertension despite two or more drugs or an estimated glomerular filtration rate of <60 mL/min/1.73 sq m based on renovascular hypertension. Both arms received optimized medical therapy (antiplatelet treatment, as well as treatment for lipids, glucose, and hypertension, including the angiotensin receptor blocker candesartan). Reported after a median of 3.6 years' follow-up, there was no difference between groups in the primary composite end point of cardiovascular or renal mortality, stroke, myocardial infarction, heart failure hospitalization, 30% fall in glomerular filtration rate, or the development of end-stage renal impairment.[25] Blood pressure response was nearly identical, and revascularization procedural complications were infrequent.

2. The CORAL trial has been critiqued because it included subjects who had modest clinical indications (two drug hypertension), and functional assessment of stenosis for physiologic significance was not part of the protocol. Moreover, as with the earlier revascularization versus medical therapy trials, the patients most likely to benefit from revascularization were not included, such as those with short duration of severe hypertension, true multidrug-resistant hypertension (average 2.1 drugs in CORAL), or recurrent flash pulmonary edema (excluded in CORAL).

3. In contrast, although not randomized, several prospective observational studies in high-risk patients showed benefit when stented. For example, when 467 such patients (some of whom had pulmonary edema, progressive renal impairment, resistant hypertension, or both resistant hypertension and progressive renal impairment) were treated by medication versus revascularization as selected by patient and physician preference, the revascularization arm subjects who had the above high-risk factors had significantly better 4-year mortality and event outcomes. When high-risk factors were absent, interestingly, there was no difference between the two treatment arms.[65]

XII. Renal Vein Thrombosis

Etiologies for renal vein thrombosis include malignancy, inferior vena cava (or vena cava filter) thrombosis, nephrotic syndrome, connective tissue diseases, and hypercoagulable states, with some reports of successful catheter-based thrombolysis or thrombectomy.[4,66,67] For this procedure, the use of a multipurpose or renal double curve guiding catheter is described, through which a glide wire and angled glide catheter are passed to cross the obstruction followed by rheolytic thrombectomy and catheter infusion of thrombolytic drug therapy, if needed.[66,67] However, in the setting of chronic renal vein occlusion, collateral venous pathways may provide adequate drainage to permit long-term viability under conservative medical therapy using anticoagulation.[68]

XIII. Renal Sympathetic Denervation for Resistant Hypertension: Theory and Early Experience

A. The prevalence of true medication-resistant hypertension has been difficult to quantify, partly because of variations in the denominators of populations examined. When resistant hypertension is defined generally as blood pressure that remains >140/90 mm Hg despite adherence to full-dose therapy for an adequate time interval using at least three drugs including a diuretic, this condition may be present in a spectrum of 3%-18% of patients depending on whether primary care practices versus tertiary clinics are considered.[1,69] In large clinical trials of hypertension treatment where drug therapy was actively titrated to prespecified targets, diastolic blood pressure <90 mm Hg was attained in 90% of instances, yet systolic blood pressure <140 mm Hg in only 60%.[1,70,71] In one specialty university hypertension clinic, only 59% of patients reached goal values of <140/90 mm Hg despite intensive titration efforts.[72] The most recently published large-scale US population data indicate that the overall prevalence of hypertension is 31% (68 million), of whom 8.9% met criteria for resistant hypertension.[32,73]

B. Early surgical experience using operative lumbar sympathectomy for uncontrollable hypertension created the theoretical basis for catheter-guided renal denervation. Initial surgical series documented improved blood pressure and survival compared against medical therapy, with enhanced diuresis and natriuresis, reduced renin release, unchanged renal blood flow, and stable glomerular filtration rate.[74] Yet orthostatic, dermatologic, pulmonary, gastrointestinal, and genitourinary adverse effects proved vexing, and the eventual extinction of the surgical approach was caused by the advent of thiazide diuretics and other effective and well-tolerated oral agents.

C. However, catheter-based denervation may provide benefits in resistant hypertension without similar side effects and is founded upon the presence of both efferent and afferent sympathetic nerves in the adventitial regions surrounding the renal arteries. The efferent nerves constitute postganglionic fibers arising from the hypothalamus and travel to the renal arteries via pre- and paravertebral sympathetic ganglia T10 through L2. The afferent nerves originate in the wall of the renal pelvis (chemo- and mechanoreceptors) and course via dorsal root ganglia L4 through T6 to central nervous system autonomic centers as well as the contralateral kidney. Increased afferent signal traffic may arise from elevated vascular pressure, renal ischemia, or renal artery stenosis. In turn, efferent sympathetic response from the central nervous system can promote direct renal vasoconstriction and augmented renin release.[75] The consequent activation of the renin-angiotensin system will manifest several actions: (1) systemic vasoconstriction, (2) augmented blood volume, (3) vascular smooth muscle hypertrophy, (4) myocardial hypertrophy, (5) salt and water retention in the kidney, and (6) overall intensification of systemic sympathetic activity. Further renal consequences can include reduced renal blood flow, increased proteinuria, and resistance to the diuretic effects of B-type natriuretic peptide. Longer range effects may encompass increased insulin resistance, impaired glucose metabolism, heart failure, generalized atherosclerosis, myocardial ischemia, increased cardiac inotropic and chronotropic responses, as well as atrial and ventricular arrhythmias.[75]

D. In terms of physiology, human studies have shown lowered blood pressure, improved renal resistive index, and lessening of proteinuria without change in glomerular filtration rate.[76] Yet it is worth considering theoretical objections to renal denervation: long-term effects are unknown, and there is a concern that treated individuals may forfeit necessary sympathetic responses to future illnesses such sepsis with distributive vasodilatory shock, allergic anaphylaxis, or life-threatening hemorrhage. For example, in an ovine model (normotensive as well as hypertensive sheep with chronic kidney disease), renal denervation versus a sham procedure was performed. Hypertension and renal function improved in the denervation kidney disease group. Experimental hemorrhage was then induced in all subjects, with greater fall in blood pressure in all denervated subjects, with attenuated heart rate and renin release responses in the denervated versus the nondenervated subjects. These responses were similar at 2 months and 5 months postprocedure, suggesting that sympathetic responses do not return over time.[77] The potential significance of these findings in humans is unknown.

XIV. Renal Sympathetic Denervation for Resistant Hypertension: Randomized Prospective Data

A. **Early Catheter-Based Trials: SymplicityHTN-1 Study** The earliest catheter-based trials of renal denervation utilized the Medtronic system, which consisted of a 6F helical radiofrequency ablating system, and which required ablation runs of 2 minutes duration each, using a maximal energy of 8 W with attainment of a temperature of 70-90°C.[78] Arteries of interest needed to be at least 4.0 mm in diameter and >20 mm in length. Subjects were excluded if they exhibited calcification, fibromuscular dysplasia, or obstructive atherosclerotic disease (need for adequate blood flow to disperse heat and avoid thermal damage to the renal artery). Using this system in a preliminary pilot trial (the SymplicityHTN-1 Study), 50 subjects were followed for 12 months, showing increasing overall improvements in blood pressure regulation after the procedure (−14/−10 mm Hg at 1 mo, advancing to −27/−17 mm Hg at 12 mo).[79] Currently there is no biomarker available to prove successful denervation.[78]

B. SymplicityHTN-2 Trial

1. The SymplicityHTN-2 Trial tested 190 subjects with resistant hypertension, of whom 106 were randomized to the renal denervation arm versus control with 12-month total follow-up duration.[80] At 6 months, control patients were permitted to crossover to renal denervation. At the 6-month point, the denervation arm showed blood pressure change of –32/–12 mm Hg versus control –1/0 mm Hg. At 12 months, the original denervation arm exhibited blood pressure change of –28/–10 mm Hg and the crossover group –24/–8 mm Hg.

2. Yet the SymplicityHTN-2 Trial was critiqued because the most dramatic improvements in blood pressure were witnessed in a cohort of subjects who had office blood pressure evaluation versus a much less impressive response in subjects who were assayed using a 24-hour ambulatory blood pressure monitor. The latter ambulatory technique (1) provides more data, (2) encompasses physiologic (or pathologic) diurnal variation, (3) eliminates transient office hypertension, (4) avoids human subjectivity in measurement, and (5) is considered a standard optimal technique for contemporary blood pressure research.

3. In addition to the question of ambulatory monitoring, other deficiencies cited included lack of a sham procedure, failure to track changes in antihypertensive medications during the follow-up period, and the relatively minimal role of therapeutic aldosterone inhibitors, shown in resistant hypertension cohorts to have nearly identical blood pressure–lowering effects as observed in the renal denervation arm over a similar time interval (for spironolactone, –21/–10 mm Hg at 6 wk, –25/–12 mm Hg at 6 mo).[81]

C. SymplicityHTN-3 Trial

1. The SymplicityHTN-3 Trial successfully addressed the above objections regarding consistent ambulatory monitoring and the inclusion of a sham procedures as the control, emphasized full doses of three antihypertensive medications for both denervation and control arms, and prohibited medication changes for the first six months postprocedure.[82] Nonetheless the trial was negative, showing a nonsignificant systolic blood pressure difference between denervation and sham procedure arms using office (–14 vs –12 mm Hg) as well ambulatory (–7 vs –5 mm Hg) measurement techniques.

2. There may be various diverse factors that explain the negative result of what had appeared to be a promising novel transcatheter method: (1) whether disorders that have strong lifestyle component can truly be studied in a randomized fashion, (2) whether the contemporary excellence of medical therapy can be matched by any interventional technique, (3) whether much of what appears to be resistant hypertension is not truly so when subjected to ambulatory monitoring, (4) whether operator-based variations contaminated the trial, (5) whether the initial trial results underscored a placebo effect rather than an objective physiologic improvement, (6) whether anatomic factors were influential, such as a potential need to perform

ablation more distally in the renal arterial tree, (7) whether there was differential postprocedure medication adherence between the two arms, and (8) finally, whether this result reflects a device-specific failure that is remediable through new catheter designs. Regarding (8), there are a multitude of novel devices in development that use diverse methods including ultrasound, alcohol ablation, and centering balloons that optimize symmetry of circumferential treatment exposure.[78,83]

D. SPYRAL HTN-OFF MED Trial

1. More recently, the SPYRAL HTN-OFF MED trial was presented and published online.[84] This study answered some of the concerns listed above,[85] showing modest yet statistically significant blood pressure lowering using renal denervation as a proof of concept exercise, where no antihypertensive medications were permitted in either renal denervation or sham-procedure control arms (denervation arm versus sham showed a difference of −5/−4 mm Hg systolic/diastolic by ambulatory monitoring, and a difference of −8/−5 systolic/diastolic by office readings, both statistically significant).[84] Although the proof of concept is scientifically interesting, it is acknowledged that this modest degree of blood pressure lowering in an untreated patient would be readily available through the simplest of medication (or even lifestyle) measures. Moreover, it is still not clear in which hypertensive clinical subsets renal denervation would be best applied.[29]
2. Of major technical interest, this study brought into play a new generation device, the Symplicity Spyral catheter. This iteration is notable for a multielectrode system that is capable of simultaneous quadrantal therapy in the main renal artery in addition to arterial branches and accessory arteries, provided these vessels are 3.0-8.0 mm in diameter. The value of branch ablation is supported by emerging data suggesting that the renal sympathetic nerves may lie closer to the vessel lumens in these more distal locations, creating heightened opportunity for ablative benefit.[86-88]

XV. Renal Sympathetic Denervation for Extrarenal Circulatory Disorders

The well-established observation that sympathetic overactivity underlies many cardiovascular and metabolic conditions, and that chemical antiadrenergic therapies (beta-adrenergic blockers, and others) have proven therapeutically useful, has given rise to several presently enrolling (or completed) studies of renal sympathetic denervation (Table 8.2). These conditions (and trials) encompass resistant hypertension (SymplicityHTN-1,2,3; SPYRAL HTN-OFF MED), atrial fibrillation (Symplicity-AF), sleep apnea,[89,90] left ventricular hypertrophy, metabolic syndrome with insulin resistance (DREAMS-Denervation of the Renal Artery

TABLE 8.2. Clinical Conditions for Which Renal Denervation has Been Proposed as Therapy
Resistant hypertension (SymplicityHTN-1,2,3)
Congestive heart failure (Symplicity-HF)
Atrial fibrillation (Symplicity-AF)
Sleep apnea
Left ventricular hypertrophy
Metabolic syndrome and insulin resistance (DREAMS)

in Metabolic Syndrome), and congestive heart failure (Symplicity-HF). A recent report describing an experimental model has linked renal sympathetic denervation with improvement in heart failure via the inhibition of neprilysin activity in the kidney.[91] Although there are plausible and attractive theoretical mechanisms by which renal denervation may benefit these disorders, as is evident from recent experience, the scientific community must await the results of well-constructed clinical trials to determine the incremental value of renal denervation beyond presently existing therapies.

XVI. Contemporary Management of Renovascular Disease and Future Directions

A. **Interventional Therapies** Interventional therapies for obstructive renovascular disease as well as hypertension (and other cardiovascular and metabolic conditions) have matured from a technical and device viewpoint over the past decades. However, more critically, there has been a refinement in the clinical diagnostic sphere: emerging investigative and practice experience is informing the community of vascular specialists with greater specificity regarding whom to treat (as well as whom not to treat) when considering evolving technologies such as renal artery stenting or denervation.

Several points, however, are clear. For individuals who have atherosclerotic renovascular disease, all should receive optimal medication and lifestyle therapy (Table 8.3). Future investigations may combine physiologic measurements with angiographic findings in testing strategies of revascularization versus optimal medical therapy.

B. Guidelines and Indications

1. Exisiting 2005 (updated 2011, 2014) guidelines continue to suggest revascularization as a **Class I** indication for hemodynamically significant renovascular disease with recurrent unexplained heart failure or flash pulmonary edema.[3,60,92]
2. **Class IIa** indications include renovascular disease with either accelerated, resistant, or malignant hypertension, or hypertension with unilateral small kidney, or hypertension with medication intolerance. Additional Class IIa indications are renal impairment with bilateral renovascular disease or renovascular disease in a solitary kidney, as well as renal artery disease and unstable angina.[3,60]

TABLE 8.3. Suggested Optimal Medical and Lifestyle Therapy for Management of Renovascular Disease
Aspirin
Clopidogrel (or other novel antiplatelet compounds)
Statin
Antihyperglycemic
Angiotensin-converting enzyme (ACE) inhibitor or angiotensin receptor blocker (if intolerant, dihydropyridine calcium blockers)
Aldosterone inhibitors (with monitoring of serum potassium)
Ideal diet
Sodium restriction
Weight control
Aerobic exercise
Smoking cessation

3. **Class IIb** indications include asymptomatic bilateral renovascular disease or solitary viable kidney with hemodynamically significant renovascular disease, asymptomatic unilateral hemodynamically significant renovascular disease in a viable kidney, and renovascular disease and renal impairment with unilateral disease in a setting where two kidneys are present.[3,60]

XVII. Summary

In the context of renovascular disease, if blood pressure regulation cannot be achieved, if loss of renal function is progressing, or if circulatory congestion is prominent, then renal revascularization is reasonable.[20] Otherwise, intensive optimized medical and lifestyle therapy should be pursued (Table 8.3).

Whether new catheter-based techniques such as renal denervation (for hypertension or numerous other adrenergically driven cardiovascular conditions) will afford true benefits must await future prospective randomized trial results and anticipated technological advances.

References

1. Moser M, Setaro JF. Resistant or difficult-to-control hypertension. *N Engl J Med.* 2006;355:385-392.
2. Singer GM, Remetz MS, Curtis JP, Setaro JF. Impact of baseline renal function on outcomes of renal artery stenting in hypertensive patients. *J Clin Hypertens.* 2009;11:615-620.
3. Hirsch AT, Haskal ZJ, Hertzer NR, et al. Executive summary. *J Am Coll Cardiol.* 2006;47:1239-1312.
4. Rogers RK, Garasic JM. Percutaneous management of renovascular diseases. In: Thompson CA, ed. *Textbook of Cardiovascular Intervention.* London: Springer-Verlag; 2014.
5. Safian RD, Madder RD. Redefining the approach to renal artery revascularization. *JACC Cardiovasc Interv.* 2009;2:161-174.
6. Lohse JR, Shore RM, Belzer FO. Acute renal artery occlusion. The role of collateral circulation. *Arch Surg.* 1982;117:801-804.
7. Goldblatt H, Lynch J, Hanzal RF, et al. Studies on experimental hypertension. I. The production of persistent elevation of systolic blood pressure by means of renal ischemia. *J Exp Med.* 1934;59:347-378.
8. Navar LG, Ploth DW. Pathophysiology of renovascular hypertension. In: Izzo JL, Sica DA, Black HR, eds. *Hypertension Primer.* 4th ed. Philadelphia: Lippincott Williams & Wilkins; 2008.
9. Nally JV. Treatment of renovascular hypertension. In: Izzo JL, Sica DA, Black HR, eds. *Hypertension Primer.* 4th ed. Philadelphia: Lippincott Williams & Wilkins; 2008.
10. Cooper CJ, Murphy TP. Is renal artery stenting the correct treatment of renal artery stenosis? The case for renal artery stenting for treatment of renal artery stenosis. *Circulation.* 2007;115:263-269.
11. Gloviczki ML, Glockner JF, Lerman LO, et al. Preserved oxygenation despite reduced blood flow in post-stenotic kidneys in human atherosclerotic renal artery stenosis. *Hypertension.* 2010;55:961-966.
12. Brewster UC, Setaro JF, Perazella MA. The renin-angiotensin-aldosterone system. Cardiorenal effects and implications for renal and cardiovascular disease states. *Am J Med Sci.* 2003;326:15-24.
13. Gloviczki ML, Keddis MT, Garovic VD, et al. TGF expression and macrophage accumulation in atherosclerotic renal artery stenosis. *Clin J Am Soc Nephrol.* 2013;8:546-553.
14. Textor SC, Lerman LO. Paradigm shifts in atherosclerotic renovascular disease. Where are we now? *J Am Soc Nephrol.* 2015;26:2074-2080.
15. Pohl MA, Novick AC. Natural history of atherosclerotic and fibrous renal artery disease. Clinical implications. *Am J Kidney Dis.* 1985;5. A120-A130.
16. Crowley JJ, Santos RM, Peter RH, et al. Progression of renal artery stenosis in patients undergoing cardiac catheterization. *Am Heart J.* 1998;136:913-918.

17. Caps MT, Perissinotto C, Zierler RE, et al. Prospective study of atherosclerotic disease progression in the renal artery. *Circulation*. 1998;98:2866-2872.
18. Caps MT, Zierler RE, Polissar NL, et al. Risk of atrophy in kidneys with atherosclerotic renal artery stenosis. *Kidney Int*. 1998;53:735-742.
19. Strandness DE. Natural history of renal artery stenosis. *Am J Kidney Dis*. 1994;24:630-635.
20. Textor SC. Renovascular hypertension. Is there still a role for stent revascularization? *Curr Opin Nephrol Hypertens*. 2013;22:525-530.
21. Bourantas CV, Loh HP, Lukaschuk EI, et al. Renal artery stenosis. An innocent bystander or an independent predictor of worse outcome in patients with chronic heart failure? A magnetic resonance imaging study. *Eur J Heart Fail*. 2012;14:764-772.
22. Olin JW, Melia M, Young JR. Prevalence of atherosclerotic renal artery stenosis in patients with atherosclerosis elsewhere. *Am J Med*. 1990;88(1N):46N-51N.
23. White CW. Catheter-based therapy for atherosclerotic renal artery stenosis. *Circulation*. 2006;113:1464-1473.
24. El-Mawardy RH, Ghareeb MA, Mahdy MM, et al. Prevalence and predictors of renal artery stenosis in hypertensive patients undergoing elective coronary procedures. *J Clin Hypertens*. 2008;10:844-849.
25. Cooper CJ, Murphy TP, Cutlip DE, et al. Stenting and medical therapy for atherosclerotic renal-artery stenosis. *N Engl J Med*. 2014;370:13-22.
26. Conlon PJ, Little MA, Pieper K, et al. Severity of renal vascular disease predicts mortality in patients undergoing coronary angiography. *Kidney Int*. 2001;60:1490-1497.
27. Safian RD, Textor SC. Renal-artery stenosis. *N Engl J Med*. 2001;344:431-442.
28. Carey RM. Resistant hypertension. *Hypertension*. 2013;61:746-750.
29. Vongpatanasin W. Resistant hypertension. A review of diagnosis and management. *JAMA*. 2014;311:2216-2224.
30. Buller CE, Norareda JG, Ramanathan K, et al. The profile of cardiac patients with renal artery stenosis. *J Am Coll Cardiol*. 2004;43:1606-1613.
31. Benjamin MM, Fazel P, Filardo G, et al. Prevalence of and risk factors of renal artery stenosis in patients with resistant hypertension. *Am J Cardiol*. 2014;113:687-690.
32. Gonzalez-Santos L, Elliott WJ, Setaro JF, Black HR. Resistant hypertension. In: Hypertension A, ed. *Companion to Braunwald's Heart Disease*. 2nd ed. Philadelphia: Elsevier Saunders; 2013.
33. Shishehbor MH, Kapadia SR. Peripheral intervention. In: Moscucci M, ed. *Grossman & Baim's Cardiac Catheterization, Angiography, and Intervention*. 8th ed. Philadelphia: Lippincott Williams & Wilkins; 2014.
34. Bax L, Woittiez AJ, Kouwenberg HJ, et al. Stent placement in patients with atherosclerotic renal artery stenosis and impaired renal function (STAR). A randomized trial. *Ann Intern Med*. 2009;150:840-848.
35. Guo H, Karla PA, Gilbertson DT, et al. Atherosclerotic renovascular disease in older US patients starting dialysis 1996–2001. *Circulation*. 2007;115:50-58.
36. Thatipelli M, Misra S, Johnson CM, et al. Renal artery stent placement for restoration of renal function in hemodialysis recipients with renal artery stenosis. *J Vasc Interv Radiol*. 2008;19:1563-1568.
37. Weber BR, Dieter DS. Renal artery stenosis. Epidemiology and treatment. *Int J Nephrol Renovasc Dis*. 2014;7:169-181.
38. Van Brussel PM, Van de Hoef TP, De Winter RJ, et al. Hemodynamic measurements for the selection of patients with renal artery stenosis. *J Am Coll Cardiol Interv*. 2017;10:973-985.
39. Makanjuola AD, Suresh M, Laboi P, et al. Proteinuria in atherosclerotic renovascular disease. *QJM*. 1999;92:515-518.
40. Scoble JE, Maher ER, Hamilton G, et al. Atherosclerotic renovascualr disease causing renal impairment. A case for treatment. *Clin Nephrol*. 1989;31:119-122.
41. Bofinger A, Hawley C, Fisher P, et al. Polymorphisms of the renin-angiotensin system in patients with multifocal renal arterial fibromuscular dysplasia. *J Hum Hypertens*. 2001;15:185-190.
42. Klein AJ, Banerjee S, Drachman DE. Peripheral arterial disease and angiography. In: Kern MJ, Sorajja P, Lim MJ, eds. *The Cardiac Catheterization Handbook*. 6th ed. Philadelphia: Elsevier; 2016.

43. Elliott WJ. Secondary hypertension. Renovascular hypertension. In: Hypertension A, ed. *Companion to Braunwald's Heart Disease.* 2nd ed. Philadelphia: Elsevier Saunders; 2013.
44. Trinquart L, Mounier-Vehier C, Sapoval M, et al. Efficacy of revascularization for renal artery stenosis caused by fibromuscular dysplasia. A systematic review and meta-analysis. *Hypertension.* 2010;56:525-532.
45. Kaplan NM, Victor RG. Renovascular hypertension. In: Kaplan NM, Victor RG, eds. *Kaplan's Clinical Hypertension.* 10th ed. Philadelphia: Lippincott Williams & Wilkins; 2010.
46. Safian RD. Transplant renal artery stenosis. What lessons should we learn? *Catheter Cardiovasc Interv.* 2011;77:294-295.
47. Jaff MR, Rundback J, Rosenfield K. Angiography of the aorta and peripheral arteries. In: Moscucci M, ed. *Grossman & Baim's Cardiac Catheterization, Angiography, and Intervention.* 8th ed. Philadelphia: Lippincott Williams & Wilkins; 2014.
48. Radermacher J, Chavan A, Bleck J, et al. Use of doppler ultrasonography to predict the outcome of therapy for renal artery stenosis. *N Engl J Med.* 2001;344:410-417.
49. Setaro JF, Saddler MC, Chen CC, et al. Simplified captopril renography in diagnosis and treatment of renal artery stenosis. *Hypertension.* 1991;18:289-298.
50. Gill-Leertouwer TC, Gussenhoven EJ, Bosch JL, et al. Predictors for clinical success at one year following renal artery stent placement. *J Endovasc Ther.* 2002;9:495-502.
51. Staub D, Zeller T, Trenk D, et al. Use of B-type natriuretic peptide to predict blood pressure improvement after percutaneous revascularization for renal artery stenosis. *Eur J Vasc Endovasc Surg.* 2010;40:599-607.
52. Subramanian R, White CJ, Rosenfield K, et al. Renal fractional flow reserve. A hemodynamic evaluation of moderate renal artery stenosis. *Catheter Cardiovasc Interv.* 2005;64:480-486.
53. Leesar MA, Varma J, Shapira A, et al. Prediction of hypertension improvement after stenting of renal artery stenosis. Comparative accuracy of translesional pressure gradients, intravascular ultrasound, and angiography. *J Am Coll Cardiol.* 2009;53:2363-2371.
54. Gruntzig A, Kuhlmann U, Vetter W, et al. Treatment of renovascular hypertension with percutaneous transluminal dilatation of a renal-artery stenosis. *Lancet.* 1978;1:801-802.
55. Van de Ven PJ, Kaatee R, Beutler JJ, et al. Arterial stenting and balloon angioplasty in ostial atherosclerotic renovascular disease. A randomized trial. *Lancet.* 1999;353:282-286.
56. Singer GM, Setaro JF, Curtis JP, Remetz MS. Distal embolic protection during renal artery stenting: impact on hypertensive patients with renal dysfunction. *J Clin Hypertens.* 2008;10:830-836.
57. Henry M, Henry I, Klonaris C, et al. Renal angioplasty and stenting under protection. The way for the future? *Catheter Cardiovasc Interv.* 2003;60:299-312.
58. Holden A, Hill A. Renal angioplasty and stenting with distal protection of the main renal artery in ischemic nephropathy. Early experience. *J Vasc Surg.* 2003;38:962-968.
59. Plouin PF, Chatellier G, Darne B, et al. Blood pressure outcome of angioplasty in atherosclerotic renal artery stenosis. A randomized trial. Essai Multicentrique Medicaments vs Angioplastie (EMMA) Study Group. *Hypertension.* 1998;31:823-829.
60. Rooke TW, Hirsch AT, Misra S, et al. 2011 ACCF/AHA focused update of the guideline for the management of patients with peripheral artery disease (updating the 2005 guideline). A report of the American College of Cardiology Foundation/American Heart Association Task Force on Practice Guidelines. *Catheter Cardiovasc Interv.* 2012;79:501-531.
61. Raman G, Adam GP, Halladay CW, et al. Comparative effectiveness of management strategies for renal artery stenosis. An updated systematic review. *Ann Intern Med.* 2016;165:635-649.
62. Webster J, Marshall F, Abdalla M, et al. Randomised comparison of percutaneous angioplasty versus continued medical therapy for hypertensive patients with atheromatous renal artery stenosis. Scottish and Newcastle Renal Artery Stenosis Collaborative Group. *J Hum Hypertens.* 1998;12:329-335.
63. Van Jaarsveld BC, Krijnen P, Pieterman H, et al. The effect of balloon angioplasty on hypertension in atherosclerotic renal-artery stenosis (DRASTIC). *N Engl J Med.* 2000;342:1007-1014.
64. Wheatley K, Ives N, Gray R, et al. Revascularization versus medical therapy for renal artery stenosis (ASTRAL). *N Engl J Med.* 2009;361:1953-1962.

65. Ritchie J, Green D, Chrysochou C, et al. High-risk clinical presentations in atherosclerotic renovascular disease. Prognosis and response to renal artery revascularization. *Am J Kidney Dis.* 2014;63:186-197.
66. Kim HS, Fine DM, Atta MG. Catheter-directed thrombectomy and thrombolysis for acute renal vein thrombosis. *J Vasc Interv Radiol.* 2006;17:815-822.
67. Jong CB, Lo WY, Hsieh MY. Catheter-directed therapy for acute renal vein thrombosis in systemic lupus erythematosus. A case report. *Catheter Cardiovasc Interv.* 2017;89:416-419.
68. Witz M, Kantarovsky A, Morag B, et al. Renal vein occlusion. A review. *J Urol.* 1996;155:1173-1179.
69. Setaro JF, Black HR. Refractory hypertension. *N Engl J Med.* 1992;327:543-527.
70. ALLHAT Collaborative Research Group. Major outcomes in high-risk hypertensive patients randomized to angiotensin-converting inhibitor or calcium channel blocker versus diuretic. The Antihypertensive and lipid-lowering Treatment to Prevent Heart Attack Trial (ALLHAT). *JAMA.* 2002;288:1981-1987.
71. Black HR, Elliott WJ, Grandits G, et al. Principal results of the Controlled Onset Verapamil Investigation of Cardiovascular Endpoints (CONVINCE) trial. *JAMA.* 2003;289:2073-2082.
72. Singer GM, Izhar M, Black HR. Goal-oriented hypertension management. Translating clinical trials to practice. *Hypertension.* 2002;40:464-469.
73. Persell SD. Prevalence of resistant hypertension in the United States, 2003-2008. *Hypertension.* 2011;57:1076-1080.
74. Smithwick RH, Thompson JE. Splanchnicectomy for essential hypertension. Results in 1,266 cases. *J Am Med Assoc.* 1953;152:1501-1504.
75. Bertog SC, Sobotka PA, Sievert H. Renal denervation for hypertension. *J Am Coll Cardiol Interv.* 2012;5:249-258.
76. Mafoud F, Cremers B, Janker J, et al. Renal hemodynamics and renal function after catheter-based renal sympathetic denervation in patients with resistant hypertension. *Hypertension.* 2012;60:419-424.
77. Singh RR, Sajeesh V, Booth LC, et al. Catheter-based renal denervation exacerbates blood pressure fall during hemorrhage. *J Am Coll Cardiol.* 2017;69:951-964.
78. Myat A, Redwood SR, Qureshi AC, et al. Renal sympathetic denervation for resistant hypertension. A contemporary synopsis and future implications. *Circ Cardiovasc Interv.* 2013;6:184-197.
79. Krum H, Schlaich M, Whitbourn R, et al. Catheter-based renal sympathetic denervation for resistant hypertension. A multicenter safety and proof-of-principal cohort study. *Lancet.* 2009;373:1275-1281.
80. Esler MD, Krum H, Schlaich M, et al. Renal sympathetic denervation for treatment of drug-resistant hypertension. One-year results from the Symplicity HTN-2 randomized, controlled trial. *Circulation.* 2012;126:2976-2982.
81. Nishizaka MK, Zaman MA, Calhoun DA. Efficacy of low-dose spironolactone in subjects with resistant hypertension. *Am J Hypertens.* 2003;16:925-930.
82. Bhatt DL, Kandzari DE, O'Neill WW, et al. A controlled trial of renal denervation for resistant hypertension. *N Engl J Med.* 2014;370:1393-1401.
83. Fischell TA, Ebner A, Gallo S, et al. Transcatheter alcohol-mediated perivascular renal denervation with the Peregrine System. *J Am Coll Cardiol Interv.* 2016;9:589-598.
84. Townsend RR, Mahfoud F, Kandzari DE, et al. Catheter-based renal denervation in patients with uncontrolled hypertension in the absence of antihypertensive medications (SPYRAL HTN-OFF MED). A randomized, sham-controlled, proof-of-concept trial. *Lancet.* 2017. doi:10.1016/S0140-6736(17)32281-X.
85. Kandzari DE, Bhatt DL, Brar S, et al. Predictors of blood pressure response in the Symplicity HTN-3 trial. *Eur Heart J.* 2015;36:219-227.
86. Mompeo B, Maranillo E, Garcia-Touchard A, et al. The gross anatomy of the renal sympathetic nerves revisited. *Clin Anat.* 2016;29:660-664.
87. Mahfoud F, Tunev S, Ewen S, et al. Impact of lesion placement on efficacy and safety of catheter-based radiofrequency renal denervation. *J Am Coll Cardiol.* 2015;66:1766-1775.
88. Fengler K, Ewen S, Höllriegel R, et al. Blood pressure response to main renal artery and combined main renal artery plus branch renal denervation in patients with resistant hypertension. *J Am Heart Assoc.* 2017;6:e006196.

89. Linz D, Mahfoud F, Schotten U, et al. Renal sympathetic denervation suppresses post-apneic blood pressure rises and atrial fibrillation in a model for sleep apnea. *Hypertension*. 2012;60:172-178.
90. Jaen-Aguilla F, Vargas-Hitos JA, Mediavilla-Garcia JD, et al. Implications of renal denervation therapy in patients with sleep apnea. *Int J Hypertens*. 2015. doi:10.1155/2015/408574.
91. Polhemus DJ, Trivedi RK, Gao J, et al. Renal sympathetic denervation protects the failing heart via inhibition of neprilysin activity in the kidney. *J Am Coll Cardiol*. 2017;70:2139-2153.
92. Parikh SA, Shishehbor MH, Gray BH, et al. Society for cardiovascular angiography and intervention expert consensus statement for renal artery stenting appropriate use. *Catheter Cardiovasc Interv*. 2014;84:1163-1171.

CHAPTER 9

Endovascular Intervention of Aortoiliac Occlusive Disease

Sasanka Jayasuriya, MBBS, FACC, FASE, RPVI, FSCAI, and William L. Bennett, MD, PhD

Key Points

- Claudication, critical limb ischemia, and erectile dysfunction are symptoms related to aortoiliac occlusive disease.
- Investigations including ABI ultrasound are performed to aid diagnosis, and CT angiography and MRA are helpful for lesion characterization and procedure planning.
- Many techniques including contralateral and ipsilateral crossing techniques could be undertaken for crossing the lesion with reentry devices used to aid access to the true lumen.
- Self-expanding stents are commonly used with 3-year primary patency being greater than 70%.

I. Introduction

Advances in transcatheter therapies have led to a shift in endovascular interventions for aortoiliac disease, even in the setting of complex lesions such as Trans-Atlantic Inter-Society Consensus Document classification (TASC) class C and D lesions in recent times.[1] Patients with peripheral arterial disease suffer from multiple comorbidities, and up to 40% suffer from significant coronary artery disease. Of these patients, the subgroup suffering from aortoiliac occlusive disease (AIOD) suffers from substantial loss of quality of life owing to claudication and critical limb ischemia.[11] Endovascular treatment options are a valuable alternative to high-risk open surgical procedures. However, the operators are encouraged to recognize the risks associated with aortoiliac interventions with attention to careful case selection, procedure planning, technical skill, and bailout strategies, which result in successful results.

II. Indications for Endovascular Intervention of Aortoiliac Occlusive Disease

A. **Claudication** is a common symptom in AIOD with complaints including claudication of the buttocks, thighs, or calf. Symptoms typically begin in the calves and proceed proximally with worsening hemodynamics. Intervention is indicated when >50% stenosis is present with lifestyle-limiting claudication (Rutherford class 2 and 3), which is not improved with medical therapy or exercise therapy. In the event of multilevel disease, inflow revascularization (treatment of AIOD) is undertaken initially.

B. **Critical Limb Ischemia** presenting as ischemic rest pain or vascular ulcers and tissue loss (Rutherford class 4, 5, and 6) is a strong indication for revascularization. Contrary to patients with claudication, patients with critical limb ischemia are treated with complete revascularization in an attempt to establish straight-line reperfusion to the affected angiosome.

C. **Erectile Dysfunction** is another indication for treatment of AIOD. The typical syndrome of buttock or thigh claudication, erectile dysfunction, and absent pulses is known as Leriche syndrome and is usually caused by AIOD.

D. **Vascular Access** for unrelated procedures such as endovascular aortic repair (EVAR) and transcatheter aortic valve replacement (TAVR) requiring large-diameter sheath introduction may require aortoiliac revascularization.

III. Diagnosis

A. **Physical Examination** performed thoroughly could suggest AIOD, although the nature and exact location of the lesion cannot be predicted. Reduced or asymmetric femoral pulses are appreciated with typical signs of chronic ischemia in the affected limb such as cold extremity, pallor, hair loss, nail atrophy, and dependent rubor.

B. The first line of **physiologic testing** includes noninvasive testing such as ankle brachial index (ABI), toe brachial pressures, segmental pressures, and pulse volume recording (PVR). If unilateral iliac stenosis is present, the ABI, segmental pressures, as well as the PVR would be reduced in the affected limb. However, in the setting of distal aortic or bilateral aortic disease, the ABI and segmental pressures may be reduced in a symmetrical fashion. Blunting of the pulse volume waveform bilaterally suggests distal aortic and bilateral iliac disease.

C. **Imaging**

1. **Duplex ultrasound** could be used as a method of imaging especially in patients with renal impairment. However, iliac ultrasound evaluation is technically challenging and time-consuming with poor images resulting due to body habitus, bowel gas, and calcification. A study by Ubbink et al suggested significant interobserver variability with iliac duplex imaging with 1/8 agreement on results.[12] Hence, alternative imaging should be considered if more precise anatomic diagnoses are needed.
2. **Computer tomography angiography (CTA)** is an excellent study modality in patients with AIOD. Current generation scanners produce accurate three-dimensional imaging and are an excellent alternative to invasive angiography for planning revascularization. Benefits of CTA evaluation include a faster scan time, high spatial resolution, and ability to visualize in-stent restenosis. However, use of iodinated contrast and radiation exposure are disadvantages, and further heavily calcified vessels may reveal inaccurately more severe stenosis due to blooming artifact.
3. **Magnetic resonance angiography (MRA)** is another effective imaging method of evaluation in AIOD. Current high-performance MR scanners produce remarkable angiography. MRA carries the benefits of not being exposed to iodinated contrast or ionizing radiation. However image acquisition takes a long time, and patients with advanced renal disease are at risk of nephrogenic systemic fibrosis. MRA also may not accurately estimate the degree of calcification, which may change the level of complexity of an intervention.
4. **Invasive angiography** is the gold standard for imaging aortoiliac disease. In assessing AIOD, the initial angiogram would comprise of an anterior-posterior distal aortic angiogram run off to include both common iliac, external iliac, and common femoral arteries (CFAs). Imaging is performed by digital subtraction angiography (DSA).

a. Evaluation of each iliac artery is performed by contralateral oblique projection, which separates the iliac bifurcation. In the event of a long-segment occlusion, the distal anastomotic site as well as below knee run off is completed to ensure the appropriate approach is undertaken and distal embolization had not occurred during intervention.

b. The hemodynamic significance of an intermediate lesion can be measured by advancing a catheter beyond the lesion with gradual pullback measurements. A more accurate method is to transduce simultaneously the side branch of the sheath and a catheter, which is at least 1 French less in diameter placed across the lesion. A peak-to-peak systolic gradient greater than 10 mm Hg is considered to be hemodynamically significant. With concomitant distal disease, a pressure gradient could be induced with intra-arterial nitroglycerin injection to induce peripheral vasodilatation.

IV. Endovascular Treatment

A. **Procedure Planning** Planning of the procedure is a key element in endovascular treatment of AIOD. Specific patient and lesion characteristics could significantly change the approach and outcomes in intervention.

1. **Lesion characteristics.** Long-segment occlusions and heavily calcified vessels should be undertaken only by the experienced operator. For early career interventionalist, backup support planning is imperative. While heavy calcification is a contraindication to aortoiliac percutaneous intervention, every lesion carries the risk of perforation. Hence the availability of bailout equipment such as occlusive balloons and covered stents should be ensured.

2. **Patient characteristics.** AIOD intervention could be relatively fast or long and complex. Hence the candidacy for conscious sedation and support from an anesthesiologist should be assessed. Considering the higher volume of iodinated contrast used, prehydration should be undertaken to reduce contrast-induced nephropathy with special attention to the patient's current volume status and left ventricular function. Low-osmolar or iso-osmolar contract agent use is also associated with a lower risk of contrast-induced nephropathy.

B. Access

1. Access site and sheath size are important decisions that lay the foundation to successful completion of the intervention. Complex aortoiliac intervention usually requires dual access. While angiography is performed through catheters advanced from one site, equipment would usually be delivered through a larger French sheath in an alterative site.

2. The most common site of access in AIOD is the ipsilateral CFA. However, in the event of complete occlusion of the external iliac artery, there may not be an adequate length in the patent vessel to advance the sheath. In this case, contralateral common femoral access or brachial access is considered. While radial access is more elegant,

in comparison to brachial access, the shaft length of current balloons and stents may not reach the external iliac vessels from a radial sheath. However, for the sole purpose of diagnostic angiography proximal to the occlusion, radial access could be obtained, through which a pigtail catheter placed in the descending aorta or a multipurpose catheter directed to the respective iliac artery would be useful to perform diagnostic angiography. However, if devices are to be delivered from above, brachial access is required. Left brachial access is preferred as the risk of cerebral embolization is less than with right brachial access in these patients with significant atherosclerotic disease.

3. In deciding sheath size, the smallest sheath, which would allow required equipment delivery, is the choice. However, in a heavily calcified vessel, a sheath that could deliver a covered stent as needed would be a wiser choice.

V. Common Femoral Disease

In the event of concurrent common femoral disease, a prior decision for the approach to managing this lesion is imperative. At the conclusion of the iliac intervention, the lesion in the CFA could be revascularized by atherectomy and drug coated balloon therapy or with hybrid revascularization with concomitant common femoral end arterectomy.

VI. Lesion Crossing

A. **External Iliac Artery and Retrograde Approach** Occlusions of the external iliac artery could be crossed by ipsilateral common femoral access, if the distal external iliac artery was patent and sheath placement was possible. Ultrasound-guided vascular access is beneficial, as femoral pulses are faint to absent. A bright-tipped sheath is used. The lesion could be crossed with an assortment of wires and backup catheters. We commonly use a 0.14″ Fielder FC (Asahi Intecc) wire with a Quickcross (Spectranetics Corp, Colorado Springs, CO) backup catheter with success in crossing the lesion in an intraluminal fashion. However, an angled Glidewire (Terumo Medical, Somerset, NJ) and a 0.35″ angled backup catheter are other options. The support catheter is advanced to the distal cap of the occlusion with gentle forward force, and the distal cap is crossed by spinning or looping the wire. As the access sheath could get displaced out of the artery when forward force is applied to cross the lesion, it should be secured manually. Subintimal crossing may be undertaken with the Glidewire, but reentering the vessel at the reconstitution site is important to prevent undue stenting and propagation of a dissection plane. Once the lesion is crossed, the backup catheter is advanced beyond the lesion and blood is aspirated to confirm intraluminal placement. A limited angiogram could be performed through the backup catheter. A stiff-bodied wire is then advanced through the backup catheter, which would be the guidewire for equipment delivery to complete the procedure. Hence this could be a 0.14″, 0.18″, or 0.35″ wire depending on the intervention planned.

B. **Antegrade Approach** An external iliac occlusion could also be crossed by the antegrade approach with access in the contralateral CFA or in the left brachial artery. With contralateral CFA access, the iliac bifurcation is crossed in standard fashion, and a

45 cm crossover sheath is advanced to the proximal cap of the occlusion. With angiography performed in the contralateral oblique position, the lesion is crossed as mentioned above.

With brachial access a 90 cm guiding sheath is advanced to the proximal cap of the lesion. The lesion is crossed with wire and a backup catheter, and the stiff guiding wire is placed in the CFA. With available landing room in the distal external iliac and CFAs, the wire advanced from the brachial position could be externalized through a sheath in the ipsilateral CFA. This could be exchanged to a stiff guiding wire, following which the intervention could be completed from the ipsilateral CFA.

C. **Common Iliac Artery Occlusions** Occlusions of the common iliac artery or common and external iliac arteries are best crossed by ipsilateral CFA access or left brachial access. Contralateral crossover sheaths usually would not be stable enough to provide the backup support or "pushability" to cross through a lesion. This is specifically true in flush occlusions of the ostial common iliac artery, although this approach could be tried as an initial strategy, as access is likely obtained for diagnostic angiography. Once the guiding sheath is usually advanced to engage the stump or in very close proximity of the lesion, which is crossed with a hydrophilic guidewire and angled backup catheter. A 0.14″ wire such as the Fielder FC (Asahi Intecc) or a 0.35″ angled Glidewire (Terumo Medical, Somerset, NJ) could be used. If brachial access was used the wire is snared out of a sheath placed in the ipsilateral CFA, thus allowing for a stiff guiding wire to be advanced to the descending aorta from the CFA, which facilitates ease of delivery of stents and correct alignment.

D. **Infrarenal and Distal Aortic Occlusions** Occlusion of the infrarenal aorta and aortoiliac bifurcation often require bilateral access due to the likely need of kissing stents. Although a retrograde crossing strategy as discussed above could be undertaken following access in bilateral CFAs, brachial access remains a reasonable alternative. If the lesions are crossed in antegrade fashion from the brachial artery access point, the wires could be externalized through the respective sheaths in the CFA. Brachial access also minimizes subintimal tracking in the descending aorta and consequently the need for reentry devices in the descending aorta. However, brachial access carries the highest risk of access site complications with hematoma, pseudoaneurysm, and thrombosis.

VII. Reentry

A. The **success of subintimal crossing** lies in reentry. Although an angled backup catheter could help to direct the wire toward the true lumen, the operator should change the angle of imaging as the lesion is crossed to ensure the wire advancement favors reentry.

B. While the majority of vessels are reentered with **standard wire and catheter strategy** some cases require more complex steps such as antegrade crossing or use of reentry devices.

C. In case of **subintimal wire-tracking of the iliac artery**, an attempt is made to cross the lesion with a second wire in an antegrade fashion. This maneuver could be undertaken with contralateral femoral access or brachial access. As the antegrade wire is advanced in a new subintimal plane and meets the retrograde wire, the retrograde wire would follow the path of the antegrade wire and advance to the true lumen.

D. However, instead of the **retrograde wire advancement technique**, one could opt to use reentry systems such as the Pioneer catheter (Medtronic, Inc., Minneapolis, MN) or Outback LTD reentry catheter (Cordis Corporation).

E. The **Pioneer catheter** is a device platform in which a curved needle is deployed under IVUS guidance. Intimal puncture is performed under direct IVUS imaging, and depending on the thickness of the subintimal flap, the operator could adjust the depth of the needle puncture. The needle traverses the intima and plaque into the true lumen, and a wire is advanced through this needle to the true lumen (Fig. 9.1).

F. Reentry with the **Outback catheter** is performed by fluoroscopy-guided alignment of markers on the catheter that indicates the location of the reentry cannula. "L" and "T" markers are used to define when the catheter was positioned in a perpendicular or inline plane of the needle, respectively. Through imaging in two orthogonal views, the orientation is confirmed to ensure the delivery catheter enters the true lumen.

G. In a study by Jacobs et al, **requirement for reentry devices** was more frequent with iliac chronic total occlusions (CTOs), in comparison with femoral CTOs (34% vs 26%). However, there was a 100% success rate in reentry with the Pioneer or Outback reentry catheters. There were no cases of bleeding from the needle deployment site or other reentry-related complications.[13]

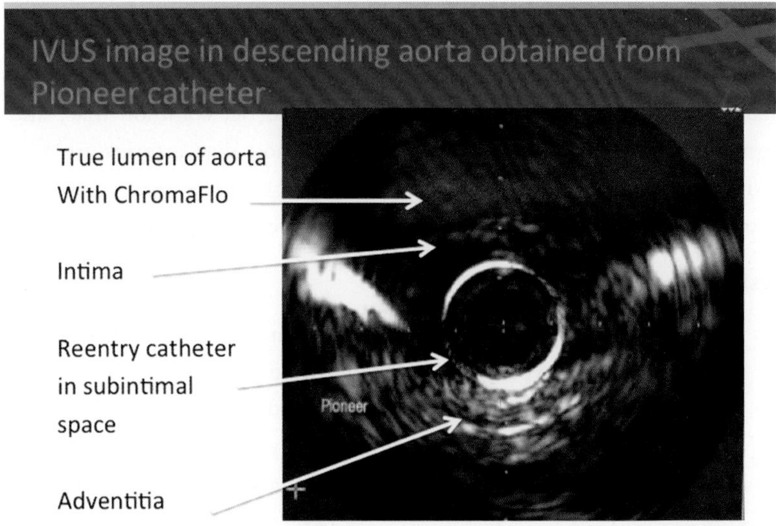

FIGURE 9.1: Intravascular ultrasound (IVUS) image with Pioneer catheter in subintimal space.

VIII. Angioplasty and Stent Placement

A. Stenting of iliac artery disease is currently **standard of practice**. However, if treatment with balloon angioplasty is undertaken for TASC A and B lesions of the external iliac artery, angiography in multiple views must be performed to exclude dissection following balloon angioplasty. Furthermore, a residual hemodynamic gradient greater than 10 mm Hg at rest or following arterial vasodilator administration warrants stent placement.

B. Several **studies** have examined the results of primary stent placement versus selective stent placement following angioplasty in iliac disease.

1. In the Dutch Iliac Stent Trial, 279 patients with >50% iliac stenosis mostly due to TASC A and B lesions were randomized to direct stent placement versus primary angioplasty with selective stent placement in case of a residual gradient >10 mm Hg.
   Almost 43% of patients in group 2 underwent selective stent placement. The primary end point, which was clinical success defined by improvement in Fontaine category, was significantly better in the selective stent group. (Hazard ratio, 0 0.8; 95% confidence limits: 0.6, 1.0.) However, long-term (5-8 year) patency rates were similar between these two groups.[14]

2. Considering endovascular intervention of TASC C and D iliac lesions, current data overwhelmingly support primary stenting. The Stents versus Angioplasty… of the Treatment of Iliac Artery Occlusions (STAG) trial randomized 112 patients to percutaneous transluminal angioplasty or primary stent placement. Technical success was higher in the primary stent group (98% vs 84%), and complications were less frequent. (5% vs 20%)

3. A meta-analysis of 16 studies with a total of 958 patients who underwent endovascular treatment for TASC C or D aortoiliac disease found better patency rates for primary stenting in comparison to selective stenting.[15]

C. **Endovascular Interventions for AIOD** Unfortunately most data on endovascular interventions for AIOD are not analyzed according to the involved segment. From an anatomical and hemodynamic standpoint the aortic, common iliac, and external iliac segments differ significantly. Aortic and common iliac arteries are straight, relatively immobile, large, and calcified. The external iliac artery is smaller in diameter and has a tortuous course. It is also exposed to external forces during the movement of the hip joint.

D. **Lesions**

1. As **lesions of the infrarenal aorta and common iliac arteries** are short and usually calcified, balloon-expandable stents are used. The balloon-expandable stents often made from stainless steel have adequate radial strength to hold a calcified lesion expanded. Ease of precise positioning during stent deployment adds value to using these stents in the aortic and common iliac positions.

2. **Lesions of the descending aorta** are seldom isolated and more frequently involves the iliac bifurcation and common iliac arteries.

3. **Isolated aortic lesions** can be treated with unilateral femoral access. Once the lesion is crossed with a low-profile hydrophilic wire and back-up catheter, a stiff 0.35″ wire such an Amplatz superstiff wire (Boston Scientific) is advanced through the backup catheter. A 12-14 mm stent is used depending on patient characteristics. IVUS examination could be undertaken to aid with sizing of the stent following which balloon-expandable stent is recommended.
4. **Lesions of the aortic bifurcation or bilateral common iliac arteries** require bilateral common femoral access. Once the lesions are crossed, balloon dilatation could be performed with a low-profile 4-5 mm compliant balloon. This would allow for the sheaths to be advanced across the iliac artery lesions. This step minimizes the risk of stent dislodgement within the calcified vessel. Use of sheaths with radiopaque markers at the tip such as the Vista brite tip (Cordis) is advantageous. Next the stents are advanced within the sheath across the lesions bilaterally, and the sheaths are retracted with the stents held in place. Simultaneous balloon expansion is undertaken for symmetric deployment of simultaneous kissing stents. A significant disadvantage of placing simultaneous kissing stents is the inability to easily access the contralateral leg by crossover of the bifurcation for future interventions necessitating an antegrade common femoral or brachial access.
5. With **isolated ostial iliac lesions**, which are less than 5 mm from the bifurcation, simultaneous kissing stents should be considered to minimize the risk of contralateral iliac occlusion owing to plaque shift and deformation of the architecture of the bifurcation.
6. When stent placement of **proximal common iliac lesions** more than 5 mm from the ostium is undertaken, simultaneous low-pressure balloon expansion of the contralateral common iliac is recommended to reduce the risk of embolization and displacement of the bifurcation.
7. **Aortoiliac lesions** are more commonly associated with thrombus formation in comparison with femoral disease. The operator would have a reasonable suspicion of thrombotic occlusions, if a wire crosses the lesion with ease. This could be managed in several ways. The intervention could be completed following several hours of catheter-assisted thrombolysis. Covered stents can be placed to minimize embolization.

E. **Occlusions** of the external iliac artery are routinely stented with self-expanding nitinol stents owing to the external forces during hip joint movement. Nitinol has a valuable feature of thermal shape memory and super elasticity, due to which the stent returns to the original shape after severe deformation. Furthermore, its ability to adapt to the tortuous path of a vessel reduces the risk of dissection and perforation in the external iliac arteries.

IX. Patency

Examining the Table 9.1, it is shown that iliac stent placement has a greater than 95% success rate and primary patency around 90% and 85% at 1-3 years, respectively.

Table 9.1. Patency Rates for Aortoiliac Stenting in TASC Class A–D Lesions

Study	Year	No. of Patients	Success Rate	Primary Patency
Uher[2]	2002	77		70% (3 y)
Leville[3]	2006	92	91%	76% (3 y)
Kashyap[4]	2008	86	100%	74% (3 y)
Higashiura[5]	2009	216		93% (3 y) 91% (5 y)
Koizumi[6]	2009	296	96%	88% (3 y) 84% (5 y)
Jaff[7]	2010	151		91% (2 y)
Ichihashi[8]	2011	533	100%	90% (1 y) 83% (5 y)
Soga[9]	2012	2601	98%	92.5% (1 y) 83% (3 y)
deDonato[10]	2013	147	100%	93% (1 y) 88% (2 y)

X. Complications

A. Ruptures

1. The most **catastrophic complication** of endovascular intervention of AIOD remains to be **vessel rupture.** Sudden complains of significant pain and hemodynamic compromise are strong warning signs of rupture. Immediate injection is performed to identify the site of the perforation, and a balloon is expanded across the site. A covered stent is called for, and rapid resuscitation should be undertaken. If the current sheath does not allow for delivery of a covered stent, contralateral femoral access should be obtained and a balloon advanced proximal to the perforation. While this balloon is inflated, the sheath can be exchanged with a view to deliver the covered stent through the original access site. Although reversal of anticoagulation is undertaken in this situation, in our institution we do not routinely use anticoagulation for nonthrombotic aortoilic interventions.

2. **Rupture is relatively rare in AIOD.** In a study including 657 iliac interventions, the rate of rupture was 0.8%.[16]

3. **Factors predisposing to rupture** include calcified vessels, occluded vessels, oversized balloons, recent endarterectomy, chronic steroid therapy, diabetes mellitus, female gender, and external iliac artery lesions.[17]

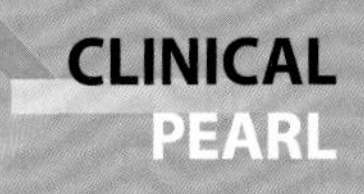

CLINICAL PEARL Before undertaking such an intervention, each operator should ensure equipment for bail out is available on the shelf, as immediate intervention is lifesaving in aortoiliac rupture.

B. **Arterial Dissection** can also occur during intervention in AIOD. As noted above, careful evaluation of final angiography in multiple views is undertaken to ensure a dissection flap is not missed. A dissection could be treated by prolonged balloon inflation across the dissection or by stenting in the setting of a flow-limiting dissection.

C. When significant **distal embolization** occurs maintaining anticoagulation, performing aspiration thrombectomy with manual aspiration or mechanical aspiration such as the Angiojet device (Boston Scientific, Marlborough, MA, USA) is the cornerstone of management. In the setting of a large thrombus, burden delivery of focal thrombolysis (10 mg of intraarterial tissue plasminogen activator) could be considered. Fresh thrombotic lesions that are resistant to above therapy may require balloon angioplasty or open thrombectomy.

D. **Acute Stent Misadventures** during iliac intervention include stent dislodgement before deployment, embolization and migration, and compression of the contralateral iliac artery. Advancing a sheath beyond the lesion before advancing the stent could minimize stent dislodgement. Embolization and migration occur in severely calcified lesions with the stents usually migrating away from calcified segments. Hence understanding the lesion and applying gentle forward or backward pressure during deployment on the stent shaft toward the calcified area of the lesion helps to reduce this complication. In the event of stent embolization, retrieval could be attempted by snaring the stent.

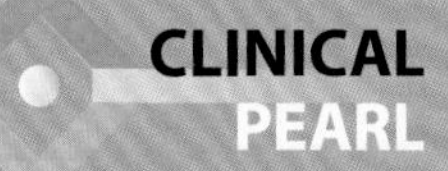

In anticipation of compression of the contralateral artery, low-pressure balloon inflation or kissing stent deployment is necessary.

E. **Late complications** include **stent thrombosis and pseudoaneurysm formation.**

1. **Stent thrombosis** is due to a mechanical reason, which often is due to an unrecognized edge dissection or poor distal runoff. Treatment with overnight thrombolytic infusion and endovascular of the flow limitation is the least complicated approach. However, if distal disease was not amenable to endovascular therapy, surgical revascularization would be undertaken.
2. **Psuedoaneurysm** formation is often due to progression of a dissection at the treatment site, which was not seen at the time of the procedure. This could be treated with an endovascular stent graft in the absence of infection.

XI. Follow-Up

A. **Medical Therapy** following intervention for AIOD usually includes aspirin for life and a second antiplatelet such as clopidogrel, prasugrel, or ticagrelor for 1 month. Aggressive risk factor management for cardiovascular disease is undertaken with treatment for diabetes mellitus, hypertension, and dyslipidemia. Smoking cessation is strongly encouraged, and walking programs are initiated.

B. Patients with AIOD should be followed at **regular intervals**. In our institution, we evaluate patients at 1-, 3-, 6-, and 12-month intervals by clinical and ultrasound evaluation. In the event of significant restenosis being noted, revascularization is recommended, as revascularization during restenosis is simpler than treating complete occlusion.

XII. Summary

AIOD is readily treatable by endovascular methods, which should be considered as first-line treatment. The success rates and patency are high. The complexity of the lesion may dictate access site and equipment needed. Each operator should be well versed in possible complications and bail out techniques in endovascular treatment of AIOD. Patients with aortoiliac disease are followed up to evaluate for clinical and ultrasound evidence of restenosis and aggressive treatment of risk factors.

References

1. Norgren L, Hiatt WR, Dormandy JA, Nehler MR, Harris KA, Fowkes FG. Inter-society consensus for the management of peripheral arterial disease (TASC II). *J Vasc Surg.* 2007;45(suppl S):S5-67.
2. Uher P, Nyman U, Lindh M, Lindblad B, Ivancev K. Long-term results of stenting for chronic iliac artery occlusion. *J Endovasc Ther.* 2002;9:67-75.
3. Leville CD, Kashyap VS, Clair DG, et al. Endovascular management of iliac artery occlusions: extending treatment to TransAtlantic Inter-Society Consensus class C and D patients. *J Vasc Surg.* 2006;43:32-39.
4. Kashyap VS, Pavkov ML, Bena JF, et al. The management of severe aortoiliac occlusive disease: endovascular therapy rivals open reconstruction. *J Vasc Surg.* 2008;48:1451-1457, 7.e1-3.
5. Higashiura W, Kubota Y, Sakaguchi S, et al. Prevalence, factors, and clinical impact of self-expanding stent fractures following iliac artery stenting. *J Vasc Surg.* 2009;49:645-652.
6. Koizumi A, Kumakura H, Kanai H, et al. Ten-year patency and factors causing restenosis after endovascular treatment of iliac artery lesions. *Circ J.* 2009;73:860-866.
7. Jaff MR, Katzen BT. Two-year clinical evaluation of the Zilver vascular stent for symptomatic iliac artery disease. *J Vasc Interv Radiol.* 2010;21:1489-1494.
8. Ichihashi S, Higashiura W, Itoh H, Sakaguchi S, Nishimine K, Kichikawa K. Long-term outcomes for systematic primary stent placement in complex iliac artery occlusive disease classified according to Trans-Atlantic Inter-Society Consensus (TASC)-II. *J Vasc Surg.* 2011;53:992-999.
9. Soga Y, Iida O, Kawasaki D, et al. Contemporary outcomes after endovascular treatment for aorto-iliac artery disease. *Circ J.* 2012;76:2697-2704.
10. de Donato G, Bosiers M, Setacci F, et al. 24-Month data from the BRAVISSIMO: a large-scale prospective registry on iliac stenting for TASC A & B and TASC C & D Lesions. *Ann Vasc Surg.* 2015;29:738-750.
11. Golomb BA, Dang TT, Criqui MH. Peripheral arterial disease: morbidity and mortality implications. *Circulation.* 2006;114:688-699.
12. Ubbink DT, Fidler M, Legemate DA. Interobserver variability in aortoiliac and femoropopliteal duplex scanning. *J Vasc Surg.* 2001;33:540-545.
13. Jacobs DL, Motaganahalli RL, Cox DE, Wittgen CM, Peterson GJ. True lumen re-entry devices facilitate subintimal angioplasty and stenting of total chronic occlusions: Initial report. *J Vasc Surg.* 2006;43:1291-1296.
14. Klein WM, van der Graaf Y, Seegers J, et al. Dutch iliac stent trial: long-term results in patients randomized for primary or selective stent placement. *Radiology.* 2006;238:734-744.

15. Goode SD, Cleveland TJ, Gaines PA. Randomized clinical trial of stents versus angioplasty for the treatment of iliac artery occlusions (STAG trial). *Br J Surg*. 2013;100:1148-1153.
16. Ballard JL, Sparks SR, Taylor FC, et al. Complications of iliac artery stent deployment. *J Vasc Surg*. 1996;24:545-553; discussion 53–5.
17. Allaire E, Melliere D, Poussier B, Kobeiter H, Desgranges P, Becquemin JP. Iliac artery rupture during balloon dilatation: what treatment? *Ann Vasc Surg*. 2003;17:306-314.

CHAPTER 10

Endovascular Interventions in Superficial Femoral Artery Disease

Qurat-ul-Aini Jelani, MD, Sasanka Jayasuriya, MBBS, FACC, FASE, RPVI, FSCAI, and Carlos Meña, MD, FACC, FSCAI

Key Points

- As a result of multiple dynamic stressors, the SFA is the most common site of involvement of atherosclerotic arterial disease in patients with PAD.
- Patients presenting with intermittent claudication should be treated with optimal medical therapy, intervention for smoking cessation, and a supervised exercise walking program.
- Patients with ongoing symptoms in spite of above therapy and patients presenting with critical limb ischemia are offered endovascular or open surgical revascularization.
- Percutaneous transluminal angioplasty with plain or drug-coated balloons and stenting with bare metal stents, drug-eluting stents, or stent grafts are endovascular treatment options in patients with femoropopliteal disease.

I. Introduction

The superficial femoral artery (SFA) is the most common site of involvement of atherosclerotic arterial disease resulting in claudication in patients with peripheral arterial disease (PAD). The SFA and the contiguous popliteal artery constitute the femoropopliteal (FP) segment which is extremely long and exposed to external compression. The SFA is exposed to multiple anatomic and dynamic challenges. There is 13% shortening of the SFA between supine and fetal positions.[1] Additionally there are 60 degrees of SFA torsion produced by simultaneous knee and hip flexion.[1] While these characteristics make it challenging to treat FP disease, FP involvement occurs in 20%-40% of patients with critical limb ischemia (CLI) and remains the most common location of disease in patients presenting with claudication.[2] The severity of symptoms from SFA disease vary considerably, based on the extent of collateralization from the profundal femoral artery. The optimal treatment of SFA disease in patients with intermittent claudication remains a matter of continuing debate. In the last decade, endovascular treatment (EVT) of infrainguinal disease has been readily adopted as an alternative to open bypass surgery. Percutaneous transluminal angioplasty (PTA) and stenting are the most commonly used EVT options for TASC (Trans-Atlantic Inter-Society Consensus) type A and B lesions.[3,4] With the advent of advanced techniques such as subintimal angioplasty, advanced devices such as those enabling reentry, availability of mechanical and laser atherectomy, even type C and D lesions are being successfully treated.[5] In most cases, endovascular procedures are also well tolerated, requiring short hospital stays, and result in rapid recovery.[6] The revised Trans-Atlantic Intersociety Consensus document[3] and the American Heart Association[7] guidelines recommend the use of EVT as first-line treatment for patients with focal and moderate disease. Open bypass is recommended for diffuse disease or long segment total occlusions. After failure of an exercise program and optimization of medical therapy, EVT may be considered. As the data for the long-term efficacy of EVT versus open surgical bypass are limited, treatment approach should be individualized and should take into account both patient and procedural risks.

II. Clinical Assessment of Peripheral Arterial Disease in Patients With Superficial Femoral Artery Disease[8]

A. Patients at Risk for Peripheral Arterial Disease

1. Patients at increased risk of PAD including SFA disease include individuals >65 years of age, patient between age 50 and 64 years with risk factors for PAD (ie, diabetes mellitus [DM], history of smoking, hyperlipidemia, and hypertension [HTN]), individuals with known atherosclerotic disease in another vascular territory (eg, coronary, carotid, subclavian, renal etc).

2. **Claudication**
   a. The majority of patients with confirmed PAD do not have typical claudication and may either have non–joint-related symptoms(atypical symptoms) or are asymptomatic.[9,10]
   b. Claudication is a classic manifestation of PAD and is defined as fatigue, discomfort, cramping, or pain of vascular origin in the muscles of the lower extremities that is consistently induced by exercise and consistently relieved by rest (within 10 min).

3. **Critical Limb Ischemia** More advanced PAD may manifest as critical limb ischemia (CLI) which is defined as chronic (>2 wk) ischemic rest pain with nonhealing wounds/ulcers or gangrene in one or both legs.

B. Examination

1. Examination of patients with PAD include pulse palpation, auscultation for femoral bruits, and inspection of the lower extremities including feet.

2. Abnormal physical examination findings may include diminished pulses, vascular bruit, nonhealing wounds/gangrene, and so forth.[8]
   a. Abnormal physical findings should be confirmed with diagnostic testing.
   b. Ankle brachial index (ABI) is generally the initial test of choice.
      i. The resting ABI is a simple, noninvasive test that is usually obtained by measuring systolic blood pressure at the brachial arteries, dorsalis pedis (DP), and posterior tibial (PT) arteries in the supine position. ABI is calculated for both legs by dividing the higher of the DP or PT pressure by the higher of the right or left arm blood pressure.
      ii. Segmental lower extremity blood pressures and pulse volume recordings are often performed along with ABIs which may be used to localize anatomic segments of disease.
      iii. A normal ABI is between 1.00 and 1.40.[11] An ABI 0.90 demonstrates 90% sensitivity and 95% specificity for PAD and is the accepted threshold for

diagnosis. Values between 0.91 and 1.00 are considered borderline; however, the cardiovascular event rate for an ABI in this range is increased by 10%-20%.

iv. At levels >1.40, the identification of PAD is not accurate because of the presence of arterial calcification and noncompressibility of the blood vessels.

v. Depending on resting ABI values, additional physiologic testing may be considered including exercise treadmill ABI testing, measurement of toe brachial index (TBI), and perfusion assessment by transcutaneous oxygen pressure ($TcPO_2$) or skin perfusion pressure (SPP).

vi. TBI is used to establish diagnosis of PAD in the setting of noncompressible arteries (ABI >1.40) and may be used in patients with suspected CLI.

vii. An abnormal ABI is consistently related with the presence of coronary and cerebrovascular disease.[12–14] In addition, it remains a predictor of cardiovascular mortality and morbidity independent of clinical risk prediction scores such as the Framingham risk score, coronary calcium score, and carotid artery intimal medial thickness.[15]

C. **Revascularization Considerations** In patients in whom revascularization is being considered, anatomic imaging may be performed including duplex ultrasound, computed tomography angiography (CTA), or magnetic resonance angiography.[16] Duplex ultrasonography is easily accessible, inexpensive, and especially useful in patients with renal failure; however, it has limited sensitivity for multilevel stenosis and in calcified vessels. CTA and MRA both allow rapid acquisition of a high-resolution, three-dimensional roadmap of the peripheral arterial tree. However, the use of CTA is limited by exposure to both iodinated contrast and ionizing radiation. MRA is associated with increased risk of nephrogenic systemic sclerosis in patients with advanced disease receiving gadolinium.

III. Medical Therapy for Patients With Peripheral Arterial Disease

A. **Exercise Programs** All patients with PAD should receive guideline-directed medical therapy including a structured exercise program. Treatment should be aimed at limb-related outcomes including improving claudication symptoms and preventing CLI and amputation. One of the goals of medical treatment is to prevent major adverse cardiovascular events including myocardial infarction (MI), stroke, and cardiovascular death. Patients with PAD continue to be undertreated[17,18] despite the benefits of multifactorial risk reduction in this patient population.[19]

B. **Pharmacotherapy** Pharmacotherapy for patients with PAD includes antiplatelets and statins and is further tailored to individual risk factors. Exercise training has been a mainstay of treatment for symptomatic PAD,[20,21] modifying several pathophysiological mechanisms including improved skeletal muscle metabolism, endothelial function, and gait abnormalities.[22] A 12-week intervention of supervised exercise program improves exercise program and quality of life in PAD.[20] In trials with follow-up ranging from 18 months to 7 years,[23–25] a persistent benefit of supervised exercise has been demonstrated. Supervised exercise program has an excellent safety profile in patients screened for absolute contraindication to exercise such as exercise-limiting cardiovascular disease, amputation or wheelchair confinement.[26–28]

C. **Smoking Cessation** Smoking remains a major risk factor for the development and progression of PAD. In a study of 739 patients undergoing lower extremity angiography, 28% were active smokers. Those who quit and continued to abstain had a significantly lower 5-year mortality and improved amputation-free survival.[29] Discontinuation of smoking is the most important lifestyle modification in preventing amputation, CLI, and MACE.

IV. Interventions for Patients With Peripheral Arterial Disease

A. Principles of Catheter-Based Interventions

1. The main treatment aim of EVT intervention in the SFA/FP circulation is to restore unobstructed flow to the tibial trifurcation. There are standard definitions for success and patency. Angiographic success refers to a residual diameter stenosis not more than 30% and subsequent patency with less than 50% recurrent stenosis.[30] Hemodynamically, the success of an intervention is indicated by an increase in ABI of at least 0.15 and an improvement in Rutherford class.[30] Restenosis occurs frequently and correlates directly with lesion length.[31]
2. Intermittent claudication (IC) may be caused by occlusive lesions in the aortoiliac segment, common femoral artery, SFA, and profundal femoral and popliteal arteries. In patients with multisegment disease, the more proximal disease should be treated first. This usually results in symptomatic improvement without extending treatment to distal arteries.[6] There are multiple EVT options for SFA/FP occlusive disease (FPOD),[6] including PTA alone,[32] angioplasty with self-expanding stents,[33] angioplasty with balloon-expandable stents,[34] angioplasty with covered stent grafts,[35,36] atherectomy,[8] antimyoproliferative drug-coated balloons (DCBs),[37–39] and drug-eluting stents (DESs).[40] Other modalities include thrombolysis that uses lytic agents acting on fibrin and thrombectomy that uses direct techniques to remove clot.

B. Overview of Guidelines[6]

1. According to the Society for Vascular Surgery (SVS) guidelines for atherosclerotic disease of the lower extremities, EVT is recommended over open surgery for focal occlusive disease of the SFA not involving the origin (class IC). For focal lesions (<5 cm), with unsatisfactory results with balloon angioplasty, selective stenting is suggested (2C). The use of self-expanding nitinol stents (with or without paclitaxel) is recommended for intermediate length lesions (1B). Surgical bypass is recommended as the initial revascularization strategy for diffuse femoropoliteal disease, small caliber (<5 mm), or extensive calcification of the SFA. According to the American College of Cardiology/American Heart Association (ACC/AHA) guidelines, revascularization of the FP segment is recommended for patients with CLI or for patients who have had a suboptimal response to a trial of exercise.[41] An endovascular

first approach is recommended for TASC A through C lesions and is a reasonable approach for TASC D lesions (Table 10.1) as determined by the experience of the operator, and the patient's comorbidities.

2. The morphological classification for SFA/FP lesions and thereby treatment is also guided by the recommendations made by the Trans-Atlantic Inter-Society Consensus document II (TASC II) (Table 10.2).[42] TASC-A and B are managed with endovascular techniques; TASC-C are treated by either endovascular revascularization or bypass based on individual risk stratification. TASC-D lesions are generally surgically managed.

3. In general the outcomes of PTA and stenting depend on both anatomic and clinical characteristics.[7] Patency after PTA is greatest for lesions in the common iliac artery, decreasing distally. Patency also decreases with increasing length, multiple and diffuse lesions, presence of comorbidities including diabetes, smoking and renal

TABLE 10.1. ACC/AHA Recommendations for Femoropoliteal Intervention in Stable Limb Ischemia

Class I, Level of Evidence: A	• Endovascular procedures are indicated for patients with a vocational or lifestyle-limiting disability • Due to intermittent claudication when clinical features suggest a reasonable likelihood of symptomatic improvement with endovascular intervention and: (1) there has been an inadequate response to exercise or pharmacological therapy, and/or (2) there is a very favorable risk-benefit ratio (eg, focal stenosis)
Class IIa, Level of Evidence: C	Stents (and other adjunctive techniques such as lasers, cutting balloons, atherectomy devices, and thermal devices) can be useful in the femoral, popliteal, and tibial arteries as salvage therapy for a suboptimal or failed result from balloon dilation (eg, persistent translesional gradient, residual diameter stenosis >50%, or flow-limiting dissection)
Class IIb, Level of Evidence: A	The effectiveness of stents, atherectomy, cutting balloons, thermal devices, and lasers for the treatment of femoral-popliteal arterial lesions is not well established (except to salvage a suboptimal result from balloon dilation)
Class III, Level of Evidence: C	Primary stent placement is not recommended in the femoral, popliteal, or tibial arteries
Class III, Level of Evidence: C	Endovascular intervention is not indicated as prophylactic therapy in an asymptomatic patient with lower extremity peripheral arterial disease (PAD)

Data from Anderson JL, Halperin JL, Albert NM, et al. Management of patients with peripheral artery disease (compilation of 2005 and 2011 ACCF/AHA guideline recommendations): A report of the American College of Cardiology Foundation/American Heart Association Task Force on practice guidelines. *Circulation.* 2013;127(13):1425-1442.

TABLE 10.2. Morphological Stratification of Femoropopliteal Lesions[42]

Lesion Type	Stenosis or Occlusion Pattern	Procedure
A	1. Single stenosis less than 3 cm of the superficial femoral artery or popliteal artery	Endovascular
B	1. Single stenosis 3-10 cm in length, not involving the distal popliteal artery 2. Heavily calcified stenoses up to 3 cm in length 3. Multiple lesions, each less than 3 cm (stenoses or occlusions) 4. Single or multiple lesions in the absence of continuous tibial runoff to improve inflow for distal surgical bypass	Endovascular
C	1. Single stenosis or occlusion longer than 5 cm 2. Multiple stenoses or occlusions, each 3-5 cm in length, with or without heavy calcification	Endovascular or surgical bypass
D	1. Complete common femoral artery or superficial femoral artery occlusions or complete popliteal and proximal trifurcation occlusions	Surgical bypass

failure.[43–49] Although there is no consensus on a diagnostic transstenotic pressure gradient, intravascular pressure measurements have been recommended to determine whether lesions are significant—for example a stenoses of 50%-75% may or may not be hemodynamically significant. Multiple criteria have been suggested including a mean gradient of 10 mm Hg before or after vasodilators or a peak systolic pressure gradient of 15% after administration of a vasodilator.[50,51]

C. Vascular Access

1. Vascular access is the most important part of any endovascular intervention (Table 10.3). The most common access vessel is common femoral artery (CFA). The brachial artery may be used in some cases; left brachial access is usually preferred, as the risk of cerebral embolization is less than access via right brachial approach. Safest approach to obtaining access is by using ultrasound guidance and using a micropuncture needle. The puncture site for CFA must be below the inguinal ligament and above the femoral bifurcation in the region overlying the femoral head. The puncture site should be confirmed fluoroscopically/angiographically. By angiography, the puncture site/needle entry site should be between the origin of the inferior epigastric artery/lateral circumflex artery and femoral bifurcation. Contralateral and ipsilateral arterial access can both be used. Generally contralateral access site is preferred which requires an up-and-over technique to cross the bifurcation. Contralateral approach may not be used in case of tortuous iliac arteries, hostile aortic bifurcations, Y-prosthesis, or abdominal stent grafts.[53] In cases of failed antegrade approach or flush SFA occlusion, ipsilateral retrograde popliteal approach may be used. Left brachial access is reserved for cases of CFA and SFA lesions in the presence of bilateral iliac artery occlusions. It is associated with the risk of vertebrobasilar stroke. Research has recently been published evaluating transradial and transulnar access in combination with transpedal access for femoral artery angioplasty.[52]

2. Once access is obtained, the micropuncture sheath is exchanged for an appropriate sized sheath (ranging from 4 to 7 French). Digital subtraction angiography of the distal aorta and iliac arteries followed by angiography of the target extremity is performed using a 5 French flush catheter.

TABLE 10.3. Access Sites Used for Superficial Femoral Artery Intervention

Access Site	
Contralateral common femoral artery (CFA)	Most commonly used. Technically feasible
Ipsilateral CFA/antegrade	In patients with significant iliac disease. Unsuitable for ostial or proximal superficial femoral artery (SFA) disease
Retrograde transpopliteal	Patients with contraindication to both contralateral and ipsilateral approach. In patients with chronic total occlusions when failure to cross proximal cap
Retrograde brachial	In patients with iliac disease or other contraindications to contralateral or ipsilateral approach. Mostly in patients with proximal or mid-SFA disease
Retrograde transpedal	Maybe combined with contralateral or ipsilateral approach. Mainly used when failure to cross proximal cap of chronic occlusions
Retrograde transradial	Maybe combined with contralateral or ipsilateral approach. Combined with transpedal approach[52]

3. After inflow assessment, the aortic bifurcation is crossed with the flush catheter and 0.035-inch angled glidewire (Terumo, Somerset, NJ). The catheter is then positioned at the inguinal ligament, and selective angiography of the lower extremity is performed. 3-5 mL injections of nonionic iso-osmolar contrast is injected to evaluate the SFA and infrapopliteal runoff. Imaging is usually done in two obliquities to fully assess areas of stenoses and visualize bifurcations. Once lesions have been identified, a 0.035 wire is then reinserted and positioned in the SFA. The flush catheter is removed, and the wire is then used to exchange the 5 French short catheter for 6-7F 45-55 cm long sheath. These sheaths provide support for lesion crossing and also allow for contrast injection.
4. Before any intervention, patients should be anticoagulated with heparin. In patients in whom heparin is contraindicated, direct thrombin inhibitors including bivalirudin, hirudin, lepiruidin, and argatroban may be used. Activated clotting time (ACT) is checked every 30-60 minutes for a goal ACT above 250 seconds. The advantage of heparin over direct thrombin inhibitors is that in case of access site complications, heparin can be reversed with protamine sulfate.
5. After anticoagulation is achieved, the lesion is traversed with a combination of a directional catheter and a 0.035-inch guidewire. If this is unable to cross lesion, a varying combination of 0.018 or 0.014 inch guidewire and catheters may be used. The catheter is positioned just proximal to the target lesions providing wire support and pushability. If these options fail due to proximal cap configuration, plaque morphology or lesion composition, subintimal angioplasty (SIA) may be attempted. SIA refers to the passage of wires and catheters into the wall of the occluded artery with reentry at a point of distal patency. This technique, first popularized by Bolia, uses a short "prolapsed loop" configuration of a hydrophilic wire extending from the tip of a guiding catheter to gain spontaneous reentry once the reconstituted artery is reached. In addition to the hydrophilic wires, multiple commercially available reentry devices are available including Outback & Pioneer (Coviden-Medtronic, Minneapolis, MN); Off-Road, Boston Scientific (Watertown, MA); and Enteer (Covidient-Medtronic). SIA or revascularization is associated with similar midterm patency rates as intraluminal therapies and can be used with excellent technical success. However, SIA should not be attempted in dense medial (Monckenberg type) calcification, absence of a reentry site, and a reentry site that is too small in diameter. Perforations or rupture maybe treated with catheter-directed occlusion or exclusion with a stent graft or surgical repair. Although SIA is the most expeditious form of intervention for long segment chronic total occlusions, it may potentially limit the use of other therapies including DCBs and atherectomy.

D. Lesion Crossing

1. Lesion crossing is central to a successful intervention. Every attempt should be made to maintain luminal position and avoid dissection into the subintimal space. Subintimal dissection increases time and complexity of the procedure. To avoid subintimal dissection, a

steerable angled wire (0.035-inch angled glidewire, Terumo), which is a hydrophilic wire is used with the help of a torque device. The angled glidewire has a floppy tip to prevent dissection with enough support to maneuver the tip. When the tip of the wire deforms, the wire is usually retracted and turned in a different direction for true lumen.

2. For high-grade stenoses, a smaller wire such as the 0.014-inch ASAHI Grand Slam (Abbott Vascular, Abbott Park, IL) may also be used. Chronic total occlusion requires more wires and catheters. In CTOs, it is difficult to ascertain whether the wire is luminal or has crossed over into the subintimal space. In those cases, 0.035-inch Stiff Angled Glidewire (Terumo) in conjunction with a 0.035-inch Angled Glide Catheter (AngioDynamics) or 0.035-inch Quick Cross catheter may be used as they provide sufficient support. The tip of the wire is usually given a J loop which then curves onto itself and creates a loop, thus allowing the body of the wire to enter subintimal space. The wire is then extended the length of the occlusion, being supported by the catheter until reentry is identified. One can then determine luminal reentry. It is essential to identify the most proximal site of target vessel reconsititution when performing interventions on CTOs. Extension beyond that jeopardizes bypass targets. Once this point is identified, catheter is advanced and wire removed. Back bleeding is then performed to confirm reentry into true lumen. Injection of 1-2 mL of contrast may also be used to confirm this. In case of multiple attempts at reentry, reentry devices such as the Pioneer Catheter (Medtronic, Minneapolis, MN) may be used to obtain luminal access. After lesion crossing, wire serves as a guide for balloon catheter and stent delivery system.

E. Percutaneous Transluminal Angioplasty for Superficial Femoral Artery Disease (Table 10.4)

1. The mechanism of angioplasty is controlled intimal dissection, disrupting luminal plaque and increasing diameter of the arterial flow. Barotrauma associated with PTA may provoke intimal hyperplasia through a combination of vessel wall inflammation and injury and altered flow due to intimal dehiscence.
   a. Specialty balloons have been developed that can "cut," "score," or "modify" inflation profile of balloons to prevent overexpansion and dissection. It has the advantage of being inexpensive and technically simpler than primary stenting. It also avoids stent fatigue and fracture which may result from torque and deformation of the FP arteries during flexion of the knee joint.
   b. Additionally, lower profile balloons may allow PTA of the SFA through sheaths as small as 4 French. PTA performs well for short lesions (<5 cm)[54] that are non-calcified; restenosis rates increase as lesion length increases.[33,37,55–58]
   c. In the VIVA objective performance criteria, the overall 12-month patency rate for lesions between 4 and 15 cm treated with PTA alone ranged from 28% to 37%.[59] PTA alone is associated with complications including flow-limiting dissection, perforation, arterial rupture, and distal embolization. In one study, stent placement for elastic recoil or significant dissection after PTA has been reported in up to 40% of cases.[33]

TABLE 10.4. Clinical Trials in Femoropoliteal Disease[60]

Clinical Trial	Device	Number of Patients	Lesion Length (cm)	IC/CLI	TLR	Restenosis
FAST[54]	PTA	121	45 ± 28	96.5/3.5	18.3	38.6
	BMS	123	45 ± 27	97.5/2.5	14.9	31.7
ABSOLUTE[61]	PTA	53	92 ± 75	87/13	31	63.0
	BMS	51	101 ± 75	88/12	28	37.0
ASTRON[62]	PTA	39	65 ± 46	97/3	–	61.1
	BMS	34	82 ± 67	91/9	–	34.4
ZILVER[63]	PTA	238	63 ± 41	90.7/8.5	17.5	67.2
	DES	241	66 ± 39	90.2/8.9	9.5	16.9
ZELLER[64]	DES	97	195 ± 65	91.7/7.2	21.5	30.4
	DCB	31	194 ± 86	81/16.8	19.3	23.9
FEMPAC[39]	PTA	54	47 ± 42	93/7	17	47.0
	DCB	48	40 ± 44	96/4	7	19.0
THUNDER[65]	PTA	54	74 ± 67	–	48	44.0
	DCB	48	75 ± 62	–	10	17.0
PACIFIER[66]	PTA	47	66 ± 55	95.7/4.3	21.4	32.5
	DCB	41	70 ± 53	95.5/4.5	7.1	8.6
IN.PACT SFA[56]	PTA	111	88 ± 51	93.7/6.3	20.6	47.6
	DCB	220	89 ± 48	95/5.0	2.4	17.8
LEVANT-2[67]	PTA	160	63 ± 40	91.9/8.1	37.5	47.4
	DCB	316	63 ± 41	92.1/7.9	38	34.8

BMS, bare metal stent; CLI, critical limb ischemia; DCB, drug-coated balloon; DES, drug-eluting stent; IC, intermittent claudication; PTA, percutaneous transluminal angioplasty; TLR, target vessel revascularization.

2. As described in the preceding section, once lesion is crossed either intraluminally or subintimally, an appropriate balloon is selected. Balloon catheters have two lumens; the lumen through which wire passes is coaxial.

a. The second lumen is connected to the balloon and permits inflation.

b. Most useful balloon catheters have low profile which allows for a small diameter when deflated, minimizing entry-site complications and allowing easy maneuverability across tight and tortuous lesions.

c. Balloon catheters should also ideally be trackable. Trackability allows for easy passage of balloon catheters over wires without pulling wires out of desired position.

d. Most current balloons are made of polyethylene terephthalate or other low compliance, strong plastic polymers.

e. Balloons are available on 0.018-0.035-inch over-the-wire (OTW) and rapid-exchange (RX or monorail) platforms. OTW catheters have more pushability while monorail balloons use a shorter wire. Generally, OTW balloons may be used as catheters.

f. Low-profile 0.018-inch systems that are compatible with 4 Fr sheath access are generally advocated to minimize the risk of bleeding. Noncompliant balloons are preferred because they inflate to a uniform diameter regardless of the amount of pressure and are less likely to cause injury to the vessel.

g. High-grade eccentric or cylindrical lesions are related to increased risk of balloon rupture during inflation.
h. The ideal balloon length is measured using an external radiopaque ruler or calibrated catheter; the proper length must treat target lesion without disruption of the normal vessel.
   i. If a semicompliant balloon is used, greater pressure will overinflate the balloon to a larger diameter. This problem is not encountered with noncompliant balloons. Balloon oversizing as well as overinflation can cause arterial injury or significant dissections. Balloon rupture can occur which may cause embolization of balloon fragments. If balloons are not properly prepared, potential air embolization may also occur. As the balloon is inflated to nominal or rated burst pressure, a narrowing is seen at the site of stenosis or occlusion which resolves when the stenosis is overcome.
   ii. Longer inflation times are often used to stabilize the luminal surface of the arterial segment; longer times may reduce the likelihood of flow-limiting dissections. We use inflation times between 60 and 180 seconds.
i. For persistent stenoses that do not resolve with standard noncompliant balloons, cutting/scoring balloons may be used; the latter are associated with less hemodynamically significant dissections

F. Percutaneous Transluminal Angioplasty for Superficial Femoral Artery Disease With Drug-Coated Balloons (See Table 10.4)

1. **Drug-Eluting Stents and Drug-Coated Balloons** The development of paclitaxel drug-eluting stents (DESs) and drug-coated balloons (DCBs) represents an evolution in the endovascular treatment of peripheral arterial disease.

2. **Clinical Trials** Randomized clinical trials have demonstrated that angioplasty with a DCB is superior to standard balloon angioplasty for moderate-length lesions in the FP region.[56,67] Multicenter registries have shown excellent primary patency of DCBs in anatomically simple and complex lesions both[68,69] with reduction in rates of restenosis, decrease in target vessel revascularization, and economic cost-savings due in part to reduced need for repeat peripheral angiograms and reintervention.[37,66,70] The principal mechanism of restenosis with PTA and bare metal stents (BMS) is thought to be neointimal hyperplasia due to mechanical injury to vessel wall. Restensosis rates are also related to distribution of PAD with longer lesions with higher restenosis rates for diffuse, infrapopliteal lesions.[19,71] CLI, representing the most severe form of PAD, is associated with long-segment FP lesions, multilevel disease, and diffuse infrapopliteal lesions.[72]

3. **United States Food and Drug Administration Approval** Two DCBs are currently approved by the United States Food and Drug Administration (FDA) for the treatment of PAD in SFA and popliteal artery. These include the Lutonix 035 DCB PTA catheter with paclitaxel and the IN.PACT Admiral DCB with paclitaxel. More recently the FDA granted premarket approval to another paclitaxel-coated balloon, the Stellarex balloon.

a. In the ILLUMENATE trial, the Stellarex balloon demonstrated consistently high patency rates and low clinically driven target revascularization rates patients with superficial femoral artery and/or popliteal artery lesions.[73,74]
b. DCB consists of a balloon catheter which is coated with an antiproliferative drug (paclitaxel) and an excipient which controls drug release. Each DCB is unique with respect to the paclitaxel dose (varying from 2 to 3.5 mg/mm^2), the carrier molecule (excipient), the balloon material, and the coating technology used. DCBs have several advantages over stents: they may be able to distribute drugs more homogenously that stents and may avoid metal or polymer-induced stent restenosis and stent fractures associated with stent implantation in the FP territory.
c. DCBs may also be used preferentially in scenarios where stent implantation is not desirable (in-stent restenosis, bifurcation carina, or diffuse FP disease).[75] Limitations of DCBs are similar to balloon angioplasty—namely lower acute gain and potentially more unstable acute results.[75] The main challenge of delivering DCBs are effective drug transfer within a specified time frame as dictated by a single balloon inflation (typically around 30 s)
d. The antiproliferative drug paclitaxel is preferred due to its lipophilicity and prolonged tissue retention rates. Paclitaxel has been shown to prevent neointimal hyperplasia by disrupting normal microtubule function, thereby inhibiting smooth muscle cell migration, proliferation, and extracellular matrix secretion. Some ongoing studies have however focused on the use of limus-based DCBs due to their efficacy in preventing neointimal hyperplasia.[76] Excipient enhances transfer of drug from balloon to tissue and vary between urea, iopromide, and polysorbate/sorbitol, which are the most commonly used.[71]

G. Trials Comparing the Use of Drug-Coated Balloon With Percutaneous Transluminal Angioplasty in Superficial Femoral Artery/Femoropopliteal Disease (See Table 10.4)

As mentioned elsewhere, there are increasing data supporting the superiority of DCB over PTA for FP as well as below-the-knee (BTK) disease. Four randomized control trials (THUNDER,[38] FemPac,[66] LEVNAT I[37] and PACIFIER[66]) demonstrated significant reduction in late lumen loss, TLR, and binary restenosis at 6-month follow-up. A meta-analysis of these trials showed no difference in their safety profiles.[77] At 24 months, TLR rate for patients in the DCB arm was one-half of that in the PTA arm in the THUNDER trial.[38] 4% of patients in the DCB arm received additional stents compared with 22% in the PTA arm. In another prospective study of DCB use for FP disease, the 2-year patency rate was 72.4% and TLR rate was reported at 14.3% ($P < .001$).[69]

V. Stenting in Superficial Femoral Artery (See Table 10.4)

A. **Bare Metal Stents** All angioplasties can be complicated by flow-limiting dissection, embolization, and acute arterial recoil. The use of self-expanding covered or bare metal stents (BMS) has been shown to improve patency and may be used to treat PTA-related complications including dissection. However, in the early studies of sirolimus- and everolimus-eluting self-expanding nitinol stent platforms for SFA, early efficacy was followed by disappointing longer term results.

B. Bare Metal Stent Studies and Trials

1. In the Sirolimus Coated Cordis Smart Nitinol Self-expandable Stent for the Superficial Femoral Artery Disease (SIROCCO) randomized trial, the sirolimus-coated stent (Cordis, Miami Lakes, FL) demonstrated improved patency in comparison with the BMS at 6 months; however, in the follow-up SIROCCO II trial, there was no significant difference in outcomes between DES and BMS at 18 months.[78,79] In the Superficial Femoral Artery Treatment with Drug-Eluting Stents (STRIDES) study, the Dynalink everolimus-eluting stent showed a 32% stent restenosis rate at 12 months.[80]
2. **Efficacy:** Several studies have demonstrated the efficacy of self-expanding stents in the treatment of longer SFA lesions. Self-expanding stents possess thermal shape memory and are more resistant to mechanical stresses by expanding on deployment at body temperature and then reexpanding after external compression.
   a. In the Vienna randomized trial, patients receiving self-expanding stents for femoral artery disease had lower rates of restenosis and better walking capacity than those treated with balloon angioplasty alone.[61]
   b. In the Randomized Study Comparing the Edwards Self-Expanding LifeStent versus Angioplasty-alone In Lesions Involving The SFA and/or Proximal Popliteal Artery (RESILIENT) study,[33] nitinol BMSs were compared with angioplasty. The observed patency rate at 1 year was 81.3% for stent versus 36.7% for angioplasty group. Post hoc analysis, however, suggested that balloon angioplasty alone was similar to self-expanding stents in short SFA lesions (<100 mm)

C. Polytetrafluoroethylene (PTFE)-Covered Stents

1. PTFE-covered stents may be used to treat long SFA lesions in patients with claudication; however, their superiority to BMS is unproven. Studies have shown no significant long-term differences in patency rates between covered stents and bare metal (nitinol) stents.[35,81] Covered stents may have a role in treatment of in-stent restenosis of SFA. However, covered stents are associated with a higher rate of acute limb ischemia[82] compared with BMS, and at this point, a clear role for covered stents in SFA lesions has not been clearly defined.

D. Drug-Eluting Stents

1. As mentioned in the preceding section, revascularization in the SFA is challenging because of extensive plaque and complex mechanical forces including elongation, torsion and flexion, and so forth. The presence of nonresorbable polymers in peripheral artery DESs induce inflammatory thrombotic reactions, which may lead to late stenosis and thrombosis.[83]

2. Zilver PTX (Cook Medical, Bloomington, IN) is the only DES to date that has demonstrated superior and sustained patency in comparison with its bare metal counterpart. It is an FDA-approved, self-expanding, nitinol stent system. The Zilver PTA is characterized by direct application of paclitaxel to the stent without use of a polymeric coating. Paclitaxel avidly binds to intracellular target proteins, allowing for drug uptake in the artery with detectable retention for up to 2 months. The ability of paclitaxel to bind target proteins avidly allows Zilver PTX to deliver paclitaxel from the abluminal surface without the aid of polymers, bindings, or carriers.[40] Its flexible z-cell design provides for wall apposition and conformability. Additionally, the presence of horizontal tiebars and z-cell decrease shortening. The Zilver 635 series (6F, 0.035 inch) and 518 series (5F, 0.018 inch) are both available in 6- to 10-mm diameter, 20- to 80-mm lengths, and 80- and 125-cm delivery systems. The indications for use allow two Zilver PTX 80-mm stents to be overlapped to treat longer lesions up to 140 mm in length.

E. Drug-Eluting Stent Studies and Trials

1. In a randomized control trial of Zilver PTX DES,[40] the stent was compared with PTA for lesions upto 14 cm in length in the SFA/proximal popliteal arteries. If bail-out stenting was needed because of suboptimal PTA or flow-limiting dissection, secondary randomization to either Zilver PTX versus bare metal Zilver stent was undertaken. At 1 year, Zilver PTZ was superior to PTA in patency rates (83% vs 33% primary patency). Provisional DES was also superior to provisional BMS with a primary patency rate of 89.9% for provisional DES versus 73.0% for provisional BMS. At 2 years, sustained superiority was demonstrated with a primary patency rate of 83.4% for DES versus 61.1% for BMS.[63] After five years of follow-up, sustained patency was again demonstrated for Zilver DES versus PTA group (64.9% vs 19% for PTA group). Similarly in the head-to-head comparison of provisional DES versus provisional BMS, sustained efficacy was demonstrated (72.4% vs 53.0%).[84] In a subgroup analysis, treatment with DES was associated with superior outcomes for complex disease, including total occlusions and longer lesions as well as high-risk cohorts such as those with diabetes or CLI (Rutherford 4-6).

2. In a European study in the economic impact of using Zilver PTX stents, net cumulative savings of € 6,807,202 were made over 5 years mainly by reducing the need for future interventions.[85] To date, no head-to-head comparisons exist between primary DES and BMS or DCB in the FP arteries. A propensity score-based comparison of DES and DCB in consecutive patients with TASC C and D lesions that were long (>10 cm) found no significant difference in 1-year patency rates.[64]

VI. Clinical Trial Update in Superficial Femoral Artery Disease

An overview of randomized controlled trials of DCBs, DES, and covered stents in FP disease is provided in Table 10.4. These trials demonstrate benefit for DES, DCB, and covered stents and may result in change in clinical practice.

A. Follow-Up

1. After intervention for lower extremity disease, aggressive follow-up to optimize medical therapy is indicated to prevent future cardiovascular events and to improve patency rates.

Counseling on risk factors modification with initiation/continuation of pharmacologic treatment is important. The mainstay of pharmacologic treatment is statins, antihypertensive agents, and antiplatelet therapy. Previous studies have indicated that patients with PAD are less likely to receive guideline-directed medical therapy than patients with other forms of cardiovascular disease including coronary artery disease.[18,86,87]

2. At least 6 months of aspirin and 1 month of clopidogrel is recommended following peripheral artery DCB use; and at least 2 months of dual antiplatelet therapy after peripheral artery drug (paclitaxel)–coated stent implantation. However, there are limited data on the duration of antiplatelet treatment after endovascular intervention, with one small study showing no differences in outcomes in 12-month follow-up between prolonged (8-12 wk) versus short duration of antiplatelet treatment (4-6 wk)[88]
3. Postoperative follow-up for patients undergoing SFA intervention is routinely performed with ABI or arterial duplex ultrasound within one month of the intervention. This is followed by imaging at 3-6 months and then yearly after. If symptoms recur, imaging may be considered earlier.

B. **ACC/AHA Recommendations** The ACC/AHA[8] has a class IA recommendation for the use of aspirin alone (range: 75-325 mg/d) or clopidogrel alone (75 mg/d) to reduce MI, stroke, and vascular death in patients with symptomatic PAD. After revascularization, it may be reasonable to initiate DAPT to reduce risk of limb-related events (Class: IIb). Treatment with statins is recommended in all patients with PAD (Class: IA, LOE: A). Similarly, antihypertensive therapy is recommended to in patients with PAD and HTN to reduce risk of MI, stroke, heart failure, and cardiovascular death (IA). Furthermore, research studies[89,90] have shown reduction in vascular events in patients with both clinical and subclinical PAD who have been treated with either an angiotensin-converting enzyme inhibitor (ACEI) or angiotensin receptor blocker (ARB) hence a class IIA, LOE A recommendation for the use of these agents.

VII. Summary

Percutaneous intervention for occlusive disease of the FP region has become the mainstay of treatment for patients with intermittent claudication and CLI. This has paralleled the development of new techniques and devices. Percutaneous interventions of the FP region are associated with low risk of mortality and morbidity. Future goals in peripheral arterial disease should focus on identifying patients with FP disease early and use of appropriate treatment strategies to prevent CLI and amputation.

References

1. Cheng CP, Wilson NM, Hallett RL, Herfkens RJ, Taylor CA. In vivo MR angiographic quantification of axial and twisting deformations of the superficial femoral artery resulting from maximum hip and knee flexion. *J Vasc Interv Radiol.* 2006;17(6):979-987.
2. Morris-Stiff G, Ogunbiyi S, Rees J, Davies CJ, Hicks E, Lewis MH. Variations in the anatomical distribution of peripheral vascular disease according to gender. *Ann R Coll Surg Engl.* 2011;93(4):306-309.

3. Norgren L, Hiatt WR, Dormandy JA, et al. Inter-society consensus for the management of peripheral arterial disease (TASC II). *Int Angiol.* 2007;26(2):S5-S67.
4. Twine CP, Coulston J, Shandall A, McLain AD. Angioplasty versus stenting for superficial femoral artery lesions. *Cochrane Database Syst Rev.* 2009;(2):CD006767.
5. Rogers JH, Laird JR. Overview of new technologies for lower extremity revascularization. *Circulation.* 2007;116(18):2072-2085.
6. Conte MS, Pomposelli FB, Clair DG, et al. Society for vascular surgery practice guidelines for atherosclerotic occlusive disease of the lower extremities: management of asymptomatic disease and claudication. *J Vasc Surg.* 2015;61(3 suppl):1S.
7. Hirsch AT, Haskal ZJ, Hertzer NR, et al. ACC/AHA 2005 practice guidelines for the management of patients with peripheral arterial disease (lower extremity, renal, mesenteric, and abdominal aortic). *Circulation.* 2006;113(11):e463-e654.
8. Gerhard-Herman MD, Gornik HL, Barrett C, et al. 2016 AHA/ACC guideline on the management of patients with lower extremity peripheral artery disease: executive summary. *Circulation.* 2016;135(2):e686-e725.
9. McDermott MMG, Mehta S, Greenland P. Exertional leg symptoms other than intermittent claudication are common in peripheral arterial disease. *Arch Intern Med.* 1999;159(4):387-392.
10. Hirsch AT, Criqui MH, Treat-Jacobson D, et al. Peripheral arterial disease detection, awareness, and treatment in primary care. *JAMA.* 2001;286(11):1317-1324.
11. Aboyans V, Criqui MH, Abraham P, et al. Measurement and interpretation of the ankle-brachial index: a scientific statement from the American Heart Association. *Circulation.* 2012;126:2890-2909.
12. Resnick HE, Lindsay RS, McDermott MM, et al. Relationship of high and low ankle brachial index to all-cause and cardiovascular disease mortality: the strong heart study. *Circulation.* 2004;109(6):733-739.
13. Jaff MR, White CJ, Hiatt WR, et al. An update on methods for revascularization and expansion of the TASC lesion classification to include below-the-knee arteries: a supplement to the inter-society consensus for the management of peripheral arterial disease (TASC II). *Vasc Med.* 2015;20(5):465-478.
14. Fowkes FGR, Rudan D, Rudan I, et al. Comparison of global estimates of prevalence and risk factors for peripheral artery disease in 2000 and 2010: a systematic review and analysis. *Lancet.* 2013;382(9901):1329-1340.
15. Ankle Brachial Index Collaboration. Ankle brachial index combined with Framingham risk score to predict. *JAMA.* 2008;300(2):197-208.
16. Pollak AW, Norton PT, Kramer CM. Multimodality imaging of lower extremity peripheral arterial disease current role and future directions. *Circ Cardiovasc Imaging.* 2012;5(6):797-807.
17. Subherwal S, Patel MR, Kober L, et al. Missed opportunities: despite improvement in use of cardioprotective medications among patients with lower-extremity peripheral artery disease, underuse remains. *Circulation.* 2012;126(11):1345-1354.
18. Pande RL, Perlstein TS, Beckman JA, Creager MA. Secondary prevention and mortality in peripheral artery disease: National Health and Nutrition examination study, 1999 to 2004. *Circulation.* 2011;124(1):17-23.
19. Armstrong EJ, Singh S, Singh GD, et al. Angiographic characteristics of femoropopliteal in-stent restenosis: association with long-term outcomes after endovascular intervention. *Catheter Cardiovasc Interv.* 2013;82(7):1168-1174.
20. Hiatt WR, Wolfel EE, Meier RH, Regensteiner JG. Superiority of treadmill walking exercise versus strength training for patients with peripheral arterial disease. Implications for the mechanism of the training response. *Circulation.* 1994;90(4):1866-1874.
21. Hiatt WR, Regensteiner JG, Hargarten ME, Wolfel EE, Brass EP. Benefit of exercise conditioning for patients with peripheral arterial disease. *Circulation.* 1990;81(2):602-609.
22. Hiatt WR, Regensteiner JG, Wolfel EE, Carry MR, Brass EP. Effect of exercise training on skeletal muscle histology and metabolism in peripheral arterial disease. *J Appl Physiol.* 1996;81(2):780-788.

23. Murphy TP, Cutlip DE, Regensteiner JG, et al. Supervised exercise versus primary stenting for claudication resulting from aortoiliac peripheral artery disease: six-month outcomes from the claudication: exercise versus endoluminal revascularization (CLEVER) study. *Circulation*. 2012;125(1):130-139.
24. Murphy TP, Cutlip DE, Regensteiner JG, et al. Supervised exercise, stent revascularization, or medical therapy for claudication due to aortoiliac peripheral artery disease: the CLEVER study. *J Am Coll Cardiol*. 2015;65(10):999-1009.
25. Fakhry F, Rouwet EV, den Hoed PT, Hunink MGM, Spronk S. Long-term clinical effectiveness of supervised exercise therapy versus endovascular revascularization for intermittent claudication from a randomized clinical trial. *Br J Surg*. 2013;100(9):1164-1171.
26. Treat-Jacobson D, Bronas UG, Leon AS. Efficacy of arm-ergometry versus treadmill exercise training to improve walking distance in patients with claudication. *Vasc Med*. 2009;14(3):203-213.
27. Gardner AW, Parker DE, Montgomery PS, Blevins SM. Step-monitored home exercise improves ambulation, vascular function, and inflammation in symptomatic patients with peripheral artery disease: a randomized controlled trial. *J Am Heart Assoc*. 2014;3(5):e001107.
28. Gardner AW, Parker DE, Montgomery PS, Scott KJ, Blevins SM. Efficacy of quantified home-based exercise and supervised exercise in patients with intermittent claudication: a randomized controlled trial. *Circulation*. 2011;123(5):491-498.
29. Armstrong EJ, Wu J, Singh GD, et al. Smoking cessation is associated with decreased mortality and improved amputation-free survival among patients with symptomatic peripheral artery disease. *J Vasc Surg*. 2014;60(6):1565-1571.
30. Stoner MC, Calligaro KD, Chaer RA, et al. Reporting standards of the society for vascular surgery for endovascular treatment of chronic lower extremity peripheral artery disease. *J Vasc Surg*. 2016;64(1):e1-e21.
31. Jones DW, Graham A, Connolly PH, Schneider DB, Meltzer AJ. Restenosis and symptom recurrence after endovascular therapy for claudication: does duplex ultrasound correlate with recurrent claudication? *Vascular*. 2015;23(1):47-54.
32. Hunink MG, Wong JB, Donaldson MC, Meyerovitz MF, Harrington DP. Patency results of percutaneous and surgical revascularization for femoropopliteal arterial disease. *Med Decis Mak*. 1994;14(1):71-81.
33. Laird JR, Katzen BT, Scheinert D, et al. Nitinol stent implantation versus balloon angioplasty for lesions in the superficial femoral artery and proximal popliteal artery: twelve-month results from the RESILIENT randomized trial. *Circ Cardiovasc Interv*. 2010;3(3):267-276.
34. Bergeron P, Pinot JJ, Poyen V, et al. A long-term results with the Palmaz stent in the superficial femoral artery. *J Endovasc Surg*. 1995;2(2):161-167.
35. Geraghty PJ, Mewissen MW, Jaff MR, Ansel GM. Three-year results of the VIBRANT trial of VIABAHN endoprosthesis versus bare nitinol stent implantation for complex superficial femoral artery occlusive disease. *J Vasc Surg*. 2013;58(2):389-395.e4.
36. Kwa AT, Yeo KK, Laird JR. The role of stent-grafts for prevention and treatment of restenosis. *J Cardiovasc Surg (Torino)*. 2010;51(4):579-589.
37. Scheinert D, Duda S, Zeller T, et al. The LEVANT I (lutonix paclitaxel-coated balloon for the prevention of femoropopliteal restenosis) trial for femoropopliteal revascularization: first-in-human randomized trial of low-dose drug-coated balloon versus uncoated balloon angioplasty. *JACC Cardiovasc Interv*. 2014;7(1):10-19.
38. Tepe G, Zeller T, Albrecht T, et al. Local delivery of paclitaxel to inhibit restenosis during angioplasty of the leg. *N Engl J Med*. 2008;358(7):689-699.
39. Werk M, Langner S, Reinkensmeier B, et al. Inhibition of restenosis in femoropopliteal arteries. Paclitaxel-coated versus uncoated balloon: femoral paclitaxel randomized pilot trial. *Circulation*. 2008;118(13):1358-1368.
40. Dake MD, Ansel GM, Jaff MR, et al. Paclitaxel-eluting stents show superiority to balloon angioplasty and bare metal stents in femoropopliteal disease: twelve-month zilver PTX randomized study results. *Circ Cardiovasc Interv*. 2011;4(5):495-504.

41. Anderson JL, Halperin JL, Albert NM, et al. Management of patients with peripheral artery disease (compilation of 2005 and 2011 ACCF/AHA guideline recommendations): a report of the American College of Cardiology Foundation/American Heart Association Task Force on practice guidelines. *Circulation.* 2013;127(13):1425-1442.
42. Norgren L, Hiatt WR, Dormandy JA, Nehler MR, Harris KA, Fowkes FGR. Inter-society consensus for the management of peripheral arterial disease (TASC II). *Eur J Vasc Endovasc Surg.* 2007;33 suppl 1: S1-S75.
43. Johnston KW, Rae M, Hogg-Johnston SA, et al. 5-year results of a prospective study of percutaneous transluminal angioplasty. *Ann Surg.* 1987;206(4):403-413.
44. Löfberg AM, Karacagil S, Ljungman C, et al. Percutaneous transluminal angioplasty of the femoropopliteal arteries in limbs with chronic critical lower limb ischemia. *J Vasc Surg.* 2001;34(1):114-121.
45. Jamsen T, Manninen H, Tulla H, et al. The final outcome of primary infrainguinal percutaneous transluminal angioplasty in 100 consecutive patients with chronic critical limb ischemia. *J Vasc Interv Radiol.* 2002;13(5):455-463.
46. Powell RJ, Fillinger M, Walsh DB, Zwolak R, Cronenwett JL. Predicting outcome of angioplasty and selective stenting of multisegment iliac artery occlusive disease. *J Vasc Surg.* 2000;32(3):564-569.
47. Stokes KR, Strunk HM, Campbell DR, Gibbsons GW, Wheeler HG, Clouse ME. Five-year results of iliac and femoropopliteal angioplasty in diabetic patients. *Radiology.* 1990;174(3 Pt 2):977-982.
48. Beck AH, Muhe A, Ostheim W, Heiss W, Hasler K. Long-term results of percutaneous transluminal angioplasty: a study of 4750 dilatations and local lyses. *Eur J Vasc Surg.* 1989;3(3):245-252.
49. Palmaz JC, Laborde JC, Rivera FJ, Encarnacion CE, Lutz JD, Moss JG. Stenting of the iliac arteries with the palmaz stent: experience from a multicenter trial. *Cardiovasc Intervent Radiol.* 1992;15(5):291-297.
50. Udoff EJ, Barth KH, Harrington DP, Kaufman SL, White RI. Hemodynamic significance of iliac artery stenosis: pressure measurements during angiography. *Radiology.* 1979;132(2):289-293.
51. Kinney TB, Rose SC. Intraarterial pressure measurements during angiographic evaluation of peripheral vascular disease: techniques, interpretation, applications, and limitations. *Am J Roentgenol.* 1996;166(2):277-284.
52. Ruzsa Z, Bellavics R, Nemes B, et al. Combined transradial and transpedal approach for femoral artery interventions. *JACC Cardiovasc Interv.* 2018;11(11).
53. Katsanos K, Tepe G, Tsetis D, Fanelli F. Standards of practice for superficial femoral and popliteal artery angioplasty and stenting. *Cardiovasc Intervent Radiol.* 2014;37(3):592-603.
54. Krankenberg H, Schlüter M, Steinkamp HJ, et al. Nitinol stent implantation versus percutaneous transluminal angioplasty in superficial femoral artery lesions up to 10 cm in length: the femoral artery stenting trial (FAST). *Circulation.* 2007;116(3):285-292.
55. Dattilo R, Himmelstein SI, Cuff RF. The COMPLIANCE 360° trial: a randomized, prospective, multicenter, pilot study comparing acute and long-term results of orbital atherectomy to balloon angioplasty for calcified femoropopliteal disease. *J Invasive Cardiol.* 2014;26(8):355-360.
56. Tepe G, Laird J, Schneider P, et al. Drug-coated balloon versus standard percutaneous transluminal angioplasty for the treatment of superficial femoral and popliteal peripheral artery disease 12-month results from the IN.PACT SFA randomized trial. *Circulation.* 2015;31(5):495-502.
57. Scheinert D, Schulte KL, Zeller T, Lammer J, Tepe G. Paclitaxel-releasing balloon in femoropopliteal lesions using a BTHC excipient: twelve-month results from the BIOLUX P-I randomized trial. *J Endovasc Ther.* 2015;22(1):14-21.
58. Liistro F, Grotti S, Porto I, et al. Drug-eluting balloon in peripheral intervention for the superficial femoral artery: the DEBATE-SFA randomized trial (drug eluting balloon in peripheral intervention for the superficial femoral artery). *JACC Cardiovasc Interv.* 2013;6(12):1295-1302.
59. Rocha-Singh KJ, Jaff MR, Crabtree TR, Bloch DA, Ansel G. Performance goals and endpoint assessments for clinical trials of femoropopliteal bare nitinol stents in patients with symptomatic peripheral arterial disease. *Catheter Cardiovasc Interv.* 2007;69(6):910-919.
60. Olin JW, White CJ, Armstrong EJ, Kadian-Dodov D, Hiatt WR. Peripheral artery disease: evolving role of exercise, medical therapy, and endovascular options. *J Am Coll Cardiol.* 2016;67(11):1338-1357.

61. Schillinger M, Sabeti S, Loewe C, et al. Balloon angioplasty versus implantation of nitinol stents in the superficial femoral artery. *N Engl J Med.* 2006;354(18):1879-1888.
62. Dick P, Wallner H, Sabeti S, et al. Balloon angioplasty versus stenting with nitinol stents in intermediate length superficial femoral artery lesions. *Catheter Cardiovasc Interv.* 2009;74(7):1090-1095.
63. Dake MD, Ansel GM, Jaff MR, et al. Sustained safety and effectiveness of paclitaxel-eluting stents for femoropopliteal lesions: 2-year follow-up from the zilver PTX randomized and single-arm clinical studies. *J Am Coll Cardiol.* 2013;61(24):2417-2427.
64. Zeller T, Rastan A, Macharzina R, et al. Drug-coated balloons vs. drug-eluting stents for treatment of long femoropopliteal lesions. *J Endovasc Ther.* 2014;21(3):359-368.
65. Tepe G, Schnorr B, Albrecht T, et al. Angioplasty of femoral-popliteal arteries with drug-coated balloons: 5-year follow-up of the THUNDER trial. *JACC Cardiovasc Interv.* 2015;8(1 Pt A):102-108.
66. Werk M, Albrecht T, Meyer DR, et al. Paclitaxel-coated balloons reduce restenosis after femoro-popliteal angioplasty: evidence from the randomized PACIFIER trial. *Circ Cardiovasc Interv.* 2012;5(6):831-840.
67. Rosenfield K, Jaff MR, White CJ. Trial of a paclitaxel-coated balloon for femoropopliteal artery disease. *J Vasc Surg.* 2016;63(3):846.
68. Micari A, Cioppa A, Vadal G, et al. Clinical evaluation of a paclitaxel-eluting balloon for treatment of femoropopliteal arterial disease: 12-month results from a multicenter Italian registry. *JACC Cardiovasc Interv.* 2012;5(3):331-338.
69. Micari A, Nerla R, Vadalà G, et al. 2-Year results of paclitaxel-coated balloons for long femoropopliteal artery disease: evidence from the SFA-long study. *JACC Cardiovasc Interv.* 2017;10(7):728-734.
70. Laird JR, Schneider PA, Tepe G, et al. Durability of treatment effect using a drug-coated balloon for femoropopliteal lesions: 24-month results of IN.PACT SFA. *J Am Coll Cardiol.* 2015;66(21):2329-2338.
71. Schmidt A, Piorkowski M, Werner M, et al. First experience with drug-eluting balloons in infrapopliteal arteries: restenosis rate and clinical outcome. *J Am Coll Cardiol.* 2011;58(11):1105-1109.
72. Conte MS. Diabetic revascularization: endovascular versus open bypass-do we have the answer? *Semin Vasc Surg.* 2012;25(2):108-114.
73. Schroë H, Holden AH, Goueffic Y, et al. Stellarex drug-coated balloon for treatment of femoropopliteal arterial disease—The ILLUMENATE global study: 12-month results from a prospective, multicenter, single-arm study. *Catheter Cardiovasc Interv.* 2018;91(3):497-504.
74. Krishnan P, Faries P, Niazi K, et al. Stellarex drug-coated balloon for treatment of femoropopliteal disease: twelve-month outcomes from the randomized ILLUMENATE pivotal and pharmacokinetic studies. *Circulation.* 2017;136(12):1102-1113.
75. Byrne RA, Joner M, Alfonso F, Kastrati A. Drug-coated balloon therapy in coronary and peripheral artery disease. *Nat Rev Cardiol.* 2014;11(1):13-23.
76. Kolachalama VB, Pacetti SD, Franses JW, et al. Mechanisms of tissue uptake and retention in zotarolimus-coated balloon therapy. *Circulation.* 2013;127(20):2047-2055.
77. Cassese S, Byrne RA, Ott I, et al. Paclitaxel-coated versus uncoated balloon angioplasty reduces target lesion revascularization in patients with femoropopliteal arterial disease: a meta-analysis of randomized trials. *Circ Cardiovasc Interv.* 2012;5(4):582-589.
78. Duda SH, Bosiers M, Lammer J, et al. Sirolimus-eluting versus bare nitinol stent for obstructive superficial femoral artery disease: the SIROCCO II trial. *J Vasc Interv Radiol.* 2005;16(3):331-338.
79. Duda SH, Pusich B, Richter G, et al. Sirolimus-eluting stents for the treatment of obstructive superficial femoral artery disease: six-month results. *Circulation.* 2002;16 suppl A:15A-19A.
80. Lammer J, Bosiers M, Zeller T, et al. First clinical trial of nitinol self-expanding everolimus-eluting stent implantation for peripheral arterial occlusive disease. *J Vasc Surg.* 2011;54(2):394-401.
81. Lammer J, Zeller T, Hausegger KA, et al. Heparin-bonded covered stents versus bare-metal stents for complex femoropopliteal artery lesions: the randomized VIASTAR trial (viabahn endoprosthesis with propaten bioactive surface [VIA] versus bare nitinol stent in the treatment of long lesions in superficial femoral artery occlusive disease). *J Am Coll Cardiol.* 2013;62(15):1320-1327.
82. Johnston PC, Vartanian SM, Runge SJ, et al. Risk factors for clinical failure after stent graft treatment for femoropopliteal occlusive disease. *J Vasc Surg.* 2012;56(4):998-1007.

83. van der Giessen WJ, Lincoff AM, Schwartz RS, et al. Marked inflammatory sequelae to implantation of biodegradable and nonbiodegradable polymers in porcine coronary arteries. *Circulation*. 1996;94(7):1690-1697.
84. Dake MD, Ansel GM, Jaff MR, et al. Durable clinical effectiveness with paclitaxel-eluting stents in the femoropopliteal artery: 5-year results of the zilver PTX randomized trial. *Circulation*. 2016;133(15):1472-1483.
85. De Cock E, Sapoval M, Julia P, de Lissovoy G, Lopes S. A budget impact model for paclitaxel-eluting stent in femoropopliteal disease in France. *Cardiovasc Intervent Radiol*. 2013;36(2):362-370.
86. Krishnamurthy V, Munir K, Rectenwald JE, et al. Contemporary outcomes with percutaneous vascular interventions for peripheral critical limb ischemia in those with and without poly-vascular disease. *Vasc Med*. 2014;19(6):491-499.
87. Selvin E, Hirsch AT. Contemporary risk factor control and walking dysfunction in individuals with peripheral arterial disease: NHANES 1999–2004. *Atherosclerosis*. 2008;201(2):425-433.
88. Kronlage M, Wassmann M, Vogel B, et al. Short vs prolonged dual antiplatelet treatment upon endovascular stenting of peripheral arteries. *Drug Des Devel Ther*. 2017;11:2937-2945.
89. Ostergren J, Sleight P, Dagenais G, et al; Investigators H study. Impact of ramipril in patients with evidence of clinical or subclinical peripheral arterial disease. *Eur Heart J*. 2004;25(1):17-24.
90. Yusuf S, Teo KK, Pogue J, et al. Telmisartan, ramipril, or both in patients at high risk for vascular events. *N Engl J Med*. 2008;10(5):343-344.

CHAPTER 11

Below Knee Revascularization

Rishi Panchal, DO

Key Points

- Below knee disease gives rise to critical limb ischemia with rest pain or ulcers.
- Below knee disease is often combined with inflow disease of the iliac and femoropopliteal segments.
- Contralateral femoral, ipsilateral femoral, and pedal access can be undertaken for infrapopliteal interventions.
- Balloon angioplasty is the main stay of treatment. Drug-coated balloon therapy and drug-eluting stents so far have not proven to be significantly beneficial in below knee disease.

I. Indications and Considerations

A. Chronic Limb Ischemia

1. Chronic limb ischemia (CLI) is defined as limb pain that occurs "at rest or impending limb loss that is caused by severe compromise of blood flow to the affected extremity."[1] In CLI, a cascade of pathophysiologic events results from a chronic lack of blood supply over several weeks to months, ultimately leading to rest pain and/or trophic lesions in the legs.[18] Rutherford and Fontaine's classification criteria place CLI at the end of the spectrum of chronic peripheral arterial disease (Table 11.1).

2. **Classic symptoms and clinical manifestations** of CLI include the following: lower extremity rest pain, nonhealing ulcers, tissue loss, gangrene, pallor of the foot, and rubor dependency.[1] CLI places patients at a significant risk for amputation and cardiovascular events, thereby making it the most important clinical indication for below-the-knee revascularization.[16] Risk factors of CLI are the same as that of general atherosclerosis and include cigarette smoking, diabetes mellitus (DM), dyslipidemia, hypertension, obesity, metabolic syndrome, hyperhomocysteinemia, increased fibrinogen, and high levels of C-reactive protein. The diagnosis of CLI is made based on clinical manifestations and objective data including the following hemodynamic parameters: ankle-brachial index of 0.4 or less, ankle systolic pressure of 50 mm Hg or less, toe systolic pressure of 30 mm Hg or less,[1] and transcutaneous oxygen less than 20 mm Hg.[12] The goal of revascularization in CLI, whether surgical or endovascular, is to provide in-line blood flow to the foot through at least 1 patent artery, in an effort to preserve a functional limb, while decreasing ischemic pain, minimizing tissue loss, facilitating wound healing,[9] improving patient function and quality of life, and prolonging survival.[18]

Table 11.1. Fontaine and Rutherford Classifications of Chronic Peripheral Arterial Disease Severity

Fontaine Classification		Rutherford Classification			
Stage	**Clinical Symptoms**	**Grade**	**Category**	**Clinical Symptoms**	
I	Asymptomatic	0	0	Asymptomatic	
IIa	Mild claudication (symptoms with walking >200 m)	I	1	Mild claudication	
IIb	Moderate to severe claudication (symptoms with walking <200 m)		2	Moderate claudication	
			3	Severe claudication	
III	Ischemic rest pain	II	4	Ischemic rest pain	
IV	Ulceration or gangrene	III	5	Minor tissue loss	Critical limb ischemia
			6	Major tissue loss	

3. The gold standard for revascularization for CLI has long included open surgical revascularization, endartectomy, and surgical infrainguinal bypass.[1]
   a. With advancements in techniques, devices, and research demonstrating the safety, efficacy, and lower cost of endovascular treatment of lower extremity peripheral arterial disease, there has been a paradigm shift over the recent years to an endovascular-first approach.[16] The endovascular-first approach to the treatment of CLI is currently considered to be the standard treatment for symptomatic infrainguinal atherosclerotic disease, with regard to good technical and clinical outcomes.[11] Endovascular revascularization is preferred over surgical revascularization in patients with comorbidities including coronary ischemia, cardiomyopathy, congestive heart failure, severe lung disease, and chronic kidney disease, which all increase risk of perioperative surgical complications.
   b. Endovascular revascularization is also indicated in patients without suitable autologous vein for bypass grafts, in patients with rest pain and disease at multiple levels who can undergo a staged intervention,[9] and in patients with severe infection near the site of planned surgical anastomosis, previously failed bypass, and short lesions. Not only does endovascular revascularization offer a less invasive and cost-effective option for the treatment of CLI but is also associated with faster recovery time, fewer complications, and shorter length of hospital stay.[16] As illustrated by the BASIL (Bypass versus Angioplasty in Severe Ischemia of the Leg) study, endovascular intervention is an effective option for treating CLI, when compared with surgical intervention, as the amputation-free survival rates were similar[9] (Fig. 11.1).

II. Anatomy

A. **Popliteal Artery** The popliteal artery divides below the knee joint into the anterior tibial artery and the tibioperoneal trunk. The anterior tibial artery descends along the interosseous membrane, becomes the dorsalis pedis artery as it crosses the ankle joint, and supplies the dorsum of the foot. The tibioperoneal trunk arises distal to the anterior tibial artery and branches into the posterior tibial artery and the peroneal artery. The posterior tibial artery continues along the tibialis posterior muscle and supplies the plantar aspects of the toes and sole, the web spaces between the toes, and the medial aspect of the heel. The posterior tibial artery has three main branches; the calcaneal branch which supplies the medial ankle and lateral plantar heel, the medial plantar artery which supplies the plantar instep, and the lateral plantar artery which supplies the lateral and plantar forefoot and plantar midfoot.[3] The peroneal artery has two main branches: the anterior perforating branch supplying part of the upper ankle and the calcaneal branch supplying the plantar aspect of the heel (Figs. 11.2 and 11.3).[13]

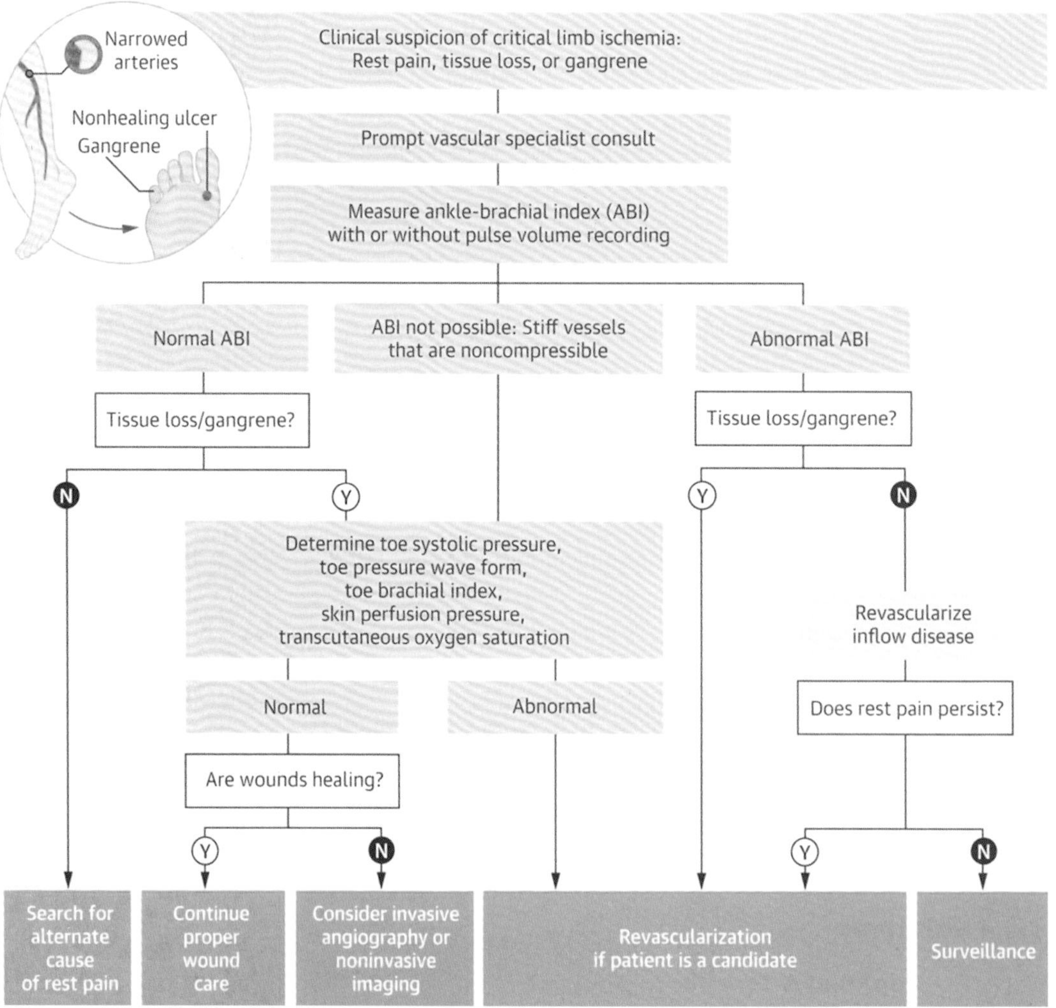

FIGURE 11.1: Management algorithm for patients with suspected critical limb ischemia. From Shishebor M, White C, Bruce G, et al. Critical limb ischemia. *JACC*. 2016;68(18):2002-2015.

B. **Approach** When determining the approach to intervention in patients with CLI, it is important to consider the concepts of angiosome-directed revascularization versus indirect revascularization. An angiosome is an anatomic unit of tissue, consisting of skin, subcutaneous tissue, fascia, muscle, and bone.[3] The foot and ankle consist of six angiosomes, with each angiosome being fed by a source artery. The posterior tibial artery feeds three angiosomes, the anterior tibial artery feeds one angiosome, and the peroneal artery feeds two angiosomes[3] (Fig. 11.3). In patients with CLI, acquiring direct flow based on the angiosome concept is important for limb salvage. Research has demonstrated a statistically significant increase in the rate of limb salvage, skin perfusion pressure, and freedom from amputation with angiosome-directed revascularization when compared with indirect revascularization in patients with CLI.[16]

III. Access

Infrapopliteal lesions can be approached from the contralateral and ipsilateral femoral artery, with the majority of stenotic infrapopliteal lesions approached from the contralateral femoral artery. Access from the contralateral femoral artery is the preferred approach when treating inflow disease and in the morbidly obese, given the propensity

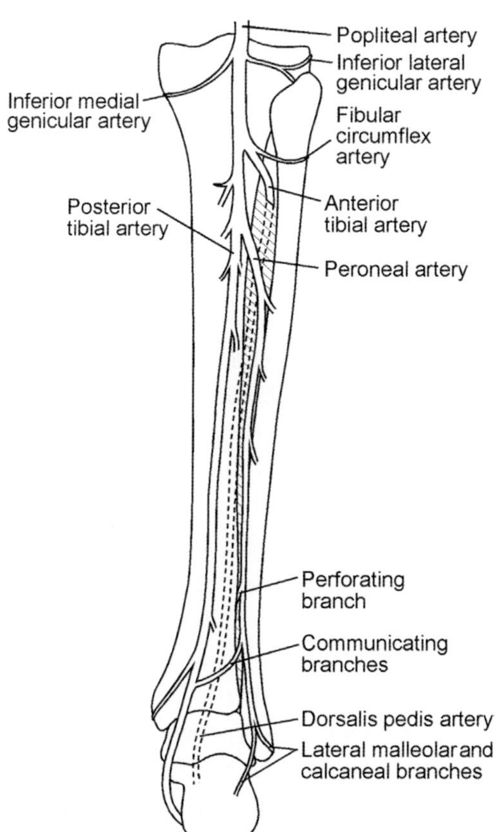

FIGURE 11.2: Arteries of the lower leg. From Silver M, Ansel G. Infrapopliteal Intervention. In: Casserly IP, Sachar R, Yadav JS, eds. *Practical Peripheral Vascular Intervention*. 2nd ed. Philadelphia, PA: Lippincott Williams & Wilkins; 2011:265-277.

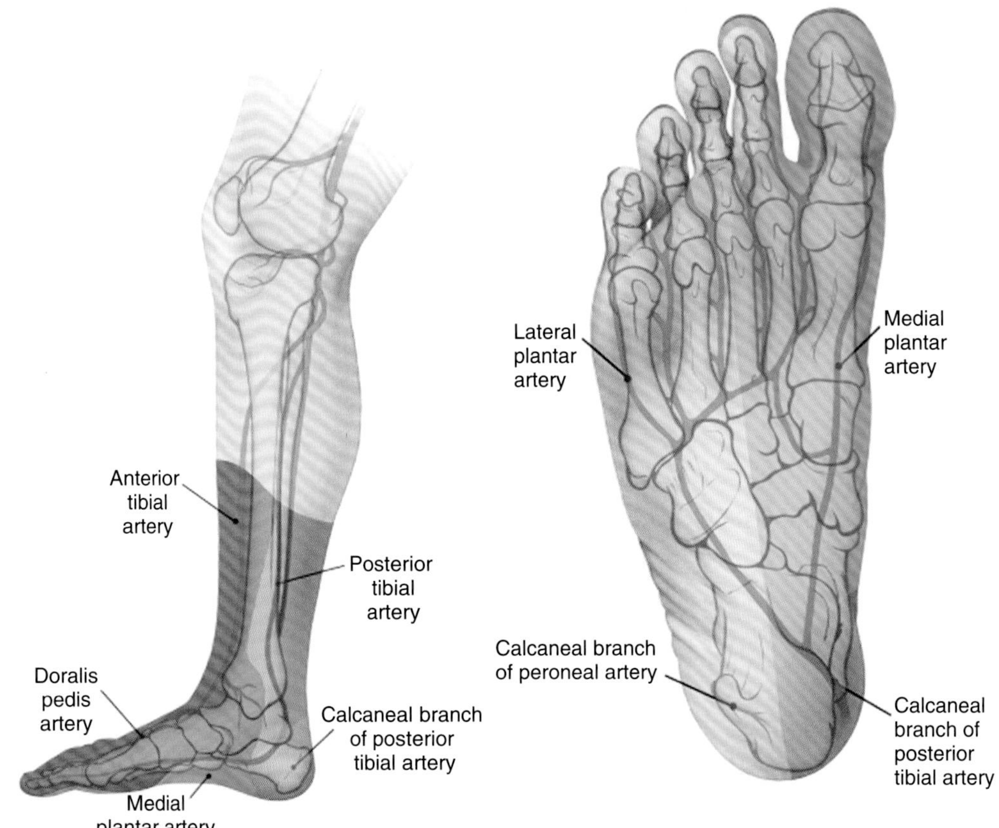

FIGURE 11.3: Angiosomes.

of the sheath to become kinked in the groin with an antegrade approach. A 5-Fr or 6-Fr crossover sheath is introduced into the contralateral artery and advanced to the distal ipsilateral iliac artery. **Antegrade access** from the ipsilateral common femoral artery is preferred when treating complex infrapopliteal disease in the absence of inflow disease. Antegrade access in the common femoral artery allows for better wire guide ability and good "**pushability**" of the catheter balloons, given the close proximity of the access site to the lesions.[11] When using a crossover approach, an increased amount of contrast is required for adequate visualization of the distal circulation given the relatively long distance from the tip of the sheath to the infrapopliteal lesion. In cases when antegrade access cannot be achieved, contralateral crossover using a 6-Fr multipurpose coronary guide catheter or a hydrophilic 5-Fr or 6-Fr guide sheath may be advanced from the contralateral common femoral artery to the distal ipsilateral superficial femoral artery or mid-popliteal artery for better maneuverability and control.[16] In patients with chronic total occlusions (CTOs), a retrograde approach, with access via the pedal, peroneal, anterior, or posterior tibial artery, can be used alone or in combination with an antegrade or crossover approach.

IV. Intervention

A. Indications

1. The most common indication for infrapopliteal endovascular intervention remains CLI with ischemic rest pain, tissue loss, and ulceration due to peripheral arterial disease. Before endovascular intervention, thorough clinical evaluation of objective data including ankle branchial index or transcutaneous oxygen pressure measurements, assessment of the width, length, and depth of ischemic ulcers should be performed.[10]
2. Noninvasive imaging modalities such as arterial duplex ultrasound, computed tomography (CT) angiography, magnetic resonance (MR) angiography can assist in preprocedural planning for below-the-knee interventions. The current standard of care remains balloon angioplasty for below-the-knee lesions. 0.014″ and 0.018″ low-profile balloon catheters are utilized to perform focal angioplasty for infrapopliteal lesions. In our experience utilizing a low-profile support catheter with a 0.014″ guidewire platform has been most successful. Selection of 0.014″ guidewire is based on plaque characteristics, calcifications, length of stenosis, and total occlusions. Focal lesions can be crossed with any commonly used 0.014″ coronary guidewires with a floppy tip.
3. However, CTO will require coronary wires with stiffer tips, such as Confianza or Fielder XT-Abbot Vascular. Once the lesion is crossed a support coronary-type guidewire (ie, V-18, V-14 Boston Scientific) can be replaced to form a scaffolding for the intervention.

B. Angioplasty Balloons

1. **Angioplasty balloons for infrapopliteal lesions** vary on size based on the location of the lesion. A 2.5 or 3 mm diameter balloon can be used for the proximal region of the infrapopliteal artery, while 2.0-2.5 mm balloons are commonly used for distal tibial and plantar arch vessels. New generation of long, low-profile 0.014″ tapered balloons with increased balloon lengths including 120-200 mm provide improved remodeling of the treated vessel, especially when employing prolonged balloon inflation times.[4] In addition, the over-the-wire platform and low compliance of these balloons allows the most effective tracking and pushing characteristics. In our practice, the Ultraverse Bard dilation catheters are well designed for tibial angioplasty.
2. **Cutting balloons and scoring balloons** additionally have facilitated below-the-knee endovascular revascularization. The AngioSculpt balloon (AngioScore Inc.) is a scoring balloon with an over-the-wire semicompliant balloon surrounded by a nitonal cage with three rectangular spiral struts. Fonesca et al, in a prospective multicenter European registry showed a 90.3% success rate and a dissection rate of 10.7%.[7] There was no need for further therapy of the treated lesions. Our experience using scoring and cutting balloons is mainly utilized for heavily calcified lesions to improve luminal gain. The primary concept is to provide intimal disruption and effective dilation requiring less wall tension.[6]

C. **Atherectomy** The basis of atherectomy underlines debulking material rather than displacement, thus decreasing distal embolization. Peripheral calcium tends to be a significant impediment to achieving revascularization, and studies show that calcium negatively impacts outcomes.[8] The Diamondback Orbital Atherectomy System (Cardiovascular Systems, Inc, St. Paul, MN) has compared below-the-knee revascularization with standard angioplasty with positive results. In a small patient study, there was increased target lesion revascularization and decreased stenosis. The system utilizes a diamond-coated crown to achieve a mechanical sanding of the vessel wall to differentially treat hard plaque while minimizing damage to the media, unlike a directional device. The low-profile technology allows treatment of distal tibial lesions, which was previously inaccessible. Our center has used this type of atherectomy device in heavily calcified lesions that are unable to be crossed by conventional crossing catheters/wires.

D. **Drug-Coated Balloons** Drug-coated balloons have shown promising results in single-center studies; however, these could not be replicated in large multicenter trials. A recent meta-analysis looked at 5 trials (*DEBATE-BTK, DEBELLUM, BIOLUX P-II Trial, IN.PACT DEEP Trial, IDEAS Trial)*, in which patients were treated with drug-eluting balloon angioplasty in a randomized trial. The majority of patients, 99.6%, had critical limb ischemia with lesion length in the intermediate range of 121 mm. At 12 month follow-up, TLR rate was 23.6% in drug-eluting balloon angioplasty versus 18.3% (RR 0.71; 95% CI 0.47-1.09; $P = 0.12$). The clinically driven total lesion revascularization rate did not differ between modalities, and there was comparable risk for amputations and major adverse events. Thus, no clinical superiority was noted in drug-eluting balloon angioplasty compared with plain old balloon angioplasty in the below-the-knee region.[17] Future results of the Lutonix below-the-knee drug-coated balloon randomized trial are currently underway. The role of drug-eluting balloons in below-the-knee revascularization remains unclear, with a need for further investigation.[5]

E. **Treatment** Infrapoplitieal arteries remain difficult to treat due to small caliber vessel, length of disease, and overall calcification burden. Bare metal stenting has been traditionally reserved as a "bailout" technique for the treatment of hemodynamically significant flow-limiting dissections post intervention along with significant elastic recoil. Siablis and colleagues showed 6 month primary patency rates at 68.1% in a small nonrandomized single center trial.[14] Drug-eluting stents appear to be promising for treatment of below-the-knee arterial disease.[2] Three major trials since 2012, ACHILLES, YUKON-BTX, and DESTINY, have shown significantly improved vessel patency compared with angioplasty alone. Endovascular interventions with drug-eluting stents may improve overall cost-effectiveness and improved quality of life outcomes in the future.[2]

V. Complications

Procedural complications include vasospasms, no-reflow, thrombosis, perforation, and flow-limiting dissection. Prevention and treatment of vasospasms may be achieved through the use of intra-arterial nitrates and calcium channel antagonists. The cause of no-reflow is often multifactorial and may result from distal embolization, vasospasm, and skeletal muscle edema.[13] When attempting to determine the cause of no-reflow, occult dissection, and thrombosis must be considered. Thrombosis that occurs during infrapopliteal intervention must be promptly addressed with catheter-based, mechanical thrombectomy. If thrombosis persists despite performing catheter-based mechanical thrombectomy, thrombolytic therapy should be considered if there are no contraindications.[13] Perforations and flow-limiting dissections commonly occur when treating long occluded segments or when using atherectomy devices. Prolonged balloon inflations are typically sufficient to achieve hemostasis. For limb-threatening perforations not controlled with balloon inflation, deployment of a coronary covered stent may be considered.[13]

References

1. Allie DE, Patlola RR, Mitran EV, Ingraldi A, Walker CM. Critical limb ischemia. In: Fogarty T, White R, eds. *Peripheral Endovascular Interventions*. 3rd ed. New York, NY: Springer; 2010:305-316.
2. Altit R, Gray WA. New innovations in drug-eluting stents for peripheral arterial disease. *Curr Cardiol Rep*. 2017;19:117.
3. Brodmann M. The angiosome concept in clinical practice. *Endovascular Today*. 2013;60-61.
4. Casserly IP, Sachar R, Yadav JS. *Manual of Peripheral Vascular Intervention*. 2nd ed. Philadelphia: Lippincott Williams & Wilkins; 2011.
5. Cassese S, Ndrepepa G, liistro F, et al. drug-coated balloons for revascularization of infrapopliteal arteries: a meta-analysis of randomized trials. *JACC Cardiovasc interv*. 2016;9:1072-1080.
6. Engelke C, Morgan RA, Belli AM. Cutting balloon percutaneous transluminal angioplasty for salvage of lower limb arterial bypass graft: feasibility. *Radiology*. 2002;223:106-114.
7. Fonseca A, Costa JR, Abizaid A, et al. Intravascular ultrasound assessment of the novel AngioSculpt scoring balloon catheter for the treatment of complex coronary lesions. *J Invasive Cardiol*. 2008;20:21-27.
8. Fitzgerald PJ, Ports TA, Yock PG. Contribution of localized calcium deposits to dissection after angioplasty. An observational study using intravascular ultrasound. *Circulation*. 1992;86(1):64-70.
9. Gerhard-Herman MD, Gornik HL, Barrett C, et al. 2016 AHA/ACC Guideline on the management of patients with lower extremity peripheral artery disease: a report of the American College of Cardiology/American heart association task force on clinical practice guidelines. *Circulation*. 2017;135(12):e726-e779. doi:10.1161/CIR.0000000000000471.
10. Got I. Transcutaneous oxygen pressure (TcP02): advantages and limitations. *Diabetes Metab*. 1998;24:379-384.
11. Higashimori A. Angiography and endovascular therapy for below-the-knee artery disease. In: Yokoi Y, ed. *Angiography and Endovascular Therapy for Peripheral Artery Disease*. Rijeka, Croatia: InTech; 2017. doi:10.5772/67179.
12. Kinlay S. Management of critical limb ischemia. *Circ Cardiovas Interv*. 2016;9:e001946.
13. Silver M, Ansel G. Infrapopliteal intervention. In: *Practical Peripheral Vascular Intervention*. 2nd ed. Philadelphia, PA: Lippincott Williams & Wilkins; 2011:265-277.
14. Siablis D. Kraniotis P, Jarnabatidis D, et al. Sirolimus-eluting versus bare stents for bailout after suboptimal infrapopliteal angioplasty for critical limb ischemia: 6-month angiographic results from a nonrandomized prospective single-center study. *J Endovasc Ther*. 2005;12:685-695.
15. Shishebor M, White C, Bruce G, et al. Critical limb ischemia. *JACC*. 2016;68(18):2002-2015. doi:10.1016/j.jacc.2016.04.071.
16. Ward C, Gamberdella J, Mena-Hurtado C. Endovascular treatment of below-the-knee arteries. In: Lanzer P, ed. *PanVascular Medicine*. 3rd ed. Springer Berlin Heidelberg; 2015:3195-3203. doi:10.1007/978-3-642-37078-6_912.
17. Van den Berg JC. Drug-eluting balloons in below the knee treatment. *J Cardiovasc Surg*. 2016;57:811-816.
18. Varu V, Hogg M, Kibbe M. Critical limb ischemia. *J Vasc Surg*. 2010;51(1):230-241.

CHAPTER 12

Drug-Coated Therapies

Madhan Shanmugasundaram, MD, FACC, FSCAI

Key Points

Endovascular interventions for peripheral artery disease (PAD) have become the corner stone of therapy.

- The prognosis and treatment strategy for PAD is dependent on the mode of presentation of each patient that includes intermittent claudication and acute or chronic limb ischemia.
- Even though PAD refers to involvement of vessels outside coronary territory, most of the disease is localized to the femoropopliteal tract.
- PAD involving femoropopliteal tract has unique characteristics including diffuse long stenosis, heavy calcification, and crossing joint lines making stent implantation suboptimal.
- Traditionally surgery was considered gold standard for lower extremity PAD, but there is significantly less morbidity and faster recovery times with endovascular therapies especially in patients with multiple medical comorbidities.
- Major criticism of endovascular therapy has been the low long-term patency rate especially for infrainguinal interventions, and the evolution of drug-coated therapy is aimed at increasing the patency rates of endovascular technologies.
- The drug-eluting stent (DES) typically consists of a scaffold, polymer matrix, and drug. Paclitaxel is the most commonly used drug in these devices and is cytotoxic, inhibiting cellular proliferation and mitosis.
- The drug-coated balloon (DCB) is the new addition to this arena and consists of standard PTA catheter, excipient that helps release the drug rapidly as soon as it comes in contact with the vessel wall and the drug itself.
- Compared with bare-metal stents or standard balloon angioplasty, both DES and DCB have shown to have better primary patency, lower binary restenosis, and lower target vessel revascularization up to 2 years.
- Combining therapies such as atherectomy and DCB have theoretical advantages and appear attractive as a treatment strategy but remains to be studied.

I. Introduction

Catheter-based revascularization strategies have rapidly evolved in the past few years and are the standard of care for patients with lower extremity peripheral artery disease (PAD). Even though PAD in general refers to involvement of any noncoronary vessel, the majority of lesions are located in the femoropopliteal tract.[1] Historically surgical intervention was the treatment of choice for patients with lifestyle-limiting claudication, critical limb ischemia (CLI) or acute limb ischemia, but with the advent of endovascular technology, the landscape of therapeutic strategies have changed. There is significantly less morbidity and faster recovery times with endovascular therapies especially in patients with multiple medical comorbidities. However, one of the major criticisms of endovascular therapy has been a poor long-term patency rate especially for infrainguinal vasculature. However, most of this evidence comes from the percutaneous transluminal angioplasty (PTA) and bare-metal stent (BMS) era. The evolution of drug-coated therapy aimed at increasing the long-term patency rates of endovascular interventions. Most of the innovations in the PAD arena for the past 5 years were in the development of an "ideal" drug-coated therapy to mimic the success of these therapies in the coronary vasculature. One could argue that this milestone is yet to be achieved, but nevertheless the explosion of cardiovascular technologies in this area cannot be ignored. The objective of this chapter is to provide a basic understanding of the drug-coated technologies in the PAD world and their current clinical implications.

II. Rationale for Drug-Coated Devices

Even though the initial success rates of endovascular revascularization in the femoropopliteal territory have improved with betterment of dedicated devices,[2] the long-term patency remains suboptimal.[3] Restenosis after endovascular therapy for PAD has been the major limitation for BMSs and PTA.[4] It is important to understand the mechanism of restenosis to expand the horizon of interventional therapies and to improve its durability. There are not a lot of pathophysiologic studies examining the mechanism of restenosis in PAD, but one can extrapolate the work done in the coronary realm. It is well recognized that the principal mechanism of restenosis is by neointimal hyperplasia.[5] The mechanical injury from angioplasty or stent implantation incites a fibroproliferative reaction initially involving the smooth muscle cells, followed by accumulation of extracellular matrix that results in neointimal thickening and eventually restenosis.[5,6] This process has been the Achilles' heel of endovascular therapy in general. Moreover in the PAD arena, femoropopliteal (FP) territory has increased biomechanical stress that results in higher in-stent restenosis with BMSs.[7] Apart from patient centric factors, there are numerous anatomic factors in PAD that predicts in-stent restenosis and hence worse long-term outcomes. CLI is usually associated with diffuse long segment FP lesions, below knee disease, or multilevel stenoses that portend higher restenosis rates.[8,9] The constant search for endovascular therapies with better long-term outcomes by reducing restenosis have resulted in the evolution of drug-coated therapies including drug-eluting stents (DESs) and drug-coated balloons (DCBs).

III. Drugs Used in Drug-Eluting Stents and Drug-Coated Balloons

It is important to have a basic understanding of the drugs used to coat the stents and balloons for better therapeutic decisions. The ideal drug would have a long tissue retention time, wide therapeutic window, and lipophilic nature to increase tissue concentration. Traditionally there have been two classes of drugs that satisfied these criteria and have been used in the treatment of CAD. These include the Rapamycin (-limus) family and paclitaxel. In PAD, paclitaxel is more commonly used. Rapamycin is a macrolide antibiotic that binds to the cellular FK-binding protein to inhibit the mammalian target of rapamycin (mTOR). This in turn inhibits the protein complexes responsible for progression of cells from G1 to S phase hence blocking smooth muscle cell migration and proliferation.[10] However, rapamycin does not cause cell death. Paclitaxel on the other hand binds to the β-subunit of tubulin heterodimer inhibiting the protein kinase essential for microtubule depolymerization. This results in the unstable microtubules that inhibit cell proliferation and mitosis.[11] Higher doses of paclitaxel can result in cell death. The manner in which these drugs are incorporated into the stent platform and balloons is uniquely different and explains the rationale of their current clinical use.

IV. Design of Drug-Eluting Stents and Drug-Coated Balloons

A. **DES Elements** The DES comprises of three basic elements: a metallic scaffold (typically nickel-titanium, platinum-chromium alloy, or stainless steel), polymer matrix that binds the drug (silicone, polyurethane, and cellulose esters), and the drug itself. The rate at which the drug elutes is proportional to the degradation of the polymer matrix, thus creating a subtle difference in the way various drug-coated therapies are used. After the initial success of DES, there were numerous issues noted with the persistence of the polymer that creates a source of delayed intimal hyperplasia and lack of endothelialization of stent surface resulting in late stent thrombosis.[12] The drug in the newer generation DES is incorporated directly into the metallic scaffold, avoiding polymer-related long term issues. A variety of biodegradable materials such as polycarbonates and polyesters have been used to make polymers and scaffolds but currently are not available in the Unites States.[13]

B. **DCB Elements** DCBs on the other hand are made of a standard PTA balloon catheter (semicompliant or noncompliant), drug (paclitaxel), and an excipient (urea or iopramide). Unlike the DES, in DCBs only paclitaxel is used, because the –limus class of drugs are susceptible to oxidation hence unstable on DCBs. Paclitaxel is lipophilic, is resistant to oxidation, and has prolonged tissue retention.[14] The hydrophilic excipient forms an important component of DCB, as it has been shown to increase the transfer of the drug into the tissue from the surface of the balloon.[9] Without the excipient, paclitaxel release from the balloon is erratic and tends to remain adhered to the balloon surface. Once the balloon is inflated and comes in contact with the vessel wall, due to the hydrophilic properties, the excipient releases the drug into the tissue, which in turn due to its lipophilic properties binds to the vessel wall. This is shown in Fig. 12.1. There are several advantages of DCB over DES, such as its utility in treating disease in "no stent zones" (bifurcations, diffusely diseased segments) and its ability to avoid stent-related long-term problems, such as restenosis or thrombosis, stent fracture, and stent-related biomechanical stress, and to be used to treat in-stent restenosis and allow more homogenous distribution of the drug.

V. Drug-Eluting Stent

A. Drug-Eluting Stent for Femoropopliteal Disease

1. **SIROCCO I and II** (A Clinical Investigation of the Sirolimus Coated Cordis Smart Nitinol Self-Expandable Stent for the Treatment of Obstructive Superficial Femoral Artery Disease) were the first randomized trials that investigated the use of DES

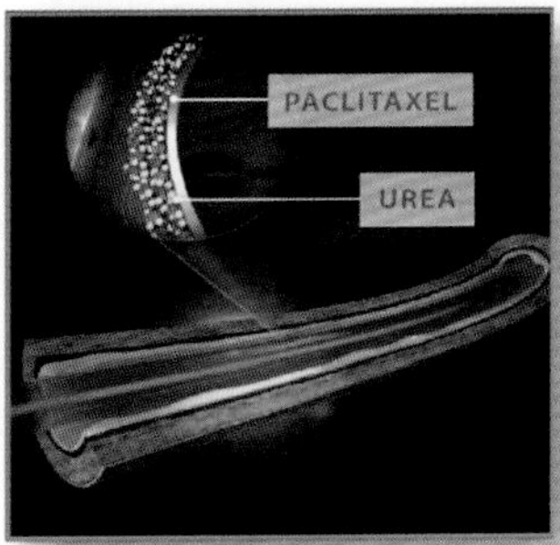

IN.PACT Admiral balloon matrix coating:
- Paclitaxel
- Urea - excipient that controls drug release

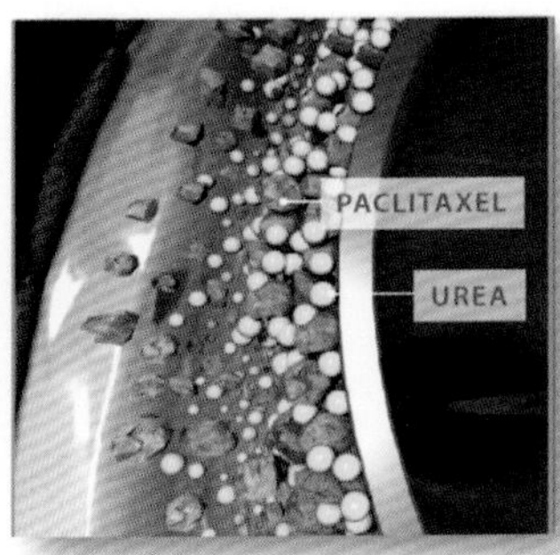

DCB inflation:
- Matrix coating contact with the blood
- Urea hydrates causing the release of paclitaxel
- Paclitaxel binds to the wall due to its hydrophobic and lipophilic properties

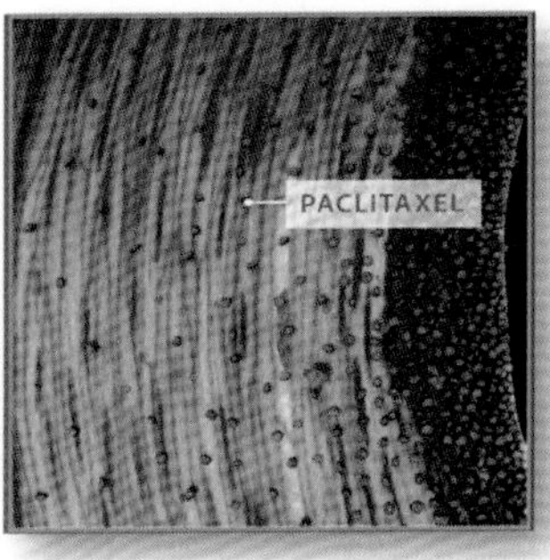

Paclitaxel penetration:
- Through vessel wall deep into the media and adventitia
- Interferes with the causes of restenosis
- Can remain in the vessel wall for over 180 days at therapeutic levels

FIGURE 12.1: Drug-coated balloon (DCB) technology. Reproduced with permission from Peterson S, Hasenbank M, Silvestro C, Raina S. IN.PACT Admiral drug-coated balloon: durable, consistent and safe treatment for femoropopliteal peripheral artery disease. *Adv Drug Deliv Rev.* 2017;112:69-77.

(Sirolimus) in the treatment of FP disease. Sirocco I had 36 patients followed for 6 months, and Sirocco II had 93 patients followed for a total of 24 months; both trials randomized patients with FP disease to either Sirolimus or BMS, and the primary outcome was Doppler measured in-stent restenosis (ISR). It was shown that there was no significant difference in the ISR rates or target lesion revascularization (TLR) at 6 or 24 months (22.6% vs 30.9%, P = NS or 22.9 vs 21.2, P = NS respectively). Two proposed reasons for the lack of difference with DES were lower than expected ISR rates in the BMS arm and late catch up effect related to stent polymer.[15,16]

2. **Everolimus-eluting stent** (Dynalink-E, Abbott) was studied in a nonrandomized trial, **STRIDES** (A Study to Evaluate the Safety and Performance of the Dynalink-E, Everolimus Eluting Peripheral Stent System for Treating Atherosclerotic de Novo or Restenotic Native Superficial Femoral and Proximal Popliteal Artery Lesions), that included 104 patients with FP disease. The 6-month primary patency rate measured by Doppler was 94% ± 2.3%, and 12-month patency rate was 68% ± 4.6%.[17]

3. **ZILVER PTX** (Evaluation of the Zilver PTX Drug-Eluting Peripheral Stent) was the largest trial that randomized over 400 patients with FP disease to either PTA or paclitaxel DES. If there was a PTA failure, the patients were then rerandomized to either BMS or DES arm. It was demonstrated that there was superior event-free survival and patency at 12 and 24 months in the DES arm compared with the PTA or BMS arm.[18,19] These results are summarized in Fig. 12.2. There was also a nonrandomized arm that included over 700 patients who underwent DES placement for FP disease with similar long-term patency rates.[18] Table 12.1 summarizes the important DES trials.

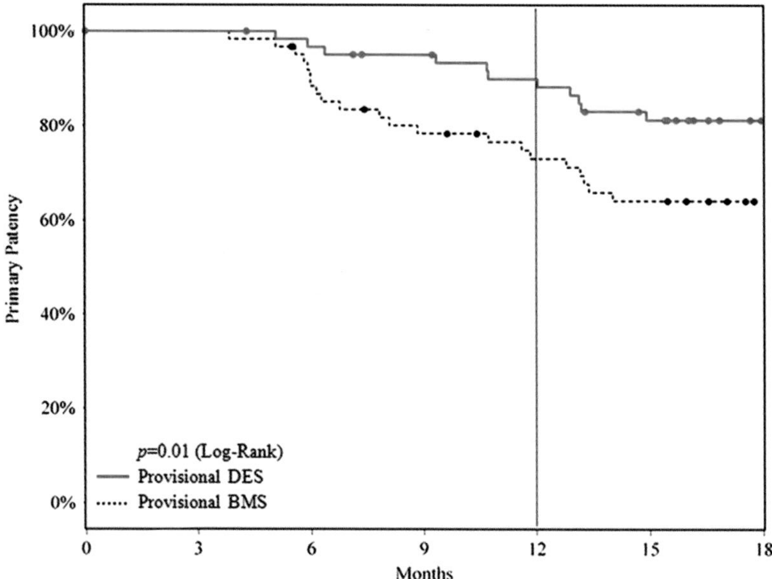

Kaplan Meier Estimates of Primary Patency, Values Represent Lesions								
Months Post-procedure	Primary Patency ± Standard Error		Cumulative Failed		Cumulative Censored		Remaining at Risk	
	Provisional BMS	Provisional DES	Provisional BMS	Provisional DES	Provisional BMS	Provisional DES	Provisional BMS	Provisional DES
0	100.0 ± 0.0%	100.0 ± 0.0%	0	0	0	1	62	62
1	100.0 ± 0.0%	100.0 ± 0.0%	0	0	0	1	62	62
6	88.4 ± 4.1%	96.7 ± 2.3%	7	2	2	2	53	59
12	73.0 ± 5.8%	89.9 ± 3.9%	16	6	5	5	41	52

FIGURE 12.2: Twelve-month primary safety outcomes. The black curve shows 82.6% event-free survival (EFS) for the percutaneous transluminal angioplasty (PTA) group, and the red curve shows the significantly higher ($P = 0.004$) 90.4% EFS for the primary drug-eluting stent (DES) group. Reproduced with permission from Dake MD, Ansel GM, Jaff MR, et al. Paclitaxel-eluting stents show superiority to balloon angioplasty and bare metal stents in femoropopliteal disease: twelve-month Zilver PTX randomized study results. *Circ Cardiovasc Interv.* 2011;4(5):495-504.

B. **Drug-Eluting Stents in Below Knee Disease** Typically, interventions for **below-the-knee (BTK) disease** are reserved for patients with CLI (rest pain or gangrene) or nonhealing ulcers as a limb-saving strategy. There are various percutaneous treatment options that have been tried for limb salvage, which include PTA, BMS, DES, and in some cases DCB.

1. The **YUKON- BTK trial** (Yukon-Drug-Eluting Stent Below-The-Knee-Prospective Randomized Double-BlindMulticenter Study) randomized 161 patients with BTK disease to either Sirolimus-eluting stent (SES) or BMS. It was shown that event-free survival and freedom from TLR were better in the SES arm at 3-year follow-up.[20]
2. The **DESTINY** (Prospective Randomized Multicenter Trial Comparing the Implant of a Drug Eluting Stent vs a Bare Metal Stent in the Critically Ischemic Lower Leg) trial used Everolimus DES in patients with BTK disease to demonstrate superior results including restenosis and freedom from TLR compared with BMS.[21] A meta-analysis by Antoniou et al. that included 4 randomized control trials

Table 12.1. DES Trials in PAD

Trial	Sample Size	Drug	Territory	Control Group	Primary Outcome	Follow-Up
SIROCCO I/II[15,16]	47	Sirolimus	FP	PTA	6-mo ISR (DUS or angio) 4.8% vs 4.5%	24 mo
STRIDES[17]	104	Everolimus	FP	N/A	6 and 12 mo patency 6 mo: 94% ± 2.3% 12 mo: 68% ± 4.6%	12 mo
ZILVER PTX[18]	479	Paclitaxel	FP	PTA and PTA + BMS	Event-free survival: 90% vs 83% ($P < 0.01$) Primary patency: 90% vs 73% ($P < 0.01$)	36 mo
YUKON BTK[20]	161	Sirolimus	BTK	BMS	12-mo event-free survival 66% vs 45% ($P = 0.02$)	36 mo
PARADISE[24]	106	Sirolimus and paclitaxel	BTK	PTA	3-y amputation free survival: 6% vs 18% ($P = 0.04$) Overall survival: 71% vs 63% ($P = 0.02$)	36 mo
DESTINY[21]	140	Everolimus	BTK	BMS	12-mo primary patency measured 85% vs 54% ($P < 0.001$)	12 mo

DES, drug-eluting stent; FP, femoropopliteal; PAD, peripheral artery disease; PTA, percutaneous transluminal angioplasty.

(RCT) showed improved patency rates, decreased restenosis with DES but with no difference in overall mortality or limb salvage rates.[22] Fusaro et al also confirmed these findings in their meta-analysis. They concluded that despite the reduction in reintervention, there was no difference in mortality or change in Rutherford class in patients with BTK disease who had DES placement.[23]

3. The **PARADISE** (Preventing Leg Amputations in Critical Limb Ischemia with Below-the-Knee Drug-Eluting Stents) trial had the largest cohort of patients with CLI and BTK disease treated with DES (Cyper ~80% and Taxus ~20%). This was a nonrandomized study, but the outcomes were compared with an historic cohort of similar patients from the BASIL (Bypass vs Angioplasty in Severe Ischemia of the Leg) trial. This trial concluded that compared with PTA, DES resulted in improved amputation-free survival in these CLI patients.[24] An updated meta-analysis published in 2013, which included around 4000 patients with BTK disease who received various therapies including PTA, BMS, and DES, demonstrated superior patency rates in short term (~1 year), freedom from TLR, and improved limb salvage with DES. However, no difference was noted between BMS and PTA.[25]

C. **Unanswered Questions in Drug-Eluting Stent Arena** DES appears to improve patency rates and reduce restenosis in both FP and BTK disease in the short term. Long-term results of DES are still questionable. Focal and short lesions (<100 mm) in the BTK territory seem to respond well to DES, but BTK disease is usually diffuse and progressive. The utility of DES to improve limb salvage in these long lesions still needs to be explored. Another lingering question is: which DES is more effective? sirolimus or paclitaxel. There is some evidence that due to shorter elution time, –limus-based DESs have better outcomes compared with paclitaxel.[10] Optimal duration of dual antiplatelet therapy after DES implantation has never been fully answered. DES is subjected to late complications such as stent thrombosis due to incomplete endothelialization.[26] There has been a lot of research into the biomechanical stress on the vessel wall caused by stents, and due to its location in the FP territory, stent fracture has been described. It has also been shown that there is nonuniform drug elution, more pronounced in the intima that is in contact with the stent. These issues make DES a less than ideal strategy for universal application in patients with PAD.

VI. Drug-Coated Balloon

A. Drug-Coated Balloons for Femoropopliteal Disease

1. DCBs have several advantages over standard PTA in regard to late lumen loss (LLL), TLR, and improved primary patency with decreased restenosis. As reviewed earlier in the chapter, paclitaxel is the most commonly used drug in DCB due to its lipophilic properties and tissue penetration. Initial proof of concept studies done in swine showed that high concentrations of paclitaxel delivered by balloon angioplasty reduced intimal hyperplasia even though the duration of exposure of the vessel wall to the drug was short.[27,28]

2. **FEMPAC** (Paclitaxel-Coated vs Uncoated Balloon: Femoral Paclitaxel Randomized Pilot Trial) trial randomized 87 patients with FP disease to either PTA or paclitaxel DCB. The primary outcome of late lumen loss at 6-months was significantly lower in the DCB group with reduction in TLR rates as well. This benefit continued to 18 months after therapy.[29] THUNDER (Local Taxane with Short Exposure for Reduction of Restenosis in Distal Arteries) trial randomized ~150 patients to standard PTA or paclitaxel DCB or paclitaxel with contrast medium DCB and demonstrated a significantly lower LLL and TLR at 6 months in both the paclitaxel arms compared with plain PTA. The addition of contrast to paclitaxel seemed to have no additional benefit in this trial. Freedom from TLR continued up to 24 months after DCB therapy.[30]

3. The **PACIFIER** (Paclitaxel-Coated Balloons in Femoral Indication to Defeat Restenosis) trial showed significant reduction in 6-month LLL and TLR in patients randomized to paclitaxel DCB. It also showed reduction in binary restenosis and fewer target limb amputations and TLR at 12 months.[31] LEVANT I (Lutonix paclitaxel-coated balloon for the prevention of FP restenosis) trial showed similar results with paclitaxel DCB in patients with FP disease although the dose used was less.[32] A meta-analysis of all these four trials showed significant reduction in TLR, binary restenosis, and LLL with paclitaxel DCB with no reduction in mortality.[33] These results are shown in Figs. 12.3 and 12.4.

4. The **IN.PACT SFA trial** (Randomized Trial of IN.PACT Admiral Drug Eluting Balloon vs Standard PTA for the Treatment of SFA and Proximal Popliteal Arterial Disease) was one of the largest randomized trials that included over 300 patients with

Target lesion revascularization

Study or Subgroup	PCB Events	PCB Total	UCB Events	UCB Total	Weight	Odds Ratio M-H, Random, 95% CI	Year
THUNDER	7	48	28	54	32.1%	0.16 [0.06, 0.42]	2008
FemPac	6	45	21	42	27.3%	0.15 [0.05, 0.44]	2008
LEVANT I	6	47	10	45	24.7%	0.51 [0.17, 1.55]	2010
PACIFIER	3	40	9	39	16.0%	0.27 [0.07, 1.09]	2011
Total (95% CI)		**180**		**180**	**100.0%**	**0.23 [0.13, 0.40]**	
Total events	22		68				

Heterogeneity: $Tau^2 = 0.02$; $Chi^2 = 3.19$, df = 3 (P = 0.36); $I^2 = 6\%$
Test for overall effect: Z = 5.09 (P < 0.00001)
$Heterogeneity_{(exact)}$: $Chi^2 = 3.26$, df = 3 (P = 0.35)
Test for overall $effect_{(exact)}$: P < 0.00001

Odds Ratio
M-H, Random, 95% CI
0.01 0.1 1 10 100
PCB Better UCB Better

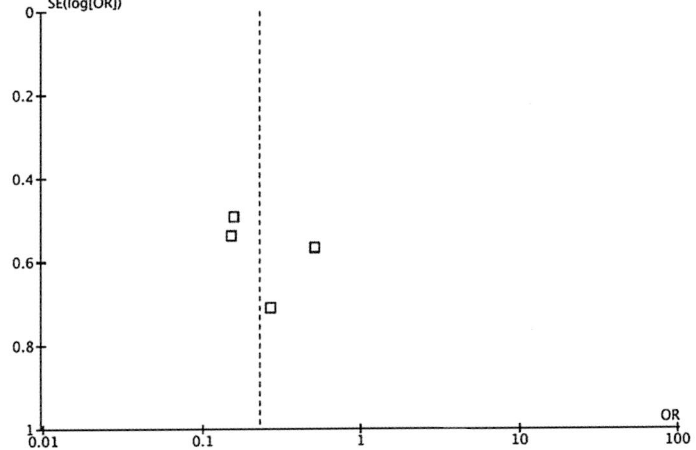

FIGURE 12.3: Target lesion revascularization in paclitaxel-coated balloon versus uncoated balloon angioplasty. Reproduced with permission from Cassese S, Byrne RA, Ott I, et al. Paclitaxel-coated versus uncoated balloon angioplasty reduces target lesion revascularization in patients with femoropopliteal arterial disease: a meta-analysis of randomized trials. *Circ Cardiovasc Interv.* 2012;5(4):582-589.

symptomatic FP disease, to either paclitaxel DCB or PTA and concluded that there was a significant increase in patency rates and reduction in clinically driven TLR at 1 year[34] These results were still favorable at the end of 2 years.[35] Table 12.2 summarizes important DCB trials.

B. **Drug-Coated Balloons in Below Knee Disease** DCBs have been used in below knee disease with mixed results. The initial study by Schmidt et al was a prospective single arm trial that examined the use of DCB in patients with below knee disease and CLI. This showed superior short- and mid-term patency rates compared with historical controls treated with PTA.[9] These findings were then confirmed in the DEBATE BTK (Drug Eluting Balloon in peripheral intervention for Below The Knee Angioplasty Evaluation) trial that randomized 132 patients with CLI (Rutherford class 4 or above) and below knee disease. It demonstrated significantly lower restenosis rates, TLR, and target vessel occlusion in the DCB arm.[36] However, the results from IN.PACT DEEP (RandomIzed AmPhirion DEEP DEB vs StAndard PTA for the treatment of below the knee CriTical limb ischemia) raised some concerns over DCB use in below knee disease. This study

A Binary restenosis

Study or Subgroup	PCB Events	PCB Total	UCB Events	UCB Total	Weight	Odds Ratio M-H, Random, 95% CI
THUNDER	7	41	21	48	38.8%	0.26 [0.10, 0.71]
FemPac	10	31	22	34	36.1%	0.26 [0.09, 0.73]
PACIFIER	4	40	12	39	25.1%	0.25 [0.07, 0.86]
Total (95% CI)		**112**		**121**	**100.0%**	**0.26 [0.14, 0.48]**
Total events	21		55			

Heterogeneity: $Tau^2 = 0.00$; $Chi^2 = 0.01$, df = 2 (P = 1.00); $I^2 = 0\%$
Test for overall effect: Z = 4.27 (P < 0.0001)
Heterogeneity$_{(exact)}$: $Chi^2 = 0.004$, df = 2 (P = 0.99)
Test for overall effect$_{(exact)}$: P < 0.00001

B Late lumen loss

Study or Subgroup	PCB Mean	PCB SD	PCB Total	UCB Mean	UCB SD	UCB Total	Weight	Mean Difference IV, Random, 95% CI
THUNDER	0.4	1.2	41	1.7	1.8	48	19.6%	-1.30 [-1.93, -0.67]
FemPac	0.5	1.1	31	1	1.1	34	25.2%	-0.50 [-1.04, 0.04]
LEVANT I	0.4	1.1	39	1.09	1	35	29.7%	-0.69 [-1.17, -0.21]
PACIFIER	-0.05	1.1	40	0.61	1.3	39	25.5%	-0.66 [-1.19, -0.13]
Total (95% CI)			**151**			**156**	**100.0%**	**-0.75 [-1.06, -0.45]**

Heterogeneity: $Tau^2 = 0.02$; $Chi^2 = 3.95$, df = 3 (P = 0.27); $I^2 = 24\%$
Test for overall effect: Z = 4.78 (P < 0.00001)

C Death

Study or Subgroup	PCB Events	PCB Total	UCB Events	UCB Total	Weight	Odds Ratio M-H, Random, 95% CI
THUNDER	2	48	1	54	19.4%	2.30 [0.20, 26.25]
FemPac	6	45	3	42	46.6%	2.00 [0.47, 8.57]
LEVANT I	1	48	3	49	21.5%	0.33 [0.03, 3.25]
PACIFIER	0	41	2	41	12.6%	0.19 [0.01, 4.09]
Total (95% CI)		**182**		**186**	**100.0%**	**1.04 [0.34, 3.18]**
Total events	9		9			

Heterogeneity: $Tau^2 = 0.15$; $Chi^2 = 3.37$, df = 3 (P = 0.34); $I^2 = 11\%$
Test for overall effect: Z = 0.06 (P = 0.95)
Heterogeneity$_{(exact)}$: $Chi^2 = 4.37$, df = 3 (P = 0.22)
Test for overall effect$_{(exact)}$: P = 0.98

FIGURE 12.4: Angiographic restenosis (A), late lumen loss (B), and mortality (C) in paclitaxel-coated balloon versus uncoated balloon angioplasty. Reproduced with permission from Cassese S, Byrne RA, Ott I, et al. Paclitaxel-coated versus uncoated balloon angioplasty reduces target lesion revascularization in patients with femoropopliteal arterial disease: a meta-analysis of randomized trials. *Circ Cardiovasc Interv.* 2012;5(4):582-589.

randomized 351 patients with CLI to either DCB or PTA and showed no significant benefit with DCB in terms of clinically driven TLR or LLL, but there was a trend toward more amputations in the DCB arm.[37]

C. **Drug-Coated Balloons for in Stent Restenosis** Another unique application for DCB is the treatment of ISR, which was explored in some trials with encouraging long-term results. A single center prospective registry included 39 patients with SFA ISR who were treated with DCB and demonstrated a 1-year patency rate of over 90% with a 10% need for bailout stenting.[38] The patency rate was still over 70% at 2 years' follow-up.[39] The DEBATE ISR (Drug-Eluting Balloon in Peripheral Intervention for In-Stent Restenosis) study showed a significant reduction in restenosis and TLR rates at 1 year

Table 12.2. DCB Trials in PAD

Trial	Sample Size	Drug	Excipient	Dose µg/mm²	Control	Territory	Primary Outcome
THUNDER[30]	154	Paclitaxel	Iopramide	3	PTA only and PTA with contrast	FP	6 mo LLL 0.4 ± 1.2 vs 1.7 ± 1.8 mm ($P < 0.001$)
LEVANT I[32]	101	Paclitaxel	Polysorbate	3	PTA	FP	6 mo LLL 0.5 ± 1.1 vs 1.1 ± 1.1 mm ($P = 0.016$)
PACIFIER[31]	91	Paclitaxel	Urea	3	PTA	FP	6 mo LLL −0.01 ± 0.3 vs 0.7 ± 0.3 mm ($P = 0.0014$)
IN.PACT SFA[34]	331	Paclitaxel	Urea	3.5	PTA	FP	12 mo primary patency 82.2% vs 52.4%; $P < 0.001$
DEBATE BTK[36]	132	Paclitaxel	Urea	3	PTA	BTK	12 mo binary restenosis 27% vs 74% ($P < 0.001$)
DEBATE SFA	110	Paclitaxel	Urea	3	PTA + BMS	BTK	12 mo binary restenosis 17% vs 47% ($P = 0.008$)

DCB, drug-coated balloon; FP, femoropopliteal; LLL, late lumen loss; PAD, peripheral artery disease; PTA, percutaneous transluminal angioplasty.

with DCB compared with historical controls treated with PTA.[40] However, at 3 years no significant difference was noted in regard to TLR.[41] Several ongoing trails aim to explore this clinical utility in a rigorous fashion.

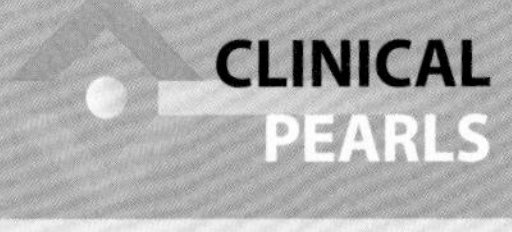

- When using DCB, adequate lesion preparation is critical before applying DCB; this may include PTA or atherectomy to enhance drug delivery to the vessel wall. It also goes without saying that one should avoid geographic miss by using anatomic landmarks and glow tape. The drug starts eluting as soon as the balloon catheter comes in contact with the blood, and although the rate of drug loss is small, it is recommended that the DCB catheter be advanced to the treatment segment as quickly as possible. Adequate inflation times are also important to ensure drug delivery, and in most cases this requires 3 minutes.
- There appears to be certain areas in which DCB would have theoretical advantage over other devices; this includes common femoral artery, ostial SFA, and bypass graft restenosis.

VII. Future Directions

There are many unanswered questions with drug-coated therapies, and consequently, there are a number of ongoing trials in this area. Bioabsorbable vascular scaffolds (BVS) may be a solution to some of the problems with drug-coated devices. It avoids the elastic recoil and

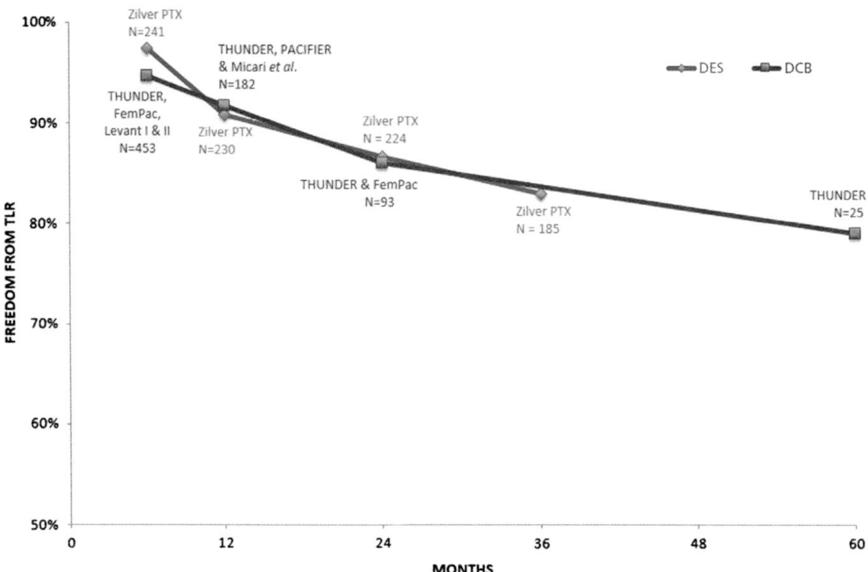

FIGURE 12.5: Freedom from target lesion revascularization (TLR) for DES compared with drug-coated balloon (DCB) in femoropopliteal trials. Reproduced with permission from Sarode K, Spelber DA, Bhatt DL, et al. Drug delivering technology for endovascular management of infrainguinal peripheral artery disease. *JACC Cardiovasc Interv.* 2014;7(8):827-839.

flow-limiting dissections seen with DCBs, and as the scaffold "disappears," there is no long-term risk of shear stress on the vessel or persistent inflammation seen with stents. After some initial success in the coronary realm, it remains to be seen if that can be reproduced in the PAD arena. The ESPRIT I trial was a single arm prospective multicenter trial that showed in carefully selected patients with predominantly focal SFA disease (30-40 mm), the BVS stent was safe and effective with 1- and 2-year binary restenosis rates of 12% and 16% and TLR rates of ~9% and 12%, respectively.[42]

There has been a considerable interest in combination therapies to overcome some of the limitations of drug-coated devices such as atherectomy followed by DCB. This was shown to be an ideal strategy with early (30-day) higher technical success and lower residual stenosis rates compared with DCB alone.[43] Several other ongoing trials are examining atherectomy or photoablative strategies combined with DCB in PAD.[44,45] There have been no direct comparison between DES and DCB, but the ongoing trials will hopefully settle the debate soon.[46,47] Fig. 12.5 shows the TLR rates for DCB and DES.

VIII. Conclusion

Drug-coated devices (DES and DCB) have been demonstrated to be safe and effective in the treatment of FP and below knee PAD. Endovascular interventions in general are limited in this territory by lower patency rates, and hence it makes perfect sense to incorporate these devices in the treatment algorithm to decrease restenosis rates. The mid-term results of DES look very promising, but the patency rates seem to be poor for longer lesions (>100 mm) and calcific stenosis. Moreover there still exist some concerns over stents causing shear stress on the vessel wall and delayed restenosis due to the scaffold. DCB can overcome most of these limitations and have shown to be an excellent addition to the PAD armamentarium. The patency rates are comparable with DES with lower restenosis rates. Moreover, this technology has the advantage of "leave nothing behind" strategy and treatment of disease in the traditional "no-stent zones." The long-term efficacy of these devices is yet to be seen. Combining DCB with atherectomy has its advantages as well. Lots of ongoing trials will shed more light in this area, and for the time being, drug-coated devices are definitely a force to be reckoned with.

References

1. Norgren L, Hiatt WR, Dormandy JA, et al. Inter-society consensus for the management of peripheral arterial disease. *Int Angiol.* 2007;26(2):81-157. PMID: 17489079.
2. Beschorner U, Sixt S, Schwarzwalder U, et al. Recanalization of chronic occlusions of the superficial femoral artery using the Outback re-entry catheter: a single centre experience. *Catheter Cardiovasc Interv.* 2009;74(6):934-938. doi:10.1002/ccd.22130. PMID: 19626685.
3. Schillinger M, Sabeti S, Loewe C, et al. Balloon angioplasty versus implantation of nitinol stents in the superficial femoral artery. *N Engl J Med.* 2006;354(18):1879-1888. doi:10.1056/NEJMoa051303. PMID: 16672699.
4. Krankenberg H, Schluter M, Steinkamp HJ, et al. Nitinol stent implantation versus percutaneous transluminal angioplasty in superficial femoral artery lesions up to 10 cm in length: the femoral artery stenting trial (FAST). *Circulation.* 2007;116(3):285-292. doi:10.1161/CIRCULATIONAHA.107.689141. PMID: 17592075.
5. Kornowski R, Hong MK, Tio FO, Bramwell O, Wu H, Leon MB. In-stent restenosis: contributions of inflammatory responses and arterial injury to neointimal hyperplasia. *J Am Coll Cardiol.* 1998;31(1):224-230. PMID: 9426044.
6. Hwang SJ, Park KW, Kwon DA, et al. High plasma interleukin-6 is associated with drug-eluting stent thrombosis: possible role of inflammatory cytokines in the development of stent thrombosis from the Korea Stent Thrombosis Registry. *Circ J.* 2011;75(6):1350-1357. PMID: 21498913.
7. Grimm J, Muller-Hulsbeck S, Jahnke T, Hilbert C, Brossmann J, Heller M. Randomized study to compare PTA alone versus PTA with Palmaz stent placement for femoropopliteal lesions. *J Vasc Interv Radiol.* 2001;12(8):935-942. PMID: 11487673.
8. Armstrong EJ, Singh S, Singh GD, et al. Angiographic characteristics of femoropopliteal in-stent restenosis: association with long-term outcomes after endovascular intervention. *Catheter Cardiovasc Interv.* 2013;82(7):1168-1174. doi:10.1002/ccd.24983. PMID: 23630047; PMCID: PMCPMC3836909.
9. Schmidt A, Piorkowski M, Werner M, et al. First experience with drug-eluting balloons in infrapopliteal arteries: restenosis rate and clinical outcome. *J Am Coll Cardiol.* 2011;58(11):1105-1109. doi:10.1016/j.jacc.2011.05.034. PMID: 21884945.
10. Duda SH, Poerner TC, Wiesinger B, et al. Drug-eluting stents: potential applications for peripheral arterial occlusive disease. *J Vasc Interv Radiol.* 2003;14(3):291-301. PMID: 12631633.
11. Katz G, Harchandani B, Shah B. Drug-eluting stents: the past, present, and future. *Curr Atheroscler Rep.* 2015;17(3):485. doi:10.1007/s11883-014-0485-2. PMID: 25651784.
12. Chen W, Habraken TC, Hennink WE, Kok RJ. Polymer-free drug-eluting stents: an overview of coating strategies and comparison with polymer-coated drug-eluting stents. *Bioconjug Chem.* 2015;26(7):1277-1288. doi:10.1021/acs.bioconjchem.5b00192. PMID: 26041505.
13. Stefanini GG, Holmes DR Jr. Drug-eluting coronary-artery stents. *N Engl J Med.* 2013;368(3):254-265. doi:10.1056/NEJMra1210816. PMID: 23323902.
14. Byrne RA, Joner M, Alfonso F, Kastrati A. Drug-coated balloon therapy in coronary and peripheral artery disease. *Nat Rev Cardiol.* 2014;11(1):13-23. doi:10.1038/nrcardio.2013.165. PMID: 24189405.

15. Duda SH, Bosiers M, Lammer J, et al. Drug-eluting and bare nitinol stents for the treatment of atherosclerotic lesions in the superficial femoral artery: long-term results from the SIROCCO trial. *J Endovasc Ther.* 2006;13(6):701-710. doi:10.1583/05-1704.1. PMID: 17154704.
16. Nakazawa G, Otsuka F, Nakano M, et al. The pathology of neoatherosclerosis in human coronary implants bare-metal and drug-eluting stents. *J Am Coll Cardiol.* 2011;57(11):1314-1322. doi:10.1016/j.jacc.2011.01.011. PMID: 21376502; PMCID: PMCPMC3093310.
17. Lammer J, Bosiers M, Zeller T, et al. First clinical trial of nitinol self-expanding everolimus-eluting stent implantation for peripheral arterial occlusive disease. *J Vasc Surg.* 2011;54(2):394-401. doi:10.1016/j.jvs.2011.01.047. PMID: 21658885.
18. Dake MD, Ansel GM, Jaff MR, et al. Sustained safety and effectiveness of paclitaxel-eluting stents for femoropopliteal lesions: 2-year follow-up from the Zilver PTX randomized and single-arm clinical studies. *J Am Coll Cardiol.* 2013;61(24):2417-2427. doi:10.1016/j.jacc.2013.03.034. PMID: 23583245.
19. Dake MD, Ansel GM, Jaff MR, et al. Paclitaxel-eluting stents show superiority to balloon angioplasty and bare metal stents in femoropopliteal disease: twelve-month Zilver PTX randomized study results. *Circ Cardiovasc Interv.* 2011;4(5):495-504. doi:10.1161/CIRCINTERVENTIONS.111.962324. PMID: 21953370.
20. Rastan A, Brechtel K, Krankenberg H, et al. Sirolimus-eluting stents for treatment of infrapopliteal arteries reduce clinical event rate compared to bare-metal stents: long-term results from a randomized trial. *J Am Coll Cardiol.* 2012;60(7):587-591. doi:10.1016/j.jacc.2012.04.035. PMID: 22878166.
21. Bosiers M, Scheinert D, Peeters P, et al. Randomized comparison of everolimus-eluting versus bare-metal stents in patients with critical limb ischemia and infrapopliteal arterial occlusive disease. *J Vasc Surg.* 2012;55(2):390-398. doi:10.1016/j.jvs.2011.07.099. PMID: 22169682.
22. Antoniou GA, Chalmers N, Kanesalingham K, et al. Meta-analysis of outcomes of endovascular treatment of infrapopliteal occlusive disease with drug-eluting stents. *J Endovasc Ther.* 2013;20(2):131-144. doi:10.1583/1545-1550-20.2.131. PMID: 23581752.
23. Fusaro M, Cassese S, Ndrepepa G, et al. Drug-eluting stents for revascularization of infrapopliteal arteries: updated meta-analysis of randomized trials. *JACC Cardiovasc Interv.* 2013;6(12):1284-1293. doi:10.1016/j.jcin.2013.08.007. PMID: 24355118.
24. Feiring AJ, Krahn M, Nelson L, Wesolowski A, Eastwood D, Szabo A. Preventing leg amputations in critical limb ischemia with below-the-knee drug-eluting stents: the PaRADISE (PReventing Amputations using Drug eluting StEnts) trial. *J Am Coll Cardiol.* 2010;55(15):1580-1589. doi:10.1016/j.jacc.2009.11.072. PMID: 20378075.
25. Yang X, Lu X, Ye K, Li X, Qin J, Jiang M. Systematic review and meta-analysis of balloon angioplasty versus primary stenting in the infrapopliteal disease. *Vasc Endovascular Surg.* 2014;48(1):18-26. doi:10.1177/1538574413510626. PMID: 24212407.
26. Finn AV, Joner M, Nakazawa G, et al. Pathological correlates of late drug-eluting stent thrombosis: strut coverage as a marker of endothelialization. *Circulation.* 2007;115(18):2435-2441. doi:10.1161/CIRCULATIONAHA.107.693739. PMID: 17438147.
27. Scheller B, Speck U, Abramjuk C, Bernhardt U, Bohm M, Nickenig G. Paclitaxel balloon coating, a novel method for prevention and therapy of restenosis. *Circulation.* 2004;110(7):810-814. doi:10.1161/01.CIR.0000138929.71660.E0. PMID: 15302790.
28. Albrecht T, Speck U, Baier C, Wolf KJ, Bohm M, Scheller B. Reduction of stenosis due to intimal hyperplasia after stent supported angioplasty of peripheral arteries by local administration of paclitaxel in swine. *Invest Radiol.* 2007;42(8):579-585. doi:10.1097/RLI.0b013e31804f5a60. PMID: 17620941.
29. Werk M, Langner S, Reinkensmeier B, et al. Inhibition of restenosis in femoropopliteal arteries: paclitaxel-coated versus uncoated balloon: femoral paclitaxel randomized pilot trial. *Circulation.* 2008;118(13):1358-1365. doi:10.1161/CIRCULATIONAHA.107.735985. PMID: 18779447.
30. Tepe G, Zeller T, Albrecht T, et al. Local delivery of paclitaxel to inhibit restenosis during angioplasty of the leg. *N Engl J Med.* 2008;358(7):689-699. doi:10.1056/NEJMoa0706356. PMID: 18272892.

31. Werk M, Albrecht T, Meyer DR, et al. Paclitaxel-coated balloons reduce restenosis after femoro-popliteal angioplasty: evidence from the randomized PACIFIER trial. *Circ Cardiovasc Interv.* 2012;5(6):831-840. doi:10.1161/CIRCINTERVENTIONS.112.971630. PMID: 23192918.
32. Scheinert D, Duda S, Zeller T, et al. The LEVANT I (Lutonix paclitaxel-coated balloon for the prevention of femoropopliteal restenosis) trial for femoropopliteal revascularization: first-in-human randomized trial of low-dose drug-coated balloon versus uncoated balloon angioplasty. *JACC Cardiovasc Interv.* 2014;7(1):10-19. doi:10.1016/j.jcin.2013.05.022. PMID: 24456716.
33. Cassese S, Byrne RA, Ott I, et al. Paclitaxel-coated versus uncoated balloon angioplasty reduces target lesion revascularization in patients with femoropopliteal arterial disease: a meta-analysis of randomized trials. *Circ Cardiovasc Interv.* 2012;5(4):582-589. doi:10.1161/CIRCINTERVENTIONS.112.969972. PMID: 22851526.
34. Tepe G, Laird J, Schneider P, et al. Drug-coated balloon versus standard percutaneous transluminal angioplasty for the treatment of superficial femoral and popliteal peripheral artery disease: 12-month results from the IN.PACT SFA randomized trial. *Circulation.* 2015;131(5):495-502. doi:10.1161/CIRCULATIONAHA.114.011004. PMID: 25472980; PMCID: PMCPMC4323569.
35. Laird JR, Schneider PA, Tepe G, et al. Durability of treatment effect using a drug-coated balloon for femoropopliteal lesions: 24-month results of IN.PACT SFA. *J Am Coll Cardiol.* 2015;66(21):2329-2338. doi:10.1016/j.jacc.2015.09.063. PMID: 26476467.
36. Liistro F, Porto I, Angioli P, et al. Drug-eluting balloon in peripheral intervention for below the knee angioplasty evaluation (DEBATE-BTK): a randomized trial in diabetic patients with critical limb ischemia. *Circulation.* 2013;128(6):615-621. doi:10.1161/CIRCULATIONAHA.113.001811. PMID: 23797811.
37. Zeller T, Baumgartner I, Scheinert D, et al. Drug-eluting balloon versus standard balloon angioplasty for infrapopliteal arterial revascularization in critical limb ischemia: 12-month results from the IN.PACT DEEP randomized trial. *J Am Coll Cardiol.* 2014;64(15):1568-1576. doi:10.1016/j.jacc.2014.06.1198. PMID: 25301459.
38. Stabile E, Virga V, Salemme L, et al. Drug-eluting balloon for treatment of superficial femoral artery in-stent restenosis. *J Am Coll Cardiol.* 2012;60(18):1739-1742. doi:10.1016/j.jacc.2012.07.033. PMID: 23040582.
39. Virga V, Stabile E, Biamino G, et al. Drug-eluting balloons for the treatment of the superficial femoral artery in-stent restenosis: 2-year follow-up. *JACC Cardiovasc Interv.* 2014;7(4):411-415. doi:10.1016/j.jcin.2013.11.020. PMID: 24630884.
40. Liistro F, Angioli P, Porto I, et al. Paclitaxel-eluting balloon vs. standard angioplasty to reduce recurrent restenosis in diabetic patients with in-stent restenosis of the superficial femoral and proximal popliteal arteries: the DEBATE-ISR study. *J Endovasc Ther.* 2014;21(1):1-8. doi:10.1583/13-4420R.1. PMID: 24502477.
41. Grotti S, Liistro F, Angioli P, et al. Paclitaxel-eluting balloon vs standard angioplasty to reduce restenosis in diabetic patients with in-stent restenosis of the superficial femoral and proximal popliteal arteries: three-year results of the DEBATE-ISR study. *J Endovasc Ther.* 2016;23(1):52-57. doi:10.1177/1526602815614555. PMID: 26511896.
42. Lammer J, Bosiers M, Deloose K, et al. Bioresorbable everolimus-eluting vascular scaffold for patients with peripheral artery disease (ESPRIT I): 2-year clinical and imaging results. *JACC Cardiovasc Interv.* 2016;9(11):1178-1187. doi:10.1016/j.jcin.2016.02.051. PMID: 27282601.
43. Endovascular Medtronic, MEDRAD Inc. *Atherectomy Followed by a Drug Coated Balloon to Treat Peripheral Arterial Disease*; 2011. https://ClinicalTrials.gov/show/NCT01366482.
44. Aljoscha Rastan, Herz-Zentrums Bad Krozingen, Medical University of Graz. *Atherectomy and Drug-Coated Balloon Angioplasty in Treatment of Long Infrapopliteal Lesions*; 2013. https://ClinicalTrials.gov/show/NCT01763476.
45. Herz-Zentrums Bad Krozingen. *Photoablative Atherectomy Followed by a Paclitaxel-Coated Balloon to Inhibit Restenosis in Instent Femoro-popliteal Obstructions*; 2011. https://ClinicalTrials.gov/show/NCT01298947.
46. Provascular GmbH, William Cook Europe. *Evaluation of Paclitaxel Eluting Stent vs Paclitaxel Eluting Balloon Treating Peripheral Artery Disease of the Femoral Artery*; 2012. https://ClinicalTrials.gov/show/NCT01728441.
47. University of Patras. *Infrapopliteal Drug Eluting Angioplasty Versus Stenting*; 2011. https://ClinicalTrials.gov/show/NCT01517997.

CHAPTER 13

Stent Therapies in the Lower Extremity: Bare-Metal, Drug-Eluting, and Reabsorbable Stents

Kwan S. Lee, MBBCh, Ahmed Harhash, MBBCh, and Tze-Woei Tan, MBBS

I. Introduction

A. **History** Percutaneous endovascular therapies for peripheral arterial disease have continued to evolve since Charles Dotter performed the first percutaneous transluminal angioplasty (PTA) of a superficial femoral artery (SFA) in 1964. In deciding optimal therapy from the myriad of devices and techniques currently available, the unique properties of specific arterial distributions must also be accounted for. Balloon angioplasty is overall effective and has the advantage of simplicity and cost-effectiveness, but results are limited by recoil, acute dissection, and significant rates of restenosis. There are numerous adjunctive therapies to angioplasty, including scoring balloon angioplasty, atherectomy in its many forms (rotational, excisional, laser), drug-coated balloons, and a variety of stents. Many permutations therefore exist for therapy and can be both confusing and complementary. Familiarity with the Inter-Society Consensus for the Management of Peripheral Arterial Disease (TASC) guidelines is important, as they categorize heterogeneous anatomical presentations of disease and guide suitability of surgical versus endovascular therapy and choice of endovascular intervention.[1]

B. **Technology** Given the central and important role of stenting in endovascular intervention, it is important to have an appreciation of the technologies involved and the relative benefits and drawbacks of each. Stents were developed to improve outcomes over angioplasty. They improve vessel patency by acting as a scaffold against recoil and dissection. The primary structural challenge in peripheral vascular disease is compressional and torsional forces acting upon the stent in specific anatomic territories during daily motion, which may crush the stent or contribute to strut fractures. In addition to the challenges posed by daily external forces, stents induce proliferative reactions, contributing to long-term restenosis.

C. **Chapter Outline** This chapter aims to provide a framework and contextual understanding of stents by discussing the technical and clinical performance of different stents used in the lower extremity. The use of stents for other vascular territories including venous intervention will be covered in their individual chapters.

II. Bare-Metal Balloon-Expandable Stents

A. **General Principles** In lower extremity arterial stenting, bare-metal balloon-expandable stents are primarily used in the iliac territory, given the lower degree of stress and torsional movement to which the iliac artery is exposed. Balloon-expandable stents should not be used in areas where repeated flexing of the artery occurs. Balloon-expandable stents are constructed from stainless steel or cobalt chromium and in general have greater radial strength and radiopacity but poorer flexibility and trackability compared with self-expanding stents. Given the mechanism of deployment, they can be positioned with greater accuracy.

B. **Common Iliac Artery** The common iliac artery is a straight and immobile vessel, being fixed to the sacral promontory, while the external iliac artery has a much more tortuous course, stretching during hip extension. Open surgical procedures have excellent patency rates but are associated with significant morbidity and mortality. Several randomized studies comparing endovascular stenting with stand-alone angioplasty demonstrated stenting to be superior in both hemodynamic parameters and Rutherford classification. A meta-analysis of iliac intervention showed that stent placement reduced the risk of long-term failure by 39% when compared with PTA alone.[2] Table 13.1 lists all current FDA (U.S. Food and Drug Administration)–approved balloon-expandable stents.

III. Balloon-Expandable Covered Stents

A. **General Principles** Covered stents can be used to treat aneurysms, perforations, and arteriovenous fistulae in the aortoiliac region. Open surgery is the preferred approach for complex and severe iliac artery occlusive disease in low-risk patients. More recently, endovascular intervention has been performed with acceptable outcomes even in TASC C and D lesions. The use of covered stents has been proposed to reduce intimal hyperplasia and to improve long-term patency by reducing restenosis. The Atrium iCAST covered stent (Maquet Getinge Group, Rastatt, Germany) and the Viabahn VBX endoprosthesis (W.L. Gore & Associates, Flagstaff, AZ) are two commercially available balloon-expandable polytetrafluoroethylene (PTFE) covered stents. Although the iCAST stent is currently approved by the FDA to treat tracheobronchial strictures, it has been used "off-label" in aortoiliac, mesenteric, and renal arterial occlusive disease. The Viabahn VBX stent was recently approved by FDA as the first balloon-expandable stent graft for use in the iliac artery.

1. The iCAST covered stent is a 316L stainless steel balloon-expandable stent, which is encapsulated entirely with a thin PTFE film. The stent graft is premounted on a noncompliant balloon and is compatible with a 6 or 7 Fr sheath. It is available in 5 to 10 mm diameter and in 16, 22, 38, and 59 mm lengths. The device is available in 80 cm and 120 cm shaft lengths and is delivered on a 0.035-in wire platform. The stent can be postdilated to 4 mm larger if necessary after deployment, but this results in stent foreshortening. The iCAST stent is stiffer than a bare-metal stent (BMS) of comparable size, and care should be taken when it is advanced through severely stenotic or occlusive lesions owing to the risk of stent dislodgement.
2. The Viabahn VBX endoprosthesis is composed of a stainless steel stent fully covered in a fluoropolymer, which is coated with bioactive heparin surface. The stent is premounted on a 0.035-in guidewire-compatible delivery system and requires a 7 or 8 Fr sheath. It is available in 5-10 mm diameter and in 15, 19, 39, and 59 mm stent lengths. Similar to the iCAST stent, the Viabahn stent can be postdilated to a larger diameter if needed.

B. **Comparison with Bare-Metal Stents** There are a few retrospective series and only one randomized controlled trial comparing the outcomes of balloon-expandable covered versus bare-metal stents (BMSs) in the treatment of severe aortoiliac occlusive lesion. One retrospective review, consisting of 54 patients showed superior patency at 2 years with the use of covered balloon-expandable stents for aortic bifurcation occlusive disease.[3] Others,

Table 13.1. FDA-Approved Balloon-Expandable Bare-Metal Stents in Lower Extremity Peripheral Arterial Disease

Device Name	Manufacturer	Material Used	Guidewire Size/ Endhole (inch)	Introducer Size (F)	Stent Diameter (mm)	Stent Length (mm)	Delivery System Length (cm)	FDA Approval
Omnilink elite	Abbott Vascular	Cobalt chromium	0.035	6, 7	6-10	12, 16, 19, 29, 39, 59	80, 135	Iliac
Express LD Iliac/Biliary Premounted	Boston Scientific	316L Stainless steel	0.035	6 (up to 8 × 37 mm), 7 (up to 10 × 57 mm)	6-10	17, 25, 27, 37, 57	75, 135	Iliac and biliary
Palmaz Iliac	Cordis	316L Stainless steel	0.035	10	8-12	30	NA	Iliac
Palmaz Iliac and Renal	Cordis	316L Stainless steel	0.035	6, 7	4-8	10, 15, 20, 29	NA	Iliac and renal
Assurant Cobalt Iliac	Medtronic	Cobalt chromium alloy	0.035	6	6, 7, 8, 9, 10	20, 30, 40, 60	80, 130	Iliac
Visi-Pro	Medtronic	316L Stainless steel	0.035	6 (5-8 mm), 7 (9-10 mm)	5, 6, 7, 8, 9, 10	12 (5-7 mm diameters), 17, 27, 37, 57	80, 135	Iliac and biliary

FDA, U.S. Food and Drug Administration.

however, showed comparable or worse outcomes of covered stents in severe iliac artery obstructive lesions.[4,5] In a retrospective series, which included 128 patients from Italy, early and midterm outcomes were comparable between covered and bare-metal balloon-expandable stents. The only benefit for covered stents was in TASC II D lesions with long lesions of the common and external iliac arteries.[4] In another series, BMS was reported to have significantly better patency compared with covered balloon-expandable stents.[5]

1. Covered Versus Balloon-Expandable Stent Trial (COBEST) The Covered Versus Balloon-Expandable Stent Trial (COBEST) enrolled 125 patients at 8 major Australian centers to determine whether covered stents were superior to BMS in the treatment of aortoiliac occlusive disease with both 1-year[6] and subsequent 5-year outcomes reported.[7] Overall, stent patency was found to be similar with covered stents and BMS. In subgroup analysis, the patency rate for covered stents was significantly higher than BMS at 18 months, and this persisted up to 60 months in TASC C and D lesions.[6,7] Although patients who received covered stents received fewer revascularization procedures in the trial, the choice of covered stent versus BMS did not affect the rate of limb amputation.[7] A recent meta-analysis that included 255 diseased arteries in 182 patients showed no significant improvement in primary patency with covered stents.[8]

C. **Summary** In summary, the results of balloon-expandable covered stents and BMS are similar in aortoiliac occlusive disease. Current literature does not support the routine use of balloon-expandable covered-stent grafts, although there is some evidence to suggest improved patency for more advanced TASC C and D lesions. They remain an important therapeutic option, however, for bailout of perforations or for complex lesions at risk of rupture during intervention.

IV. Self-Expanding Stents

A. Wallstent

1. Self-expanding Wallstents (Boston Scientific, Marlborough, MA) were first deployed in the SFA in the late 1990s but were quickly shown to be inferior to nitinol self-expanding stents with a relatively high rate of strut fracture.[9] Wallstents are made of Elgiloy, a "superalloy" combining cobalt, chromium, nickel, molybdenum, manganese, and a relatively small amount of iron. It is therefore nonferromagnetic and magnetic resonance imaging (MRI) compatible. The platinum core renders this stent radiopaque. It has a braided, tubular woven-mesh design, which imparts flexibility and an outward self-expanding force to the stent. These unique design characteristics impart an ability to recapture the stent even when 87% deployed, allowing it to be repositioned during deployment. The woven-mesh configuration of the Wallstent causes it to adapt its diameter to the width of the vessel lumen compared with nitinol stents, which expand to a predetermined diameter. The length of a deployed Wallstent is more variable, being dependent on the vessel diameter, therefore susceptible to foreshortening or the opposite.

B. Nitinol Self-Expanding Stents

1. The introduction of nitinol self-expanding stents changed the treatment of femoropopliteal endovascular disease, moving stent implantation from primarily a bailout procedure after failed balloon angioplasty to a reasonable initial approach. Nitinol is a metal alloy of nickel and titanium, which exhibits two unique and closely related properties: shape memory effect and superelasticity. Shape memory is the ability of nitinol to undergo deformation at one temperature and then recover its original shape at a higher temperature. Nitinol stents have improved radial strength and reduced foreshortening and crush resistance owing to the above unique properties, making them well suited for use in the SFA, the longest artery in the human body, subject to flexion, extension, lateral compression, and torsional forces during daily activity.

2. Nitinol self-expanding stents have not been shown to be superior over angioplasty for short, focal lesions. The FAST (Femoral Artery Stenting Trial) randomized 244 patients with lesions between 1 and 10 cm to angioplasty versus primary stent implantation. Despite higher initial technical success, no differences were seen at 12-month follow-up in ultrasound-assessed binary restenosis rates, target lesion revascularization, or Rutherford category.[10]

3. For lesions of intermediate length, however, self-expanding nitinol BMSs have been shown to be superior to balloon angioplasty. An important early trial, the Vienna Absolute study, randomized 104 patients to primary nitinol stenting versus balloon angioplasty with optional secondary stenting. Mean lesion length was 13.2 cm in the stent group, and secondary stenting was performed in the angioplasty group in 32% of patients. The restenosis rate and treadmill walk distance were significantly superior in the primary stented group at 6- and 12-month follow-up.[11] Subsequent studies have supported this initial finding.[12,13]

C. **Summary** In routine clinical practice, many patients have much longer SFA lesions than those studied in randomized trials, which are associated with high restenosis rates.[14] Restenosis is difficult to treat and associated with worse clinical outcome. For this reason, self-expanding nitinol BMSs are currently mainly used in conjunction with plain balloon angioplasty or drug-coated balloon angioplasty to spot stent segments with unsatisfactory angioplasty results in external iliac, superficial femoral, or popliteal arteries. All self-expanding, FDA-approved stents for the lower extremities are listed in Table 13.2.

V. Self-Expanding Covered Stents

A. **General Principles** Despite continued advances in SFA endovascular intervention, TASC II C and D lesions remain a technical challenge with poor primary patency rates due to in-stent restenosis and stent fracture. The length and complexity of an SFA lesion are the most important factors linked to such failure. Theoretically, a stent graft in the SFA with continuous exclusion of the vessel wall from luminal flow may prevent neointimal tissue growth, reducing the risk of in-stent restenosis and thrombosis commonly

Table 13.2. FDA-Approved Self-Expandable Bare-Metal Stents in Lower Extremity Peripheral Arterial Disease

Device Name	Manufacturer	Material Used	Guidewire Size/ Endhole (inch)	Introducer Size (F)	Stent Diameter (mm)	Stent Length (mm)	Delivery System Length (cm)	FDA Approval
Absolute Pro	Abbott Vascular	Nitinol	0.035	6	6, 7, 8, 9, 10	20, 30, 40, 60, 80, 100	80, 135	Iliac
Supera	Abbott Vascular	Nitinol	0.018	6	4.5, 5, 5.5, 6, 6.5	20, 30, 40, 60, 80, 100, 120, 150	120	SFA and proximal popliteal
E-Luminexx Vascular and Biliary	Bard Peripheral Vascular	Nitinol	0.035	6	7, 8, 9, 10	20, 30, 40, 60, 80, 100	80, 135	Iliac and biliary
LifeStar Vascular and Biliary	Bard Peripheral Vascular	Nitinol	0.035	6	7, 8, 9, 10	20, 30, 40, 60, 80, 100	80, 135	Iliac and biliary
LifeStent Solo Vascular	Bard Peripheral Vascular	Nitinol	0.035	6	6, 7	200	100, 135	SFA and full popliteal
LifeStent and LifeStent XL Vascular	Bard Peripheral Vascular	Nitinol	0.035	6	5, 6, 7	20, 30, 40, 60, 80, 100, 120, 150, 170	80, 130	SFA and full popliteal
Astron	Biotronik (distribued by Getinge/Macquet)	Nitinol	0.035	6	7, 8, 9, 10	30, 40, 60, 80	72, 130	Iliac
Epic	Boston Scientific	Nitinol	0.035	6	6, 7, 8, 9, 10, 12	20, 30, 40, 50, 60, 70, 80, 100, 120	75, 120	Iliac
Innova	Boston Scientific	Nitinol	0.035	6	5, 6, 7, 8	20, 40, 60, 80, 100, 120, 150, 200	75, 130	SFA
Wallstent Endoprosthesis	Boston Scientific	Elgiloy	0.035	6	6, 7, 8, 9, 10	18, 20, 23,24, 34, 35, 36, 38, 39, 46, 47, 49, 52, 55, 59, 61, 66, 67, 69	75, 135	Iliac
Zilver 518	Cook Medical	Nitinol	0.018	5	6, 7, 8, 9, 10	20, 30, 40, 60, 80	125	Iliac
Zilver 635	Cook Medical	Nitinol	0.035	6	6, 7, 8, 9, 10	20, 30, 40, 60, 80	80, 125	Iliac
Smart Control Iliac	Cordis	Nitinol	0.035	6	9, 10	20, 30, 40, 60	80, 120	Iliac
Smart Control Vascular	Cordis	Nitinol	0.035	6	6, 7, 8	20, 30, 40, 60, 80, 100	80, 120	Iliac and SFA
Smart Vascular	Cordis	Nitinol	0.035	6	6, 7, 8	120, 150	120	SFA
Gore Tigris	Gore	Nitinol/ ePTFE	0.035	6	5, 6, 7	40, 60, 80, 100	120	SFA and proximal popliteal up to 240 mm in length
Complete SE	Medtronic	Nitinol	0.035	6	5, 6, 7, 8, 9, 10	20, 40, 60, 80, 100, 120, 150	80, 130	Iliac, SFA, and proximal popliteal
EverFlex—SFA and PPA	Medtronic	Nitinol	0.035	6	6, 7, 8	20, 30, 40, 60, 80, 100, 120, 150, 200	80, 120	SFA and proximal popliteal
EverFlex—Iliac	Medtronic	Nitinol	0.035	6	6, 7, 8	20, 30, 40, 60, 80, 100, 120	80, 120	Iliac
Protege GPS	Medtronic	Nitinol	0.035	6	9, 10, 12	20, 30, 40, 60, 80	80, 120	Iliac
Misago RX	Terumo	Nitinol	0.035	6	6, 7, 8	40, 60, 80, 100, 120, 150	135	SFA and proximal popliteal

FDA, U.S. Food and Drug Administration; *PPA*, proximal popliteal artery; *SFA*, superficial femoral artery.

seen with BMSs in addition to providing protection from distal embolization during deployment. One potential drawback of a stent graft, however, is the possible exclusion of important collateral branches, which may worsen pretreatment symptoms or lead to limb ischemia in the event of a graft thrombosis. This property of exclusion is used specifically, however, in the treatment of popliteal artery aneurysms.

B. Clinical Use in Peripheral Arterial Disease

1. FDA Approval

a. The only **FDA-approved self-expanding stent graft** in the treatment of lower extremity peripheral arterial disease is the Viabahn Endoprosthesis (W.L. Gore & Associates, Flagstaff, AZ), a flexible, self-expanding covered-stent graft. The expanded polytetrafluoroethylene (ePTFE) lining is supported externally by a nitinol stent throughout its entire length and is now available with a heparin-bonded surface, which may decrease the likelihood of stent thrombosis.[15] A non–heparin-bonded version is also available for patients with a history of heparin-induced thrombocytopenia. It first became available in the United States in 2002 and was subsequently approved by the FDA in 2005 for SFA intervention.

b. It is available in 5-8 mm diameters with a length between 2.5 and 25.0 cm. The device is deployed either through a 6- to 8-French sheath on a 0.018″ wire platform or through a 7- to 8-French sheath over a 0.035″ platform. Larger devices intended for the iliac artery are available in 9-13 mm diameters and 2.5-15.0 cm lengths. These larger devices are built on a 0.035″ guidewire platform and require a 9-French or larger sheath.

2. Randomized Controlled Trials

a. To date, a number of published randomized controlled trials have evaluated the use of a Viabahn stent graft in the treatment of SFA occlusive disease.[16-19] The first trial, reported in 2009, compared the efficacy of Viabahn stent grafts with a prosthetic femoral to above-knee popliteal bypass in patients with TASC-II A through D lesions. Primary patency (59% vs 58%, P = .81) and secondary patency (74% vs 71%, P = .89) of the stent graft and surgical bypass were comparable up to 4 years[16] Two other randomized control trials compared the efficacy of a covered-stent graft and a BMS in complex femoropopliteal arterial lesions.[17,19] In the first, the VIASTAR trial, the 12-month primary patency was similar between the stent graft and the BMS (70.9% and 55.1%, respectively, P = .11), based on an intention-to-treat analysis.[19] The benefit of the stent graft was more prominent in long SFA lesions. The 12-month patency for patients with a >20 cm SFA lesion was significantly better for the stent graft than BMS, (71.3% vs 36.8%, respectively, P = .01). Updated in 2015, 2-year results for the VIASTAR trial showed sustained benefit of the stent graft over BMS, especially in patients with long SFA lesions. Interestingly, freedom-from-reintervention and bypass surgery rates were similar after the stent graft and BMS for lesions <20 and ≥20 cm. The second trial, the VIBRANT trial, showed no significant differences in primary patency rates at 3 years between the Viabahn stent graft and BMS, respectively

(24.2% vs 25.9%), for TASC-II C and D lesions.[17] Although both the stent graft and the BMS had reasonable outcomes in the first year after device implantation, long-term primary patency was generally poor in patients with complex SFA lesions.

b. The Viabahn stent graft has been evaluated for treatment of SFA in-stent restenosis.[20] Eighty-three patients with SFA in-stent restenosis and Rutherford category 2-5 ischemia were enrolled in 7 European sites and randomized to receive the Viabahn stent graft or standard balloon angioplasty. For treatment of in-stent restenosis 12-month patency rates were significantly better in the stent graft group (74.8% vs 28% respectively, $P < .001$), for treatment of in-stent restenosis. Likewise, a meta-analysis, which included four prospective randomized trials, one retrospective trial, and nine case series, showed that at 1 year, a covered-stent graft in the SFA has better outcomes than other interventions, including balloon angioplasty and BMS.[21] The rate of stent fractures in long lesions was significantly lower with stent grafts.

C.

1. **Antiplatelet and Antithrombotic Therapy** Despite the lack of consensus guidelines on antiplatelet or antithrombotic therapy post peripheral stenting, there have been theoretical concerns of increased stent thrombosis in covered grafts. Optimal post–stent graft medical therapy is unknown and has not been studied in a randomized fashion. Evaluation of a nonrandomized retrospective series of patients treated with aspirin and clopidogrel for 6 weeks post intervention versus aspirin and clopidogrel indefinitely in the absence of bleeding complications versus triple therapy (aspirin, clopidogrel, and anticoagulation) in patients with other indications for anticoagulation showed no difference in patency with the different aspirin and clopidogrel treatment strategies. There was, however, a significant benefit with triple therapy in comparison to temporary clopidogrel in long-term patency, which was, however, off-set by bleeding complications.[22]

2. **Summary** Covered-stent grafts are used as a safe option for the treatment of symptomatic SFA lesions, with reasonable technical success and reasonable short-term patency outcomes. Although long-term patency is equivalent to a BMS, the stent graft might have the theoretical benefit of reducing in-stent restenosis and stent fracture. Finally, it is useful for the treatment of in-stent restenosis and perforation and may be a less-invasive option for patients who need a prosthetic above-the-knee bypass. The technical characteristics and features of both Viabahn stent grafts are listed in Table 13.3.

VI. Supera Nitinol Self-Expanding Bare Metal Stent

A. **Peipheral Stents and Risk of Strut Fracture** Strut fracture is a common issue with traditional laser-cut nitinol tube self-expanding stents in the infrailiac vessels of the lower extremity owing to significant rotational and flexional stressors encountered in normal movement. Strut fractures predispose toward restenosis and lead to a reduction in primary patency post peripheral intervention. To address this common issue, the Supera stent (Abbott

Table 13.3. FDA-Approved Self-Expanding Stent Grafts in Lower Extremity Peripheral Arterial Disease

Device Name	Manufacturer	Material Used	Guidewire Size (inch)	Introducer Size (F)	Stent Diameter (mm)	Stent Length (mm)	Delivery System Length (cm)	FDA Approval
Gore Viabahn Endoprosthesis	Gore	Nitinol/ePTFE, gold	0.035	7-12	5, 6, 7, 8, 9, 10, 11, 13	25, 50, 100, 150	75, 120	Iliac, SFA, and AV access grafts
Gore Viabahn Endoprosthesis with heparin bioactive surface	Gore	Nitinol/ePTFE, gold	0.018/0.014 (5-8 mm), 0.035 (5-13 mm)	6-12	5, 6, 7, 8, 9, 10, 11, 13	25, 50, 75, 100, 150, 250	75 (0.035 inch endhole only), 120	Iliac, SFA, and AV access grafts

AV, arteriovenous; *FDA*, U.S. Food and Drug Administration; *SFA*, superficial femoral artery.

Vascular, Santa Clara, CA), an interwoven, braided nitinol, helical self-expanding BMS, was developed with design features, which dramatically reduce the fracture rate, increase multidimensional flexibility, and result in excellent radial strength. The biomimetic properties of the stent enable the stent to flex, bend, and move with the vessel, distributing stress evenly.

B. Supera Stent

1. The Supera stent is available in 4.5-6.5 mm diameters and lengths ranging between 20 and 150 mm, delivered via a 6-French catheter and a 0.018″ end-hole system. It is primarily used clinically in the treatment of superficial femoral and popliteal stenosis on either de novo or restenotic lesions.

2. Owing to its unique characteristics, deployment requires careful vessel preparation techniques, specific to the stent. The vessel should be predilated to achieve a 1:1 match between the stent outer diameter and the postdilation vessel caliber. There should not be more than 1-mm oversizing of the stent. The delivery catheter mechanism allows for precise release of the helical coils via thumb movements, allowing for control of the deployed length. This also leads to the ability to increase the density of deployed coils if desired to increase radial strength in specific sections of the stent. The stent is much longer within the delivery catheter compared with the deployed length, occasionally leading to compressed or elongated deployment of the stent length in untrained hands. This feature makes it unsuitable for use in ostial lesions.

3. **SUPERB Trial**

   a. The clinical performance of the Supera stent is best represented by the SUPERB trial, the SUPERSUB study, and the Leipzig registries. Notably, no strut fractures have been recorded in any of the reported clinical trials to date during follow-up. The SUPERB trial was a nonrandomized, prospective, multicenter, investigational device exemption, single-arm trial, which enrolled 264 patients undergoing treatment of de novo or restenotic lesions of the SFA or proximal popliteal artery. Almost all lesions in the study were in the SFA with an average lesion length of 78 mm. Early safety as evaluated by freedom from death, target vessel revascularization, or any amputation of the index limb at 30 days postprocedure was achieved in 99.2% of patients. Primary patency at 12 months was 86.3%.[23] The Leipzig SUPERA 500 registry reported 2-year single-center outcomes on 492 limbs in 439 unselected patients treated with the Supera stent. Primary patency was 83.3% at 12 months and 72.8% at 2 years. Secondary patency was 98.1% and 92.0%, respectively. No difference was noted in SFA versus popliteal lesions.[24] SUPERSUB was a single-center, prospective, single-arm study, which reported 1-year outcome in the use of Supera stents in long femoropopliteal complete TASC C and TASC D occlusions treated via subintimal revascularization with an average lesion length of 279 mm. Primary patency at 1 year was 94.1%, and freedom from TLR was 97.1%.[25] The Leipzing SUPERA popliteal artery stent registry reported 12-month retrospective outcomes on 101 patients undergoing 125 stents with an average lesion length of 84 mm. The 6- and 12-month primary patency rates were 94.6% and 87.7% with secondary patency rates of 97.9% and 96.5%, respectively.[26]

b. These findings have been borne out in several real-world registries, additionally confirming the total absence of strut fractures.[27-30] Although exceedingly rare, a single case report in the literature suggests that when strut fractures do occur, the peculiar design of the stent may predispose the break to result in the complete loss of integrity of the stent.[31]

In conclusion, although the Supera stent has not been studied in a randomized fashion, it constitutes an important advance in stent design, with its extreme flexibility, higher radial strength, and dramatically lower strut fracture rate. These design features make it ideal and preferred for use in the popliteal artery, when stents are indicated due to the extreme biomechanical forces imposed on this segment from repetitive knee flexion.[32] Careful attention must be paid to deployment of the stent, due to its unique features, and operators should be well-versed in deployment technique.

VII. Drug-Eluting Self-Expanding Stents

Given the high rates of intimal proliferation following PTA with or without deployment of BMSs and high rate of in-stent-restenosis, antiproliferative therapies have been used in peripheral arterial diseases with drug-coated balloons and drug-eluting stents (DES).

A. First-Generation Peripheral Drug-Eluting Stents (DES)

First-generation drug-eluting stents (DES) using sirolimus did not provide additional clinical benefit when compared with BMSs. The failure of first-generation DES delivering two different doses of sirolimus was attributed in part to rapid uncontrolled drug release.[33] This led to the development of the everolimus-eluting stent, incorporating a copolymer for slower more efficient drug release. Although initial nonrandomized studies confirmed the safety and efficacy of the technology, it only achieved 68% patency at 1 year.[34]

B. Paclitaxel Peripheral Self-Expanding Stents (Zilver PTX)

1. While initial first-generation DES achieved discouraging outcomes in peripheral artery disease (PAD), the use of paclitaxel-eluting DES was on the rise in coronary arteries with superior outcomes compared with BMS. Despite both paclitaxel- and limus-type drugs expressing antiproliferative properties, paclitaxel is highly lipophilic, which permits high protein binding and excellent transmembrane passage, resulting in high intracellular concentrations in the subintimal layers.[35] Following the successful use of paclitaxel as an antiproliferative therapy in drug-coated balloon systems for femoropopliteal territories, two novel stent systems for the lower extremity have been developed using the same agent, with only one system currently FDA-approved for clinical use. The Zilver PTX (Cook Medical, Bloomington, IN) is an open-cell, flexible, self-expanding nitinol stent with a polymer-free paclitaxel coating. The stent is enclosed within a sheath before deployment at the target vessel location and is coated only on the outer surface, which traps paclitaxel between the stent struts and the vessel wall after deployment. Unlike standard DES used in coronary arteries, the Zilver PTX structure does not include a copolymer, with rapid drug release peaking typically within the initial 14 days after deployment followed by a dramatic decrease.[36]

2. **Zilver PTX**
   a. The Zilver PTX is currently available in diameters from 5 to 10 mm and lengths from 20 to 80 mm, delivered via a 6-French system. It is designed for use in above-the-knee femoropopliteal arteries having reference vessel diameter from 4 to 9 mm, either de-novo or restenotic lesions, typically after balloon angioplasty. Predilatation before stent placement is routinely required. Given the absence of polymer binding paclitaxel to the stent and the outer coating of the stent surface, manual handling of the stent is contraindicated, and care must be taken while handling the stent not to wash out the paclitaxel coating before stent deployment.
   b. The Zilver PTX randomized clinical study tested the effectiveness of Zilver PTX in SFA lesions, randomizing 439 patients either to primary DES implantation or to PTA alone. Compared with the PTA group, the primary DES group exhibited superior 12-month event-free survival (90.4% vs 82.6%; P = .004) and primary patency (83.1% vs 32.8%; P = .001). Of note, 120 patients had acute PTA failure and underwent secondary randomization to provisional DES (n = 61) or BMS (n = 59). Compared with BMS, provisional DES exhibited superior primary patency (89.9% vs 73.0%; P = .01) and superior clinical benefit (90.5% and 72.3%, P = .009).[37] Recently, 5-year follow-up confirmed the sustainability of earlier findings, with primary patency at 5 years of 64.9% for the primary DES group in comparison with 19% for the PTA group.[38] The device features of the Zilver PTX stent are listed in Table 13.4.

C. Drug-Eluting Self-Expanding Stents In-Development A new DES system is currently being tested for use in the femoropopliteal arteries. The Eluvia DES (Boston Scientific, Marlborough, MA) is a nitinol self-expanding stent. However, unlike the Zilver

Table 13.4. FDA-Approved Drug-Eluting Stents in Lower Extremity Peripheral Arterial Disease

Device Name	Manufacturer	Material Used	Drug Delivered	Guidewire Size (inch)	Introducer Size (F)	Stent Diameter (mm)	Stent Length (mm)	Delivery System Length (cm)	FDA Approval
Zilver PTX	Cook medical	Nitinol	Paclitaxel	0.035	6	6, 7, 8	40, 60, 80, 100, 120	125	SFA

FDA, U.S. Food and Drug Administration; *SFA*, superficial femoral artery.

PTX, this system design includes an active layer of the fluoropolymer PVDF-HFP (poly[vinylidene fluoride-co-hexafluoropropylene]), which is the coating polymer on the Promus Element coronary stent (Boston Scientific, Marlborough, MA) to control paclitaxel release over longer periods. Initial data reported a stunning primary patency of 96% at 12-month follow-up.[39] Randomized trials with longer term follow-up are currently in progress.

VIII. Bioresorbable Scaffolds

A. **General Principles** With unsatisfactory primary patency rates after endovascular therapy with angioplasty or stents, bioresorbable scaffold (BRS) systems are being developed for their theoretical benefits of maintaining further diagnostic and therapeutic options in the long term, such as follow-up MRI, repeated revascularization via endovascular approach, or bypass surgery.

1. The most common scaffold system is composed of poly-L-lactide (PLLA), which typically resorbs to carbon dioxide and water over 2-3 years.[40] The second, less popular BRS system is metal based (magnesium and other minerals) and has been used below the knees with unfavorable outcomes, mostly related to very rapid resorption and lower radial strength.[41] Newer PLLA BRS incorporate the antiproliferative agent everolimus, with a BRS copolymer to control drug release into the subintimal layer similar to the recently discontinued ABSORB (Abbott Vascular, Santa Clara, CA), bioabsorbable coronary stent.

2. The unique aspects of BRS stents are not only limited to their composition and the advantage of resorption, as such advantage comes at a great cost of strut thickness. Typically, BRS struts are about twice as thick as traditional metal stents with lower radial strength and flexibility, leading to lower deliverability. As most BRSs are radiolucent, fluoroscopic visualization of the actual stent is impossible, and most stents have radiopaque markers to facilitate visualization. These factors contribute to a deployment process, which tends to be less forgiving, requiring careful technique and training. Other technical aspects include problems with overlapping multiple stents, secondary to thicker struts, causing longer overlapping segments to increase the likelihood of stent thrombosis. Postdilation of BRS should be limited, as they do not provide comparable radial strength to metal stents and are more susceptible to fracture if postdilated beyond their prespecified nominal pressures. These factors significantly impact outcomes of BRS technology.[42]

B. Lower Extremity Clinical Trials

1. A systematic review of seven small trials investigating the use of non–drug-eluting BRS in lower extremities demonstrated high procedural success. However, mean primary patency rates were not encouraging at 61.6% in femoral arteries after 6-12 months compared with 50.3% in below-the-knee lesions.[43] Currently, two BRS stents carry the CE mark for use in the lower extremity, the Igaki-Tamai stent (Kyoto Medical Planning Co., Kyoto, Japan) and the REMEDY stent (Kyoto Medical Planning Co., Kyoto, Japan). Both, however, have been shown to be inferior compared with nitinol stents.[44,45] An unsuccessful attempt to improve performance using drug-coated balloon deployment before BRS implantation was studied in a small cohort of 20 patients, with a low rate of primary patency and high rate of target lesion revascularization.[44]

2. Given these suboptimal results, the use of non–drug-coated BRS stents has been limited, with a shift toward using antiproliferative coated BRS. The ESPRIT scaffold system (everolimus-eluting PLLA scaffold) was tested in 35 patients with lesions located in the superficial femoral artery (88.6%) and external iliac artery (11.4%). At 1 and 2 years, binary restenosis rates were 12.1% and 16.1%, respectively.[46] The Absorb everolimus-eluting bioresorbable vascular scaffold was the only FDA-approved BRS in coronary artery disease. The feasibility and efficacy of their use in arteries below the knee was tested in 33 patients with excellent 12-month primary patency of 96% and 84.6% at 24 months.[47]

C. Summary

BRSs are a promising arena for endovascular therapy in PAD, despite the technical challenges they pose for endovascular operators. Currently, no BRS is FDA approved for clinical use in peripheral vessels. This may change in the near future with promising data from everolimus-eluting BRS stents. With newer generation BRSs with thinner struts and providing more radial strength, these scaffolds may reshape the future of endovascular intervention.

References

1. Norgren L, Hiatt WR, Dormandy JA, et al. Inter-society consensus for the management of peripheral arterial disease (TASC II). *J Vasc Surg.* 2007;45(suppl S):S5-67.
2. Bosch JL, Hunink MG. Meta-analysis of the results of percutaneous transluminal angioplasty and stent placement for aortoiliac occlusive disease. *Radiology.* 1997;204:87-96.
3. Sabri SS, Choudhri A, Orgera G, et al. Outcomes of covered kissing stent placement compared with bare metal stent placement in the treatment of atherosclerotic occlusive disease at the aortic bifurcation. *J Vasc Interv Radiol.* 2010;21:995-1003.
4. Piazza M, Squizzato F, Spolverato G, et al. Outcomes of polytetrafluoroethylene-covered stent versus bare-metal stent in the primary treatment of severe iliac artery obstructive lesions. *J Vasc Surg.* 2015;62:1210-1218 e1.
5. Humphries MD, Armstrong E, Laird J, Paz J, Pevec W. Outcomes of covered versus bare-metal balloon-expandable stents for aortoiliac occlusive disease. *J Vasc Surg.* 2014;60:337-343.
6. Mwipatayi BP, Thomas S, Wong J, et al. A comparison of covered vs bare expandable stents for the treatment of aortoiliac occlusive disease. *J Vasc Surg.* 2011;54:1561-1570.
7. Mwipatayi BP, Sharma S, Daneshmand A, et al. Durability of the balloon-expandable covered versus bare-metal stents in the Covered versus Balloon Expandable Stent Trial (COBEST) for the treatment of aortoiliac occlusive disease. *J Vasc Surg.* 2016;64:83-94 e1.

8. Hajibandeh S, Hajibandeh S, Antoniou SA, Torella F, Antoniou GA. Covered vs uncovered stents for aortoiliac and femoropopliteal arterial disease: a systematic review and meta-analysis. *J Endovas Ther.* 2016;23:442-452.
9. Schlager O, Dick P, Sabeti S, et al. Long-segment SFA stenting–the dark sides: in-stent restenosis, clinical deterioration, and stent fractures. *J Endovas Ther.* 2005;12:676-684.
10. Krankenberg H, Schluter M, Steinkamp HJ, et al. Nitinol stent implantation versus percutaneous transluminal angioplasty in superficial femoral artery lesions up to 10 cm in length: the femoral artery stenting trial (FAST). *Circulation.* 2007;116:285-292.
11. Schillinger M, Sabeti S, Loewe C, et al. Balloon angioplasty versus implantation of nitinol stents in the superficial femoral artery. *N Engl J Med.* 2006;354:1879-1888.
12. Dick P, Wallner H, Sabeti S, et al. Balloon angioplasty versus stenting with nitinol stents in intermediate length superficial femoral artery lesions. *Catheter Cardiovasc Interv.* 2009;74:1090-1095.
13. Laird JR, Katzen BT, Scheinert D, et al. Nitinol stent implantation versus balloon angioplasty for lesions in the superficial femoral artery and proximal popliteal artery: twelve-month results from the RESILIENT randomized trial. *Circ Cardiovasc Interv.* 2010;3:267-276.
14. Davaine JM, Azema L, Guyomarch B, et al. One-year clinical outcome after primary stenting for Trans-Atlantic Inter-Society Consensus (TASC) C and D femoropopliteal lesions (the STELLA "STEnting Long de L'Artere femorale superficielle" cohort). *Eur J Vasc Endovasc Surg.* 2012;44:432-441.
15. Begovac PC, Thomson RC, Fisher JL, Hughson A, Gallhagen A. Improvements in GORE-TEX vascular graft performance by Carmeda BioActive surface heparin immobilization. *Eur J Vasc Endovasc Surg.* 2003;25:432-437.
16. McQuade K, Gable D, Hohman S, Pearl G, Theune B. Randomized comparison of ePTFE/nitinol self-expanding stent graft vs prosthetic femoral-popliteal bypass in the treatment of superficial femoral artery occlusive disease. *J Vasc Surg.* 2009;49:109-115, 116 e1-9; discussion 116.
17. Geraghty PJ, Mewissen MW, Jaff MR, Ansel GM, Investigators V. Three-year results of the VIBRANT trial of VIABAHN endoprosthesis versus bare nitinol stent implantation for complex superficial femoral artery occlusive disease. *J Vasc Surg.* 2013;58:386-395 e4.
18. Saxon RR, Chervu A, Jones PA, et al. Heparin-bonded, expanded polytetrafluoroethylene-lined stent graft in the treatment of femoropopliteal artery disease: 1-year results of the VIPER (Viabahn Endoprosthesis with Heparin Bioactive Surface in the Treatment of Superficial Femoral Artery Obstructive Disease) trial. *J Vasc Interv Radiol.* 2013;24:165-173; quiz 174.
19. Lammer J, Zeller T, Hausegger KA, et al. Heparin-bonded covered stents versus bare-metal stents for complex femoropopliteal artery lesions: the randomized VIASTAR trial (Viabahn endoprosthesis with PROPATEN bioactive surface [VIA] versus bare nitinol stent in the treatment of long lesions in superficial femoral artery occlusive disease). *J Am Coll Cardiol.* 2013;62:1320-1327.
20. Bosiers M, Deloose K, Callaert J, et al. Superiority of stent-grafts for in-stent restenosis in the superficial femoral artery: twelve-month results from a multicenter randomized trial. *J Endovas Ther.* 2015;22:1-10.
21. Zhang L, Bao J, Zhao Z, Lu Q, Zhou J, Jing Z. Effectiveness of viabahn in the treatment of superficial femoral artery occlusive disease: a systematic review and meta-analysis. *J Endovascular Ther.* 2015;22:495-505.
22. Ullery BW, Tran K, Itoga N, Casey K, Dalman RL, Lee JT. Safety and efficacy of antiplatelet/anticoagulation regimens after viabahn stent graft treatment for femoropopliteal occlusive disease. *J Vasc Surg.* 2015;61:1479-1488.
23. Garcia L, Jaff MR, Metzger C, et al. Wire-interwoven nitinol stent outcome in the superficial femoral and proximal popliteal arteries: twelve-month results of the SUPERB Trial. *Circ Cardiovasc Interv.* 2015;8.
24. Werner M, Paetzold A, Banning-Eichenseer U, et al. Treatment of complex atherosclerotic femoropopliteal artery disease with a self-expanding interwoven nitinol stent: midterm results from the Leipzig SUPERA 500 registry. *EuroIntervention.* 2014;10:861-868.
25. Palena LM, Diaz-Sandoval LJ, Sultato E, et al. Feasibility and 1-year outcomes of subintimal revascularization with supera(R) stenting of long femoropopliteal occlusions in critical limb ischemia: the "Supersub" study. *Catheter Cardiovasc Interv.* 2017;89:910-920.

26. Scheinert D, Werner M, Scheinert S, et al. Treatment of complex atherosclerotic popliteal artery disease with a new self-expanding interwoven nitinol stent: 12-month results of the Leipzig SUPERA popliteal artery stent registry. *JACC Cardiovasc Interv.* 2013;6:65-71.
27. Leon LR, Dieter RS, Gadd CL, et al. Preliminary results of the initial United States experience with the Supera woven nitinol stent in the popliteal artery. *J Vasc Surg.* 2013;57:1014-1022.
28. Myint M, Schouten O, Bourke V, Thomas SD, Lennox AF, Varcoe RL. A real-world experience with the supera interwoven nitinol stent in femoropopliteal arteries: midterm patency results and failure analysis. *J Endovascular Ther.* 2016;23:433-441.
29. Montero-Baker M, Ziomek GJ, Leon L, et al. Analysis of endovascular therapy for femoropopliteal disease with the Supera stent. *J Vasc Surg.* 2016;64:1002-1008.
30. George JC, Rosen ES, Nachtigall J, VanHise A, Kovach R. SUPERA interwoven nitinol stent outcomes in above-knee intErventions (SAKE) study. *J Vasc Interv Radiol.* 2014;25:954-961.
31. Cambiaghi T, Spertino A, Bertoglio L, Chiesa R. Fracture of a supera interwoven nitinol stent after treatment of popliteal artery stenosis. *J Endovas Ther.* 2017;24:447-449.
32. Kroger K, Santosa F, Goyen M. Biomechanical incompatibility of popliteal stent placement. *J Endovas Ther.* 2004;11:686-694.
33. Duda SH, Bosiers M, Lammer J, et al. Sirolimus-eluting versus bare nitinol stent for obstructive superficial femoral artery disease: the SIROCCO II trial. *J Vasc Interv Radiol.* 2005;16:331-338.
34. Lammer J, Bosiers M, Zeller T, et al. First clinical trial of nitinol self-expanding everolimus-eluting stent implantation for peripheral arterial occlusive disease. *J Vasc Surg.* 2011;54:394-401.
35. Levin AD, Vukmirovic N, Hwang CW, Edelman ER. Specific binding to intracellular proteins determines arterial transport properties for rapamycin and paclitaxel. *Proc Natl Acad Sci USA.* 2004;101:9463-9467.
36. Dake MD, Van Alstine WG, Zhou Q, Ragheb AO. Polymer-free paclitaxel-coated Zilver PTX stents–evaluation of pharmacokinetics and comparative safety in porcine arteries. *J Vasc Interv Radiol.* 2011;22:603-610.
37. Dake MD, Ansel GM, Jaff MR, et al. Paclitaxel-eluting stents show superiority to balloon angioplasty and bare metal stents in femoropopliteal disease: twelve-month Zilver PTX randomized study results. *Circ Cardiovasc Interv.* 2011;4:495-504.
38. Dake MD, Ansel GM, Jaff MR, et al. Durable clinical effectiveness with paclitaxel-eluting stents in the femoropopliteal artery: 5-year results of the zilver PTX randomized trial. *Circulation.* 2016;133:1472-1483; discussion 1483.
39. Muller-Hulsbeck S, Keirse K, Zeller T, Schroe H, Diaz-Cartelle J. Twelve-month results from the MAJESTIC trial of the eluvia paclitaxel-eluting stent for treatment of obstructive femoropopliteal disease. *J Endovas Ther.* 2016;23:701-707.
40. Patel N, Banning AP. Bioabsorbable scaffolds for the treatment of obstructive coronary artery disease: the next revolution in coronary intervention? *Heart.* 2013;99:1236-1243.
41. Bosiers M, Peeters P, D'Archambeau O, et al. AMS INSIGHT–absorbable metal stent implantation for treatment of below-the-knee critical limb ischemia: 6-month analysis. *Cardiovasc Intervent Radiol.* 2009;32:424-435.
42. Varcoe RL, Thomas SD, Rapoza RJ, Kum S. Lessons learned regarding handling and deployment of the absorb bioresorbable vascular scaffold in infrapopliteal arteries. *J Endovas Ther.* 2017;24:337-341.
43. van Haelst ST, Peeters Weem SM, Moll FL, de Borst GJ. Current status and future perspectives of bioresorbable stents in peripheral arterial disease. *J Vasc Surg.* 2016;64:1151-1159 e1.
44. Werner M, Schmidt A, Scheinert S, et al. Evaluation of the biodegradable Igaki-Tamai scaffold after drug-eluting balloon treatment of de novo superficial femoral artery lesions: the GAIA-DEB study. *J Endovascular Ther.* 2016;23:92-97.
45. Bontinck J, Goverde P, Schroe H, Hendriks J, Maene L, Vermassen F. Treatment of the femoropopliteal artery with the bioresorbable REMEDY stent. *J Vasc Surg.* 2016;64:1311-1319.
46. Lammer J, Bosiers M, Deloose K, et al. Bioresorbable everolimus-eluting vascular scaffold for patients with peripheral artery disease (ESPRIT I): 2-year clinical and imaging results. *JACC Cardiovasc Interv.* 2016;9:1178-1187.
47. Varcoe RL, Schouten O, Thomas SD, Lennox AF. Experience with the absorb everolimus-eluting bioresorbable vascular scaffold in arteries below the knee: 12-month clinical and imaging outcomes. *JACC Cardiovasc Interv.* 2016;9:1721-1728.

CHAPTER 14

Atherectomy for Peripheral Arterial Disease

Bennett Cua, MD, FACC, Mahmoud Abdelghany, MD, and Robert R. Attaran, MD, FACC, FASE, FSCAI, RPVI

Key Points

- The principles and goals of atherectomy include plaque modification, debulking, vessel preparation, and minimizing the need for stent deployment.
- The mechanisms of atherectomy by excimer laser include plaque debulking by photochemical, photothermal, and photomechanical for plaque ablation.
- Orbital atherectomy, directional atherectomy, and forward-cutting atherectomy are other FDA-approved methods of atherectomy.

I. Introduction

A. **Percutaneous Interventions for Peripheral Artery Disease** Percutaneous interventions for peripheral artery disease (PAD) continue to rapidly evolve providing a variety of tools to restore lower extremity blood flow. However, the paucity of randomized control trials comparing these different revascularization techniques has left us without an evidence-based roadmap to guide treatment. Although the advent of nitinol stents has greatly reduced early restenosis after balloon angioplasty by addressing complications such as vessel dissection and elastic recoil during the index procedure, its long-term success remains hampered by in-stent restenosis (ISR). Drug-coated technology including stents and balloons, scoring balloons, and atherectomy devices are all potential tools for prevention and treatment of ISR. Current practices are based predominantly on evidence gathered from small safety trials and single-center experiences with a few selective randomized control trials.

B. **Zilver PTX DES** The Zilver PTX paclitaxel-coated nitinol drug-eluting stent (DES) (Cook Medical, Bloomington, IN) has gained popularity for the treatment of femoropopliteal arterial stenoses with a proven superior 12-month event-free survival and patency rates compared with balloon angioplasty with provisional bare metal stent (BMS), but it is important to note that the average lesion length was only 6.5 cm.[1] More recently, 5-year follow-up data were published[2] comparing Zilver PTX with balloon angioplasty. The Zilver PTX DES demonstrated sustained superiority in freedom from reintervention compared with balloon angioplasty.

C. **Treatment** Nevertheless, the optimal treatment strategy for longer lesions that are more frequently seen in real-world practice remains unclear, and the role for atherectomy remains to be seen.

II. Principles of Atherectomy

The fundamental aim of atherectomy is (1) plaque modification to facilitate passage of other endovascular equipment and balloon expansion, (2) debulking of atherosclerotic and calcium burden to maximize luminal diameter gain, (3) vessel preparation to avoid suboptimal balloon angioplasty, and (4) to minimize the need for stent deployment. There are several different types of atherectomy devices designed to cut, shave, sand, or vaporize plaques in diseased arteries. Current data do not support use of atherectomy devices alone in de novo lesions but instead may be a helpful adjunct to revascularization. For example, vessel preparation by directional atherectomy (DA) before balloon angioplasty with drug-coated balloon (DCB) was effective and safe. Although the DEFINITIVE AR study (Directional Atherectomy Followed by a Paclitaxel-Coated Balloon to Inhibit Restenosis and Maintain Vessel Patency—A Pilot Study of Anti-Restenosis Treatment) did not show a significant difference between DA plus DCB in comparison with DCB only for the treatment of femoropopliteal artery disease at 1 year; patients treated with DA plus DCB had higher technical success rate (89.6% vs 64.2%; $P = .004$) and lower flow-limiting dissection rate (2% vs 19%; $P = .01$) compared with DCB only.[3]

III. Excimer Laser Atherectomy

Spectranetics is the manufacturer of four excimer laser atherectomy devices for infrainguinal lower extremity arteries: (1) Turbo-Elite (previously CliRpath), (2) Turbo-Booster, (3) Turbo-Tandem, and (4) Turbo-Power (Fig. 14.1). The first device is used for both above- and below-the-knee arteries, whereas the latter three devices are for above-the-knee lesions.

A. ELA System Mechanics

The Spectranetics (Maple Grove, MN) excimer laser atherectomy devices emit a xenon chloride (XeCl) ultraviolet light from the fiberoptic catheter tip at a wavelength of 308 nm, ablating atherosclerotic plaque and vaporizing thrombi at a penetration depth of 50 μm by a combination of photochemical, photothermal, and photomechanical effects while minimizing damage to surrounding tissue.[4] Through the photochemical process, the high-energy, monochromatic laser beams directly break the molecular carbon-carbon bonds of atherosclerotic plaque or thrombus with subsequent dissipation of energy. The released energy, through the photomechanical effect, evaporates the intracellular water ahead of the tip of the laser catheter, producing a steam bubble that rapidly expands and contracts resulting in tissue breakdown. The laser emission is pulsed rather than continuous like its Argon predecessors, minimizing the photothermal process as excessive heating promotes aneurysm formation, late perforations, and a high restenosis rate. Each pulse is 125 ns with 80 pulses delivered per second. This calculates to less than 1 mm of atherosclerotic plaque ablated per second necessitating slow advancement of the laser to ensure that the advancement rate does not exceed the tissue removal rate in to maximize

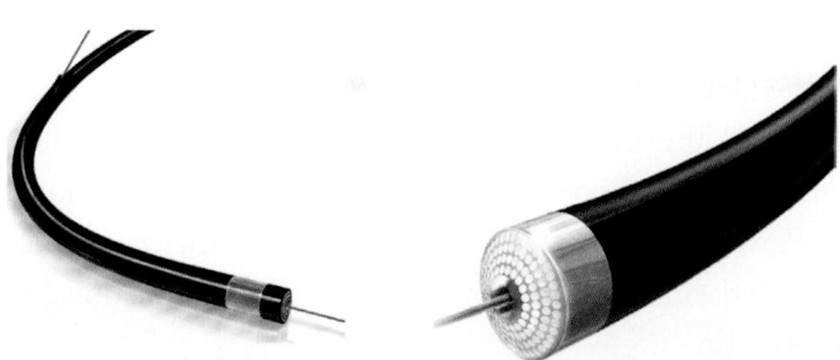

FIGURE 14.1: Turbo-Elite Laser Atherectomy Catheter. Courtesy of Royal Philips.

luminal diameter gain of the vessel. The residual particles measure less than 10 microns in diameter conferring minimal risk of distal embolization.[5] The laser should only be activated after saline flush to remove iodinated contrast material from the target blood vessel, because contrast and hemoglobin absorb the excimer laser light at 308 nm, yielding cavitation bubbles, vapor bubbles, and percussive waves, which can lead to dissections or perforations.[6]

B. ELA for Critical Limb Ischemia

1. The **L**aser **A**ngioplasty in **C**ritical Limb **I**schemia (LACI) Belgium trial published in 2005 demonstrated the safety and efficacy of the Turbo-Elite (previously CliRpath) for treatment of critical limb ischemia (defined as Rutherford category 4, 5, or 6) in poor surgical bypass candidates.[6] There was fairly even distribution of lesions between femoropopliteal, infrapopliteal, and multilevel lesions. The standard endovascular method of crossing the lesion with a guidewire followed by over-the-wire lasing was successfully executed in 84% (43 of 51) of cases with the remainder 16% (8 of 51) of lesions requiring a step-by-step technique to achieve recanalization. The step-by-step technique involves sequential advancement of the guidewire and activation of the laser catheter in a telescoping fashion until the entire length of the occlusion is crossed. Adjunctive PTA, stenting, and a combination of PTA with stenting were used in 33%, 6%, and 47%, respectively. Limb salvage of the treated limb at 6 months (study primary endpoint) was 90.5% and freedom from critical limb ischemia was 86%.
2. The LACI Phase 2 trial also studied the Turbo-Elite enrolling patients in the United States and Germany with the same inclusion and exclusion criteria as LACI Belgium but comparatively resulted in a cohort with a higher incidence of diabetes and non-healing ulcers (Rutherford category 5-6). Reflective of the cohorts' poor protoplasm, there was a 10% mortality rate at 6 months almost exclusively from cardiac causes. The primary endpoint of 6-month limb salvage was achieved in 93% of surviving legs. The step-by-step technique was used in 17% (26 of 145) of cases with minimal additional risk while significantly increasing the success rate of crossing total occlusions. Adjunctive PTA and stent placement were required in 96% and 45% of cases, respectively.[7]

C. ELA in Claudicants

1. The Turbo-Elite laser catheter's en face, concentric laser orientation limited its ability to optimally treat femoral-popliteal lesions as it was unable to create a lumen much larger than the nominal diameter of the ablation catheter.[8] Directional lasing allowed for more complete removal of atherosclerotic plaque, neointimal hyperplasia, and thrombus by off-axis lasing, which was incorporated into the Turbo-Elite with the addition of a bias guide catheter.[9] This first directional lasing catheter was known as the Turbo-Booster. The Turbo-Tandem followed as the second-generation directional ELA catheter. The Turbo-Power is the newest generation ELA catheter that has removed the bias guide catheter while still preserving its directional functionality with a newly designed eccentric tip.

2. **C**li**R**path **E**xcimer **L**aser System to Enlarge **L**umen **O**penings (CELLO) was a single-arm, prospective registry published in 2009 studying the efficacy and safety of using the Turbo-Booster with the Turbo-Elite to increase luminal diameter of the superficial femoral and popliteal artery above the knee joint in patients with intermittent claudication. The average lesion length was 5.6 cm with 61.5% with moderate-to-severe calcification. The tandem use of Turbo-Elite followed by Turbo-Booster achieved both efficacy and safety primary endpoints with a reduction in index lesion percent diameter stenosis prior to any adjunctive therapy from 77% + 15% at baseline to 34.7% + 17.8% with no major adverse events (MAEs) at 6 months. Intravascular ultrasound (IVUS) data from CELLO showed that luminal diameter gain achieved with ELA had equal contribution from plaque debulking and vessel enlargement demonstrated by an increase in external elastic membrane circumference.[8]

D. ELA for In-Stent Restenosis (Table 14.1)

1. The Turbo-Booster, Turbo-Tandem, and Turbo-Power are the only atherectomy devices approved for treatment of femoral-popliteal ISR lesions (level 1 clinical evidence).
2. The **P**hoto**a**blation Using the **T**urbo-Booster and **E**xcimer Laser for **In**-Stent Restenosis **T**reatment (PATENT) study in 2014 used the Turbo-Elite to create a pilot channel followed by a mean of 5.7 passes with the Turbo-Booster to treat symptomatic femoropopliteal ISR, which achieved a high procedure success rate but with only primary patency at 6 and 12 months of 64.1% and 37.8%, respectively.[10]
3. The **EXCI**mer Laser Randomized Controlled Study for Treatment of Femoropopli**TE**al **I**n-**S**tent **R**estenosis (EXCITE-ISR) trial in 2015 is the first large, prospective, randomized control trial that demonstrates superiority in terms of procedural success (93.5% vs 82.7%; $P = .01$) with significantly less procedural complications (major dissections, residual stenosis >30%, or need for bailout stenting), 6-month freedom from target lesion revascularization (TLR) (73.5% vs 51.8%; $P < .005$), and 30-day MAE rates (5.8% vs 20.5%; $P < .001$) when using ELA in addition to percutaneous transluminal angioplasty (PTA) versus PTA alone to treat bare nitinol in-stent restenosis.[11] The average lesion length was 19.6 cm in the ELA plus PTA group and 19.3 cm in the PTA-only group. There was a statistically significant difference in the presence of severe calcification with 27.1% and 9.1% in the ELA plus PTA and PTA-only group, respectively. The combination of ELA and PTA offers a 52% reduction in TLR (HR 0.48; 95% CI: 0.31-0.74). Similar to the PATENT study, ELA was performed using

Table 14.1. ELA and IVUS Key Points
• The three main mechanisms by which ELA works are photochemical, photothermal, and photomechanical.
• The Turbo-Tandem and Turbo-Power are the only two FDA-approved atherectomy devices approved for treatment of femoropopliteal ISR with level 1 clinical data.
• Limited distal embolization with rates comparable to angioplasty and stenting but with rates lower compared to SilverHawk directional atherectomy.
• IVUS studies show that increase in vessel luminal diameter with ELA is equally attributed to plaque debulking and expansion of vessel wall circumference.

the Turbo-Elite to create a pilot channel if needed and then followed with 4 quadrant passes with the Turbo-Tandem for maximal plaque debulking. Prior treatment for ISR in the target limb, increased lesion length, decreased reference vessel diameter, and treatment with PTA alone without ELA were associated with an increase in TLR occurrence with lesion length as the only significant interaction term. There were no reported stent fractures due to laser-stent interactions. IVUS studies have demonstrated a 35% reduction in stenosis and a 112% luminal area gain, 60% of which is attributed to vessel expansion with the Turbo-Tandem.

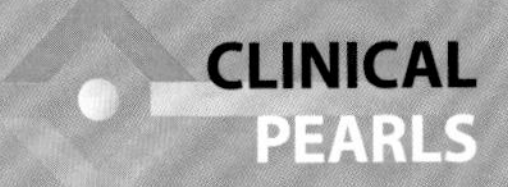

- Lasing should never be initiated until saline flush is used to remove iodinated contrast and blood from the target vessel.
- Slow advancement of the laser to ensure that the advancement rate does not exceed the tissue removal rate in to maximize luminal gain of the vessel.
- The Turbo-Elite is the only ELA device that can be used to cross occlusions with the step-by-step technique.
- After a pilot channel has been made in a difficult-to-cross lesion with the Turbo-Elite, follow up with the Turbo-Power or Turbo-Tandem to obtain maximal luminal diameter.

IV. Rotational Atherectomy (Table 14.2)

A. **RA Device: Jetstream XC** The Boston Scientific (Marlborough, MA) Jetstream (Fig. 14.2) is a rotational, front-cutting atherectomy device that offers (1) differential-cutting targeting plaque while avoiding damage to normal endothelium and (2) continuous active aspiration to reduce embolization potentially allowing for better treatment of lesions with mixed morphology such as calcium, soft plaque, fibrous plaque, and thrombus. The Jetstream XC catheter made for above-the-knee lesions has an expandable blade technology that can create two lumen sizes with the same atherectomy device while the Jetstream SC for below-the-knee lesions only has one blade size. The expandable blade modes are known as blades down (BD; minimal tip) and blades up (BU; maximum tip).

B. Rotational Atherectomy for Infrainguinal PAD

1. The Multicenter Pathway PVD trial[12] published in 2009 studied the safety and efficacy of the Pathway PV system utilized by the Boston Scientific's Jetstream. The study included 172 patients with Rutherford Class 1-5 lower limb ischemia. This

Table 14.2. RA Key Points

- The Jetstream provides concomitant atherectomy and continuous aspiration.
- Despite having a continuous aspiration feature, distal emboli remain a concern and embolic protection devices must be considered.
- The Jetstream has been shown to be safe and effective in short, calcified femoral-popliteal lesions.
- Increase in vessel lumen size is predominantly due to atherosclerosis and calcium debulking.
- The role for rotational atherectomy below the knee remains unclear.

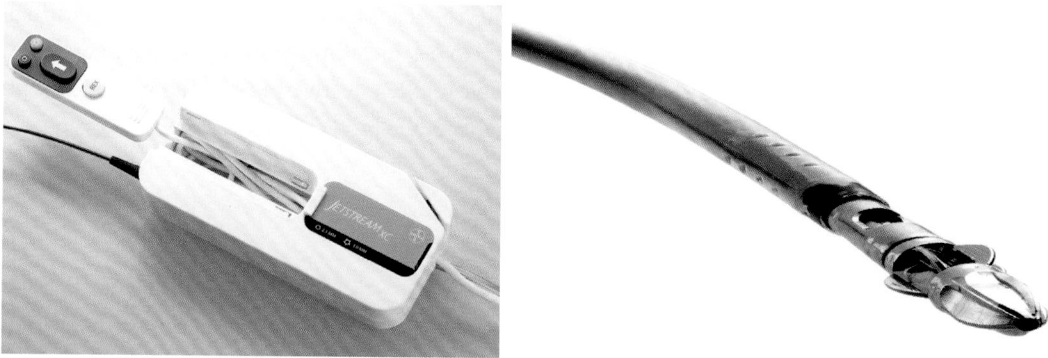

FIGURE 14.2: Medical EXPO Boston Scientific. Cutting Atherectomy Catheter/Arterial Jetstream. Image provided courtesy of Boston Scientific.

trial's cohort had a higher proportion of diabetic patients and vessels with smaller reference diameters compared with the SilverHawk atherectomy cohorts. Lesion inclusion criteria included an atherosclerotic stenosis >70% and up to 10 cm lesion length in the femoropopliteal segment or up to 3 cm lesion length in infrapopliteal vessels. Ninety two percent of the lesions were located in the SFA or popliteal artery, whereas only 8% were in the tibial arteries. The average treated lesion length was only 2.7 cm, 51% of patients had moderate-to-high calcium scores, and 31% had total occlusions. Despite having a continuous active aspiration component, there were 9.9% (n = 17) reported distal embolic events. A separate small study by Boiangiu et al[13] comprising 22 participants undergoing Jetstream atherectomy with a distal embolic device showed that macroscopic debris was recovered in 95.4% (21 of 22). Debris analysis revealed collagen material, fibrin, macrophages, calcification and cholesterol-rich material measuring 1 to 10 mm in size, which is capable of occluding tibial vessels that are 1 to 3 mm in size. Compared with the SilverHawk atherectomy cohort, Jetstream atherectomy was associated with a higher occurrence of clinically significant distal emboli at 72.7% versus 46.7%.

2. The Multicenter Pathway PVD trial's[12] primary study endpoint of MAE rates at 1 and 6 months were 1% and 20%, respectively, which are comparable to the uncontrolled studies of SilverHawk atherectomy. MAE was primarily driven by restenosis rates with a 1-year rate of 38.2%, and this was also similar to SilverHawk atherectomy's 1-year restenosis rates of 35.4% and 37.8%. The 1-year limb salvage rate was 100% despite 15% of the cohort having Rutherford class 4-5 limb ischemia. Atherectomy was performed as stand-alone therapy in 33% of patients with adjunctive balloon angioplasty in 59% and stenting in 7%. Based on these limited data, the Jetstream seems to be effective and safe in those with short, calcified femoral-popliteal lesions.[12] In a separate study, the Jetstream was shown to successfully increase lumen dimensions in moderately to severely calcified femoral-popliteal lesions from an average area of 6.6-10.0 mm^2 (P = .001) by IVUS. Debulking of calcium is the main mechanism by which luminal area gain was achieved in contrast to ELA.[14] To date, there are no

randomized trials available comparing the use of Jetstream atherectomy with balloon angioplasty or drug-coated technologies including stenting. These atherectomy devices have been shown to be safe and highly effective in reducing embolic events when used in conjunction with a distal embolic protection device.[15]

V. Orbital Atherectomy (Table 14.3)

A. OA Device: Diamondback 360

1. CSI (St Paul, MN) Diamondback 360 (DB360) (Fig. 14.3) is an orbital atherectomy device with an eccentrically mounted diamond-coated crown that sits on a flexible drive shaft and rotates over a proprietary 0.014-in guidewire (ViperWire) to treat de novo, calcified lower extremity lesions.
2. DB360 utilizes centrifugal force and differential sanding to modify calcified and fibrotic plaque while protecting the vessel media.[16,17] As the crown's rotational speed increases, the centrifugal force is amplified creating a larger orbit diameter. Healthy compliant arterial tissues flex away from the crown while diseased fibrocalcific and calcific plaques remain adherent to the spinning crown. Cross-sectional histological analysis of porcine arteries post DB360 treatment showed minimal damage to the internal elastic lamina, media, and external elastic lamina, which is thought to reduce arterial restenosis rates.[16] The unique orbital motion of the crown also allows for continuous blood and saline flow across the lesion, maintaining continuous perfusion to the distal limb and constant heat dissipation. There are also a variety of crown sizes and shapes (solid, classic, and micro crown) available to facilitate treating vessels of different caliber as well as morphological lesions.
3. Because the debris washed downstream from the atherectomy site has an average diameter that is much smaller than that of the average capillary size (2-3 vs 9.5 μm), the vast majority of particles are flushed through the capillary bed and ultimately absorbed by the body via the reticuloendothelial system. The combination of strict treatment intervals of 20-30 seconds with alternating rest periods of similar duration, smaller crowns, and liberal administration of vasodilators prevents procedural complications such as slow flow, vessel closure, and spasm.[18] Nevertheless, it is our practice to utilize a distal embolic protection device when utilizing orbital atherectomy above the popliteal artery.

Table 14.3. OA Key Points
• Orbital atherectomy (DB360) can be used for modification of calcified lesions in to decrease the need for bailout stenting when balloon angioplasty is complicated by dissection, vessel closure, or spasm. • Adhere to strict treatment intervals with equal rest time, use smaller crown sizes, and administer vasodilators liberally to prevent slow flow, vessel closure, or spasm. • DB360 should not be used for in-stent restenosis, bypass grafts, and when thrombus or dissection is present. • Atherectomy debris measures on the of 2 μm and is flushed through the capillary system ultimately being absorbed by the reticuloendothelial system.

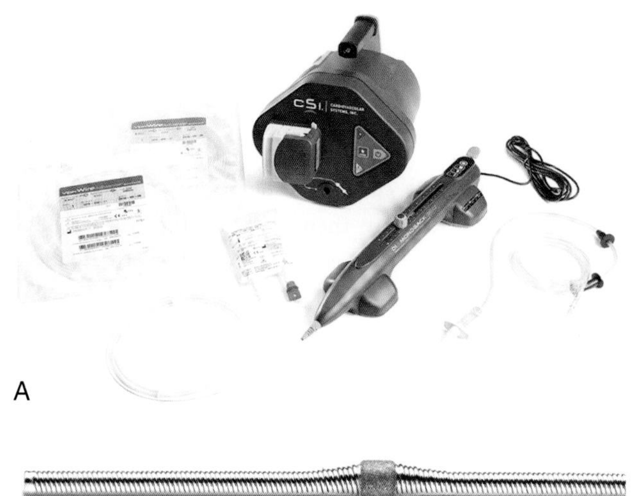

FIGURE 14.3: CSI Cardiovascular System, INC. Diamondback 360 Peripheral Orbital Atherectomy System. A, Depicts the catheter setup, (B) shows a magnified image of the orbital atherectomy catheter tip. ©2019 Cardiovascular Systems, Inc. CSI®, Diamondback 360®, GlideAssist®, ViperWire Advance® and ViperSlide® are registered trademarks of Cardiovascular Systems, Inc., and used with permission.

B. **Orbital Atherectomy for Popliteal, Peroneal, and/or Tibial Arteries in CLI** CALCIUM 360 was a multicenter study that comprised 50 patients with Rutherford classification 4-6 limb ischemia randomized 1:1 to OA with balloon angioplasty (BA) versus BA alone. The vessels treated included popliteal, peroneal, and/or tibial arteries that had an angiographic stenosis >50%, fluoroscopically visible calcium >25% of treated segment, and a main target vessel reference diameter >1.5 mm. The average lesion length in the DB360 arm was greater than the BA arm (9.1 vs 6.9 cm). Primary endpoints were restoration of normal lumen defined as a residual stenosis <30% with no bailout stenting or dissection. The OA group had numerically less dissections, bailout stenting, and residual stenosis, but none reached statistical significance.[19]

C. **Orbital Atherectomy for Above-the-Knee PAD** The COMPLIANCE 360 trial compared treatment of calcified femoropopliteal disease with OA with BA and BA only. The hypothesis for performing OA before BA is that a reduction in calcification burden may translate into more compliant vessels resulting in fewer dissections and hopefully less adjunctive stenting. When compared with BA alone, OA plus BA yielded greater luminal gain. The primary endpoint of freedom from TLR (including adjunctive stenting) or restenosis was achieved in 77.1% of lesions in the OA group versus only 11.5% in the BA group ($P < .001$) at 6 months, but there was no difference at 12 months when adjunctive stenting was excluded from being considered a TLR event (81% vs 78.3%, $P > .99$).[20] Although the occurrence of TLR at 12 months was the same, there was a significantly lower number of stents deployed in the OA group.

VI. Directional Atherectomy (Table 14.4)

A. DA Devices and Trials

1. The Medtronic (Fridley, MN) SilverHawk and TurboHawk (Fig. 14.4) are forward-cutting devices utilizing a high-speed cutting blade to shred obstructing arterial atheroma into ribbons of plaque that are then collected into the catheter nose cone. Multiple passes are taken through the lesion during which the blade is redirected sequentially in all quadrants in to obtain full circumferential coverage and maximize plaque debulking. Both DA devices are produced in multiple sizes so that femoropopliteal and tibial-peroneal arteries can be accommodated.

2. DEFINITIVE LE is a prospective, multicenter nonrandomized study testing the safety and efficacy of Medtronic's SilverHawk and TurboHawk DA catheters. There were 800 subjects enrolled with claudication/chronic limb-threatening ischemia (CLI) and at least a 50% stenosis or occlusion in their femoropopliteal and/or tibial-peroneal vessels.[21] Multilevel lesions within the target leg were included as long as each discrete lesion length was <20 cm, but severely calcified vessels were excluded. The average length of the longest lesion in each individual was 8.3 + 5.5 cm. Prespecified endpoints included primary patency in claudicants and freedom from major unplanned amputation in CLI patients at 12 months. The overall primary patency in claudicants at 12 months was 78% (95% CI: 74%-80.6%), which is similar to and even better than the outcomes of BMS, DES, and DCB for lower extremity revascularization. The 12-month limb salvage rate of 95% achieved in the CLI group was higher than the 75% patency rate achieved with DES in ACHILLES.[21,22] Although prior small, single-center studies had demonstrated lower patency rates in diabetics, the authors' showed that diabetic claudicants who underwent DA have noninferior 12-month primary patency rates compared with their nondiabetic counterparts. Periprocedural complications from DA included embolization (3.8%), perforation (5.3%), abrupt closure (2.0%), and need for bailout stenting (3.2%). DA objectively increases the vessel diameter and has an added advantage of being able to avoid implantation of a foreign intravascular scaffold while maintaining similar and even superior efficacy compared with other revascularization techniques.

B. DA for Moderate-to-Severe Vessel Calcification

1. The majority of atherectomy studies, including the DEFINITIVE LE, excluded patients with severe arterial calcification in part to avoid lesion morphologies that

Table 14.4. DA Key Points
• Slow passes and frequent interruption of passes for decreased embolization rates.
• The use of DA resulted in similar 12-mo primary patency rates compared with other revascularization techniques (BMS, DES, DCB) but with a unique benefit of being able to avoid stent placement.
• Diabetics have noninferior primary patency rates compared with nondiabetics when revascularized with DA.
• DA is effective and safe for femoropopliteal lesions with moderate and severe calcifications but should be used with a distal embolic protection device, whenever possible.

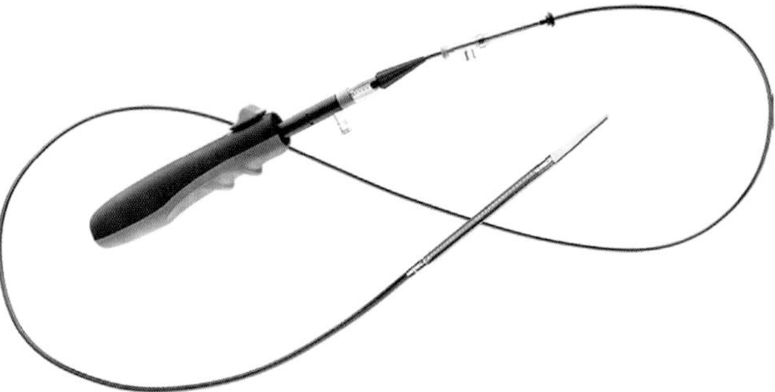

FIGURE 14.4: Medtronic. HawkOne Directional Atherectomy System. Atherectomy of Peripheral Vasculature. Medtronic. Used with permission by Medtronic ©2019.

are prone to complications such as dissections, vessel perforation, and atherosclerotic embolization. Balloon angioplasty of severely calcified lesions has been shown to be associated with early elastic recoil and both poor acute and long-term outcomes. Stenting severe calcified lesions can result in suboptimal stent expansion ultimately jeopardizing stent patency.[23]

2. The DEFINITIVE CA++ registry demonstrated that directional atherectomy when used with the SpiderFX distal embolic protection device was safe and effective in those with moderately to severely calcified femoropopliteal lesions and Rutherford clinical category 2-4 ischemia.[15] The treated lesion's mean length was short measuring 3.9 + 2.6 cm with 17.9% of lesions occluded and 81% classified as severely calcified. The 30-day freedom from MAE rate was 93.1% and a <50% residual diameter stenosis was achieved in 92% of lesions. The ideal SpiderFX filter position was in the popliteal artery just proximal to the anterior tibial take-off. Debris was recovered in 88.4% of filters with a 2.3% embolic rate that is comparable to stenting and PTA data.[24]

VII. Phoenix Atherectomy Device (Table 14.5)

A. The Philips (Volcano Corporation, San Diego, California) Phoenix atherectomy system (Fig. 14.5) is an over-the-wire front-cutting device that has a metal element at the tip of the catheter for treatment of peripheral arterial diseases. The device is available in multiple sizes including 1.8 mm 5F, 2.2 mm 6F, and 2.4 mm 7F sheath. Both 1.8 and 2.2-mm catheters are used for below- and above-the-knee intervention, whereas the 2.4-mm catheter is only used for femoropopliteal interventions. There are 2 versions of the 2.4 mm catheter, the tracking catheter (130 cm in length) and the deflection catheter (127 cm in length). The latter is the only Phoenix atherectomy device that has the directional cutting ability that allows debulking of arterial diameters that are larger than the catheter's diameter.[25]

Table 14.5. Phoenix Atherectomy Device Key Points
• The Phoenix atherectomy device is a front-cutting atherectomy device that is available in three sizes. • Size 1.8 and 2.2 mm can be used for both above- and below-the-knee interventions while 2.4 mm is only for femoropopliteal interventions. • Usage of 2.4 mm catheter for below-the-knee was associated with increased risk of dissection and perforation. • Phoenix atherectomy device showed an acceptable safety and efficacy in a prospective, single-arm, nonrandomized trial.

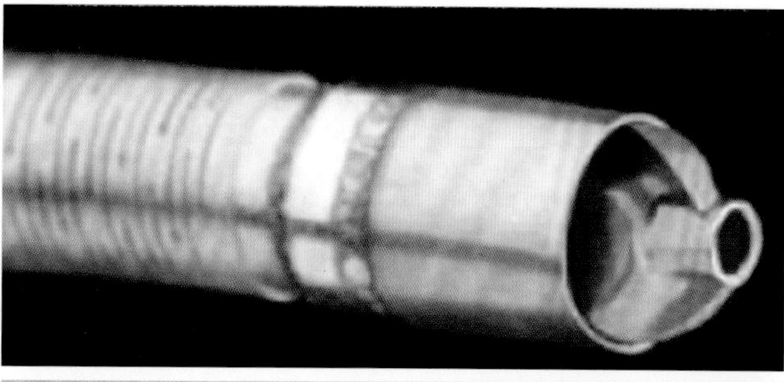

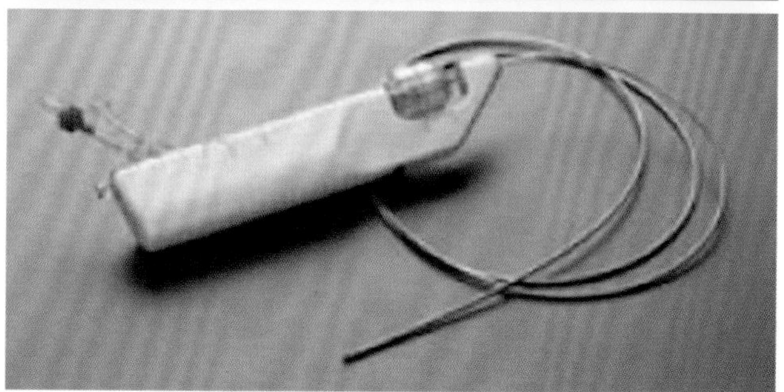

FIGURE 14.5: Phoenix atherectomy system Courtesy of Royal Philips.

B. The Phoenix atherectomy system was studied in the prospective, multicenter, nonrandomized, single-arm Endovascular Atherectomy Safety and Effectiveness Study (EASE) trial in the United States and Germany.[25] The trial was intended to study the safety and efficacy of the Phoenix device in treatment of the below-the-knee peripheral arterial disease. One hundred and twenty-eight patients were enrolled with abnormal resting or exercise ankle-brachial index with Rutherford class 2-5 and ≥70% stenosis for a total treated lesion length ≤10 cm. The primary efficacy endpoint was technical success defined as post-atherectomy stenosis ≤50%, whereas the secondary efficacy endpoint included procedure success, defined as the proportion of target lesions with residual stenosis ≤30%, and clinical success, defined as ≥1 Rutherford grade improvement at 30 days and 6 months. The primary safety endpoint was absence of MAE at 30 days. The study showed 95.1% (117/123) technical success. The residual stenosis post-atherectomy was ≤30% in 99.2% (122/123). The clinical success was achieved in 74.5% of patients at 30 days and for 80% at 6 months. MAEs occurred in 5.7% (6/105) through 30 days, and 16.8% at 6 months with 1% rate of dissection and symptomatic distal embolization and 2% rate of perforation. Of importance distal protection was used in 4.7% of procedures in the per protocol group, but none of these embolic protection devices were used in the treatment of target lesions. The 6-month freedom of target vessel revascularization and target lesion revascularization was 88.0% and 86.1%, respectively. In the subgroup analysis, patients without CLI achieved a significant clinical success compared with patients with CLI.[25]

References

1. Dake MD, Ansel GM, Jaff MR, et al. Paclitaxel-eluting stents show superiority to balloon angioplasty and bare metal stents in femoropopliteal disease: twelve-month Zilver PTX randomized study results. *Circ Cardiovasc Interv*. 2011;4(5):495-504.
2. Dake MD, Ansel GM, Jaff MR, et al. Durable clinical effectiveness with paclitaxel-eluting stents in the femoropopliteal artery: 5-year results of the Zilver PTX randomized trial. *Circulation*. 2016;133(15):1472-1483.

3. Zeller T, Langhoff R, Rocha-Singh KJ, et al. Directional atherectomy followed by a paclitaxel-coated balloon to inhibit restenosis and maintain vessel patency: twelve-month results of the DEFINITIVE AR study. *Circ Cardiovasc Interv.* 2017;10(9). pii:e004848.
4. Das TS. Excimer laser-assisted angioplasty for infrainguinal artery disease. *J Endovasc Ther.* 2009;16(2 suppl 2):II98-II104.
5. Hamburger J. *New Aspects of Excimer Laser Coronary Angioplasty: Physical Aspects and Clinical Results.* Rotterdam: Jaap N. Hamburger; 1999.
6. Bosiers M, Peeters P, Elst FV, et al. Excimer laser assisted angioplasty for critical limb ischemia: results of the LACI Belgium study. *Eur J Vasc Endovasc Surg.* 2005;29(6):613-619.
7. Laird JR, Zeller T, Gray BH, et al. Limb salvage following laser-assisted angioplasty for critical limb ischemia: results of the LACI multicenter trial. *J Endovasc Ther.* 2006;13(1):1-11.
8. Dave RM, Patlola R, Kollmeyer K, et al. Excimer laser recanalization of femoropopliteal lesions and 1-year patency: results of the CELLO registry. *J Endovasc Ther.* 2009;16(6):665-675. doi:10.1583/09-2781.1.
9. Rastan A, Sixt S, Schwarzwälder U, et al. Initial experience with directed laser atherectomy using the CLiRpath photoablation atherectomy system and bias sheath in superficial femoral artery lesions. *J Endovasc Ther.* 2007;14(3):365-373.
10. Schmidt A, Zeller T, Sievert H, et al. Photoablation using the turbo-booster and excimer laser for in-stent restenosis treatment: twelve-month results from the PATENT study. *J Endovasc Ther.* 2014;21(1):52-60.
11. Dippel EJ, Makam P, Kovach R, et al. Randomized controlled study of excimer laser atherectomy for treatment of femoropopliteal in-stent restenosis: initial results from the EXCITE ISR trial (EXCImer Laser Randomized Controlled Study for Treatment of FemoropopliTEal In-Stent Restenosis). *JACC Cardiovasc Interv.* 2015;8(1 Pt A):92-101.
12. Zeller T, Krankenberg H, Steinkamp H, et al. One-year outcome of percutaneous rotational atherectomy with aspiration in infrainguinal peripheral arterial occlusive disease: the multicenter pathway PVD trial. *J Endovasc Ther.* 2009;16(6):653-662.
13. CBoiangiu, MFissha, KKaid, et al. Analysis of Retrieved Particulate Debris After Superficial Femoral Artery (SFA) Atherectomy Using the Pathway Jetstream G3 Device. Paper presented at: SCAI 2011 Scientific Sessions; Baltimore, Maryland.
14. Maehara A, Mintz GS, Shimshak TM, et al. Intravascular ultrasound evaluation of JETSTREAM atherectomy removal of superficial calcium in peripheral arteries. *EuroIntervention.* 2015;11(1):96-103.
15. Roberts D, Niazi K, Miller W, et al. Effective endovascular treatment of calcified femoropopliteal disease with directional atherectomy and distal embolic protection: final results of the DEFINITIVE Ca^{++} trial. *Catheter Cardiovasc Interv.* 2014;84(2):236-244.
16. Adams GL, Khanna PK, Staniloae CS, et al. Optimal techniques with the Diamondback 360 System achieve effective results for the treatment of peripheral arterial disease. *J Cardiovasc Transl Res.* 2011;4(2):220-229.
17. Sotomi Y, Shlofmitz RA, Colombo A, Serruys PW, Onuma Y. Patient selection and procedural considerations for coronary orbital atherectomy system. *Interv Cardiol.* 2016;11(1):33-38.
18. Das T, Mustapha J, Indes J, Vorhies R. Technique optimization of orbital atherectomy in calcified peripheral lesions of the lower extremities: the CONFIRM series, a prospective multicenter registry. *Catheter Cardiovasc Interv.* 2014;83(1):115-122.
19. Shammas NW, Lam R, Mustapha J, et al. Comparison of orbital atherectomy plus balloon angioplasty vs. balloon angioplasty alone in patients with critical limb ischemia: results of the CALCIUM 360 randomized pilot trial. *Endovasc Ther.* 2012;19(4):480-488.
20. Dattilo R, Himmelstein SI, Cuff RF. The COMPLIANCE 360° Trial: a randomized, prospective, multicenter, pilot study comparing acute and long-term results of orbital atherectomy to balloon angioplasty for calcified femoropopliteal disease. *J Invasive Cardiol.* 2014;26(8):355-360.
21. McKinsey JF, Zeller T, Rocha-Singh KJ, et al. Lower extremity revascularization using directional atherectomy: 12-month prospective results of the DEFINITIVE LE study. *JACC Cardiovasc Interv.* 2014;7(8):923-933.
22. Scheinert D, Katsanos K, Zeller T, et al. A prospective randomized multicenter comparison of balloon angioplasty and infrapopliteal stenting with the sirolimus-eluting stent in patients with ischemic peripheral arterial disease: 1-year results from the ACHILLES trial. *J Am Coll Cardiol.* 2012;60:2290-2295.

23. Rocha-Singh KJ, Zeller T. Jaff MR. Peripheral arterial calcification: prevalence, mechanism, detection, and clinical implications. *Catheter Cardiovasc Interv.* 2014;83(6):E212-E220.
24. Schillinger M, Sabeti S, Loewe C, et al. Balloon angioplasty versus implantation of nitinol stents in the superficial femoral artery. *N Engl J Med.* 2006;354:1879-1888.
25. Davis T, Ramaiah V, Niazi K, et al. Safety and effectiveness of the Phoenix Atherectomy System in lower extremity arteries: early and midterm outcomes from the prospective multicenter EASE study. *Vascular.* 2017;25(6):563-575.

CHAPTER 15

Current Use and Availability of Reentry Devices

Samit M. Shah, MD, PhD and
Carlos Meña, MD, FACC, FSCAI

Key Points

- Chronic total occlusions of the superficial femoral artery are a common presentation of peripheral arterial disease, and subintimal crossing has become a mainstay of infrainguinal intervention. However, failure to reenter the true lumen is the primary limitation to procedural success.
- True lumen reentry devices have been shown in multiple trials to facilitate true lumen reentry and increase initial procedural success, but these devices are associated with increased financial cost and risk of vessel injury.

I. Chronic Total Occlusions

1. Chronic total occlusions (CTO) are present in nearly 50% of patients with peripheral arterial disease and most commonly affect the superficial femoral artery (SFA).[1]
2. Revascularization of CTO lesions can be technically challenging, and the presence of a CTO is associated with decreased procedural success.[2] Specifically, CTO refers to occlusive lesions that have been present for greater than or equal to three months or stable lesions that completely prevent contrast opacification of the distal vessel.[3,4] These lesions are composed of a proximal and distal fibrocalcific cap, mixed luminal plaque with thrombin and fibrin, and localized inflammation in the adjacent vascular wall.[5]
3. The goal of endovascular intervention for CTO is to cross the proximal cap, traverse the occluded lumen, and reenter the distal vessel to reestablish antegrade flow.[6] However, the proximal cap may be heavily calcified, and lesions affecting the SFA may span over 20 cm in length.[7] In many cases, crossing the true lumen may not be possible and a subintimal method can be used. This was first described by Amman Bolia in 1987 when an iatrogenic popliteal artery dissection was used to circumvent a 10 cm occlusion with recanalization of the true lumen distal to the lesion.[8]
4. The key aspects of the subintimal approach include accessing the subintimal space with a hydrophilic wire, crossing the lesion with a wire loop, and reentering the true lumen beyond the occluded segment. Angioplasty is performed in the subintimal space to create a neolumen between the intimal and adventitial layers of the vessel. The success of the subintimal approach hinges on the ability of the operator to reenter the true lumen distal to an occlusive lesion. Failure to reenter the true lumen has been cited as the primary limitation to procedural success in up to 15% of cases.[9–11]
5. True lumen reentry and the specialized devices that have been developed for this purpose are the focus of this chapter.

II. Pioneer Plus Catheter

A. **First Reentry Device** The first reentry device that was used in clinical practice was the CrossPoint.

B. TransVascular Systems (Palo Alto, CA) was subsequently purchased by Medtronic Inc. (Minneapolis, MN) in 2003, and the device was renamed the Pioneer catheter.

C. In 2013, the device was purchased by the Philips-Volcano Corporation (Rancho Cordova, CA) and rereleased as the Pioneer Plus catheter (Fig. 15.1A).

1. This dual-lumen catheter uses intravascular ultrasound (IVUS) to localize the true lumen of the vessel, and an extendable hollow 24G nitinol needle up to 7 mm long is deployed through the subintimal tissue to facilitate placement of a noncoated 0.014″ guidewire in the true lumen of the vessel.[12,13] Notably, the device was recalled by Medtronic in 2011 owing to failure of the nitinol needle to retract back into the device.[14]

2. The device has an outer diameter of 6Fr and is advanced over a monorail 0.014″ guidewire into the subintimal space (Fig. 15.1B). A 20 MHz IVUS transducer at the tip of the device is used to orient the true lumen of the vessel at "12 o'clock" (Fig. 15.2) and the nitinol hypotube is then deployed to a fixed distance (from 3 to 7 mm). A second 0.014″ can then be advanced into the true lumen of the vessel, allowing for

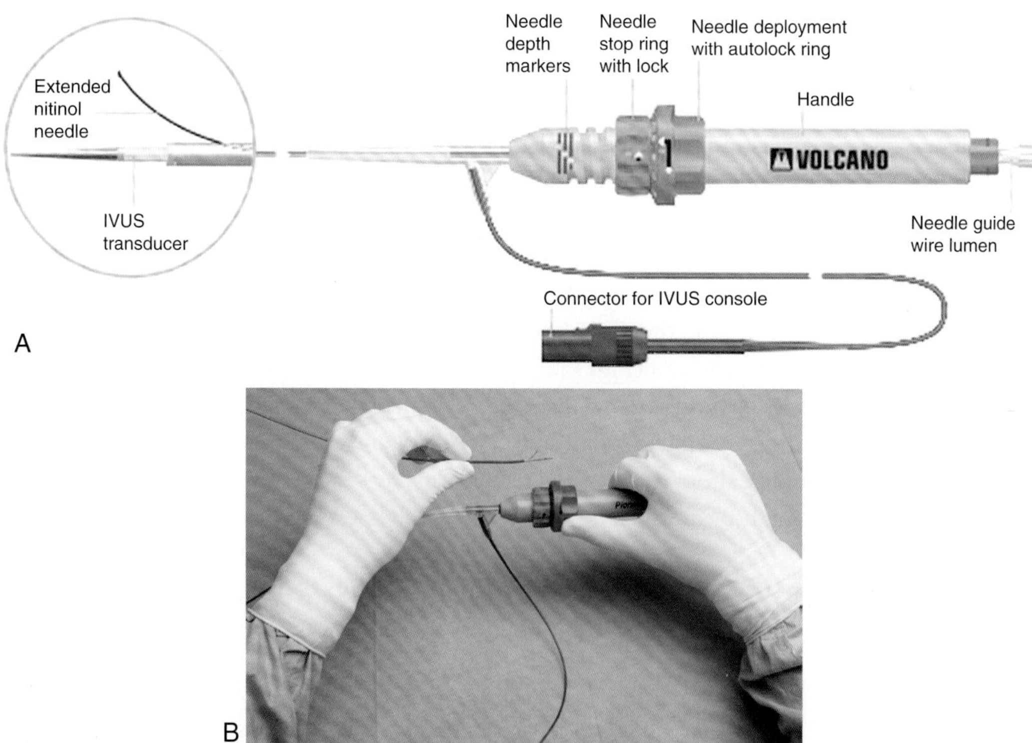

FIGURE 15.1: A, The Philips-Volcano Pioneer Plus rentry catheter is shown with a distal 20 MHz IVUS (intravascular ultrasound) transducer, nitinol needle for intimal plane puncture, and control handle. B, Pioneer Plus device with needle extended and hand on the control wheel. Courtesy of Royal Philips.

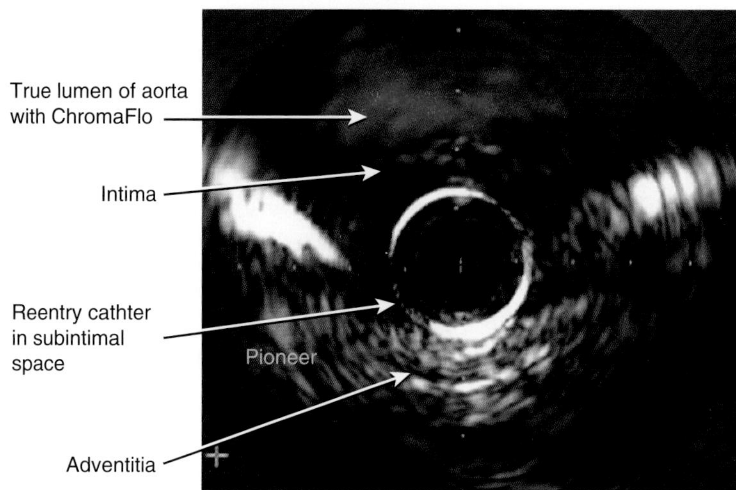

FIGURE 15.2: IVUS (intravascular ultrasound) image of true lumen from Pioneer Plus Catheter.

the retraction of the needle, removal of Pioneer catheter, and subsequent angioplasty of the subintimal space. This method has been used successfully in both iliac[15] and femoropopliteal lesions[16] with a reported success rate greater than 95%.[17,18] The length of the catheter is 120 cm which limits use of the device in infrapopliteal disease.

III. Outback Re-Entry Catheter

The LuMend (Redwood City, CA) Outback catheter was the first reentry device to gain Food and Drug Administration approval in 2001. In 2005, Cordis Corporation (Warren, NJ) purchased LuMend and released the second-generation Outback LTD reentry catheter. The current product is marketed as the Outback Elite reentry catheter. This catheter is 6Fr and uses an extendable 22G nitinol needle that exits a fenestration that is demarcated by radiopaque markers on the catheter. The true lumen is aligned using orthogonal views under fluoroscopic guidance, and the nitinol hypotube is deployed,[19] allowing an 0.014″ wire to be advanced into the true lumen (Fig. 15.3). The Outback device has been used successfully in femoropopliteal lesions and external iliac disease.[20] The reported procedural success rate with the Outback catheter has ranged from 65 to >95%,[20–22] and the primary reasons for failure are failure to recannalize the true lumen and inability to cross the iliac bifurcation.[22] The catheter length is 80 cm or 120 cm which limits use below the knee.

IV. Boston Scientific Offroad Reentry Catheter System

The Boston Scientific (Marlborough, MA) Offroad reentry catheter system uses a positioning balloon catheter with a semicompliant 5.4 mm conical balloon that positions with an outlet toward the true lumen of the vessel. Theoretically, the media and adventitia provide greater resistance to balloon inflation allowing the catheter to orient toward the softer initima of the true lumen. A 20 mm lancet-tipped microcatheter is then inserted through the balloon catheter and used to cross the intimal plane into the true lumen, allowing passage of a non-coated 0.014″ wire (Fig. 15.4). The balloon catheter is 5Fr but requires a 6Fr guiding sheath.

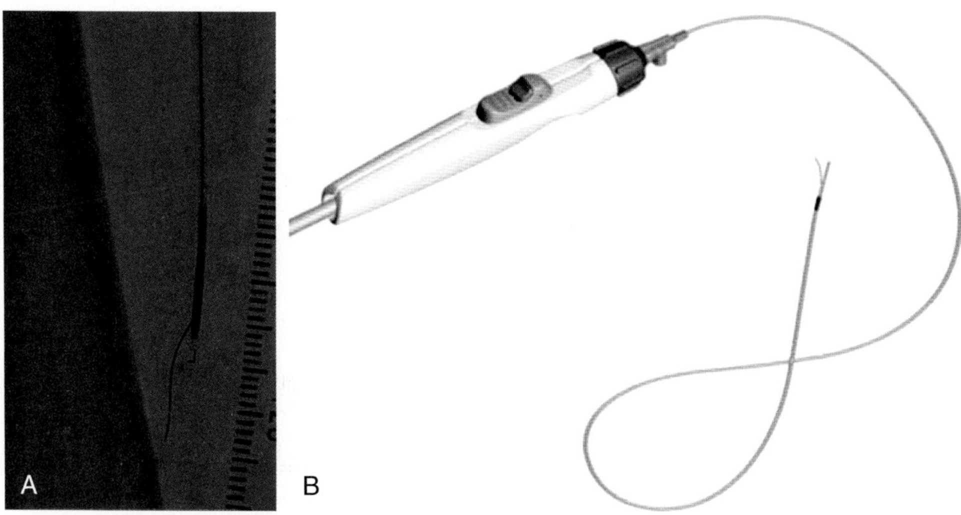

FIGURE 15.3: A, Fluoroscopic image of the Cordis Outback LTD reentry catheter with 0.014″ wire entering the true lumen of the superficial femoral artery (SFA) and radiopaque "L" marker. B, Cordis Outback Elite reentry catheter with needle extended. A, From Schneider PA, Caps MT, Nelken N. Re-entry into the true lumen from the subintimal space. *J Vasc Surg*. 2013;58(2):529-534. B, Courtesy of Cordis, a Cardinal Health Company.

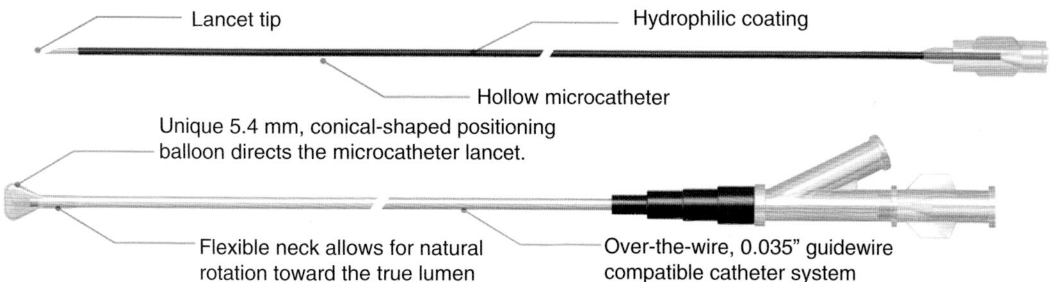

FIGURE 15.4: Boston Scientific Offroad system with 5Fr over-the-wire balloon catheter and inner lancet-tipped microcatheter. Image provided courtesy of Boston Scientific.

This device was studied in the multicenter Re-ROUTE trial which enrolled 92 patients in European centers with CTO lesions between 1 and 30 cm (average length 17.5 mm). The technical success rate was 85% with a major adverse event rate of 3.3% rate due to thrombus embolization.[23] This device has been available since 2013, and the catheter shaft length is 70 cm or 100 cm.

V. Mantaray Balloon Catheter

BridgePoint Medical (Minneapolis, MN) developed the Mantaray balloon catheter and received FDA approval in 2011. An exclusive licensing agreement was reached with Covidien and the device is now marketed as the Enteer reentry system. This platform is similar to the Stingray coronary CTO device. A flat, noncompliant balloon is advanced into subintimal

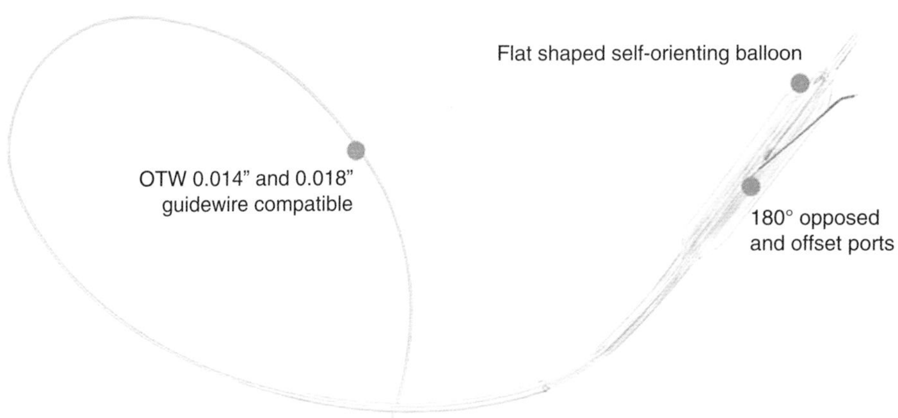

FIGURE 15.5: Covidien Enteer reentry system with 5Fr shaft, flat noncompliant balloon, and offset port for guidewire exit into the intimal plane. Used with permission by Medtronic ©2019.

space and expanded, orienting a port toward the intima and true lumen. A stiff 0.014″ guide wire can then be advanced through the port to gain true lumen entry (Fig. 15.5). Unlike the three previously discussed systems that use sharp needles or lancets, the Enteer relies on the ability for a stiff guidewire to penetrate the intima. Technical success has been reported from 82% to 86% in two studies, including the Peripheral Facilitated Antegrade Steering Technique in Chronic Total Occlusions (PFAST-CTO) trial.[24] This device can be used in 5Fr sheaths and is available in 135 cm and 150 cm catheter shaft lengths, making it useful for infrapopliteal disease.

VI. Conclusion

True lumen reentry is a pivotal aspect of endovascular CTO intervention, and these reentry devices have been demonstrated to improve rates of success and reduce procedure time. Device costs are significant and can range from over $1500 to greater than $3000,[17] and use of a reentry device is not currently reimbursed by payer sources. However, this added expense may be offset by higher overall procedural success. The risks to the patient of reentry device use include vessel injury or perforation from needle, lancet, or wire trauma. In outcome analyses for each device the rates of major adverse events are typically less than 5% and rarely related to device use.[17,18,20–22,24] Use of a specific reentry device requires operator familiarity with the device characteristics (sheath size, catheter shaft length, guidewire requirements), IVUS or fluoroscopic landmarks, and maneuvers for troubleshooting device failure or malfunction. There are no randomized trials comparing one device against another, so operators must choose the equipment that is best suited for a particular situation. In summary, specialized true lumen reentry devices are a major technological advancement in the field of peripheral intervention and subintimal angioplasty, and these devices have become an essential tool for complex CTO intervention.

References

1. Mahmud E, Cavendish JJ, Salami A. Current treatment of peripheral arterial disease: role of percutaneous interventional therapies. *J Am Coll Cardiol.* 2007;50(6):473-490.
2. Sethi S, Mohammad A, Ahmed SH, et al. Recanalization of popliteal and infrapopliteal chronic total occlusions using Viance and CrossBoss crossing catheters: a multicenter experience from the XLPAD Registry. *J Invasive Cardiol.* 2015;27(1):2-7.
3. Banerjee S, Pershwitz G, Sarode K, et al. Stent and non-stent based outcomes of infrainguinal peripheral artery interventions from the multicenter XLPAD registry. *J Invasive Cardiol.* 2015;27(1):14-18.
4. Banerjee S, Sarode K, Patel A, et al. Comparative assessment of guidewire and microcatheter vs a crossing device-based strategy to traverse infrainguinal peripheral artery chronic total occlusions. *J Endovasc Ther.* 2015;22(4):525-534.
5. Roy T, Dueck AD, Wright GA. Peripheral endovascular interventions in the era of precision medicine: tying wire, drug, and device selection to plaque morphology. *J Endovasc Ther.* 2016;23(5):751-761.
6. Safian RD. CTO of the SFA: what is the best approach? *Catheter Cardiovasc Interv.* 2013;82(3):493-494.
7. Gallagher KA, Meltzer AJ, Ravin RA, et al. Endovascular management as first therapy for chronic total occlusion of the lower extremity arteries: comparison of balloon angioplasty, stenting, and directional atherectomy. *J Endovasc Ther.* 2011;18(5):624-637.
8. Bolia A, Miles KA, Brennan J, Bell PR. Percutaneous transluminal angioplasty of occlusions of the femoral and popliteal arteries by subintimal dissection. *Cardiovasc Intervent Radiol.* 1990;13(6):357-363.
9. Banerjee S, Thomas R, Sarode K, et al. Crossing of infrainguinal peripheral arterial chronic total occlusion with a blunt microdissection catheter. *J Invasive Cardiol.* 2014;26(8):363-369.
10. Jacobs DL, Motaganahalli RL, Cox DE, Wittgen CM, Peterson GJ. True lumen re-entry devices facilitate subintimal angioplasty and stenting of total chronic occlusions: Initial report. *J Vasc Surg.* 2006;43(6):1291-1296.
11. London NJ, Srinivasan R, Naylor AR, et al. Subintimal angioplasty of femoropopliteal artery occlusions: the long-term results. *Eur J Vasc Surg.* 1994;8(2):148-155.
12. Krishnamurthy VN, Eliason JL, Henke PK, Rectenwald JE. Intravascular ultrasound-guided true lumen reentry device for recanalization of unilateral chronic total occlusion of iliac arteries: technique and follow-up. *Ann Vasc Surg.* 2010;24(4):487-497.
13. Saket RR, Razavi MK, Padidar A, Kee ST, Sze DY, Dake MD. Novel intravascular ultrasound-guided method to create transintimal arterial communications: initial experience in peripheral occlusive disease and aortic dissection. *J Endovasc Ther.* 2004;11(3):274-280.
14. Food and Drug Administration ODE. *Class 2 Device Recall Pioneer Plus Catheter PPlus 120. Recall Number Z-0864–2011 [Internet].* 2011. Available from: https://www.accessdata.fda.gov/scripts/cdrh/cfdocs/cfRES/res.cfm?id=91085
15. Rezq A, Aprile A, Sangiorgi G. Pioneer re-entry device for iliac chronic total occlusion: truly a paradigm shift. *Catheter Cardiovasc Interv.* 2013;82(3):495-499.
16. Al-Ameri H, Shin V, Mayeda GS, et al. Peripheral chronic total occlusions treated with subintimal angioplasty and a true lumen re-entry device. *J Invasive Cardiol.* 2009;21(9):468-472.
17. Smith M, Pappy R, Hennebry TA. Re-entry devices in the treatment of peripheral chronic occlusions. *Tex Heart Inst J.* 2011;38(4):392-397.
18. Saketkhoo RR, Razavi MK, Padidar A, Kee ST, Sze DY, Dake MD. Percutaneous bypass: subintimal recanalization of peripheral occlusive disease with IVUS guided luminal re-entry. *Tech Vasc Interv Radiol.* 2004;7(1):23-27.
19. Schneider PA, Caps MT, Nelken N. Re-entry into the true lumen from the subintimal space. *J Vasc Surg.* 2013;58(2):529-534.
20. Aslam MS, Allaqaband S, Haddadian B, Mori N, Bajwa T, Mewissen M. Subintimal angioplasty with a true reentry device for treatment of chronic total occlusion of the arteries of the lower extremity. *Catheter Cardiovasc Interv.* 2013;82(5):701-706.

21. Gandini R, Fabiano S, Spano S, et al. Randomized control study of the outback LTD reentry catheter versus manual reentry for the treatment of chronic total occlusions in the superficial femoral artery. *Catheter Cardiovasc Interv.* 2013;82(3):485-492.
22. Shin SH, Baril D, Chaer R, Rhee R, Makaroun M, Marone L. Limitations of the outback LTD re-entry device in femoropopliteal chronic total occlusions. *J Vasc Surg.* 2011;53(5):1260-1264.
23. Schmidt A, Keirse K, Blessing E, Langhoff R, Diaz-Cartelle J, European Study G. Offroad re-entry catheter system for subintimal recanalization of chronic total occlusions in femoropopliteal arteries: primary safety and effectiveness results of the re-route trial. *J Cardiovasc Surg (Torino).* 2014;55(4):551-558.
24. Wosik J, Shorrock D, Christopoulos G, et al. Systematic review of the bridgepoint system for crossing coronary and peripheral chronic total occlusions. *J Invasive Cardiol.* 2015;27(6):269-276.

CHAPTER 16

Acute Limb Ischemia: Thrombectomy and Thrombolysis

S. Elissa Altin, MD and Senthilraj Ganeshan, MD

Key Points

- Acute limb ischemia is a vascular emergency when viability of limb is threatened, and revascularization is recommended within 3-6 hours for acute presentations.
- Clinical symptoms and signs include the 6 P's: pain out of proportion to examination, diminished pulses, pallor, poikilothermia, paresthesias, and paralysis.
- Limb loss at 30 days is reported to be as high as 30%-50%.
- Endovascular revascularization with catheter-directed thrombolysis, rheolytic thrombectomy, and aspiration thrombectomy are common treatment options.
- Surgical embolectomy and bypass are more invasive treatment methods.

I. Introduction

Acute limb ischemia (ALI) is a vascular emergency that occurs when the viability of an extremity and the life of the affected individual are threatened owing to a sudden interruption in arterial perfusion to a limb. It is most commonly the result of thromboembolic pathology.[1] Many patients who develop ALI have occlusive peripheral arterial disease, but in the absence of preexisting atherosclerosis, ALI can still occur from embolic sources. Patients may present with profound symptoms, including disabling pain in the setting of acute vascular and neurologic deficits.[2] The systemic release of inflammatory mediators as a result of ischemic injury may result in multiorgan dysfunction, which can become life-threatening.[3] Patients with ALI are at high risk of amputation and death, making it crucial that practitioners establish the diagnosis early. Although mortality due to ALI has decreased, it is still estimated at 15% within the 30-day period from diagnosis.[4,5] By definition, patients with ALI have a decrease in limb perfusion for less than 14 days. The Rutherford classification has assigned clinical categories useful for determining the severity of the threat to viability, urgency to revascularize, and the optimal approach to management.[6]

II. Epidemiology

A. Peripheral Arterial Disease

1. Despite the substantial clinical burden, there are limited data evaluating the epidemiology of ALI in a given population of patients with peripheral arterial disease (PAD). A population-based prospective cohort study of approximately 93,000 people in the United Kingdom recently described an incidence of ALI events in 10 per 100,000 per year, which is consistent with the findings of a prior large scale Swedish registry data set.[7,8] Importantly, this study population was predominantly white (94%), making it difficult to use the findings to predict outcomes for other ethnic groups. Overall

survival at 30 days was 75.3% and 55.9% at 5 years. Amputation-free survival was 59.1% at 3 months, and future limb loss at 1 year was 7.5%. Among patients with ALI, 41.9% had prior PAD and 69% had a history of one or more forms of atherosclerotic cardiovascular disease. The investigators also found that when compared with the prospective registry data they collected over a 10-year period, routine hospital episode and death coding data missed approximately half of all acute ischemic episodes (combination of ALI, chronic limb ischemia, and acute visceral ischemia) and, in other cases, incorrectly labeled an event as an ischemic episode indicating that the incidence and prevalence rates derived from coding data may be inaccurate.[8]

2. According to the 2007 Trans-Atlantic Inter-Society Consensus (TASC), 30-day amputation rates have been reported to be 10%-30%, despite use of modern endovascular methods and mortality rates for ALI ranging from 15%-20%. The cause of death is not reported in most studies.[9] In the TOPAS trial, 1-year mortality was 13.3% after catheter-directed thrombolysis and 15.7% after surgical revascularization.[10]

B. **Thrombosis** Importantly, over the past few decades, rates of thrombosis have risen while rates of embolism have declined without any significant change in the overall incidence of ALI.[7,11,12] It is possible that this is partly due to improvements in the treatment of conditions responsible for embolic phenomena, including atrial fibrillation and valvular heart disease. With an aging population and an increase in the prevalence of the metabolic syndrome, peripheral arterial disease is an expanding epidemic, and a continued rise in the rate of thrombosis and the overall incidence of ALI can be anticipated owing to increasing disease burden and as a complication of endovascular and surgical treatment of the disease.

III. Etiology

A. **Mechanisms of ALI** Thrombosis and embolism are the two major mechanisms of ALI. In-situ thrombosis occurs in patients with underlying PAD or prior bypass grafting.[13] Acute thrombosis of a limb artery often occurs at sites of prior stenosis owing to atherosclerotic disease, but can also occur at arterial aneurysms. Venous bypass grafts often develop anastomotic thrombosis, whereas prosthetic grafts may thrombose anywhere along the length of the conduit.[13]

B. **Origin** An estimated 85% of acute embolisms are of cardiac origin. Risk factors for embolic ALI include atrial fibrillation, apical myocardial infarction with subsequent ventricular thrombus formation, prosthetic heart valves, patent foramen ovale in association with paradoxical embolism, and thrombophilias. Extracardiac emboli arise from sources including aneurysms, atherosclerotic plaque debris, and venous thromboembolisms which enter the arterial system through intracardiac shunting. Aneurysm walls, due to abnormal or slow flow, often contain thrombus which can embolize distally. In particular, aneurysms of the aorta and popliteal artery are the most common sources of embolic ALI. Hematologic and thrombophilic conditions can additionally predispose to arterial thrombosis, including the antiphospholipid syndrome and heparin-induced thrombocytopenia.[9] Atherosclerotic plaque debris due to dislodgement is a major source of embolism during catheterization, as well as procedural catheter based thromboembolism.[9] Emboli most commonly lodge at the bifurcation of the femoral artery, trifurcation of the popliteal, and aortic bifurcation.

IV. Clinical Presentation

A. Presentation

1. A classic presentation of ALI includes a constellation of signs and symptoms described as the classic six "P's": acute onset of pain out of proportion to examination, diminished pulses, early skin mottling (pallor), coolness to touch (poikilothermia), distal paresthesias, and paralysis. However, there are many factors which can alter the clinical presentation, including the location and duration of the arterial occlusion, the degree of collateral circulation, the extent of preexisting arterial disease (presence of collaterals), and the metabolic consequences of tissue ischemia.[13]

2. Patients are often easily able to recall the precise timing of the onset of pain, especially for those whose ALI is due to an embolization. Pain is usually severe but over time can relent because nerve damage ensues as ischemia progresses. Patients with PAD who have arterial thrombosis can present with a more gradual or stuttering presentation, as the severity of clinical ischemia is reduced owing to the formation of collaterals. Pallor or paleness below the level of obstruction occurs, and pulses may be absent or diminished when compared with the contralateral side. Temperature dysregulation occurs, causing the limb to be cool (poikilothermia), as the transfer of heat to the extremity is interrupted by inadequate blood flow. Most commonly these findings are located one joint distal to the level of occlusion. Late symptoms include paresthesias and paralysis which occur secondary to neural and muscular ischemia and death, respectively. Livedo reticularis may be seen if the embolization is to the more distal vessels.

B. Physical Examination

1. A thorough physical examination is necessary in the diagnosis of ALI and determination of its severity and the patient's prognosis. The initial evaluation should include vital signs, the external appearance of the patient, the temperature of the skin, a detailed vascular examination including palpation of pulses in the femoral, popliteal, dorsalis pedis, and posterior tibial arteries of the affected and contralateral limb, and a neuromotor evaluation for sensation and muscle strength. A Doppler instrument should be used to establish if flow is present in distal arteries when a palpable pulse is absent.

2. In the event of a normal vascular examination on the contralateral limb, an embolic etiology of ALI is likely. In a patient presenting with symptoms consistent with thrombosis but no known history of PAD, physical findings to suggest underlying PAD include diminished extremity pulses, scant hair growth, atrophic skin, hypertrophied nails, and ischemic ulcers.

C. **Rutherford Classification of Acute Limb Ischemia** Patients should be categorized into a Rutherford stage of ALI based on their clinical presentation and physical findings which can guide decisions on their immediate management. Stage I includes those with typical presenting symptoms, audible arterial and venous Doppler signals, and preserved sensation and muscle strength on examination. Patients categorized as stage I have no immediate threat to limb viability. Stage II indicates that limb viability is threatened. In stage IIa the threat is marginal, with the limb considered salvageable if promptly treated. These patients have minimal sensory loss usually involving the toes, and the arterial Doppler signal is frequently inaudible. In stage IIb, there is an immediate threat to limb viability, and the limb may be salvageable with immediate revascularization. Sensory loss is more extensive and spreads proximally along the feet, muscle weakness is also present at a mild or moderate severity, and the arterial Doppler signal is usually absent. In stage III, the limb is considered irreversibly damaged with major tissue loss or permanent nerve damage. Sensory loss is profound, paralysis is present, and arterial as well as venous Doppler signals are absent.[6]

V. Diagnostic Evaluation

A. **Differential Diagnosis** The differential diagnosis for ALI includes direct arterial trauma, vasospasm, extrinsic compression, decreased systemic perfusion, acute neurologic syndromes, deep venous thrombosis, vasculitis, and chronic limb ischemia. The history and physical examination are typically sufficient to arrive at a leading diagnosis of ALI. Once conditions mimicking acute limb ischemia have been excluded, nonatherosclerotic causes of acute limb ischemia should be evaluated. In most cases, with the exception of arterial trauma, dissection, and compartment syndrome, the initial management is often unchanged.

B. Imaging

1. Noninvasive diagnostic imaging available to determine the nature and extent of the occlusion includes duplex ultrasonography, computed tomographic (CT) angiography, and magnetic resonance (MR) angiography. The role of these imaging modalities in patients with Rutherford IIb ALI is limited as revascularization is required within 3-6 hours for limb salvage[14]; although CT or MR angiography may delineate vascular anatomy and assist in treatment planning, it is important that these tests do not delay intervention.

2. Duplex ultrasound is a useful test to perform preprocedurally on most patients, as it can be done quickly and entails little risk to the patient. In patients planned to undergo surgery, CT or MR angiography is useful to ensure an accurate diagnosis and determine the extent of arterial occlusion.[15,16] In patients who are planned to receive endovascular therapies, digital subtraction arteriography can be performed immediately before the procedure to provide the information necessary to plan the intervention.[17]

VI. Treatment

Treatment strategies for acute limb ischemia are directed at clot removal and treatment of any underlying vessel lesion to include atherosclerotic disease, dissection, aneurysm, thrombosis, intimal hyperplasia, and other predisposing factors. These include medical therapy with anticoagulation, endovascular treatment with catheter-directed thrombolysis and mechanical thrombectomy, and surgery for embolectomy or bypass. The decision regarding which treatment strategy to pursue depends on patient characteristics as well as classification of the threatened limb, including candidacy for anticoagulation and thrombolysis based on clinical history and suitability for surgery based on careful medical assessment of cardiac and respiratory risk. It is important to understand before choosing therapy whether the patient can tolerate the type and length of treatment and whether the thrombus is accessible by the modality chosen and to perform an assessment of the risk-benefit profile of anticoagulation and thrombolysis.

A. **Anticoagulation** Systemic unfractionated heparin (or low-molecular-weight heparin) should be administered at first presentation with ALI once diagnosis is made for goal aPTT 1/5-2x control.[18] Early data from surgical literature suggest that early first-line high-dose heparin treatment results in a significant decrease in the mortality rate without an increase in the amputation rate. This not only prevents propagation of thrombus distally induced by stasis but also proximally induced by turbulence of incoming blood abutting thrombus. In addition to beneficial effects on stalling clot propagation, heparin helps to prevent catheter thrombosis during endovascular treatment of thrombus without a significant difference in bleeding complications combined with urokinase or rt-PA administration.[6,19]

B. Thrombolysis

1. In 1974, Dotter et al reported the initial study in 17 patients of efficacy of low-dose streptokinase thrombolysis in acute thrombus, with a 35% success rate of clot lysis balanced by a 24% rate on major bleeding.[20] He described positioning side-hole catheters into the obstructive clot to perfuse streptokinase proximal or into the lesion, using a dose 1/100th of the systemic therapeutic dose in the first report of catheter-directed thrombolysis. Thrombolysis is commonly performed now, with decades of data supporting its use as first-line therapy in acute limb ischemia in the absence of patient-based contraindications as long as expected time to restoration of flow to the jeopardized limb is sufficient for limb salvage.
2. Once arterial access is obtained, diagnostic angiography of the lower extremity vasculature can be performed to identify the level of the thrombotic occlusion not only to formulate the endovascular approach but also for surgical planning if revascularization fails. The "guidewire traversal test" has been shown to be an important predictor of technical success of thrombolysis therapy.[19] Cautious manipulation of the guidewire to avoid vascular injury while crossing the thrombus is paramount. In the event the guidewire cannot be advanced through the lesion entirely, the catheter may

be positioned within the proximal portion of the thrombus. Although many catheters exist on the market for thrombolysis, essentially any multi–side-hole catheter that reaches the lesion may be used for lytic drug delivery to the thrombus (Cragg-McNamara; ev3 Endovascular Inc, Plymouth, MN and Unifuse: AngioDynamics, Latham, NY).

3. Techniques for infusing thrombolytic agents into the clot vary based on where the catheter is initially positioned (proximal to clot, inside of clot, or at distal end), whether the catheter is moved proximally or distally during the course of infusion, and whether lytic dose is constant, graded, or periodically forced to optimize delivery of drug to the lesion. *Intrathrombus infusion* involves passing the infusion catheter through the thrombus to release lytic into the thrombus, which is most commonly employed and yields improved clot dissolution. *Intrathrombus lacing* involves use of a catheter positioned within the clot with gradual withdrawal as thrombolysis occurs to administer lytic throughout the lesion. These two techniques are favored based on the balance between most effective and least demanding.[21]

4. With the catheter in place and secured, the patient can be monitored in intensive care unit (ICU) or step down to assess for any signs of bleeding, hematologic abnormality until repeat angiogram is performed within 12-24 hours of initiation of lysis. If there is resolution of thrombus, any underlying vascular lesion that predisposed to thrombus can be treated at that time.

C. Mechanism of Action and Dosing of Thrombolytic Agent

1. Thrombolytic agents are serine proteases that work by converting plasminogen to plasmin. Plasmin acts to break the cross-links between fibrin molecules, which subsequently lyses the clot. Currently available thrombolytic agents for lower extremity lysis are recombinant tissue plasminogen activators, including alteplase (Genentech), reteplase (EKR therapeutics), and tenecteplase (Genentech). Streptokinase, although it was the first thrombolytic agent available, has limited clinical use in the United States owing to antigenicity, higher bleeding rates, and lesser efficacy. Urokinase, a direct plasminogen activator, is no longer available in the United States owing to manufacturing issues.

2. There are no data to support the routine monitoring of laboratory values during thrombolysis. Serum fibrinogen level is thought to predict bleeding, but this has not been validated. In the PURPOSE trial (Prourokinase vs urokinase for recanalization of peripheral occlusions, safety, and efficacy), Ouriel et al. found that 81% of patients with serum fibrinogen <100 mg/dL had a bleeding complication (major or minor) compared with patients with fibrinogen >100 mg/dL who had a bleeding complication rate of 59%.[22] Another study of 36 patients receiving reteplase showed that there was significant fibrinogen depletion and that the percent decrease in level correlated to bleeding complications. Major bleeding complications were associated with a mean 72% decrease in fibrinogen while minor complications were associated with a 46% decrease in fibrinogen.[23]

D. **Contraindications to Thrombolysis** Bleeding is a major concern with the use of any fibrinolytic therapy. The contraindications to catheter-directed thrombolysis originate from experience with the use of systemic thrombolysis. Data are available which show in comparison that less bleeding events occur with catheter-directed thrombolysis, making it important to individualize the risk-benefit ratio of endovascular intervention in patients presenting with ALI.[24] Absolute contraindications include ongoing bleeding, intracranial hemorrhage, compartment syndrome, and severe limb ischemia that requires immediate surgical intervention.[17] Other considerations which may serve as relative contraindications include the following: within the past 3 months, a history of eye surgery, neurosurgery, or intracranial trauma; within the past 2 months, a history of stroke or transient ischemic attack; within the past 10 days, a history of major surgery, major trauma, or gastrointestinal bleeding; and lastly, a history of an intracranial neoplasm or severe contrast allergy should also be taken into account.[17]

1. **Randomized Controlled Trials of CDT** Early randomized control data supporting the use of catheter-based thrombolysis comes from the Rochester trial, STILES trial, and the TOPAS trial, which are reviewed below. A recent meta-analysis of literature from 1990 to 2014 including these trials to compare open surgical versus endovascular management of ALI shows overall that limb salvage and amputation rates are similar and acceptable by both modalities and are probably complementary in restoring adequate flow to the threatened limb.[25] In the selected patient, data support catheter directed thrombolysis (CDT) as first-line therapy in Rutherford class I, IIa, and possibly IIb limb ischemia given similarity in early outcomes to include limb salvage, amputation free survival, and survival despite possibility of future interventions.[26]

2. **Rochester Trial** 114 patients with signs and symptoms of ALI <7 days were randomized to catheter-directed thrombolysis (urokinase) versus surgery.[27] Thrombolysis resulted in resolution of thrombus in 70% of cases, with the remainder proceeding to surgery. At 30 days, the catheter-directed thrombolysis group had superior amputation-free survival, but at one year limb salvage rates were similar between groups. Not unexpectedly, the surgical group had more cardiopulmonary complications (49% vs 16% in the CDT group), possibly driving the early survival benefit of the endovascular strategy. Median length of hospital stay was similar between groups (11 d), with slightly higher hospital cost in the thrombolysis group ($15,672 vs $12,253).

E. **TOPAS (Thrombolysis or Peripheral Arterial Surgery)** Ouriel et al. published the results of 544 patients with lower extremity native or bypass graft occlusions of <14 days duration randomized to CDT with r-UK versus surgery.[10] In phase 1, 213 patients compared r-UK doses versus surgery, showing that 4000 IU/min of recombinant UK for 4 hours followed by 2000 IU/min for max 48 hours balanced the maximal lytic effect (71% achievement of lysis of thrombus) with the lowest rate of bleeding. Phase 2 looked at 544 patients with ALI <14 days and showed that at 6 months and 1 year, the amputation-free survival rate was not significantly different between the groups with similar median hospital stays. Followed to 1 year, amputation-free survival and mortality remained similar. In the CDT group, bypass graft occlusion patients showed better amputation-free survival rates than native vessel thrombosis. The thrombolysis major intracranial hemorrhage rate was 12% compared with 5% in the surgery group.

F. **STILE (Surgery vs Thrombolysis for Ischemia of the Lower Extremity) Trial** The STILE investigators published the results of 393 patients with nonembolic ALI, who were randomized to thrombolysis (rt-PA or urokinase) or surgery with post hoc stratification of symptoms into <14 days duration and >14 days duration.[28] 30% of patients had ischemic symptoms for <14 days. CDT in patients symptomatic <14 days had lower rates of amputation, improved limb salvage, and shorter lengths of stay than surgical patients or CDT patients with symptoms >14 days. In this group, rt-PA and urokinase were similarly effective and safe, but rt-PA showed shorter lysis time. For the patients with symptoms >14 days, the surgical group had lower amputation rates at 6 months.

G. Percutaneous Mechanical Thrombectomy

1. Percutaneous mechanical thrombectomy (PMT) encompasses a group of techniques and devices aimed at removing thrombus with a combination of mechanical disruption, dissolution, and aspiration. Success of catheter-directed thrombolysis depends on size, composition, location, and age of the thrombus, as well as inflow and outflow from the lesion. Contraindications to thrombolysis may preclude its use in some patients, and PMT represents an adjunctive therapy for clot removal and even first-line therapy in some cases.

2. An underlying principal of PMT treatment is recirculation with hydrodynamic maceration of thrombus and removal via aspiration based on the Bernoulli principle and Venturi effect. There are three principal categories of recirculation for thrombus evacuation: rheolytic, ultrasonic, and mixing devices.

3. The AngioJet rheolytic thrombectomy system (Medrad Interventional/Possis, Minneapolis, MN) includes single use catheter and pump sets with multiuse drive unit and functions to remove clot via high-pressure saline injection at the distal catheter tip to form a low pressure zone via the Bernoulli effect that macerates the thrombus. Following this, the clot is sucked back into the catheter for removal. This system is FDA approved for infrainguinal arterial cases and has been shown to aspirate >75% of thrombus in ALI of native vessels or grafts.[29] In one experience of 21 patients with ALI (52% of who had contraindications to lysis), AngioJet resulted in 91% removal of thrombus with 89% of patients achieving limb salvage at 6 months.[30] The power-pulse spray technology has been reported to have a 90% success rate with infusion of thrombolytic infusion through the catheter to optimize clot disruption and removal.[29]

4. Possible complications from this system include distal embolization, theoretical hemolysis with repeated passes of the device, and fluid overload potential owing to continuous device irrigation.[31] In addition, the risk of distal embolization remains but can be mitigated by use of a filter.

H. **Percutaneous Aspiration Thrombectomy** Percutaneous aspiration thrombectomy is based on the simple concept of a negative pressure syringe attached to a catheter to aspirate thrombus. The Pronto catheter (Vascular Solutions, Inc, Minneapolis, MN) is a rapid exchange aspiration thrombectomy catheter with a 0.035-in crossing profile and hydrophilic coating. The volume of thrombus aspiration potential is limited compared with rheolytic catheters, but this is balanced by the small profile of the device and deliverability. There are no formal studies on the use of the Pronto device in ALI, only reports in the literature of its use in managing embolization during peripheral intervention.[32] The Export catheter (Medtronic, Inc, Minneapolis, MN) is a similar catheter to the Pronto, but there are no published reports of its use in ALI.

I. **Percuataneous Ultrasonography-Assisted Fibrinolysis** Percutaneous ultrasonography-assisted fibrinolysis was developed as an alternative to CDT to decrease the bleeding complication rate associated with thrombolytics by augmenting enzymatic clot lysis with low-intensity ultrasound to loosen fibrin strands and increase clot permeability to expose more plasminogen receptors for binding.[33-35] The DUET study (Dutch randomized trial comparing standard catheter-directed thrombolysis and ultrasound-accelerated thrombolysis for arterial thromboembolic infrainguinal disease) evaluated whether ultrasound-assisted lysis can reduce therapy time compared with standard CDT. Sixty patients with Rutherford I and IIa acute limb ischemia (average duration of ischemia being 19 days) were randomized to standard CDT or ultrasound-assisted thrombolysis. The primary outcome measured was the duration of thrombolysis for uninterrupted flow. They found that ultrasound-assisted thrombolysis showed a significantly faster time to flow restoration (17.7 vs 29.5 h).[36] Hourly thrombolytic dose rate of urokinase was the same in both groups, but the ultrasound-assisted group received lower total dose of thrombolysis given the shorter infusion time necessary for flow restoration. DUET II is a nonrandomized trial being planned to investigate lower hourly dose to decrease bleeding risks owing to thrombolysis.

VII. Surgical Revascularization

Ultimately, a surgical strategy using location centered approach may be necessary with an ischemic thrombus. These include balloon catheter thrombectomy and bypass surgery, with adjunctive endarterectomy and intraoperative lysis. For acute limb ischemia of <14 days duration, catheter-based thrombolytic therapies are reasonable first-line treatment, but based on the TOPAS trial, surgical revascularization is generally preferred as first-line therapy in patients with symptomatic occlusion >14 days.

VIII. Reperfusion Injury

Reperfusion injury is a clinical diagnosis that must be suspected in any patient after revascularization who presents with severe pain, weakness, and decreased sensation in the affected limb. Patients should be carefully monitored postprocedure for any change in symptoms. Laboratory result abnormalities can include myoglobinuria and CK elevation.[37] The anterior compartment is most vulnerable, and it is critical to assess for peroneal nerve function by foot dorsiflexion and to assess for decreased sensation between the first and second toes. Ultimately, this is a clinical diagnosis, but measurement of compartment pressures confirms the diagnosis. Treatment is surgical fasciotomy to decompress elevated compartment pressure.

IX. Summary

Acute limb ischemia is associated with high rates of hospital mortality and limb loss, with 15%-20% of patients dying within 1 year of initial presentation owing to underlying morbid conditions.[13] Timely diagnosis is critical to limb salvage. Clinical assessment of limb temperature, pulses, motor, and sensory function is necessary to classify the limb as viable, threatened, or nonviable. Administration of intravenous unfractionated heparin is appropriate after diagnosis. Patients with a viable or marginally threatened limb can proceed to imaging, but those with a threatened limb should proceed to angiogram to guide treatment with catheter-based therapies (thrombolysis and thrombectomy) or surgical revascularization.

References

1. Patel NH, Krishnamurthy VN, Kim S, et al; CIRSE and SIR Standards of Practice Committees. Quality improvement guidelines for percutaneous management of acute lower-extremity ischemia. *J Vasc Interv Radiol.* 2013;24(1):3-15. doi:10.1016/j.jvir.2012.09.026.
2. Braun R, Lin M. Acute limb ischemia: a case report and literature review. *J Emerg Med.* 2015;49(6):1011-1017. doi:10.1016/j.jemermed.2015.03.008.
3. Jaffery Z, Thornton SN, White CJ. Acute limb ischemia. *Am J Med Sci.* 2011;342(3):226-234. doi:10.1097/MAJ.0b013e31820ef345.
4. Earnshaw JJ, Whitman B, Foy C. National Audit of Thrombolysis for Acute Leg Ischemia (NATALI): clinical factors associated with early outcome. *J Vasc Surg.* 2004;39(5):1018-1025. doi:10.1016/j.jvs.2004.01.019.
5. Eliason JL, Wainess RM, Proctor MC, et al. A national and single institutional experience in the contemporary treatment of acute lower extremity ischemia. *Ann Surg.* 2003;238(3):382-389; discussion 389-390. doi:10.1097/01.sla.0000086663.49670.d1.
6. Rutherford RB, Baker JD, Ernst C, et al. Recommended standards for reports dealing with lower extremity ischemia: revised version. *J Vasc Surg.* 1997;26(3):517-538.
7. Dryjski M, Swedenborg J. Acute ischemia of the extremities in a metropolitan area during one year. *J Cardiovasc Surg (Torino).* 1984;25(6):518-522.
8. Howard DP, Banerjee A, Fairhead JF, et al. Population-based study of incidence, risk factors, outcome, and prognosis of ischemic peripheral arterial events: implications for prevention. *Circulation.* 2015;132(19):1805-1815. doi:10.1161/CIRCULATIONAHA.115.016424.
9. Norgren L, Hiatt WR, Dormandy JA, et al. Inter-society consensus for the management of peripheral arterial disease. *Int Angiol.* 2007;26(2):81-157.
10. Ouriel K, Veith FJ, Sasahara AA. Thrombolysis or peripheral arterial surgery: phase I results. TOPAS investigators. *J Vasc Surg.* 1996;23(1):64-73; discussion 74-75.
11. Byrne RM, Taha AG, Avgerinos E, Marone LK, Makaroun MS, Chaer RA. Contemporary outcomes of endovascular interventions for acute limb ischemia. *J Vasc Surg.* 2014;59(4):988-995. doi:10.1016/j.jvs.2013.10.054.
12. Ouriel K, Veith FJ, Sasahara AA. A comparison of recombinant urokinase with vascular surgery as initial treatment for acute arterial occlusion of the legs. Thrombolysis or Peripheral Arterial Surgery (TOPAS) investigators. *N Engl J Med.* 1998;338(16):1105-1111. doi:10.1056/NEJM199804163381603.
13. Creager MA, Kaufman JA, Conte MS. Clinical practice. Acute limb ischemia. *N Engl J Med.* 2012;366(23):2198-2206. doi:10.1056/NEJMcp1006054.

14. Rutherford RB. Clinical staging of acute limb ischemia as the basis for choice of revascularization method: when and how to intervene. *Semin Vasc Surg.* 2009;22(1):5-9. doi:10.1053/j.semvascsurg.2008.12.003.
15. Roh BS, Park KH, Kim EA, et al. Prognostic value of CT before thrombolytic therapy in iliofemoral deep venous thrombosis. *J Vasc Interv Radiol.* 2002;13(1):71-76.
16. Sharafuddin MJ, Wroblicka JT, Sun S, Essig M, Schoenberg SO, Yuh WT. Percutaneous vascular intervention based on gadolinium-enhanced MR angiography. *J Vasc Interv Radiol.* 2000;11(6):739-746.
17. Karnabatidis D, Spiliopoulos S, Tsetis D, Siablis D. Quality improvement guidelines for percutaneous catheter-directed intra-arterial thrombolysis and mechanical thrombectomy for acute lower-limb ischemia. *Cardiovasc Intervent Radiol.* 2011;34(6):1123-1136. doi:10.1007/s00270-011-0258-z.
18. Blaisdell FW, Steele M, Allen RE. Management of acute lower extremity arterial ischemia due to embolism and thrombosis. *Surgery.* 1978;84(6):822-834.
19. McNamara TO, Fischer JR. Thrombolysis of peripheral arterial and graft occlusions: improved results using high-dose urokinase. *AJR Am J Roentgenol.* 1985;144(4):769-775. doi:10.2214/ajr.144.4.769.
20. Dotter CT, Rosch J, Seaman AJ. Selective clot lysis with low-dose streptokinase. *Radiology.* 1974;111(1):31-37. doi:10.1148/111.1.31.
21. Kessel DO, Berridge DC, Robertson I. Infusion techniques for peripheral arterial thrombolysis. *Cochrane Database Syst Rev.* 2004;(1):CD000985. doi:10.1002/14651858.CD000985.pub2.
22. Ouriel K, Kandarpa K, Schuerr DM, Hultquist M, Hodkinson G, Wallin B. Prourokinase versus urokinase for recanalization of peripheral occlusions, safety and efficacy: the PURPOSE trial. *J Vasc Interv Radiol.* 1999;10(8):1083-1091.
23. Hull JE, Hull MK, Urso JA. Reteplase with or without abciximab for peripheral arterial occlusions: efficacy and adverse events. *J Vasc Interv Radiol.* 2004;15(6):557-564.
24. Dormandy JA, Rutherford RB. Management of peripheral arterial disease (PAD). TASC working group. TransAtlantic Inter-Society Consensus (TASC). *J Vasc Surg.* 2000;31(1 Pt 2):S1-S296.
25. Berridge DC, Kessel DO, Robertson I. Surgery versus thrombolysis for initial management of acute limb ischaemia. *Cochrane Database Syst Rev.* 2013;(6):CD002784. doi:10.1002/14651858.CD002784.pub2.
26. Wang JC, Kim AH, Kashyap VS. Open surgical or endovascular revascularization for acute limb ischemia. *J Vasc Surg.* 2016;63(1):270-278. doi:10.1016/j.jvs.2015.09.055.
27. Ouriel K, Shortell CK, DeWeese JA, et al. A comparison of thrombolytic therapy with operative revascularization in the initial treatment of acute peripheral arterial ischemia. *J Vasc Surg.* 1994;19(6):1021-1030.
28. Weaver FA, Comerota AJ, Youngblood M, Froehlich J, Hosking JD, Papanicolaou G. Surgical revascularization versus thrombolysis for nonembolic lower extremity native artery occlusions: results of a prospective randomized trial. The STILE investigators. Surgery versus thrombolysis for ischemia of the lower extremity. *J Vasc Surg.* 1996;24(4):513-521; discussion 521-513.
29. Rogers JH, Laird JR. Overview of new technologies for lower extremity revascularization. *Circulation.* 2007;116(18):2072-2085. doi:10.1161/CIRCULATIONAHA.107.715433.
30. Silva JA, Ramee SR, Collins TJ, et al. Rheolytic thrombectomy in the treatment of acute limb-threatening ischemia: immediate results and six-month follow-up of the multicenter AngioJet registry. Possis peripheral AngioJet study AngioJet investigators. *Cathet Cardiovasc Diagn.* 1998;45(4):386-393.
31. Ansel GM, George BS, Botti CF, et al. Rheolytic thrombectomy in the management of limb ischemia: 30-day results from a multicenter registry. *J Endovasc Ther.* 2002;9(4):395-402. doi:10.1583/1545-1550(2002)009<0395:RTITMO>2.0.CO;2.
32. Zafar N, Prasad A, Mahmud E. Utilization of an aspiration thrombectomy catheter (Pronto) to treat acute atherothrombotic embolization during percutaneous revascularization of the lower extremity. *Catheter Cardiovasc Interv.* 2008;71(7):972-975. doi:10.1002/ccd.21561.
33. Braaten JV, Goss RA, Francis CW. Ultrasound reversibly disaggregates fibrin fibers. *Thromb Haemost.* 1997;78(3):1063-1068.
34. Hardig BM, Persson HW, Olsson SB. Low-energy ultrasound exposure of the streptokinase molecule may enhance but also attenuate its fibrinolytic properties. *Thromb Res.* 2006;117(6):713-720. doi:10.1016/j.thromres.2005.05.027.

35. Siddiqi F, Odrljin TM, Fay PJ, Cox C, Francis CW. Binding of tissue-plasminogen activator to fibrin: effect of ultrasound. *Blood*. 1998;91(6):2019-2025.
36. Schrijver AM, van Leersum M, Fioole B, et al. Dutch randomized trial comparing standard catheter-directed thrombolysis and ultrasound-accelerated thrombolysis for arterial thromboembolic infrainguinal disease (DUET). *J Endovasc Ther*. 2015;22(1):87-95. doi:10.1177/1526602814566578.
37. Valdez C, Schroeder E, Amdur R, Pascual J, Sarani B. Serum creatine kinase levels are associated with extremity compartment syndrome. *J Trauma Acute Care Surg*. 2013;74(2):441-445; discussion 445-447. doi:10.1097/TA.0b013e31827a0a36.

CHAPTER 17

Hybrid Lower Extremity Revascularization

Sameer Nagpal, MD,
Carlos Meña, MD, FACC, FSCAI, and
Bauer E. Sumpio, MD, PhD

I. Introduction

Patients with chronic limb ischemia often have multilevel aortoiliac and infrainguinal disease. These patients usually require complete revascularization to alleviate symptoms and improve wound healing or prevent amputation in the case of critical limb ischemia. While some lesions are best treated using an endovascular catheter based approach, others, such as flow-limiting atherosclerosis of the common femoral artery, are best suited for surgical management. Patients requiring both modalities of intervention are often treated in a staged fashion, but there is increasing appreciation for using a single, simultaneous, hybrid procedure which makes up 5%-21% of current lower extremity revascularization procedures.[1] Hybrid procedures combine wire- and catheter-based therapies with surgery into a single procedure to improve revascularization completeness and efficiency and patient satisfaction and reduce the overall risk associated with performing multiple procedures.

II. Preprocedure Assessment

A. **Imaging and Labs** Preprocedure planning with noninvasive imaging such as computed tomography angiography, magnetic resonance angiography, or invasive angiography assists the operator in developing an optimal hybrid surgical and endovascular plan. Specifically, appropriate operatory or interventional laboratory requirements, patient positioning, suitability of various access points, appropriate equipment selection, and any case-specific anatomic complexities can be reviewed before intervention. Previously, less complex lesions were targeted for endovascular interventions with surgical management reserved for more complex disease or lengthy chronic total occlusions. However, with advancement in endovascular-based technologies and operator skill set, percutaneous interventions are often used even for complex Trans-Atlantic Intersociety Consensus (TASC) C or D lesions.

B. **Drugs** Typically, hybrid procedures are performed with general anesthesia in an operating room with a mobile fluoroscopy unit capable of performing digital subtraction angiography. Dual-antiplatelet loading is usually delayed until after the intervention to lower immediate surgical bleeding risk, especially in case of unforeseen complications. Preoperative prophylactic intravenous antibiotics are typically provided to prevent infection. After surgical exposure of the vessels and before vessel clamping or sheath insertion, intravenous heparin is administered to target an activated clotting time of twice the upper limit of normal.

III. Concomitant Iliac and Common Femoral Arterial Disease

A. **Endarterectomy** In the case of occlusive aortoiliac disease extending into the ipsilateral common femoral bifurcation, surgical common femoral endarterectomy is typically performed first. A longitudinal common femoral arteriotomy is made and can be extended proximally into the distal external iliac artery or distally into the proximal superficial and deep femoral arteries just beyond the bifurcation. After endarterectomy is performed and the obstructing plaque is removed, the arteriotomy is closed with a patch angioplasty (using autogenous vein graft or synthetic or biologic material) or interposition synthetic graft.

B. **Endovascular Technique** Following surgical endarterectomy, the inflow iliac lesion is then approached via endovascular technique. Contralateral standard retrograde femoral access is obtained percutaneously, and a distal aortic angiogram is pursued if one has not been obtained previously. For lesions involving the external iliac artery, contralateral access may be sufficient if there is enough length over the bifurcation to allow positioning of a long sheath with adequate support. For lesions involving the proximal or ostial common iliac artery, a sheath is placed into the ipsilateral surgically exposed and reconstructed femoral artery to perform the endovascular intervention, which typically is successful using solely a wire and catheter technique for lesion crossing. Bare-metal balloon-expandable stents are generally used within the common iliac segment given their stronger radial force and use in ostial lesions, whereas self-expandable bare-metal stents are often used within the external iliac segment, particularly in tortuous vessels, given their conformability.

IV. Concomitant Iliac and Infrainguinal Disease

Iliac artery stenting may be combined with infrainguinal bypass in a single hybrid procedure. In this case, surgical cut down is used to expose the common femoral artery, through which retrograde stenting of the ipsilateral iliac artery is performed via an endovascular approach. After successful restoration of adequate inflow, infrainguinal bypass is then carried out in the usual surgical fashion, favoring nonreversed saphenous vein graft (over synthetic grafting) from the common femoral artery to above or below the knee vessels as dictated by the patient's anatomy and atherosclerotic disease burden.

V. Severe Bilateral Iliac Disease

Patients with unilateral complete occlusion of the iliac system and contralateral iliac disease amenable to catheter-based therapy may undergo stenting of the contralateral iliac artery followed by cross-femoral bypass during a single hybrid procedure. This hybrid procedure obviates the need for an aorto-bifemoral bypass, which carries a larger operative morbidity and mortality, particularly in higher risk patients. The hybrid procedure begins with surgical exposure of the femoral arteries ipsilateral to the targeted iliac lesion. After retrograde sheath insertion and stenting of the iliac lesion, cross-femoral bypass can be performed beginning with the synthetic graft anastomosis to the already exposed femoral artery and tunneling of the graft across the pelvis with end to side anastomosis to the contralateral femoral artery.

VI. Infrainguinal Multilevel Disease

In patients with multilevel infrainguinal disease who do not have adequate veins for a single long bypass graft and in whom catheter-based management failed to provide adequate outflow, endovascular therapy of superficial femoral arterial disease can be combined with distal popliteal to calf vessel bypass grafting. In such cases, percutaneous access of the contralateral femoral artery can be used for the endovascular portion of the procedure unless common femoral endarterectomy is also being performed, in which case direct antegrade access via the arteriotomy is preferred.

VII. Common Femoral and Infrainguinal Disease

The combination of common femoral and distal infrainguinal disease may be treated with femoral endarterectomy to begin with as described above, followed by antegrade sheath insertion into the exposed vessel. Antegrade access allows for better support, feedback, and pushability of wires, catheters, and other devices, which may be necessary for distal below-the-knee lesions or chronic total occlusions with calcified proximal caps.

VIII. Hybrid Revascularization Outcomes

Hybrid interventions are becoming increasingly common place given their benefits as summarized in Table 17.1 along with preliminary data to suggest their noninferiority to staged interventions with respect to major outcomes and overall risk. Several studies have demonstrated limb salvage and intervention patency rates to be equivalent for hybrid procedures compared with lone endovascular or surgical treatment strategies. One large retrospective study of 654 patients undergoing lower extremity revascularization with endovascular, surgical, or hybrid strategies showed comparable 3-year limb salvage rates in excess of 80% and similar primary and secondary patency rates along with long term survival.[2] A second study of 162 patients (248 limbs) with iliofemoral occlusive disease undergoing either hybrid iliac stenting and common femoral endarterectomy or surgical aortoiliac and femoral reconstruction demonstrated similar 30-day mortality (1.1% vs 1.4%, $P = .85$) and primary patency at 3 years (91% vs 97%, $P = .29$) which was maintained regardless of TASC lesion status. Overall long-term survival was lower for those undergoing hybrid revascularization (40% vs 74%, $P = .007$), likely owing to the higher risk cardiac status of the patients undergoing hybrid revascularization.[3] Finally, Chang et al., retrospectively studied 171 patients undergoing simultaneous iliac artery stenting or stent grafting with common femoral endarterectomy. Complete iliac artery occlusion was present in 41% of cases, and stent grafts were also used in 41% of cases. The immediate technical success rate was 98%. Five-year primary and secondary patency rates were 60% and 98%, respectively. Endovascular reintervention was required in 14% and inflow surgical bypass in 10% of patients.[4]

IX. Summary

Patients with chronic limb ischemia and multilevel occlusive disease are often treated with a combination of endovascular and surgical techniques to improve claudication or for limb salvage in critical limb ischemia. Performing these procedures in a staged fashion can delay care, reduce patient satisfaction, and increase procedure- and anesthesia-related risks.

Table 17.1. Benefits of Hybrid Lower Extremity Revascularization
1. Complete inflow and outflow revascularization *without delay* inherent in staged procedures
2. Immediate surgical back-up in case of failed or complicated endovascular attempt
3. Reduced femoral access site complications in cases of surgical cut down
4. Reduced overall procedure and anesthesia related risks
5. Improved cost-effectiveness by reducing hospitalization length
6. Immediate angiographic flow assessment of surgical treatment/graft

Consolidating treatment into a single hybrid procedure incorporating both endovascular and surgical therapies provides complete revascularization with improved efficiency and patient satisfaction, lower cumulative procedure-related risks and costs, and equivalent limb salvage outcomes to a staged approach based on the available data. Careful preprocedure planning is necessary and often requires advanced noninvasive imaging to define anatomy and other complexities.

References

1. Ebaugh JL, Gagnon D, Owens CD, Conte MS, Raffetto JD. Comparison of costs of staged versus simultaneous lower extremity arterial hybrid procedures. *Am J Surg.* 2008;196(5):634-640.
2. Dosluoglu HH, Lall P, Cherr GS, Harris LM, Dryjski ML. Role of simple and complex hybrid revascularization procedures for symptomatic lower extremity occlusive disease. *J Vasc Surg.* 2010;51(6):1425-1435.e1.
3. Piazza M, Ricotta JJ, Bower TC, et al. Iliac artery stenting combined with open femoral endarterectomy is as effective as open surgical reconstruction for severe iliac and common femoral occlusive disease. *J Vasc Surg.* 2011;54(2):402-411.
4. Chang RW, Goodney PP, Baek JH, Nolan BW, Rzucidlo EM, Powell RJ. Long-term results of combined common femoral endarterectomy and iliac stenting/stent grafting for occlusive disease. *J Vasc Surg.* 2008;48(2):362-367.

CHAPTER 18

Pharmacotherapy in Peripheral Artery Disease

Faisal Hasan, MD,
Khwaja Yousuf Hasan, MBBS,
William L. Bennett, MD, PhD, and
Sameh Mohareb, MD

Key Points

- Treatment of hypertension with ACEI has been shown to have antiatherogenic properties as well as reduced clinical events in patient with peripheral arterial disease (PAD).
- Aspirin monotherapy has been shown to be of benefit in treatment of secondary prevention patient with peripheral arterial disease.
- Statin therapy is known to improve morbidity and mortality in patients with peripheral arterial disease.
- Smoking cessation and supervised walking programs have shown benefit in patients with PAD.

I. Introduction

Peripheral artery disease (PAD) is a manifestation of systemic atherosclerosis. It is associated with a reduction in functional capacity and quality of life, but more importantly, presence of PAD is associated with an increased risk of cardiovascular and cerebrovascular morbidity and mortality compared with the general population.[1] Treatment of PAD is based on lifestyle modification, relief of symptoms, and aggressive treatment of risk factors of atherosclerosis. This includes aggressive management of hypertension, dyslipidemia, diabetes mellitus, antiplatelet therapy, cessation of smoking, and graded exercise prescription. Guideline-directed medical therapy (GDMT) has been shown to reduce cardiovascular events and improve functional status of patients with PAD. However, these patients are less likely to receive GDMT than patients with other forms of cardiovascular disease such as coronary artery disease.[2]

Medical management of PAD has a proven role in improving cardiovascular outcomes and functional capacity. Therapy with antiplatelet agents has been shown to improve cardiovascular and lower extremity atherosclerotic disease outcomes among patients with symptomatic or asymptomatic PAD irrespective of revascularization. Treatment of hypertension with ACE inhibitors has been shown to decrease clinical events in patients with PAD. ACE inhibitors have also been shown to have antiatherogenic properties that would have favorable effects in PAD. Statins have been shown to lower the risk of adverse limb outcomes of revascularization and amputation as well as reduce symptoms in PAD.

II. Antithrombotic Therapy

A. **Antiplatelet Agents** Antiplatelet agents have been studied extensively in cardiovascular diseases. The Antithrombotic Trialists' Collaboration studies have shown that antiplatelet therapy is associated with a mortality benefit that is driven primarily by a significant reduction in myocardial infarction, stroke, and vascular death among patients with PAD.[3] The recently published American Heart Association/American College of Cardiology and European Society of Cardiology guidelines on PAD endorse the long-term use of single antiplatelet agents (aspirin or clopidogrel) in patients with symptomatic

PAD for prevention of major adverse cardiac events.[4,5] Their role in asymptomatic patients with PAD (that is ABI <0.9) or with atypical symptoms is uncertain; however, it is still recommended, as aspirin has been shown to reduce the risk of vascular events in this population as well.[6]

1. **Aspirin** acts by irreversibly inhibiting cyclooxygenase-2 and prevents formation of thromboxane A2 from arachidonic acid.[7] It has been shown to reduce the risk of myocardial infarction, stroke, and death from cardiovascular events in patients with symptomatic and asymptomatic PAD. The use of aspirin for secondary prevention has been well established by the Antithrombotic Trialists' Collaboration studies. A meta-analysis of 287 studies involving more than 200,000 patients compared different antiplatelet regimens or antiplatelet agents with controls. Antiplatelet therapy resulted in a reduction in outcomes of myocardial infarction by 33%, reduction in stroke by 25% and reduction in vascular death by 17% without any apparent side effects.[3] Similarly in a meta-analysis of 60 studies (mostly aspirin alone or in combination with dipyridamole) antiplatelet therapy was associated with a significant reduction in arterial or venous graft occlusion among patients undergoing any form of a vascular procedure.[8] The role of aspirin in primary prevention has been less well established. The Aspirin for Asymptomatic Atherosclerosis (AAA) trial examined the role of aspirin in patients with subclinical PAD (ABI [ankle-brachial index] <0.95). The primary endpoint of the study was an initial fatal or nonfatal myocardial infarction, stroke, or need for revascularization. There was no difference in the primary endpoint among patients who received aspirin or placebo over a follow-up of 8.2 years.[9] The POPAD trial similarly compared use of aspirin and antioxidants versus placebo among diabetic patients with subclinical PAD. Again, no difference was found in the primary endpoints of nonfatal or fatal cardiovascular events despite the high-risk profile of the patients.[10]

2. The **adenosine diphosphate** (ADP) P2Y12 receptor antagonists include the **thienopyridines (ticlopidine, clopidogrel, prasugrel)** and **ticagrelor**. Thienopyridines are irreversible antagonists, whereas ticagrelor is a reversible antagonist of the ADP receptor.[11,12] Ticlopidine was found to be very effective in prevention of vascular events; however, its use has been discontinued because significant hematologic side effects. Only clopidogrel and ticagrelor have been studied in patients with PAD. The CAPRIE (Clopidogrel versus Aspirin in Patients at Risk of Ischemic Events) was a large multicenter double-blinded randomized controlled trial that compared aspirin with clopidogrel for secondary prevention in patients who had evidence of atherosclerotic disease.[13] The PAD cohort included patients who had intermittent claudication with an ABI of <0.85 or those who had intermittent claudication and had undergone a peripheral vascular intervention in the form of surgical or percutaneous revascularization. Generally, the results of the trial favored the use of clopidogrel over aspirin monotherapy for PAD; however, the absolute benefit was small, albeit statistically significant. The PLATO (ticagrelor versus clopidogrel in patients with acute coronary

syndrome) trial established the superiority of ticagrelor over clopidogrel in acute coronary syndrome.[14] In light of these findings, it was hypothesized that similar findings could be extrapolated among patients with PAD. The EUCLID (Examining Use of Ticagrelor in Peripheral Artery Disease) trial was carried out to test this hypothesis; however, it failed to establish the superiority of ticagrelor over clopidogrel in PAD.[15] There were no significant differences in the primary and secondary endpoints among both drugs; however, there was a higher rate of discontinuation of ticagrelor due to side effects (mainly dyspnea and minor bleeding). Both the ACC and ESC guidelines to date recommend the use of clopidogrel or aspirin as single antiplatelet therapy for prevention of major adverse cardiac events in patients with PAD.[4,5]

B. **Benefits of Antiplatelet Therapy** The overall benefit of dual antiplatelet therapy for symptomatic PAD is uncertain. A post hoc analysis of the Clopidogrel for High Atherothrombotic Risk and Ischemic Stabilization, Management and Avoidance (CHARISMA) trial failed to demonstrate a significant benefit of dual antiplatelet therapy with clopidogrel and aspirin over aspirin alone in prevention of major adverse cardiac events with an increase in the risk of minor bleeding.[16,17] However, a small randomized controlled trial demonstrated a decrease in the risk of revascularization among patients who had undergone endovascular revascularization with use of dual antiplatelet therapy.[18,19] Similarly, a decrease in limb-related events was noted among patients who had undergone below-knee prosthetic bypass grafts.[20] Therefore dual antiplatelet therapy may only be reasonable in a small subset of patients with PAD who have had surgical or endovascular revascularization.

C. **Vorapaxar** Vorapaxar is a novel PAR-1 receptor antagonist, which is the principle thrombin receptor on platelets and is also present on vascular endothelium. The TRA2°P-TIMI 50 was a double-blind randomized controlled trial that tested the efficacy of vorapaxar on top of standard antiplatelet therapy for secondary prevention among patients with stable atherosclerotic disease and evidence of lower extremity arterial disease.[21] Vorapaxar did not reduce the risk of myocardial infarction, death, or stroke; however, it significantly reduced the incidence of acute limb ischemia and peripheral revascularization. The trial demonstrated a reduction in risk of both native artery and bypass graft thrombosis. This benefit was offset by an increase in the risk of moderate and severe bleeding including intracranial hemorrhage. Vorapaxar may provide some clinical benefit among patients with acute limb ischemia; however, its overall efficacy on top of existing antiplatelet therapy among patients with symptomatic PAD is unclear and warrants further research.

D. **Heparin** Systemic anticoagulation with heparin or a direct thrombin inhibitor is indicated in patients who present with acute limb ischemia. Anticoagulation with heparin prevents thrombus propagation and reduces inflammation.[22,23] Anticoagulation with warfarin for PAD is not recommended. Warfarin has been demonstrated to increase risk of bleeding and subsequently increase mortality among patients with PAD when added to aspirin. The guidelines do not recommend the routine use of warfarin or vitamin K antagonists in addition to aspirin in PAD.

E. **Oral Anticoagulation Agents** Recently, there has been a lot of interest in the role of novel oral anticoagulation agents in secondary cardiovascular prevention. These agents have been extensively studied and approved for prevention of thromboembolism associated with nonvalvular atrial fibrillation. They include rivaroxaban, edoxaban, dabigatran, and apixaban. Rivaroxaban is a powerful factor Xa inhibitor; it binds to free factor Xa and factor Xa associated with prothrombinase complex. The recently published COMPASS trial is an international, double-blind randomized controlled trial that compared low-dose rivaroxaban in combination with aspirin (rivaroxaban 2.5 mg twice a day plus aspirin 100 mg), rivaroxaban (5 mg twice a day) alone, and aspirin (100 mg) alone for secondary cardiovascular prevention. The trial was stopped prematurely at 23 months because of superiority of the low-dose rivaroxaban and aspirin group.[24] The trial enrolled 7470 patients with lower extremity PAD and carotid artery disease. Among patients with PAD, addition of low-dose rivaroxaban to aspirin when compared with aspirin alone resulted in a 28% reduction in major adverse cardiovascular events and a 46% reduction in limb-threatening ischemia including amputation. However, there was an increase in the risk of major nonfatal bleeding in the rivaroxaban and aspirin combination group. Therefore, the role of novel oral anticoagulation agents in PAD is not yet completely established. Further trials are needed to clarify the role of these agents in the prevention and treatment of PAD.

III. Statins

A. **Hyperlipidemia** Hyperlipidemia is closely associated with the atherosclerosis. Statins are HMG-CoA reductase inhibitors, the principal enzyme involved in endogenous cholesterol synthesis. Statins inhibit cholesterol biosynthesis, increase uptake and degradation of low-density lipoproteins, decrease the secretion of lipoproteins, and inhibit LDL oxidation. Statins also modulate intracellular processes that reduce accumulation of esterified cholesterol in macrophages, increase activity of nitric oxide synthetase, decrease the inflammatory process, and increase stability of atherosclerotic plaques.[25] Lipid-lowering therapy with statins is associated with a reduction in symptoms, morbidity, and mortality associated with cardiovascular disease.

B. **Trials** Trials with simvastatin and atorvastatin have demonstrated an improvement in walking distance in patients with PAD.

1. In the Heart Protection Study (HPS Study), simvastatin therapy was associated with a 17% reduction in vascular mortality, 24% reduction in coronary artery events, and a 27% reduction in stroke among patients with PAD at 5 years, regardless of their presenting cholesterol levels.[26] Conversely, similar trials with bezafibrate and high-dose niacin failed to demonstrate a reduction in fatal and nonfatal cardiovascular events. This proves that it is not just the lipid-lowering effects of statins but also the pleiotropic effects that may be responsible for the mortality benefit that statins provide for cardiovascular diseases. Treatment with statin therapy is also associated with improvement in symptoms of claudication.

2. A Cochrane systematic review of 18 trials involving more than 10,000 patients demonstrated that lipid-lowering with statins is associated with a reduction in cardiovascular morbidity and mortality and an improvement in local symptoms.[27]

3. Results from the REACH registry also demonstrate that statin therapy is associated with a reduction in adverse limb outcomes, including worsening symptoms, need for revascularization, and amputation-free survival. In another study, use of statins was associated with a reduction in major adverse cardiac events and all-cause mortality among patients with asymptomatic patients with PAD.[28] Therefore, all patients with PAD should be treated with statins.

IV. Antihypertensive Therapy

Trials The angiotensin-converting enzyme inhibitors have vasculo-protective, antiproliferative, and antiatherogenic properties. They promote the degradation of bradykinin, which increases the endothelial release of nitrous oxide and decreases endothelial oxidative stress.

1. The HOPE (Heart Outcomes Prevention Evaluation) trial was a large multicenter randomized control trial of more than 9000 patients.[29] It demonstrated that use of ramipril in high-risk cardiovascular patients, who did not have a low ejection fraction or evidence of heart failure, was associated with a 25% reduction in risk of myocardial infarction, death, and stroke. The HOPE study prompted an interest in the use of ACE inhibitors for patients with symptomatic PAD. A small study of 212 patients demonstrated that after 6 months of treatment with ramipril, patients with PAD and intermittent claudication were able to walk significantly longer distances pain free as compared with patients who received placebo.[30]

2. The ONTARGET trial compared use of telmisartan, ramipril, and combination therapy in patients with PAD.[31] The trial established the efficacy of telmisartan in PAD and demonstrated it to be an acceptable alternative to ramipril. Patients who received a combination of ramipril and telmisartan had a higher rate of side effects, which included hypotension, renal failure, and syncope; thus combined use of an ACE inhibitor and an angiotensin receptor blocker is not recommended.

V. Symptomatic Therapy for Claudication

Cilostazol

1. Cilostazol is a selective phosphodiesterase-3 inhibitor. It is very effective in improving walking distance and symptoms of claudication. It increases the amount of cyclic AMP (cAMP) resulting in an increase in protein kinase A, which inhibits activation of myosin light-chain kinase. This prevents smooth muscle contraction in the arterial vascular bed, causing vasodilation. Cilostazol has been studied extensively in PAD and its use is associated with a decrease in the symptoms of claudication without an improvement in cardiovascular outcomes or an improvement in quality of life.[32] Its important side effects include abdominal diarrhea, headache, and dizziness. Cilostazol is contraindicated in patients with congestive heart failure.

2. Therapies such as pentoxifylline and chelation therapy have proven to be ineffective in PAD and are not recommended.[33,34] Management of PAD would be incomplete without having a comprehensive approach toward maintaining a healthy lifestyle that would include good glycemic control, maintaining optimal blood pressure, quitting smoking, and following a supervised home-based or hospital-based exercise regimen.

References

1. Grenon SM, Vittinghoff E, Owens CD, Conte MS, Whooley M, Cohen BE. Peripheral artery disease and risk of cardiovascular events in patients with coronary artery disease: insights from the Heart and Soul Study. *Vasc Med.* 2013;18(4):176-184.
2. Krishnamurthy V, Munir K, Rectenwald JE, et al. Contemporary outcomes with percutaneous vascular interventions for peripheral critical limb ischemia in those with and without poly-vascular disease. *Vasc Med.* 2014;19(6):491-499.
3. Collaboration AT. Collaborative meta-analysis of randomised trials of antiplatelet therapy for prevention of death, myocardial infarction, and stroke in high risk patients. *BMJ.* 2002;324(7329):71-86.
4. Aboyans V, Ricco JB, Bartelink MEL, et al. 2017 ESC guidelines on the diagnosis and treatment of peripheral arterial diseases, in collaboration with the European Society for Vascular Surgery (ESVS): document covering atherosclerotic disease of extracranial carotid and vertebral, mesenteric, renal, upper and lower extremity arteries Endorsed by: the European Stroke Organization (ESO) the task force for the diagnosis and treatment of peripheral arterial diseases of the European Society of Cardiology (ESC) and of the European Society for Vascular Surgery (ESVS). *Eur Heart J.* 2017;39(9):763-816.
5. Gerhard-Herman MD, Gornik HL, Barrett C, et al. 2016 AHA/ACC guideline on the management of patients with lower extremity peripheral artery disease: a report of the American College of Cardiology/American Heart Association Task Force on Clinical Practice Guidelines. *J Am Coll Cardiol.* 2017;69(11):e71-e126.
6. Diehm C, Allenberg JR, Pittrow D, et al. Mortality and vascular morbidity in older adults with asymptomatic versus symptomatic peripheral artery disease. *Circulation.* 2009;120(21):2053-2061.
7. Catella-Lawson F, Reilly MP, Kapoor SC, et al. Cyclooxygenase inhibitors and the antiplatelet effects of aspirin. *N Engl J Med.* 2001;345(25):1809-1817.
8. Collaboration AT. Collaborative overview of randomised trials of antiplatelet therapy-II: Maintenance of vascular graft or arterial patency by antiplatelet therapy. *BMJ.* 1994;308(6922):159-168.
9. Fowkes FG, Price JF, Stewart MC, et al. Aspirin for prevention of cardiovascular events in a general population screened for a low ankle brachial index: a randomized controlled trial. *JAMA.* 2010;303(9):841-848.
10. Belch J, MacCuish A, Campbell I, et al. The prevention of progression of arterial disease and diabetes (POPADAD) trial: factorial randomised placebo controlled trial of aspirin and antioxidants in patients with diabetes and asymptomatic peripheral arterial disease. *BMJ.* 2008;337:a1840.
11. Capodanno D, Dharmashankar K, Angiolillo DJ. Mechanism of action and clinical development of ticagrelor, a novel platelet ADP P2Y12 receptor antagonist. *Expert review of cardiovascular therapy.* 2010;8(2):151-158.
12. Savi P, Nurden P, Nurden AT, Levy-Toledano S, Herbert JM. Clopidogrel: a review of its mechanism of action. *Platelets.* 1998;9(3-4):251-255.
13. Committee CS. A randomised, blinded, trial of clopidogrel versus aspirin in patients at risk of ischaemic events (CAPRIE). CAPRIE Steering Committee. *Lancet.* 1996;348(9038):1329-1339.
14. Wallentin L, Becker RC, Budaj A, et al. Ticagrelor versus clopidogrel in patients with acute coronary syndromes. *N Engl J Med.* 2009;361(11):1045-1057.
15. Hiatt WR, Fowkes FG, Heizer G, et al. Ticagrelor versus Clopidogrel in symptomatic peripheral artery disease. *N Engl J Med.* 2017;376(1):32-40.
16. Cacoub PP, Bhatt DL, Steg PG, Topol EJ, Creager MA, Investigators C. Patients with peripheral arterial disease in the CHARISMA trial. *Eur Heart J.* 2009;30(2):192-201.

17. Bhatt DL, Fox KA, Hacke W, et al. Clopidogrel and aspirin versus aspirin alone for the prevention of atherothrombotic events. *N Engl J Med.* 2006;354(16):1706-1717.
18. Tepe G, Bantleon R, Brechtel K, et al. Management of peripheral arterial interventions with mono or dual antiplatelet therapy–the MIRROR study: a randomised and double-blinded clinical trial. *Eur Radiol.* 2012;22(9):1998-2006.
19. Strobl FF, Brechtel K, Schmehl J, et al. Twelve-month results of a randomized trial comparing mono with dual antiplatelet therapy in endovascularly treated patients with peripheral artery disease. *J Endovasc Ther.* 2013;20(5):699-706.
20. Belch JJ, Dormandy J, Biasi GM, et al. Results of the randomized, placebo-controlled clopidogrel and acetylsalicylic acid in bypass surgery for peripheral arterial disease (CASPAR) trial. *J Vasc Surg.* 2010;52(4):825-833, 33.e1-2.
21. Bonaca MP, Scirica BM, Creager MA, et al. Vorapaxar in patients with peripheral artery disease: results from TRA2°P-TIMI 50. *Circulation.* 2013;127(14):1522-1529. doi:10.1161/CIRCULATIONAHA.112.000679.
22. Blaisdell F, Steele M, Allen R. Management of acute lower extremity arterial ischemia due to embolism and thrombosis. *Surgery.* 1978;84(6):822-834.
23. Turba UC, Bozlar U, Simsek S. Catheter-directed thrombolysis of acute lower extremity arterial thrombosis in a patient with heparin-induced thrombocytopenia. *Catheter Cardiovasc Interv.* 2007;70(7):1046-1050.
24. Eikelboom JW, Connolly SJ, Bosch J, et al. Rivaroxaban with or without Aspirin in stable cardiovascular disease. *N Engl J Med.* 2017;377(14):1319-1330.
25. Stancu C, Sima A. Statins: mechanism of action and effects. *J Cell Mol Med.* 2001;5(4):378-387.
26. Group HPSC. Randomized trial of the effects of cholesterol-lowering with simvastatin on peripheral vascular and other major vascular outcomes in 20,536 people with peripheral arterial disease and other high-risk conditions. *J Vasc Surg.* 2007;45(4):645-654; discussion 53-4.
27. Taylor F, Huffman MD, Macedo AF, et al. Statins for the primary prevention of cardiovascular disease. *Cochrane Database Syst Rev.* 2013;(1):CD004816.
28. Kumbhani DJ, Steg PG, Cannon CP, et al. Statin therapy and long-term adverse limb outcomes in patients with peripheral artery disease: insights from the REACH registry. *Eur Heart J.* 2014;35(41):2864-2872.
29. Yusuf S, Sleight P, Pogue J, et al. Effects of an angiotensin-converting-enzyme inhibitor, ramipril, on cardiovascular events in high-risk patients. *N Engl J Med.* 2000;342(3):145-153.
30. Kurklinsky AK, Levy M. Effect of ramipril on walking times and quality of life among patients with peripheral artery disease and intermittent claudication: a randomized controlled trial. *J Am Med Assoc.* 2013;309:453-460. *Vasc Med.* 2013;18(4):234-236.
31. Yusuf S, Teo KK, Pogue J, et al. Telmisartan, ramipril, or both in patients at high risk for vascular events. *N Engl J Med.* 2008;358(15):1547-1559.
32. Bedenis R, Stewart M, Cleanthis M, Robless P, Mikhailidis DP, Stansby G. Cilostazol for intermittent claudication. *Cochrane Database Syst Rev.* 2014;(10):CD003748.
33. Salhiyyah K, Senanayake E, Abdel-Hadi M, Booth A, Michaels JA. Pentoxifylline for intermittent claudication. *Cochrane Database Syst Rev.* 2012;1:CD005262.
34. Villarruz MV, Dans A, Tan F. Chelation therapy for atherosclerotic cardiovascular disease. *Cochrane Database Syst Rev.* 2002(4):CD002785.

CHAPTER 19

Vascular Access Complications

Sameer Nagpal, MD and Young Erben, MD

I. Introduction

The dramatic increase in endovascular procedures by 317% from 2000 to 2009 has led us to encounter procedural complications in greater frequency.[1] Furthermore, the development of newer endovascular technologies have uncovered a newer set of complications related to these techniques. We can classify these complications into (1) access site complications, (2) complications related to the use of wires and catheters, (3) intervention specific complications, and (4) miscellaneous.

II. Access Site Complication

A. **Hematoma** Access site bleeding is the most common complication of endovascular procedures, with an incidence of groin hematoma reported as high as 23%, dependent on a variety of procedure- and patient-related circumstances.[2,3] Modifiable risk factors include puncture technique, chosen access site, larger sheath size and indwelling time, and the aggressive use of antiplatelet and anticoagulant medications. Nonmodifiable risk factors include obesity, anatomic anomalies, hypertension, chronic renal insufficiency, female gender, low body weight, obesity, coagulopathy, and inability to cooperate with postprocedural restrictions.[4]

Bleeding is most commonly an immediate complication; however, it may occur up to 48 hours after the procedure in cases requiring ongoing use of anticoagulants. Localized hematoma is the most common presentation, resulting from extravasation of blood from the arteriotomy site into the surrounding soft tissue. Ultrasound is occasionally used to confirm the diagnosis if physical examination findings are equivocal (Fig. 19.1), most often in obese patients. In cases of access site hematoma with significant pain, ultrasound may be necessary to exclude associated pseudoaneurysm or arteriovenous fistula. In the vast majority of cases, extended manual or device-assisted compression of the arteriotomy site and gentle manual diffusion of the hematoma is all that is needed. Transfusion is generally reserved for cases of significant blood loss, evidence of new or worsening myocardial ischemia, or hemodynamic instability.

1. **Femoral Access Site Bleeding** Femoral access site bleeding is correlated with a longer hospitalization and higher rates of morbidity and mortality at 30 days post procedure, especially when transfusion is required.[2,5]

   The modified Seldinger technique is the most commonly used method of gaining femoral arterial access. Technical and anatomic precision are critical to minimizing the risk of bleeding. Arterial puncture should occur within the common femoral artery (CFA), below the inguinal ligament and above its bifurcation, directly over the middle one-third of the femoral head. Puncture at this site allows for manual compression against a noncompliant structure to achieve adequate hemostasis. Superficially, this location is approximately 1-2 cm below the inguinal ligament half way between the anterior superior iliac crest and the pubic symphysis. The inguinal skin crease should not be used as a landmark for arterial puncture as it is located below the femoral artery bifurcation in 70% of patients. Fluoroscopy is routinely used

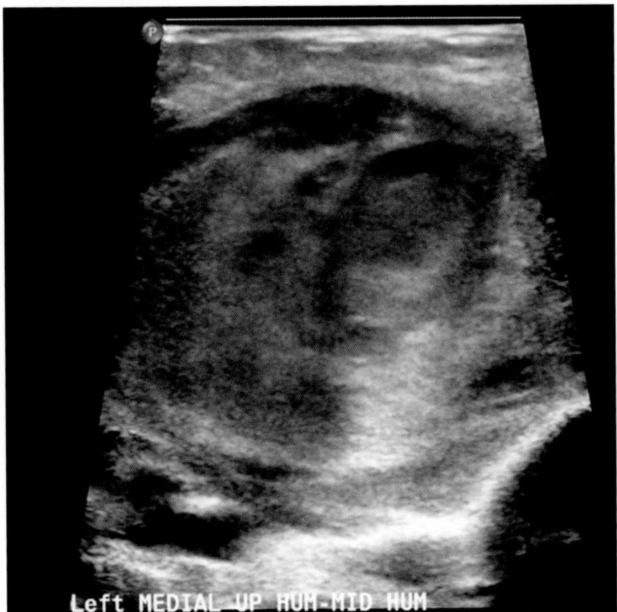

FIGURE 19.1: Ultrasound image of a soft tissue hematoma.

to locate the femoral head and assist in guiding anatomically precise CFA cannulation. Care must also be taken to avoid puncture of the posterior wall of the femoral artery from which bleeding may be less readily apparent. The use of a micropuncture needle is generally preferred to reduce arterial trauma in case multiple attempts at access are needed.

2. **Retroperitoneal Hemorrhage** Retroperitoneal (RP) hemorrhage is a rare but dreaded complication of high femoral arterial puncture above the inguinal ligament and occurs in approximately 0.3%-0.8% of cases involving femoral arterial access.[2,6,7] The etiology is usually injury to a suprainguinal vessel or puncture of the posterior wall of the femoral or external iliac artery. Other than this, traditional risk factors include (1) female gender, (2) peripheral vascular disease, and (3) low body surface area.[4,6] RP hemorrhage has two potential manifestations. First, the hemorrhage may be contained within the fascia of the iliopsoas muscle, which can be associated with compression neuropathy involving the lumbar plexus. Second, the RP hemorrhage may occur within the space between the peritoneum and RP structures, which is large enough to accommodate life threatening amounts of blood loss (Fig. 19.2). One report classified the most common presenting signs and symptoms of RP hemorrhage in 26 patients, which were hypotension (92%), diaphoresis (58%), groin discomfort (46%), abdominal or flank pain (42%), bradycardia (31%), and back pain (23%).[6] Bruising of the flanks, described as "Grey Turner" sign, or the umbilicus, known as "Cullen" sign is typically a late manifestation. Occasionally, RP bleeding can present as a "vagal" reaction with bradycardia and diaphoresis, typically thought of as a benign response to pain or sheath removal, but only transiently responsive to intravenous fluids and atropine. Noncontrast abdominal and pelvic computed tomography

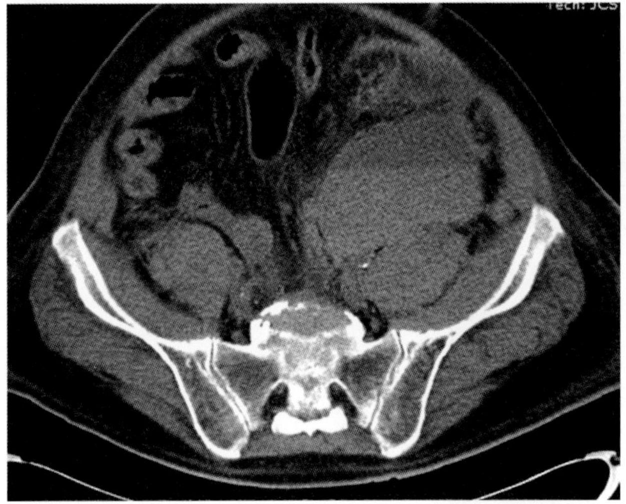

FIGURE 19.2: Axial cut of a computed tomography with a left retroperitoneal hematoma.

scan is highly sensitive and specific for confirming the diagnosis and is also helpful in identifying possible hydronephrosis due to ipsilateral ureter or bladder compression. Successful management depends on early recognition, supportive care with intravenous fluids, blood products, and optimizing the coagulation and platelet profile is all that is usually required until hemostasis is naturally achieved. In uncommon cases of extreme hemodynamic consequence consideration should be given to urgent angiography with prolonged percutaneous balloon inflation at the arteriotomy site, use of a covered stent, or surgical exploration and direct repair of the arteriotomy site.

3. **Radial, Brachial, and Distal Lower Extremity Access Site Hemorrhage** Compared with femoral arterial access, rates of major bleeding (OR = 0.53), all-cause mortality (OR = 0.71), and major adverse cardiovascular events (OR = 0.84) are lower with radial arterial access in patients undergoing percutaneous coronary intervention according to a 2016 meta-analysis of over 22,000 patients.[8] This is due to the radial artery's smaller caliber and superficial course, limiting internal bleeding and allowing easy compression of external bleeding. Localized hematomas may require extended manual compression of the arteriotomy site, arm elevation, and application of ice. If unrecognized, however, hematoma formation within the wrist may spread briskly from local infiltration of the soft tissue to involvement of a significant portion of the forearm. Rarely, signs of vascular compromise including pain, pallor, paresthesia, and paralysis may ensue, signifying compartment syndrome and requiring surgical evacuation to prevent tissue necrosis and restore vascular integrity.

B. **Arteriovenous Fistula** An arteriovenous fistula (AVF) is an abnormal communication between an artery and a vein. The incidence of clinically detected postcatheterization femoral AVF ranges from 0.006% to 0.86% from published data including one large prospective study surveying over 10,000 patients for 3 years.[9-14] When routine duplex scanning is used post procedure, the reported incidence in one study was 2.8%, with all patients being asymptomatic.[15] The main etiology is proximate puncture of an artery and vein such as with simultaneous right and left heart catheterization or through-and-through puncture of an artery into its accompanying vein. Risk factors include low femoral puncture (below the bifurcation), left-sided or multiple femoral punctures, simultaneous arterial and venous access, higher levels of anticoagulation, hypertension, and female gender.[16]

The average shunt volume of an iatrogenic fistula is 160-510 mL/min, less than that needed to cause cardiac impairment, which typically occurs when shunt volume is approximately 30% of resting cardiac output.[9] Arterial insufficiency and venous hypertension are the two main consequences of arterial-venous shunting. Flow within the distal artery is diminished or reversed when the area of the fistula exceeds the diameter of the inflow artery by threefold and flow in the proximal artery increases up to 8-fold.[17,18] The proximal vein diameter increases with increasing flow with no change in antegrade flow in the distal vein.[19] Over time, the proximal artery enlarges, and thinning of the arterial wall with aneurysmal dilation occurs. The proximal vein, exposed to pulsatile flow, also enlarges and the wall of the vein becomes arterialized.[20]

1. **Diagnosis** The history and physical examination may indicate the presence of an AVF. Most patients are asymptomatic, and the most common presenting sign is the presence of a palpable thrill or bruit heard on auscultation, or a pulsatile mass. Rarely, large fistulas with high shunt volumes may present with symptoms related to arterial insufficiency, venous hypertension, or high-output congestive heart failure.

   Confirmation and characterization of an AVF can reliably be made with Doppler ultrasonography. Findings include visualization of turbulent bidirectional flow at the level of the fistula, loss of triphasic waveforms in the proximal artery with high peak systolic velocities, decreased flow in the distal artery, and elevated pulsatile venous outflow peak systolic velocities.

2. **Management** The natural history of iatrogenic AVFs is that many will close spontaneously. One study with a 3-year follow-up of postcatheterization femoral AVFs demonstrated a spontaneous closure rate of 38%, all occurring within 1 year. The median time to closure was 3 months.[9] A second study reported an 81% spontaneous closure rate, 90% of which were closed within 4 months.[21] Anticoagulation was the only identified risk factor for persistence of an AVF, which inhibits thrombus formation required for closure.[9] In light of this, asymptomatic small or medium-sized AVFs may be conservatively managed with close surveillance by duplex ultrasonography.

   For symptomatic patients, or those with large AVFs unlikely to spontaneously close or likely to result in symptoms, intervention is indicated. The goal is closure of the fistula, normalization of cardiac and circulatory hemodynamics, and reestablishment of vascular continuity. The use of duplex ultrasound-guided compression therapy has been generally unsuccessful, rendering this an unfavorable noninvasive treatment option. Endovascular and open surgical management are the mainstays of therapy. Endovascular techniques are generally reserved for high surgical risk patients or those with challenging anatomic considerations such as marked obesity, prior groin surgeries, or significant venous collaterals, which increase bleeding risk.

Endovascular options include embolization (using autologous clot, gelatin sponge, microfibrillar collagen, polyvinyl alcohol particles, metal coils, detachable balloons, and liquid agents such as N-butyl cyanoacrylate) and, more commonly, covered stent-grafting. The use of intra-arterial covered stents in the femoral position poses the risk of occluding side branches and limiting future percutaneous access sites. SFA stent grafts for iatrogenic femoral AVFs have a reported 1 year patency rate of greater than 80%.[22-25] Surgical repair for acute or chronic AVFs is often the treatment of choice for good surgical candidates with favorable anatomy. In chronic AVF with significant venous hypertension, preoperative endovascular placement of arterial or venous balloons may minimize blood loss. Repair of the fistula usually requires proximal and distal control of both vessels. Vein patch angioplasty or interposition bypass grafts are used for repair of a large AVF.

C. **Pseudoaneurysm** Pseudoaneurysms (PSAs), also known as false aneurysms, result from a contained rupture of the arterial wall, and they form when the arteriotomy site has not sealed after sheath removal or when hemostasis is disrupted. Arterial injury allows for pulsatile blood flow into the confined adjacent perivascular space, which communicates with the arterial lumen through a narrow channel, commonly referred to as a neck. Unlike true aneurysms, PSAs do not involve all three layers of the arterial wall and therefore are prone to rupture. In the femoral artery, PSAs are usually caused by low arterial puncture, as the spatial constraints of the thigh contain the arterial rupture. Most PSAs occur within 3 days of sheath removal. PSAs may be complicated by distal embolization and extrinsic compression on adjacent neurovascular structures, potentially causing neuropathy, deep venous thrombosis, and rarely, local tissue or limb ischemia.

The incidence of PSA after diagnostic catheterization ranges from 0.05% to 2% and rises as high as 8% when complex interventions are performed, especially when antithrombotic and antiplatelet therapy is administered.[7,26-28] One study reported that 83% of PSAs were related to interventional procedures.[28]

Several patient and procedural risk factors contribute to the formation of PSAs, the most important of which are inadequate period of manual compression and low femoral arterial puncture (within the superficial femoral artery). Other risk factors include large bore sheaths (>8F), use of anticoagulant and antiplatelet therapy, obesity, hypertension, peripheral arterial disease, hemodialysis, complexity of interventions, and advanced age (>65 y old).[29]

1. **Diagnosis** Patients with postcatheterization femoral artery PSA commonly present with pain and swelling in the affected groin. Signs or symptoms of neuropathy, deep venous thrombosis, local soft tissue ischemia, or acute limb ischemia due to distal thromboembolism may be present if the PSA is large enough to compress neurovascular structures. Physical examination may demonstrate a pulsatile mass with a systolic bruit. Some patients present with pain out of proportion to that which is expected from an endovascular procedure, and in these cases, PSA should be definitively excluded. Some patients, however, may be entirely asymptomatic and with a benign physical examination in the setting of a small PSA.

The diagnosis is confirmed by the use of duplex ultrasonography, which carries a sensitivity of 94% and specificity of 97% for the detection of PSA.[30] PSAs are identified as an echo lucent sac communicating with the arterial lumen through a luminal channel (neck). Color Doppler may demonstrate pulsatile swirling flow into the sac (ying-yang sign), and pulsed-wave Doppler interrogation of the neck typically demonstrates blood flow into and out of the PSA sac and arterial lumen. The size of the PSA, the presence and size of chambers, associated neck, and venous and arterial flow both proximal and distal to the PSA should all be assessed carefully by duplex ultrasound. In cases where duplex ultrasound (Fig. 19.3) is unavailable or the results are equivocal, intravenous contrast enhanced computed tomography (CT) imaging can be used to diagnose PSA.

2. **Management** Strategies widely available for the treatment of postcatheterization PSA include observation, ultrasound-guided compression, ultrasound-guided thrombin injection, surgical repair, and in rare instances, endovascular repair.

   In most cases of small (<2 cm) and asymptomatic PSA, spontaneous thrombosis and resolution often occurs within 1 month.[21] Surveillance duplex ultrasound is required to ensure resolution. Possible activity restriction, uncertainty of clinical course, and repeated ultrasound testing are downsides to this approach.

   Ultrasound-guided compression is a noninvasive treatment for uncomplicated PSAs with a success rates between 72% and 88%.[31,32] The technique is contraindicated in suprainguinal femoral artery and anastomotic PSAs. The ultrasound transducer is used to apply direct pressure over the neck of the PSA, which obstructs flow into the aneurysmal sac, and this is immediately confirmed with Doppler imaging. Compression is applied on average for 30-50 minutes until thrombosis within the

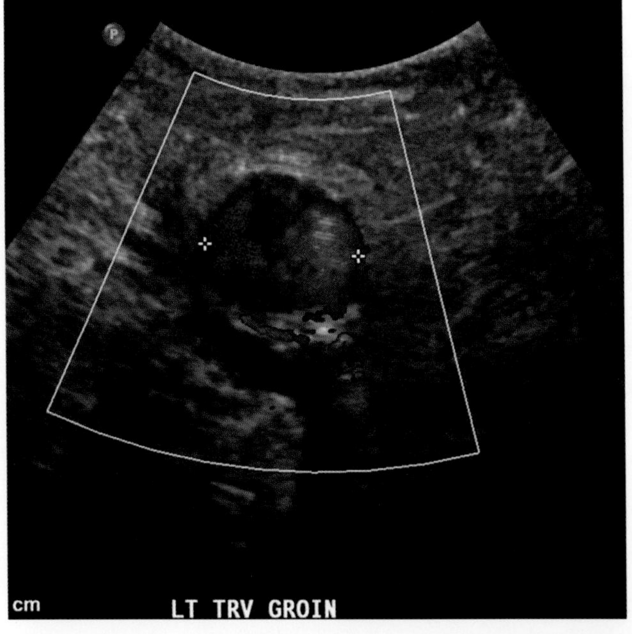

FIGURE 19.3: Common femoral artery PSA. Notice the "yin-yang" sign.

sac is achieved. This technique is challenging in patients who are obese, on chronic anticoagulation, and/or dual anti-platelet therapy, and those with large sized PSA (>4 cm). The presence of one or more of these factors dramatically reduces the success rate and raises complication rates.

Ultrasound-guided thrombin injection is a minimally invasive method widely accepted as the treatment of choice for uncomplicated postcatheterization PSA with an average success rate of over 95% as reported by numerous studies.[29] The technique involves the percutaneous injection of thrombin (as an off-label use) into the PSA sac using ultrasound guidance. Compared with ultrasound-guided compression, thrombin injection is better tolerated, carries a higher procedural success rate, and remains effective in those on anticoagulation, with large PSAs, or when used in cases involving the suprainguinal femoral artery. Arterial thrombosis is a rare but known complication, with the majority occurring in small PSAs.

Surgical repair of postcatheterization PSA was a mainstay of therapy until the 1990s when percutaneous thrombin injection was introduced. However, surgery remains critical in the management of PSAs that are rapid expanding, ruptured, infected, compressing adjacent neurovascular structures resulting in neuropathy, limb or local tissue ischemia, or venous thrombosis, or for those located at an anastomotic site. Surgical repair is often performed for postcatheterization suprainguinal femoral and upper extremity PSAs due to the higher rate of associated neuropathy in brachial artery PSAs. Repair of the arterial wall defect with interrupted polypropylene suture is most often performed, although patch angioplasty or interposition bypass grafting may be required in the case of significant injury.

D. Arterial Occlusion

1. **Femoral** Acute femoral artery occlusion complicates endovascular procedures in less than 0.8% of cases. Limb ischemia is commonly due to embolism of wire-, catheter-, or sheath-associated thrombus, often when the instrument is removed from the patient. The use of vascular closure devices with intra-arterial components may result in arterial occlusion by physical obstruction of a small caliber arterial lumen, footplate-induced dislodgement of vascular plaque, or suture-mediated subintimal dissection and subsequent thrombosis.

   Risk factors include the presence and extent of vascular disease, small caliber arteries (women, diabetics), low puncture site (superficial femoral or profunda femoris artery), larger sheath size and indwelling time, prolonged manual compression, low-flow state, and hypercoagulable disorder.

   a. Diagnosis

      Abrupt onset of any of the "6 P's" should raise suspicion for acute limb ischemia: pain, pallor, pulselessness, paresthesia, poikilothermia, and paralysis. Thromboembolic events, including cholesterol emboli from the use of wires and catheters in diseased vessels, may result in distal arterial occlusion resulting in blue toe syndrome, indicative of digital ischemia. The diagnosis of arterial thrombosis can be confirmed with Doppler ultrasonography in uncertain and low-risk cases. Otherwise, prompt angiography is often required to precisely localize the lesion and for swift intervention. Acute limb ischemia is a medical emergency and carries significant morbidity and mortality if not expeditiously diagnosed and accordingly treated.

b. Management

Immediate management includes initiation of systemic anticoagulation, usually intravenous unfractionated heparin, and contralateral access with either endovascular thrombectomy, catheter directed fibrinolysis, or angioplasty and stenting. If percutaneous techniques fail, swift surgical thrombectomy or bypass may be necessary to restore blood flow and avoid amputation.

Cannulation of the radial artery commonly results in arterial occlusion, with a reported incidence of approximately 10%.[33] Fortunately, the dual blood supply to the hand via the ulnar artery and palmar arch renders nearly all patients asymptomatic, although there are rare instances of ischemic complications. Published data suggest that approximately half of all radial artery occlusions may spontaneously recanalize within 1 month.[34]

Nonmodifiable risk factors include female gender, young age, and peripheral vascular disease. The use of smaller profile sheaths, intra-operative anticoagulation, and avoidance of occlusive hemostasis can mitigate the risk of radial occlusion. Repeated access attempts raise the risk of thrombosis slightly. One study of 455 patients undergoing transradial access showed a reduction in the rate of radial occlusion by color Doppler ultrasound before discharge from 30.5% to 13.7% in those patients who received a 5F compared with 6F sheath.[35] None of the patients developed critical limb ischemia. On sheath removal, application of the minimal amount of pressure required to achieve hemostasis but maintaining antegrade blood flow, or patent hemostasis, significantly reduces the rate of radial occlusion based on two clinical trials. It is important to prevent radial occlusion to preserve the access site for future procedures, and for its utility in dialysis fistulas and coronary bypass grafting.

To prevent ischemic complications, some operators may perform the modified Allen test or Barbeau test to assess the patency of the ulnar and palmar vessels. The Allen test is performed by maintaining occlusive manual pressure on the radial and ulnar arteries while asking the patient to clench his or her fist several times until the palm is blanched. Releasing pressure from the ulnar artery should return maximal blush to the palm within 9 seconds. The Barbeau test is a more objective test or ulnopalmar arch patency and is reported to be more sensitive than the Allen test. It is performed by first placing a pulse oximeter on the thumb or index finger of the hand to be tested and ensuring a normal baseline oximetery reading. Then, occlusive pressure is applied to the radial artery, and the oximetry waveform is continually assessed for 2 minutes. The response can be classified into 4 types: Type A, no change in oximetry waveform; Type B, damping and eventual recovery of the oximetry waveform by 2 minutes; Type C, loss of a waveform with recovery (even if damped) by 2 minutes; and Type D, permanent loss of a waveform. Patients with a Type C response have recruitment of collateral flow and would likely have been excluded from radial access based on an Allen test alone. Patients with a Type D response (1.5% of patients) have no collateral pulsatile flow and should not undergo radial artery catheterization.

The diagnosis of radial artery occlusion is readily made when a previously detected radial artery pulse is no longer palpable. Only rarely do patients develop symptomatic ischemia with pain, pallor, paresthesia, poikilothermia, or paralysis. Uncertain cases can be confirmed with duplex ultrasonography.

Treatment is not necessary for asymptomatic patients. Patients with signs of critical limb ischemia should undergo urgent attempt at percutaneous revascularization via an antegrade brachial artery approach using thrombectomy and coronary balloons as needed. Surgical revascularization may be necessary in cases where an endovascular approach is not feasible or unsuccessful.

2. **Brachial Artery** The overall rate of major brachial complications (2.3%) has been reported to be equivalent to that seen with femoral access (2.0%) but higher than with radial access (0%), in one randomized controlled trial of 900 patients.[36] However, because of its anatomic position as a terminal artery and smaller lumen size, it is rarely the preferred site of access.

   Thrombosis of the brachial artery will almost always lead to the devastating complication of limb threatening ischemia. Rates of brachial artery occlusion in the literature are reported to be as high as 6%; however, with the recent use of lower profile sheaths, they now average 1% and are more common in those with small vessels such as women or those with extensive vascular disease.[37] As in all cases of acute limb ischemia, prompt revascularization is necessary to prevent limb loss, and in the brachial position, surgical therapy is usually required.

III. Intervention-Specific Complications

A. **Infection** Access site infection following closure with manual compression is a rare complication of endovascular procedures. Those that do occur most often involve the femoral site at a rate of <0.1%.[26] Although rare, they are potentially serious given the pathogen's immediate access to the bloodstream and subsequent widespread dissemination. Risk factors include prolonged use of indwelling sheath, early reaccess, presence of hematoma or PSA, diabetes, obesity, overlying skin or soft tissue infection, and immune-compromised state. The use of a vascular access closure device raises the incidence of infection as high as 5%. Retained intravascular foreign material may serve as a nidus for infection, which carries a high rate of morbidity and mortality. Mycotic PSA is the most common complication.

1. **Diagnosis** Patients may present with fever, pain, tenderness, erythema, swelling, or discharge at the infected access site. Laboratory data often reveal leukocytosis. Blood cultures and duplex ultrasonography may assist in making the diagnosis. Access site infections in the setting of closure device use present after an average of 7-10 days with the most commonly isolated organism being *Staphylococcus Aureus* (75%).[38]

2. **Management** Prompt administration of intravenous antibiotics is the mainstay of treatment. In the case of severe infection, commonly in the setting of an access closure device, surgical debridement with removal of any indwelling foreign material may be necessary. In one retrospective review of patients with an access closure device infection, all patients underwent surgical debridement, half of whom required reconstructive surgery with a 6% mortality rate.[38]

In summary vascular access complication are rare but could lead to significant morbidity and mortality. Hence operators should be familiar with risk factors, clinical symptoms and signs, and treatment options for complications of vascular access.

References

1. https://www.advisory.com/research/cardiovascular-roundtable/cardiovascular-rounds/2015/02/making-millions-stenting-legs-what-are-the-facts.
2. Doyle BJ, Ting HH, Bell MR, et al. Major femoral bleeding complications after percutaneous coronary intervention: incidence, predictors, and impact on long-term survival among 17,901 patients treated at the Mayo Clinic from 1994 to 2005. *JACC Cardiovasc Interv*. 2008;1(2):202-209.
3. Koreny M, Riedmüller E, Nikfardjam M, Siostrzonek P, Müllner M. Arterial puncture closing devices compared with standard manual compression after cardiac catheterization: systematic review and meta-analysis. *JAMA*. 2004;291(3):350-357.
4. Wiley JM, White CJ, Uretsky BF. Noncoronary complications of coronary intervention. *Catheter Cardiovasc Interv*. 2002;57(2):257-265.
5. Manoukian SV, Feit F, Mehran R, et al. Impact of major bleeding on 30-day mortality and clinical outcomes in patients with acute coronary syndromes: an analysis from the ACUITY trial. *J Am Coll Cardiol*. 2007;49(12):1362-1368.
6. Farouque HM, Tremmel JA, Raissi Shabari F, et al. Risk factors for the development of retroperitoneal hematoma after percutaneous coronary intervention in the era of glycoprotein IIb/IIIa inhibitors and vascular closure devices. *J Am Coll Cardiol*. 2005;45(3):363-368.
7. Applegate RJ, Sacrinty MT, Kutcher MA, et al. Trends in vascular complications after diagnostic cardiac catheterization and percutaneous coronary intervention via the femoral artery, 1998 to 2007. *JACC Cardiovasc Interv*. 2008;1(3):317-326.
8. Ferrante G, Rao SV, Jüni P, et al. Radial versus femoral access for coronary interventions across the entire spectrum of patients with coronary artery disease: a meta-analysis of randomized trials. *JACC Cardiovasc Interv*. 2016;9(14):1419-1434.
9. Kelm M, Perings SM, Jax T, et al. Incidence and clinical outcome of iatrogenic femoral arteriovenous fistulas: implications for risk stratification and treatment. *J Am Coll Cardiol*. 2002;40(2):291-297.
10. Ricci MA, Trevisani GT, Pilcher DB. Vascular complications of cardiac catheterization. *Am J Surg*. 1994;167(4):375-378.
11. McCann RL, Schwartz LB, Pieper KS. Vascular complications of cardiac catheterization. *J Vasc Surg*. 1991;14(3):375-381.
12. Messina LM, Brothers TE, Wakefield TW, et al. Clinical characteristics and surgical management of vascular complications in patients undergoing cardiac catheterization: interventional versus diagnostic procedures. *J Vasc Surg*. 1991;13(5):593-600.
13. Oweida SW, Roubin GS, Smith RB, Salam AA. Postcatheterization vascular complications associated with percutaneous transluminal coronary angioplasty. *J Vasc Surg*. 1990;12(3):310-315.
14. Glaser RL, McKellar D, Scher KS. Arteriovenous fistulas after cardiac catheterization. *Arch Surg*. 1989;124(11):1313-1315.
15. Kresowik TF, Khoury MD, Miller BV, et al. A prospective study of the incidence and natural history of femoral vascular complications after percutaneous transluminal coronary angioplasty. *J Vasc Surg*. 1991;13(2):328-333. discussion 333-335.

16. Perings SM, Kelm M, Jax T, Strauer BE. A prospective study on incidence and risk factors of arteriovenous fistulae following transfemoral cardiac catheterization. *Int J Cardiol.* 2003;88(2-3):223-228.
17. Holman E, Taylor G. Problems in the dynamics of blood flow. II. Pressure relations at site of an arteriovenous fistula. *Angiology.* 1952;3(6):415-430.
18. Ramacciotti E, Galego SJ, Gomes M, Goldenberg S, De Oliveira Gomes P, Pinto Ortiz J. Fistula size and hemodynamics: an experimental model in canine femoral arteriovenous fistulas. *J Vasc Access.* 2007;8(1):33-43.
19. Holman E. Clinical and experimental observations on arteriovenous fistulae. *Ann Surg.* 1940;112(5):840-878.
20. Stehbens WE. Blood vessel changes in chronic experimental arteriovenous fistulas. *Surg Gynecol Obstet.* 1968;127(2):327-338.
21. Toursarkissian B, Allen BT, Petrinec D, et al. Spontaneous closure of selected iatrogenic pseudoaneurysms and arteriovenous fistulae. *J Vasc Surg.* 1997;25(5):803-808. discussion 808-809.
22. Waigand J, Uhlich F, Gross CM, Thalhammer C, Dietz R. Percutaneous treatment of pseudoaneurysms and arteriovenous fistulas after invasive vascular procedures. *Catheter Cardiovasc Interv.* 1999;47(2):157-164.
23. Ruebben A, Tettoni S, Muratore P, Rossato D, Savio D, Rabbia C. Arteriovenous fistulas induced by femoral arterial catheterization: percutaneous treatment. *Radiology.* 1998;209(3):729-734.
24. Thalhammer C, Kirchherr AS, Uhlich F, Waigand J, Gross CM. Postcatheterization pseudoaneurysms and arteriovenous fistulas: repair with percutaneous implantation of endovascular covered stents. *Radiology.* 2000;214(1):127-131.
25. Baltacioglu F, Cimşit NC, Cil B, Cekirge S, Ispir S. Endovascular stent-graft applications in latrogenic vascular injuries. *Cardiovasc Intervent Radiol.* 2003;26(5):434-439.
26. Nasser TK, Mohler ER, Wilensky RL, Hathaway DR. Peripheral vascular complications following coronary interventional procedures. *Clin Cardiol.* 1995;18(11):609-614.
27. Tavris DR, Wang Y, Jacobs S, et al. Bleeding and vascular complications at the femoral access site following percutaneous coronary intervention (PCI): an evaluation of hemostasis strategies. *J Invasive Cardiol.* 2012;24(7):328-334.
28. Katzenschlager R, Ugurluoglu A, Ahmadi A, et al. Incidence of pseudoaneurysm after diagnostic and therapeutic angiography. *Radiology.* 1995;195(2):463-466.
29. Webber GW, Jang J, Gustavson S, Olin JW. Contemporary management of postcatheterization pseudoaneurysms. *Circulation.* 2007;115(20):2666-2674.
30. Coughlin BF, Paushter DM. Peripheral pseudoaneurysms: evaluation with duplex US. *Radiology.* 1988;168(2):339-342.
31. Lange P, Houe T, Helgstrand UJ. The efficacy of ultrasound-guided compression of iatrogenic femoral pseudo-aneurysms. *Eur J Vasc Endovasc Surg.* 2001;21(3):248-250.
32. Eisenberg L, Paulson EK, Kliewer MA, Hudson MP, DeLong DM, Carroll BA. Sonographically guided compression repair of pseudoaneurysms: further experience from a single institution. *AJR Am J Roentgenol.* 1999;173(6):1567-1573.
33. Zankl AR, Andrassy M, Volz C, et al. Radial artery thrombosis following transradial coronary angiography: incidence and rationale for treatment of symptomatic patients with low-molecular-weight heparins. *Clin Res Cardiol.* 2010;99(12):841-847.
34. Stella PR, Kiemeneij F, Laarman GJ, Odekerken D, Slagboom T, van der Wieken R. Incidence and outcome of radial artery occlusion following transradial artery coronary angioplasty. *Cathet Cardiovasc Diagn.* 1997;40(2):156-158.
35. Uhlemann M, Möbius-Winkler S, Mende M, et al. The Leipzig prospective vascular ultrasound registry in radial artery catheterization: impact of sheath size on vascular complications. *JACC Cardiovasc Interv.* 2012;5(1):36-43.
36. Kiemeneij F, Laarman GJ, Odekerken D, Slagboom T, van der Wieken R. A randomized comparison of percutaneous transluminal coronary angioplasty by the radial, brachial and femoral approaches: the access study. *J Am Coll Cardiol.* 1997;29(6):1269-1275.
37. Armstrong PJ, Han DC, Baxter JA, Elmore JR, Franklin DP. Complication rates of percutaneous brachial artery access in peripheral vascular angiography. *Ann Vasc Surg.* 2003;17(1):107-110.
38. Sohail MR, Khan AH, Holmes DR, Wilson WR, Steckelberg JM, Baddour LM. Infectious complications of percutaneous vascular closure devices. *Mayo Clin Proc.* 2005;80(8):1011-1015.

CHAPTER 20

Limb Salvage From a Podiatric Standpoint

Michael I. Gazes, DPM, MPH, FACFAOM, AACFAS and Peter A. Blume, DPM, FACFAS

I. Introduction

Salvaging the lower extremity for functional, efficient, and low energy ambulation is the ultimate goal after ischemia, trauma, or infection in the lower extremity. Surgical emergencies exist, including gas gangrene, septic joints, a necrotizing fasciitis, which can lead to dramatic tissue loss, complicating limb salvage efforts (Fig. 20.1). Peripheral neuropathy, leading to ulcerations, deep soft tissue foot infections, and osteomyelitis also require special and dedicated care to avoid loss of limb and/or life.

Peripheral neuropathy is the most common cause of foot ulcerations, with diabetes mellitus being the most common cause of neuropathy.[1] Other causes also exist, including metabolic, toxins, viral and bacterial infections, genetics, ischemia, and inflammatory conditions. Patients with diabetes have a 15% lifelong incidence of developing foot ulcers, resulting in over 50% of nontraumatic lower limb amputations.[2-6] Reduced vascular perfusion and decreased oxygen to the lower limb diminishes the body's ability to heal suffocated wound sites, leading to prolonged exposure of open tissue to bacteria and increased likelihood of bone and soft tissue infection. Additionally, abnormal perfusion of blood to the foot can lead to weakening of bones. Combining weakened bones and neuropathy can lead to Charcot neuroarthropathy and major deformities at risk for wounds and infections, increasing the threat for major lower extremity amputation.[7,8]

II. Infection Control

A. **Risk Factors** Infection, particularly of an ulcer site, is a significant risk factor for lower extremity amputation.[4,5] Infections can cause a delay in wound healing with deterioration of the surrounding tissue.[9] Causes for lower extremity infections include vascular impairment, neuropathy, and decreased resistance to infection.[9-12]

B. **Antibiotics** Control of infection is typically via culture-guided antibiotics. Severe infections require intravenous antibiotics with prophylactic polymicrobial coverage prior to culture results including gram-positive and gram-negative anaerobes and aerobes.[13] As

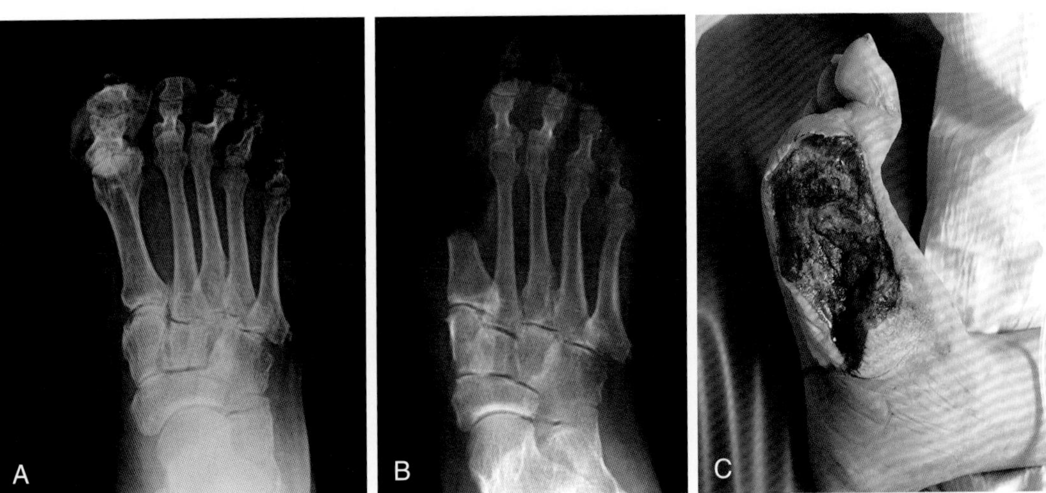

FIGURE 20.1: A, Gas gangrene visible with radiolucency by first metatarsophalangeal joint. B, Status post partial first ray resection with excisional debridement of all nonviable soft tissue and bone. C, Postoperative day 2.

deep wound cultures become available, antibiotic coverage can be narrowed depending on growth. Mild soft tissue infections generally require 2 weeks of therapy.[14] Deeper soft tissue infections may require up to 2 months of treatment.[14] Osteomyelitis requires 6 weeks or longer of an antibiotic regimen in addition to surgical bone debridement.[15] Prolonged ulcerations over osseous prominences should be evaluated for osteomyelitis. Improper footwear is the most common cause of neuropathic ulcerations, particularly when bony prominences or foot deformities exist.[16]

C. **Examinations** A biomechanical examination and wound offloading removes abnormally high-pressure areas in a neuropathic patient. Techniques for offloading include accommodative inserts, total contact casting, braces, and the use of felt. Computerized gait analysis effectively assesses high pedal pressure locations, leading to increased orthotic customization. Studies found that total contact casting heals ulcerations faster than half shoes and removable casts.[17] Patients given a removable cast were found to wear it for only 28% of their steps.[18] Patients undergoing total contact casting have increased healing as demonstrated histologically with evidence of angiogenesis and formation of granular tissue as compared with patients treated with debridement alone.[19] Contraindications to nonremovable casts include infection and/or ischemic wounds. Offloading via surgical procedures, such as exostectomies, tendon lengthenings or transfers, fusions, osteotomies, application of external fixation, and/or amputations may be required for adequate offloading of sites and ultimate wound reduction and prevention. Advanced wound healing products can also be attempted.

D. **Osteomyelitis**

1. Osteomyelitis, which on the foot typically occurs at ulcerative sites with bone prominences or at deep infection sites, is a highly destructive complication often necessitating long-term intravenous antibiotics, surgical debridement, or amputation. The average 5-year patient survival rate after amputation in the diabetic population is 39%.[20] Surgically, eliminating the source of infection is the primary goal. The secondary goal involves salvaging the extremity for functional, efficient, and low energy ambulation. During resection, specimens should be obtained of both the infected site and clean margins for pathological and microbiological evaluation. Next, "dead space" must be managed to avoid further complications, including hematomas and creation of areas allowing further infectious reactions.
2. Sharp debridement of ulcerations off-loads sites by removing hyperkeratosis, necrotic tissue, foreign material, and infectious organisms.[15,21] Sharp debridement should include the removal of all nonviable soft tissue and bone until healthy granular wound beds are obtained. Once infection has been eradicated, wounds can be closed or covered with primary wound closure, split thickness skin grafts, local flaps, or free flaps. If vascular perfusion to tissues are not adequate, clostridial collagenase is used for enzymatic debridement of the wound site.[22] Hydrocolloid and hydrogel dressings lead to autolysis of necrotic tissues.
3. A variety of dressing options for ulcerations are available and are dependent upon wound etiology and patient characteristics. Treatment of peripheral edema is also beneficial.

4. Negative pressure wound therapy (NPWT) can be used to stimulate angiogenesis and the formation of granular tissue, decreasing overall healing time of wounds.[23,24]

5. If vascular flow is the chief issue delaying wound healing, revascularization should be attempted. Vascular assessment includes Doppler ultrasound, duplex ultrasound, ankle brachial index, toe brachial index, and angiography.[25,26] Prakash et al found that the presence of neuropathy increases foot ulcerations and the ischemia worsens the overall presentation.[27,28] Peripheral vascular disease in patients with diabetes typically involves occlusive arterial lesions involving the femoral-popliteal segment and the tibial arteries below the knee.[28] In the diabetic population, chronic hyperglycemia leads to endothelial cell dysfunction, resulting in an increase in thromboxane A2 and a decrease in vasodilators, leading to hypercoagulation and vasoconstriction.[29] In patients with peripheral arterial disease, grafts and bypasses may be indicated. If vascular interventions are indicated, the procedures should be performed as soon as possible to avoid further tissue degeneration distally. In situations that vascular interventions are not feasible, amputation of the limb may be warranted.[1]

III. Advanced Wound Healing

A. **Phases** Wound healing consists of three phases: acute inflammatory, proliferative, and maturation. The acute inflammatory phase consists of vasoconstriction of arterioles and capillaries, platelet aggregation, and the inflammatory cell cascade. The proliferative phase includes fibroblastic activity, extracellular matrix reorganization, and angiogenesis.[30-32] The maturation phase involves the formation of scar tissues in addition to the synthesis and breakdown of collagen. Numerous advanced wound healing therapies exist, ranging from complex biologic dressings, stem cells, laser treatments, hyperbaric oxygen therapies, negative pressure wound therapies (NPWT), splint thickness skin grafts and flaps.[30,31]

B. **Extracellular Matrix** Collagen-based modalities provide collagen, the major protein in the extracellular matrix. Sustainable extracellular scaffolds are compromised in ulcerations, and treatment with collagen provides a structural scaffold matrix to support extracellular components, increase fibroblast proliferation, mediate cell migration and organization, and inhibit excessive MMPs.[15,33,34]

C. **Noninvasive Vascular Studies**

1. When there is concern for limb ischemia or vascular insufficiency in the face of a chronic nonhealing wound, noninvasive vascular studies can be obtained. Noninvasive vascular studies with preferred parameters include ankle brachial index (ABI) of <0.7, toe brachial index (TBI) <0.4, or transcutaneous oxygen tension (TcPO2) levels <30 mm Hg. Abnormal values increase wound complications.[35-37] Arteriography can be performed for evaluation of the arterial tree. Six angiosomes exist in the foot and ankle[38]: three from the posterior tibial artery, two from the peroneal artery, and one from the dorsalis pedis artery.[38] Arteriography can determine if an angiosome is not perfused at an area of ulceration. It also assists with location of flap formation or incision placement. If revascularization can be performed, direct

revascularization of an ulceration's angiosome yields a higher healing rate of wound healing.[39] If revascularization cannot be achieved, hyperbaric oxygen therapy can be attempted with ischemic wounds. It exposes patients to 100% oxygen at 2-3 times the normal atmospheric pressure, increasing the saturation of oxygen in the blood to decrease hypoxia and edema and promote wound healing.[40]

2. After revascularization, when a healthy and granular wound bed is achieved, split thickness skin grafting (STSG) can be performed. The procedure includes harvesting skin from a donor site and transplanting it to a recipient site. During this process, the harvested skin is separated from its local blood supply and is completely dependent on the recipient site's blood supply for survival (Fig. 20.2).[41] If the type of wound does not indicate STSG for closure and direct closure cannot be attained, flap closure can be attempted.

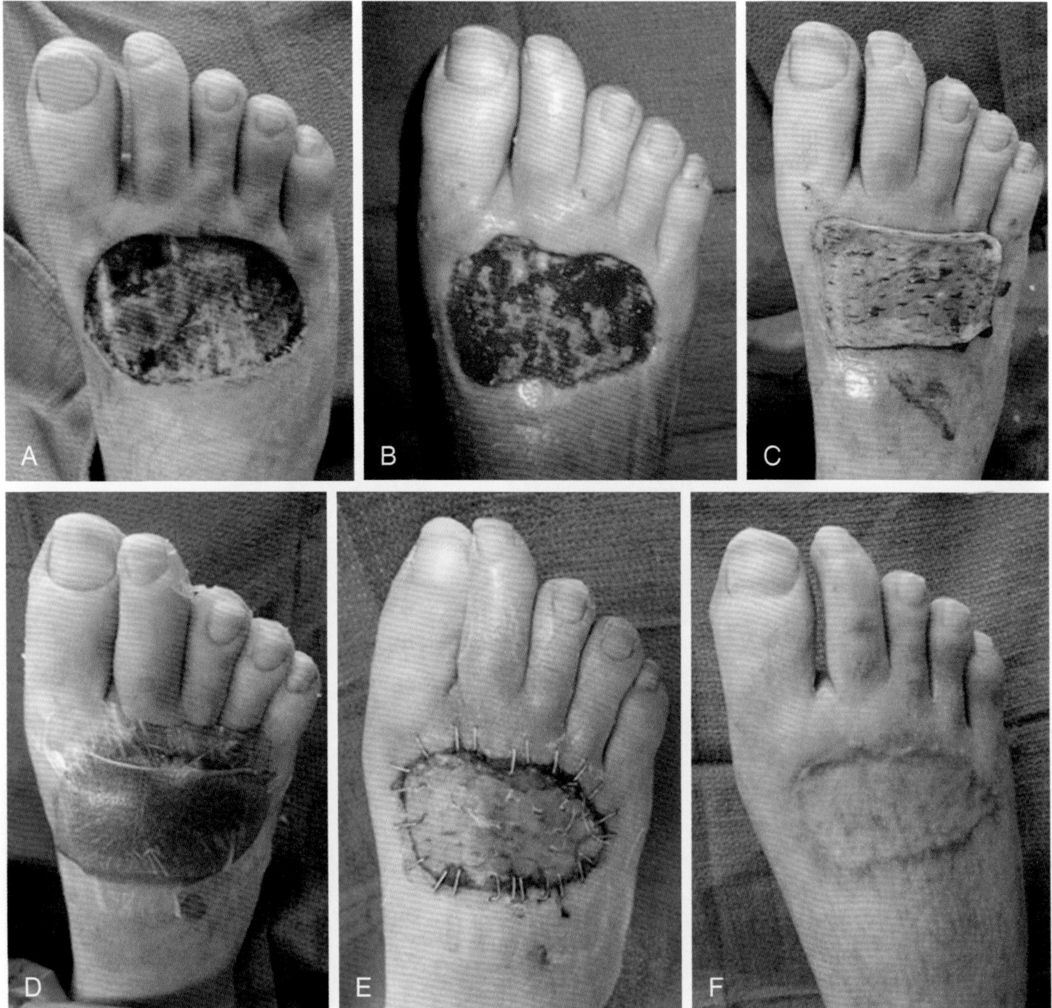

FIGURE 20.2: Dorsal right foot wound treated with excisional debridement, STSG application, and negative pressure therapy. A, Dorsal foot wound, (B) postsurgical debridement, (C) application of STSG, (D) negative pressure therapy, (E,F) completion of wound closure.

3. Flaps are tissues utilized for transplantation vascularized by a stem or pedicle.[42] Flaps may include epidermis, dermis, subcutaneous tissue, underling fascia, or muscle. Different flap techniques utilized in plastic and reconstructive interventions for wounds include advancement, rotational, and transpositional flaps (Fig. 20.3). Four main features for consideration in determining incisions for flap formation include adequate exposure, adequate blood supply, sparing of sensory and motor nerves, and attention to skin tension lines.[43] Skin incisions placed perpendicular to skin tension lines can increase scar contractures. These types of flaps are perfused by a perforator artery from the dermis to the subdermal plexus and differ from an axial flap, which has a direct cutaneous vascular supply. Angiosomes evaluation is essential as random flaps rely on perforators for survival.[44]

4. Choke vessels link adjacent angiosomes and can be used to enhance perfusion to an angiosome.[44] The delay phenomenon results in the dilation of existing choke vessels within the flap rather than an ingrowth of new vessels, increasing overall perfusion to the site.[45] Raising the flap causes a local sympathectomy in the delay phenomenon, leading to vasodilation.[44] Distant axial flaps, tissue expansion, and free flaps can be performed when split thickness skin grafting and local random flaps are not suitable. These techniques are more complex with increased risk for morbidity.

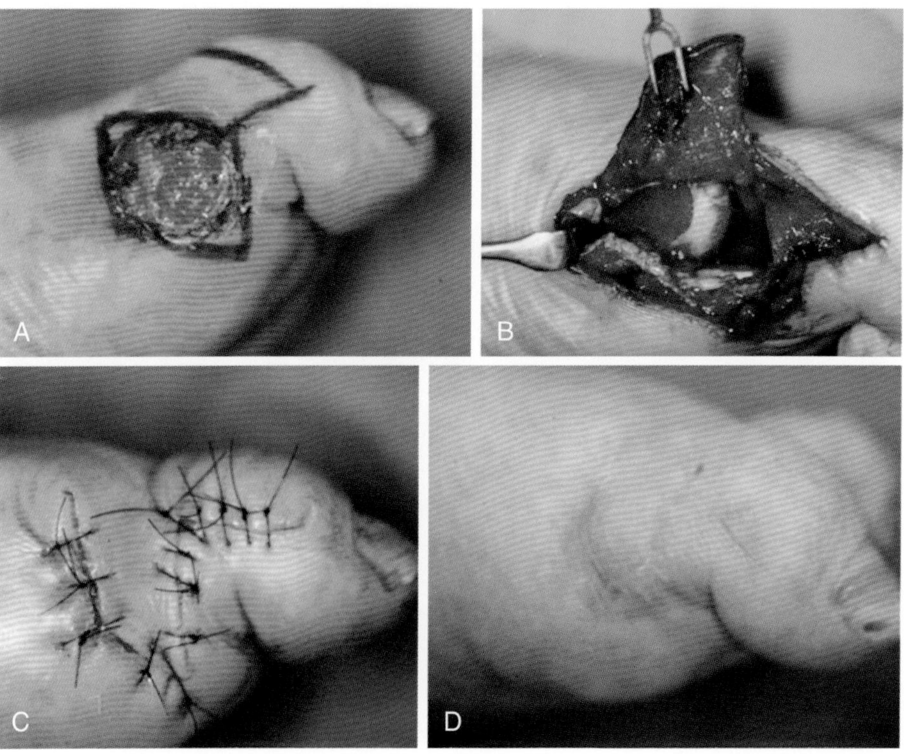

FIGURE 20.3: Rhomboid transpositional flap. A, Drawing flap out prior to incision to ensure appropriate skin tension for closure and measurements for coverage, (B) raising the flap full thickness to level of bone, (C) flap inset with closure, (D) final closure appearance.

IV. Summary

Ischemia, trauma, gas gangrene, septic joints, necrotizing fasciitis, and deformities and ulcerations leading to infections and osteomyelitis can have detrimental effects of the lower extremity. Salvaging the lower extremity for functional, efficient, and low energy ambulation is the ultimate goal after treating the primary source for an at risk foot. When ischemia is leading to the pedal complications, the limb requires evaluation to determine whether efficient blood flow exists for tissue oxygenation. If inefficient flow exists, revascularization should be attempted. If revascularization is unable to be attempted or is ineffective, modalities, including hyperbaric oxygen, can be used. When open wounds exist without infection and are delayed in closure, negative pressure wound therapy, collagen-based modalities, skin grafts, and skin flaps can be utilized to attempt closure prior to new infection again putting the foot at risk for amputation. Limb salvage is not typically a one-stage surgical procedure and may require multiple interventions before desired results are attained. Ultimately, in addition to a skilled multispecialty health care team, extensive amounts of time and compliant patients with postoperative protocols are necessary to achieve limb salvage.

References

1. Sumpio BE. Foot ulcers. *N Engl J Med.* 2000;343:787-793.
2. Boulton AJ, Armstrong DG, Albert SF, et al. Comprehensive foot examination and risk assessment: a report of the task force of the foot care interest group of the American diabetes association, with endorsement by the American association of clinical endocrinologists. *Diabetes Care.* 2008;31(8):1679-1685.
3. Reiber GE, Lipsky BA, Gibbons GW. The burden of diabetic foot ulcers. *Am J Surgery.* 1998;176(suppl 2A):5S-10S.
4. Reiber GE, Vileikyte L, Boyko EJ, et al. Causal pathways for incident lower-extremity ulcers in patients with diabetes from two settings. *Diabetes Care.* 1999;22:157-162.
5. Pecoraro RE, Reiber G, Burgess EM. Pathways to diabetic limb amputation: basis for prevention. *Diabetes Care.* 1990;13:513-521.
6. Eneroth M, Apelqvist J, Stenstrom A. Clinical characteristics and outcome in 223 diabetic patients with deep foot infections. *Foot Ankle Int.* 1997;18:716-722.
7. Lee L, Blume PA, Sumpio B. Charcot joint disease in diabetes mellitus. *Ann Vasc Surg.* 2003;17(5):571-580.
8. Knox RC, Dutch W, Blume P, Sumpio BE. Diabetic foot disease. *Int J Angiol.* 2000;9(1):1-6.
9. Lipsky BA, Berendt AR. Principles and practice of antibiotic therapy of diabetic foot infections. *Diabetes Metab Res Rev.* 2000;16:(suppl 1):S42-S46.
10. Laing P. The development and complications of diabetic foot ulcers. *Am J Surg.* 1998;176(2A suppl):11S-9S.
11. Caputo GM, Cavanagh PR, Ulbrecht JS, Gibbons GW, Karchmer AW. Assessment and management of foot disease in patients with diabetes. *N Engl J Med.* 1994;331:854-860.
12. [a] Shah BR, Hux JE. Quantifying the risk of infectious diseases for people with diabetes. *Diabetes Care.* 2003;26:510-513.
    [b] Lipsky BA, Berendt AR, Deery G, et al. Diagnosis and treatment of diabetic foot infections. IDSA Guidelines for Diabetic Foot Infections CID. 2004;39:885-910.
13. Joshi N, Caputo GM, Weitekamp MR, Karchmer AW. Infections in patients with diabetes mellitus. *N Eng J Med.* 1999;273:721-723.
14. Sumpio BE. Contemporary evaluation and management of the diabetic foot. *Scientifica.* 2012:435487.
15. Lipsky BA, Berendt AR, Cornia PB, et al. 2012 Infectious disease society of America clinical practice guidelines for the diagnosis and treatment of diabetic foot infections. *Clin Infect Dis.* 2012;54(12):e132-e173.
16. Macfarlane RM, Jeffcoate WJ. Factors contributing to the presentation of diabetic foot ulcers. *Diabet Med.* 1997;14:867-870.

17. Armstrong DG, Nguyen HC, Lavery LA, van Schie CH, Boulton AJM, Harless LB. Off-loading the diabetic foot wound: a randomized clinical trial. *Diabetes Care.* 2001;24:1019-1022.
18. Armstrong DG, Lavery LA, Kimbriel HR, Nixon BP, Boulton AJM. Activity patterns of patients with diabetic foot ulceration: patients with active ulceration may not adhere to a standard pressure off-loading regimen. *Diabetes Care.* 2003;26:2595-2897.
19. Piaggesi A, Viacava P, Rizzo L, et al. Semi-quantitative analysis of the histopathological features of the neuropathic foot ulcer: effects of pressure relief. *Diabetic Care.* 2003;26:3123-3128.
20. Tentolouris N, Al-Sabbagh S, Walker MG, Boulton AJ, Jude EB. Mortality in diabetic and nondiabetic patients after amputations performed from 1990 to 1995: a 5-year follow-up study. *Diabetes Care.* 2004;27(7):1598-1604.
21. Steed DL, Donohoe D, Webster MW, Lindsley L. Effect of extensive debridement and treatment on the healing of diabetic foot ulcers. *J Am Coll Surg.* 1996;183:61-64.
22. Tallis A, Motley TA, Wunderlich RP, et al. Clinical and economic assessment of diabetic foot ulcer debridement with collagenase: results of a randomized controlled study. *Clin Ther.* 2013;35(11):1805-1820.
23. Wagner FW. The diabetic foot. *Orthopedics.* 1987;10(1):163-174.
24. Bus SA. Offloading the diabetic foot; evidence and clinical decision making. *EWMA J.* 2012;12(3);13-15.
25. Sumpio B, Thakor P, Mahler D, Blume P. Negative pressure wound therapy as postoperative dressing in below knee amputation stump closure of patients with chronic venous insufficiency. *Wounds.* 2011;23(10):301-308.
26. Park SC, Choi CY, Ha YI, Yang HE. Utility of toe-brachial index for diagnosis of peripheral arterial disease. *Arch Plast Surg.* 2012;39(3):227-231.
27. Prakash SS, Krishnakumar, Prabha C. The influence of peripheral neuropathy and peripheral vascular disease in the outcome of diabetic foot management – a prospective study. *Int J Med Res Health Sci.* 2014;4(2):258-264.
28. LoGerfo FW. Peripheral arterial occlusive disease and the diabetic: current clinical management. *Heart Dis Stroke.* 1992;1(6):395-397.
29. Paraskevas KJ, Baker DM, Pompella A, Mikhailidis DP. Does diabetes mellitus play a role in restenosis and patency rates following lower extremity peripheral arterial revascularization? A critical overview. *Ann Vasc Surg.* 2008;22(3):481-491.
30. Snyder RJ, Kirsner RS, Warriner RA, Lavery LA, Hanft JR, Sheehan P. Consensus recommendations on advancing the standard of care for treating neuropathic foot ulcers in patients with diabetes. *Ostomy Wound Manage.* 2010;56(4 suppl):S1-S24.
31. Garwood C, Steinberg J, Kim P. Bioengineered alternative tissues in diabetic wound healing. *Clin Podiatr Med Surg.* 2015;32(1):121-133.
32. Ennis WJ, Lee C, Gellada K, Corbiere TF, Koh TJ. Advanced technologies to improve wound healing. *Plast Reconstr Surg.* 2016;138:94-104.
33. Amber M, Gazes M, Blume P. Assessing collagen-based modalities for diabetic foot ulcerations. *Podiatry Today.* 2016;29(5).
34. Bakker K, Apelqvist J, Lipsky B, Van Netten J. The 2015 IWGDF guidance documents on prevention and management of foot problems in diabetes: development of an evidence-based global consensus. *Diabetes Metab Res Rev.* 2016;32(suppl 1):2-6.
35. Attinger CE. Use of soft tissue techniques for salvage of the diabetic foot. In: Kominsky S, ed. *Medical and Surgical Management of the Diabetic Foot.* St. Louis: Mosby; 1994:323-366.
36. Attinger C, Bulan EJ, Blume PA. Pharmacological and mechanical management of wounds. In: Mathes SJ, ed. *Plastic surgery.* Vol. 1. St. Louis: Elsevier; 2006:863-899.
37. Benitez E, Sumpio B, Chin J, Sumpio B. Contemporary assessment of foot perfusion in patients with critical limb ischemia. *Semin Vasc Surg.* 2014;27:3-15.
38. Attinger C, Evans K, Bulan E, Blume P, Cooper P. Angiosomes of the foot and ankle and clinical implications for limb salvage: reconstruction, incisions, and revascularization. *Plast Reconstr Surg.* 2006;117(7S):261S-293S.

39. Neville R, Attinger C, Bulan E, Ducic I, Thomassen M, Sidawy A. Revascularization of a specific angiosome for limb salvage: does the target artery matter? *Ann Vasc Surg*. 2009;23:367-373.
40. Lipsky B, Berendt R. Hyperbaric oxygen therapy for diabetic foot wounds. *Diabetes Care*. 2010;33(5):1143-1145.
41. Barratt GE, Koopmann CF. Skin grafts: physiology and clinical considerations. *Otolaryngol Clin North Am*. 1984;17:335-351.
42. Alnaeb ME, Boutin A, Crabtree VP, et al. Assessment of lower extremity peripheral arterial disease using a novel automated optical device. *Vasc Endovascular Surg*. 2007;41(6):522-527.
43. Brobyn TJ, Cramer LM, Hulnick SJ. Facial resurfacing with the limberg flap. *Clin Plast Surg*. 1976;3(3):481-490.
44. Blume P, Donegan R, Schmidt B. The role of plastic surgery for soft tissue coverage of the diabetic foot and ankle. *Clin Podiatr Med Surg*. 2014;31:127-150.
45. Dhar S, Taylor I. The delay phenomenon: the story unfolds. *Plast Reconstr Surg*. 1999;104:2079.

CHAPTER 21

Pulmonary Vascular Diseases and Interventions

Eileen M. Harder, MD and Wassim H. Fares, MD, MSc

Key Points

- Depending on patient comorbidities and the severity of the insult, PEs may cause a wide variety of symptoms, ranging from none to dyspnea to sudden death.
- PEs can be classified by mortality risk: high (massive), intermediate (submassive), and low (nonsubmassive). These groups are defined clinically by certain prognostic factors.
- PE treatment depends on the risk group.
- PH has many different etiologies, and the World Health Organization (WHO) separates this disease into five different classes.
- The best screening test for any suspected PH is transthoracic echocardiography (TTE).
- WHO group 1 PH is pulmonary arterial hypertension (PAH). It can be idiopathic, heritable, drug or toxin related, or associated with certain conditions including congenital heart disease or portal hypertension.
- If TTE suggests PAH, definitive diagnosis is made by right heart catheterization (RHC).
- PAH treatment depends on the cause of PH and disease severity. It often involves advanced medical therapy; certain forms of PAH may require surgery.
- WHO group 4 PH is caused by chronic pulmonary emboli (CTEPH).

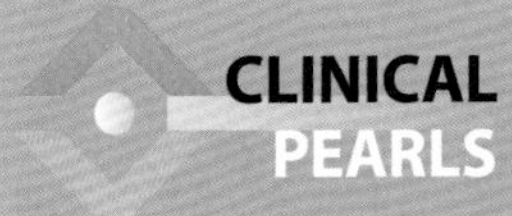

- High-risk PEs are defined by hemodynamic instability (sustained hypotension or shock).
- Intermediate PEs are hemodynamically stable but have evidence of RV dysfunction and/or myocardial injury. All of these features are absent in low-risk PEs.
- In hemodynamically unstable patients, PE can be diagnosed by TTE. Stable patients should undergo CT pulmonary angiogram (CTPA).
- Patients with high-risk PEs should receive urgent treatment with systemic thrombolysis, surgical embolectomy, or catheter-based methods, as appropriate.
- Intermediate and low-risk PEs should receive anticoagulation.
- PAH on RHC is defined as a mean PAP ≥25 mm Hg with pulmonary artery wedge pressure (PAWP) ≤15 mm Hg and pulmonary vascular resistance (PVR) >3 Wood units.
- Treatment of PAH may entail calcium channel blockers (for the small number of vasoreactive patients) or advanced therapy.
- Uncorrected atrial septal defects (ASDs) may also cause PAH. Patients with ASD-PAH should undergo early closure, provided that they do not have Eisenmenger syndrome.

- Portopulmonary hypertension is a form of PAH associated with portal hypertension. Liver transplant is indicated in patients with mPAP <35 mm Hg and PVR <5 Wood units.
- CTEPH should be considered in acute PE patients whose dyspnea and other symptoms do not resolve after 3-6 months.
- In suspected CTEPH, a positive TTE is followed by a ventilation/perfusion scan. RHC and/or pulmonary angiography are required to confirm the diagnosis.
- The only definitive treatment for CTEPH is pulmonary endarterectomy (PEA). Balloon pulmonary angioplasty or advanced therapy may be considered in non-PEA candidates.

I. Pulmonary Vascular Disease

Pulmonary vascular disease (PVD) refers to any disease that affects the pulmonary vessels. The two most common conditions are pulmonary emboli and pulmonary hypertension, and this chapter will focus on these diseases and their management.

II. Acute Pulmonary Emboli

A. **Epidemiology** An acute pulmonary embolus (PE) occurs when a pulmonary artery (PA) or one of its branches becomes obstructed, most commonly by thrombus. The incidence of PEs is unknown, and this may be due partly to underdiagnosis—silent PEs may occur in up to 30%-50% of deep venous thrombosis (DVT) cases, and they are often only noted incidentally on autopsy.[1-3] Recent estimates suggest that there are approximately 600,000 PEs in the United States per year, and it may contribute to death in up to one-third of these patients.[4-7]

B. **Risk Factors** There are many inherited and acquired PE risk factors. Inherited factors include hypercoagulable states, such as factor V Leiden or prothrombin mutations, protein C or S deficiencies, and antithrombin deficiency. Important acquired risk factors include older age, major or orthopedic surgery, leg or hip fractures, cancer, immobility, spinal cord injury, prior PE/DVT, obesity, pregnancy, oral contraceptive or hormone replacement therapy, and antiphospholipid antibody syndrome, among others.[2,8] For patients with DVTs, PE risk is particularly high with proximal thigh clots.

C. **Pathophysiology** PEs and DVTs are types of venous thromboembolism, in which clot formation is based on Virchow triad of venous stasis, hypercoagulability, and endothelial injury. In normal lungs, perfusion matches ventilation—hypoxic vasoconstriction occurs in poorly ventilated areas, and well-oxygenated regions remain perfused. PEs create a ventilation-perfusion mismatch. In the most severe cases, perfusion is completely absent and systemic shunting of deoxygenated blood occurs.[5,9] This results in hypoxemia, which is further worsened by cytokines that promote inflammation and vasocontriction.[9] Compensatory hyperventilation occurs and as a result, respiratory alkalosis with low P_{CO2} is usually present.[9] Hypercapnia should increase suspicion for a massive embolism.[9]

PEs also cause circulatory dysfunction. Generally, hemodynamic abnormalities occur only when ≥30%-50% of the pulmonary arterial system is occluded, although even a small clot can cause dysfunction in patients with heart and lung disease.[8,10,11] Obstructed vessels and the accompanying vasoconstriction of normal vasculature cause a sudden rise in pulmonary vascular resistance (PVR) and acute pulmonary hypertension (PH). The increased afterload dilates the right ventricle (RV), decreases myocardial contractility, and diminishes coronary vessel perfusion.[12] A normal, nonweakened RV can generate a systolic pressure up to 40 mm Hg, but above this in the acute setting, RV failure occurs.[11] Right-sided stroke volume (SV) and cardiac output (CO) are reduced. As the RV further stretches, the septum moves into the left ventricle (LV). The end result is decreased left-sided filling, preload, and CO.[13]

The body triggers a complex compensatory cascade including sympathetic activation to increase PA flow and preserve systemic circulation.[8] Depending on the severity of the insult, a PE can manifest as a wide spectrum of findings ranging from no hemodynamic abnormalities to RV failure, hypotension, and shock. In the most severe cases, compensation is inadequate and sudden death occurs, often by pulseless electrical activity or asystole.[8,11]

D. **Classification** Although PEs can be classified in multiple different ways, the most clinically relevant system stratifies disease severity based on mortality risk—high, intermediate, or low.[2,11] These terms correspond to massive, submassive, and nonsubmassive PEs, respectively.

High-risk (massive) disease is defined by the presence of sustained hypotension or shock in the setting of an acute PE that is not due to another cause. Some guidelines also suggest pulseless or persistent bradycardia (<40 beats per minute) as alternative inclusionary criteria.[14] Hypotension is generally defined as a systolic blood pressure <90 mm Hg, a systolic drop ≥40 mm Hg for >15 minutes or the requirement for vasopressor support.[2,11,14,15] Evidence of tissue hypoperfusion, such as a lactic acidosis, suggests a progression to shock.

Low (nonsubmassive) and intermediate (submassive) risk PEs are hemodynamically stable. These classes are separated by RV dysfunction and/or myocardial injury—one or two of these features are present in intermediate disease, but both are lacking in low-risk PEs. RV dysfunction is defined by the presence of RV dilation, elevated NT-proBNP or BNP, or ECG changes (represented by new right bundle branch block; anteroseptal ST elevation or depression; or anteroseptal T-wave inversion).[14] Myocardial injury is reflected as elevated troponin I or T.[14]

E. **Presentation** PE can manifest with a wide variety of symptoms—ranging from none to sudden death—depending on disease severity and patient comorbidities. Symptoms are usually nonspecific, including dyspnea, pleuritic chest pain, cough, and/or lower extremity swelling.[16] Physical examination may reveal tachypnea, tachycardia, decreased breath sounds, decreased arterial oxygen saturation, and/or hypotension.[16]

F. **Diagnosis** Risk category dictates workup and treatment. Patients with suspected high-risk (massive) PEs should be immediately stabilized, including with vasopressors if necessary. Early diagnosis is crucial, as time to treatment affects the risk of mortality. If patients become stable enough for transport to radiology, immediate CT pulmonary angiogram (CTPA) should be done. Bedside echocardiography should be performed, particularly if patients are unable to undergo CTPA. Findings of severe RV dilation, decreased systolic function, septal bowing, RV wall hypokinesis or McConnell sign (RV mid-free wall akinesia with normal apical motion), visualized right-heart thrombi, and/or inspiratory lack of inferior vena cava (IVC) collapse suggest high-risk PE.[17] When stable, patients should undergo confirmatory CTPA.

Hemodynamically stable patients with suspected low- or intermediate-risk PE should undergo further workup. D-dimer may be high, although this occurs in many other conditions including infection, pregnancy, and cancer. Arterial blood gas may reveal hypoxemia, alveolar-arterial gradient, or respiratory alkalosis. Other findings may be elevated leukocytosis, BNP, or troponin. ECG usually shows sinus tachycardia and nonspecific ST- and T-wave changes; less common findings include new arrhythmia, right bundle branch block, RV strain, right axis deviation, or inferior Q-waves, among others. Chest X-ray rarely shows Hampton hump or Westermark sign.

After assessment, the pretest probability of PE should be evaluated in hemodynamically stable patients. This can be done by either clinical suspicion or predictive calculators, such as the modified Wells or Geneva scores.[11,18,19] If PE is likely, CTPA is the initial step in diagnostic workup. If it reveals clots, treatment should begin; if it is negative, other diagnoses should be considered. If scoring suggests that PE is unlikely, D-dimer testing may be done, followed by CTPA if the level is high. In patients with a contrast allergy, renal failure, or pregnancy, the initial imaging test should be ventilation/perfusion (V/Q) scan. Echocardiography may be useful in some hemodynamically stable patients to evaluate for RV strain, but it is not required.

G. **Treatment** Treatment depends on PE risk. Hemodynamically unstable patients with high-risk (massive) disease are at increased risk for early death. Supportive measures should be initiated while a treatment decision is made; these include vasopressors and oxygen as necessary.[11] Definitive reperfusion treatment can be performed with systemic thrombolysis, catheter-directed interventions, or surgical embolectomy.

1. **High-Risk (massive) PE**
   a. Thrombolysis

   Thrombolysis rapidly breaks down clots to improve perfusion and off-load the RV. In high-risk PE, it is associated with decreased mortality and improved hemodynamics compared with anticoagulation alone.[20,21] The most commonly used thrombolytics are recombinant tissue-type plasminogen activation (tPA, alteplase), streptokinase, and urokinase.[14] Of these, tPA is usually chosen for its short infusion time (the general standard dose is 100 mg tPA over 2 h).[14] If anticoagulation was started, it may be temporarily stopped during thrombolytic infusion.

   The major side effect of thrombolysis is increased bleeding risk, and so it should not be used in many patients. Absolute contraindications include active bleed; known intracranial malignancy or vascular lesion; any prior intracranial hemorrhage; suspected aortic dissection; and recent (ie, within the past 3 mo) ischemic stroke, brain or spine surgery, or significant closed-head and/or facial trauma.[14] Relative contraindications vary between guidelines but generally include history of and/or current severe poorly controlled hypertension, prolonged CPR (>10 min) or major surgery in the previous 3 weeks, ischemic stroke >3 months ago, internal bleeding within the past 2-4 weeks, active peptic ulcer, dementia, noncompressible vascular puncture, pregnancy, current anticoagulant use, age >75 years, infective endocarditis, advanced liver disease, or diabetic retinopathy.[11,14] Based on these contraindications, approximately 50%-60% of patients do not receive systemic thrombolysis.[22]

b. Catheter-Directed Management

1. Catheter-Directed Embolectomy

Catheter-based PE treatment may consist of mechanical, thrombolytic, or combined interventions to off-load the RV and improve perfusion.[23] For patients with absolute contraindications to thrombolysis, a mechanical procedure, such as thrombus fragmentation, rheolytic thrombectomy, suction thrombectomy, or rotational thrombectomy, may be used.[11] These methods are generally recommended only for clots in the main or lobar PAs.[14] Evidence for some of them is limited, and there are little data comparing their effectiveness and outcomes. A 2007 systematic review demonstrated approximately equal success rates for the first three techniques (fragmentation 82%, rheolytic 75%, and suction [aspiration] 81%); however, technology has significantly improved since this time.[24] Given the required technical skill, these interventions should be performed only at expert centers.

i. Thrombus Fragmentation

Thrombus fragmentation mechanically breaks the thrombus into smaller fragments. This immediately reduces main PAP by displacing these small fragments to the distal branches.[23] In this procedure, a sheath is placed and a rotatable pigtail catheter is introduced over a guidewire. The catheter is manually rotated to break up the thrombus. It may also be performed with balloon angioplasty catheters or other devices.[14] Given that it is inexpensive, this is the most common technique; it can also be combined with other mechanical methods to improve outcomes.[25]

ii. Rheolytic Thrombectomy

Rheolytic thrombectomy employs the Bernoulli principle through the use of high-pressure saline jets.[26] In this technique, a sheath is placed, a guidewire is introduced, and the device is inserted over it. Saline jets are used to create a low-pressure zone around the catheter, which macerates the thrombus and pulls the fragments back for removal via a suction port. Local thrombolytics can also be injected and removed via this system. Of note, at least one of the rheolytic thrombectomy systems has been associated with intraprocedure bradycardia that may necessitate short treatment times, temporary breaks, or transvenous pacing.[26] Other side effects may include hemoptysis, hemoglobinuria, and renal insufficiency.

iii. Suction Embolectomy

Suction embolectomy uses suction to remove thrombus and can be done alone or in combination with other techniques. In this procedure, a specific aspiration sheath with a special hemostatic valve is advanced into the thrombus.[23] A syringe is used to apply suction while the catheter is moved gently over a short distance in the pulmonary artery. Clot is cleared when blood enters the syringe, and this procedure may require multiple advancements of the suction catheter over the guidewire. Alternatively, suction embolectomy can be performed with newer devices that incorporate aspiration and filtration with dual-venous access. This extracorporeal circulation bypass system aspirates blood, clears it of clot, and then reintroduces it.[26]

iv. Rotational Thrombectomy

Rotational thrombectomy uses rotating coils to treat PEs. A high-speed rotating metallic coil in a catheter lumen creates a negative pressure that disrupts the thrombus, macerates it, and then aspirates it. A small study has suggested this method is effective in clearing thrombus and improving PAP.[27]

2. Catheter-Directed Thrombolysis

Catheter-directed thrombolysis (CDT) denotes the local infusion of thrombolytics, either alone or with mechanical interventions.[23] In this procedure, a simple catheter with multiple side holes is placed into the pulmonary artery and the drug is passively infused. The thrombolytic dose used in CDT is only a small amount of that used for systemic treatment, and so bleeding risk is decreased.[26]

The combination of local thrombolysis with mechanical interventions is referred to as pharmacomechanical thrombolysis (PMT). Studies suggest that the best outcomes come from PMT—one analysis demonstrated a 95% success rate when fragmentation, suction, or rheolytic therapy was used with local thrombolysis, compared with 81% when a mechanical intervention was used without CDT.[14,24] Ultrasound has also been successfully combined with CDT. In this method, a specific device is used that consists of a catheter with multiple side holes and a central ultrasonic core wire. The catheter is placed into the thrombus and then the ultrasonic core is inserted and locked into place. The high-frequency waves disrupt the thrombus and promote better thrombolytic penetration.

c. Surgical Embolectomy

Surgical embolectomy is recommended in centrally located, high-risk (massive) PE with thrombolytic contraindications or failure.[28] It also is useful in patients with right atrial (RA) and RV clots or a large patent foramen ovale.[28] Mortality was historically around 30%; however, it has decreased to as low as 4%-6% in more recent years.[11,14]

PE embolectomy is a variation of the modified Tredenlenburg operation.[28,29] Median sternotomy is made and normothermic cardiopulmonary bypass (CPB) is established. Intravenous (IV) unfractionated heparin is the preferred anticoagulation for better control and easier reversal. Arteriotomy is made into the main PA between the pulmonic valve and PA bifurcation.[28] This allows for saddle and left PE access; clot is extracted by forceps whole if possible or with suction if necessary.[30] If clot is in the right PA, an incision can be made in this vessel between the aorta and superior vena cava.[28] Incisions can be extended distally as necessary. Certain centers use lung massage for clot extraction and others do not because of an increased risk of pulmonary damage. All main PA branches should be inspected by direct visualization or flexible surgical angioscopy. The RA and RV should also be explored and cleared; any patent foramen ovale should be closed. Of note, an inferior vena cava filter may be inserted preoperatively or within the first 24 hours postoperatively to prevent reembolization.[29]

2. **Intermediate-Risk (submassive) and Low-Risk (nonsubmassive) Pulmonary Embolus** Hemodynamically stable patients should receive supportive care as needed during diagnostic workup. Patients with intermediate-risk (submassive) PE should start anticoagulation with IV unfractionated heparin or subcutaneous low-molecular-weight (LMW) heparin. When fully anticoagulated, they can be transitioned to an oral agent, namely either a direct factor Xa inhibitor, direct thrombin inhibitor, or warfarin.[11,31] For the majority of patients with their first provoked PE, anticoagulation should be continued for 3 months.[14] Those with unprovoked clots may benefit from a longer treatment course, depending on their risk factors.[11,14] Patients with cancer or pregnancy are considered to be a special population; LMW heparin is preferred over an oral agent.[11]

   Thrombolysis is generally not recommended in hemodynamically stable patients with intermediate-risk (submassive) PE.[31] Thrombolysis improves hemodynamics in this population (compared with anticoagulation alone), but major bleeding is more frequent, and it is generally considered that the risks outweigh the benefits.[11,31] Patients with intermediate-risk disease—particularly those with significant RV dysfunction on echocardiography or borderline blood pressure—should be monitored carefully for decompensation, in the event that thrombolysis becomes necessary.[14]

   Thrombolysis should not be used in low-risk (nonsubmassive) disease. Hospitalization may not be required in this population, but anticoagulation should be initiated.

III. Pulmonary Hypertension

A. **Definition** PH refers to an elevated PA pressure, defined as a mean PA pressure (mPAP) ≥25 mm Hg at rest as measured by a right heart catheterization (RHC).[32] Based on the etiology, the World Health Organization (WHO) divides PH into five major groups. The first is pulmonary arterial hypertension (WHO group 1 PH). The other four include PH due to left heart disease (group 2), chronic lung disease or hypoxemia (group 3), chronic thromboemoli (group 4), and miscellaneous conditions (group 5). PH may also be named based on the site of elevated pressure—if only arterial, it is "precapillary" but if "venous" as defined by a high mean pulmonary arterial wedge pressure (PAWP), then it may be referred to as "postcapillary." As these terms are the ends of a wide spectrum of vasculopathic changes that can be present in PH, the disease may not always be easily classifiable into one of these two distinct entities.[33]

B. **Epidemiology** Because of the many causes of PH, its prevalence is difficult to determine. Estimates suggest that it affects 1% of the global population, although this increases to 10% in those older than 65 years.[34] The most common cause is left heart disease (WHO PH group 2).[35] Prognosis and treatment differ vastly between the WHO PH groups, and so it is essential that disease is correctly classified, particularly in patients with multiple risk factors.[35]

C. Pulmonary Arterial Hypertension (WHO PH Group 1)

1. **Introduction** PAH (WHO group 1 PH) encompasses PH that is idiopathic (IPAH), heritable (HPAH), drug or toxin related, or associated with certain conditions (connective tissue disease [CTD], congenital heart disease [CHD], portal hypertension, human immunodeficiency virus-1 [HIV-1], or schistosomiasis). The prevalence of PAH is unknown but is believed that there may be 15 cases per 1 million people.[35] IPAH is most common (approximately 40%-60%), followed by PAH associated with CTD, CHD, and portal hypertension.[36,37] Historically, PAH was most frequent in young females. Recent data still reveal a female predominance (60%-80%), but the mean age at diagnosis has increased to the mid-50s.[38]

2. **Presentation** PAH presents with nonspecific symptoms including dyspnea, fatigue, and exercise intolerance; initially, these are only with exertion but occur at rest as the disease progresses.[35] Later symptoms include angina, syncope, peripheral edema, and palpitations. Because of the vague presentation, the median time from symptom onset to RHC is 1.1 years in the United States.[38] Twenty percent of patients report symptoms for >2 years before diagnosis.[39]

   PH symptom severity is graded with the WHO functional assessment, which is a modification of the New York Heart Association system for heart failure. WHO functional class (WHO-FC) I corresponds to no limitation of physical activity. Class II denotes a slight activity limitation (dyspnea, fatigue, chest pain, near syncope with ordinary activity) but no symptoms at rest. Class III indicates symptoms with less than ordinary physical activity. Class IV indicates symptoms at rest, and these patients may have evidence of right heart failure.

3. **Diagnosis** Given the nonspecific presentation, PAH should be considered in any patient with dyspnea that cannot be fully explained by any present heart or lung disease. The best screening test for any suspected PH is transthoracic Doppler echocardiography. There is no defined PH cutoff, but individual guidelines suggest that a systolic pulmonary artery pressure (sPAP) of ≥40 or ≥50 mm Hg requires further workup.[40,41] Other suspicious findings on echocardiography include RA or RA enlargement, PA dilation, or septal flattening.

Additional evaluation should be done to identify any underlying cause of PH.[35] History may suggest familial inheritance, drugs/toxins, or left heart disease.[35] Laboratory testing should include HIV-1, rheumatologic studies (eg, antinuclear antibody), liver and thyroid function, coagulation studies, and complete blood count. Chest X-ray should be performed; in advanced disease, this may reveal an enlarged RA or RV, dilated pulmonary arteries, or pruned peripheral pulmonary vessels.[42] Pulmonary function tests and sleep studies should be done in all patients to evaluate for WHO group 3 PH, with the addition of high-resolution chest CT if clinical history suggests interstitial lung disease. PH workup for CHD, portal hypertension, and chronic thromboemboli are discussed in the following sections.

RHC is required for definitive PH diagnosis and classification. PAH is characterized by an mPAP ≥25 mm Hg with PAWP ≤15 mm Hg and PVR >3 Wood units.[32] Of note, heart failure with preserved ejection fraction (HFpEF) may infrequently present with a similar hemodynamic profile to PAH with low PAWP. In this instance, clinical context including comorbidities and left heart function should be assessed; left heart catheterization may be useful. Volume challenge during RHC to assess for PAWP increase is controversial and is not recommended by the most recent guidelines because of lack of standardization.[32,43]

During RHC and unless contraindicated (eg, because of systemic hypotension or cardiac shock), vasoreactivity should be tested in all PAH patients to determine candidacy for high-dose calcium channel blocker (CCB) treatment.[42] This test is particularly important in patients with IPAH, HPAH, and drug-related PAH; those with other associated PAH forms are extremely unlikely to be vasoreactive. It is performed with inhaled nitric oxide, IV epoprostenol, or IV adenosine. Vasoreactivity is present if the mean pulmonary artery pressure (mPAP) decreases ≥10 mm Hg and to <40 mm Hg without decrease in cardiac output or systolic blood pressure.[44]

4. **Treatment** PAH is a progressive and complex disease.[45] Treatment has multiple goals: decrease symptoms to WHO-FC I/II, increase six-minute walk distance (6MWD), decrease BNP, normalize RV size and function on echocardiography, and normalize hemodynamics.[46] Notably, many of these factors—WHO-FC, BNP, 6MWD, and certain hemodynamic parameters, among others—correlate with survival, which has increased over recent years. None of the current drugs, however, are approved for the specific indication of decreasing mortality.[47,48]

   At diagnosis, PAH patients should be counseled on general measures including directed physical activity, pregnancy avoidance, psychosocial support, medication adherence, and vaccinations.[42,49] A referral to an expert center should be made. Supportive therapy should include oxygen for low arterial oxygen saturations and diuretics for decompensated right heart failure.[42,49] Warfarin is sometimes recommended in IPAH, as well as patients on IV prostanoid analogues, although the evidence supporting its routine use is not robust.[40,42] Digoxin may be useful to control tachyarrythmias.[40]

Disease risk dictates the need for PAH therapy. Risk is based on signs of RV failure, time to symptom progression, syncope, WHO-FC, 6MWD, cardiopulmonary exercise test (if done), NT-proBNP, echocardiography, and hemodynamics.[40,50] WHO-FC I patients do not require therapy, but they should be closely monitored for disease progression.[51]

WHO-FC II and III patients should start treatment. In IPAH, HPAH, or drug-related PAH, initial therapy depends on the vasoreactivity test. The small vasoreactive subset should be started on a CCB, provided that they do not have right heart failure or other contraindications.[51] Nifedipine, diltiazem, or amlodipine can be used.[40] Long-term responders—even among vasoreactive patients—are infrequent and high-dose CCBs may have significant side effects, so this population should be reassessed for response approximately 3 months after starting therapy.[44,52]

The foundation of PAH treatment is advanced therapy. Three contributing pathways can be targeted by one of five drug classes: endothelin receptor antagonists (ERAs), guanylate cyclase stimulators, phosphodiesterase-5 inhibitors (PDE5), prostacyclin analogues, and receptor agonists. Initial monotherapy has historically been favored, although interest has increased in upfront treatment with ≥2 drugs. Recently, the Ambrisentan and Tadalafil in Patients with Pulmonary Arterial Hypertension (AMBITION) trial examined the use of initial combination therapy in the treatment-naïve population.[53] Patients treated with ambrisentan and tadalafil had decreased PAH-related clinical failures (a composite of measures including death, disease progression, unsatisfactory long-term response), compared with those treated with either drug alone. Patients who received combination therapy also had better 6MWDs, NT pro-BNP reductions, and clinical responses.[53] Currently, the European Society of Cardiology (ESC)/European Respiratory Society recommend initial combination therapy as an option in WHO-FC II to IV disease.[42] Of note, in treatment-naïve patients with WHO-FC IV or rapidly progressive WHO-FC III, continuously infused prostacyclin analogues should be started (in addition to another drug, if combination therapy is to be utilized).[46,51]

Patients should be monitored closely with repeat echocardiography and 6MWT.[42,48,54] Double or triple sequential combination therapy is used in patients who have inadequate response to monotherapy or dual-drug treatment.[46]

In WHO-FC IV patients with inadequate clinical response or severe syncope despite maximal medical therapy, balloon atrial septostomy (BAS) may be considered.[42] The interatrial septum is punctured with a guidewire and then successive dilations are performed with graded balloon catheters of increasing sizes.[42,55] This creates a right-to-left shunt that off-loads the RV; despite the decreased oxygen saturation, systemic flow is increased and so overall oxygenation is improved.[56,57] This is a palliative procedure—potentially useful in bridging to lung transplant—but small studies demonstrate improved hemodynamics and 6MWD.[42] This method can be associated with significant mortality and so should not be performed in end-stage patients, as it may worsen their disease.[56,57] The Potts shunt—an anastomosis between the left PA and descending aorta—may be useful in children with severe refractory WHO-FC IV PAH.

D. Atrial Septal Defects

1. **Epidemiology** WHO group 1 PH may also develop from congenital heart disease (CHD) including atrial septal defects (ASDs). Worldwide, ASDs occur in 1.6 per 1000 live births and account for 13% of CHD.[58,59] Based on the defect site, there are different types: secundum (70%), primum (15%), sinus venous (15%), and coronary sinus (1%). Secundum ASDs are more common in women.

2. **Presentation** Most small ASDs (≤4 mm) spontaneously close or shrink, but larger defects ≥8-12 mm are at risk for enlarging.[60] Most patients are asymptomatic until adulthood but develop symptoms after their 40s including fatigue, dyspnea, palpitations, and exercise intolerance.[61] As PAH develops, patients may have cyanosis, syncope, hemoptysis, atrial arrhythmias, or RV failure.[62] Exam may reveal fixed splitting of the second heart sound or a systolic flow murmur.[61]

3. **Pathogenesis** Estimates suggest that PAH (with or without Eisenmenger syndrome) occurs in 5%-10% of adults with untreated ASDs.[60] Small defects have minimal left-to-right shunting, but it may be significant in larger ASDs (>10 mm).[60] This causes progressive vessel remodeling, increased PVR, and ultimately PH.[63] Eisenmenger syndrome (ES) occurs when PH forces shunt reversal to right-to-left flow, causing cyanosis at rest.[35] Patients with ES have worse outcomes than ASD-PAH alone, and they were historically considered to be better than those in IPAH. Recent data, however, suggest that survival between IPAH and ES cohorts is similar, although it is not clear if this perceived better prognosis is due to improved medical therapy or to survivor bias.[64]

4. **Diagnosis** In suspected PAH-CHD, transthoracic Doppler echocardiography should be used to assess the atrial septum. Agitated saline may reveal right-to-left flow, but it should not be used in known large shunts because of air embolus risk. If transthoracic imaging is not revealing, transesophageal echocardiography (TEE) should be done.[62] Cardiac MRI may be useful if echocardiography is inconclusive.[62] Cardiac catheterization is required for ASD-PAH diagnosis.

5. **Treatment** After ASD-PAH diagnosis is made, patients should be referred to an expert PAH center. General supportive measures should be initiated, with the addition of dehydration and strenuous exercise avoidance.[42] Anti-arrhythmics and anticoagulation should be used for atrial arrhythmias as appropriate; however, anticoagulation without arrhythmia is not indicated because of bleeding risk, especially hemoptysis.[63]

   ASD treatment depends on the defect size and associated PAH severity. Patients with small shunts and normal RV size should be monitored for RV enlargement and/or PAH with routine ECG and echocardiography.[62] Early closure is essential to prevent PAH. Guidelines recommend that it should be done in patients with RV overload—despite symptoms—who have not progressed to severe PAH.[61,62] The ESC guidelines recommend that PVR be <5 Wood units to undergo closure, although it can be considered in patients with a left-to-right shunt and PVR <2/3 of systemic vascular resistance or PAP <2/3 systemic pressure (baseline or postvasodilator).[61,62] Closure should also be considered in patients with paradoxical embolism or orthodeoxia-platypnea.[61,62] Of note, outcomes are best when age at repair is <25 years; however, closure can be performed at any age and it is thought to be the optimal management even in adults (vs. medical therapy).[61,65] It should not be done in ES—pulmonary remodeling is likely extensive and repair may worsen PAH, leading to RV failure and death.[62,63,66]

a. Atrial Septal Defect Closure Methods

Closure of an ASD can be done surgically or percutaneously. Percutaneous transcatheter intervention is recommended for secundum defects that are <36-40 mm diameter and that have adequate margins off valves (except the aorta).[60-62] Outcomes are excellent with closure rates of 93%-99% and a major complication rate of 1%.[60] This procedure is performed under TEE and fluoroscopic guidance. Briefly, the left atrium is catheterized and a guidewire is inserted. ASD size can be estimated with a balloon catheter and the "stop-flow" technique, in which the balloon is placed across the defect, inflated with contrast until the shunt disappears by echocardiography, deflated, and then reinflated. An ASD closure device that is of equal size or one size larger than the defect is selected and soaked in saline to prevent air embolus. The delivery system is advanced into an upper pulmonary vein (usually the left), and the wire and dilator are removed while allowing free blood flow from the sheath to decrease air embolus risk. The device is inserted, the left atrial disc is deployed, and this is checked with fluoroscopy and TEE. The sheath is pulled back and then the right atrial disc is then deployed. Its position is verified; the discs should be parallel and separated by the atrial septum. If the device position is correct, the delivery cable is released. TEE should reveal no or minimal residual shunt.

Surgery was the preferred intervention but now is used for nonclosable or nonsecundum ASDs.[62] Pericardial patch closure is preferred, although direct suturing is possible for small defects. It can be done by open or minimally invasive approaches. Success rates are similar to percutaneous repair, although complications are higher and hospitalizations tend to be longer.[60]

Patients with residual shunt, PAH, arrhythmias, or age >40 years should be followed after closure with echocardiography and ECG.[61] Antiplatelet therapy and endocarditis prophylaxis are advised after percutaneous intervention.[61]

b. Medical Therapy

Patients with ES should not undergo ASD closure. In WHO-FC III and IV disease, guidelines suggest advanced pharmacologic therapy. European guidelines recommend bosentan; small studies suggest that other agents may also improve outcomes but these are not recommended.[61] Combination therapy can be considered, but its efficacy is unknown.

E. **Other Forms of PAH-CHD** In addition to ASD, other forms of CHD may result in PAH. Some of them may be addressed by palliative atrial septostomy. The Potts shunt procedure may also be used for transposition of the great arteries, and although beyond the scope of this chapter, the Glenn or Fontan shunt creation can address hypoplastic left heart syndrome and/or tricuspid atresia.

F. **Portopulmonary Hypertension** Portopulmonary hypertension (PoPH) is WHO group 1 PAH associated with portal hypertension, with or without underlying liver disease. Estimates of PoPH vary widely, but it appears to account for approximately 10% of all PAH diagnoses.[67,68] Risk is increased in females and autoimmune hepatitis.[67]

The pathogenesis of PoPH is not well understood. Multiple mechanisms have been proposed including volume overload causing shear stress, systemic inflammatory changes, and portosystemic shunts circulating nonmetabolized circulating toxins.[69] PVR increases and ultimately leads to pulmonary vascular remodeling. No correlation has been identified between the severity of liver disease and of PoPH.[35]

Like IPAH, PoPH presents with nonspecific symptoms, and patients are usually in their 40s or 50s at diagnosis.[70] TTE is the best screening test, but the gold standard for diagnosis, like all other PAH subgroups, is RHC. All patients undergoing liver transplant evaluation should receive at least TTE, with RHC if needed based on the TTE findings.

Treatment options for PoPH are limited. Diuretics should be initiated. Anticoagulation is not recommended, given that this population is already at increased risk of bleeding due to coagulopathy. CCBs should also be avoided, as they could worsen portal hypertension. If advanced therapy is required, IV epoprostenol or sildenafil can be used, although there may be a role for other PAH-specific medications.[70,71] Of note, transjugular intrahepatic portosystemic shunt (TIPS) placement increases preload, CO, and mPAP and is therefore contraindicated in PoPH.[72]

Liver transplantation (LT) is a curative option for certain PoPH patients. Guidelines suggest it is indicated in candidates with mPAP <35 mm Hg and PVR <5 Wood units.[73] Patients with worse hemodynamics who undergo LT have higher mortality. In this group, a trial of advanced vasodilator therapy should be attempted, and patients should be listed for LT if mPAP and PVR fall to <35 mm Hg and <5 Wood units, respectively. In the United States, this well-controlled PoPH group is granted an exception from the traditional Model for End-Stage Liver Disease (MELD) system, thus raising their scores and hopefully decreasing time to transplant.[74] Of note, not all PoPH patients who undergo liver transplant have resolution of PoPH—some may continue to require vasodilator therapy, although the reasons for this are not clear.

G. **Chronic Thromboembolic Pulmonary Hypertension**

1. **Introduction** Chronic thromboembolic PH (CTEPH) results from chronic obstruction of pulmonary arteries and arterioles. It is a form of precapillary PH defined as mPAP ≥25 mm Hg with PAWP ≤15 mm Hg in the setting of chronic flow-limiting pulmonary artery thrombi after ≥3 months of effective anticoagulation.[75,76] CTEPH develops in 1%-4% of acute PE patients, although this is likely an underestimate.[75,77,78]

Interestingly, it appears that approximately 25%-63% of CTEPH patients have never had a known or documented acute PE, although these events may have simply not been detected.[79,80] CTEPH risk is particularly high in those acute PE patients who are young or who have an idiopathic presentation.[79,81] Other risk factors are similar to those for PEs, with of the addition of splenectomy, hypothyroidism, or ventriculoatrial shunt.

2. **Diagnosis** CTEPH should be considered in acute PE patients whose symptoms (ie, dyspnea, etc.) do not resolve after 3-6 months.[78] TTE should be performed; if it is suggestive of PH, a V/Q scan is done next.[75] If this imaging demonstrates a high probability of PE, both RHC and pulmonary angiography are needed to confirm CTEPH, determine severity, and evaluate surgical candidacy.[75] If the V/Q scan is indeterminate but the suspicion for CTEPH is still high, guidelines suggest either pulmonary angiography and/or RHC.[75,82] CTEPH is unlikely with a normal V/Q scan. CTPA may be useful before surgery, but it is less sensitive than V/Q and is not recommended for diagnosis.[83]

   Certain patterns on angiography are associated with CTEPH: pouch defects; intimal irregularities; pulmonary artery bands or webs; abrupt or angular narrowing of the major pulmonary arteries; and obstructed main, lobar, or segmental vessels at their point of origin with absent downstream flow.[84-86] Two or more of these patterns tend to be present in CTEPH.[84]

3. **Treatment** At diagnosis, CTEPH patients should be referred to an expert center. The only curative option is pulmonary endarterectomy (PEA), and the majority of patients are candidates for this procedure.[78] In nonsurgical candidates (owing to comorbidities and/or clot accessibility), balloon pulmonary angioplasty (BPA) or medical therapy may be considered. At diagnosis, lifelong anticoagulation should be started to prevent pulmonary clot propagation and DVT. It can be initiated with either IV unfractionated heparin or subcutaneous low-molecular-weight heparin. After full therapeutic anticoagulation is achieved, patients can be transitioned to warfarin with an international normalized ratio goal of 2.0-3.0.[87] Inferior vena cava (IVC) filter placement is controversial, and its use varies between centers.

   a. Pulmonary Endarterectomy

      PEA is the only definitive treatment for CTEPH.[82] Mortality is <5% at expert facilities, and most patients experience significant symptom and hemodynamic improvement.[87] Mortality increases with PVR; residual/recurrent PH after surgery is the major predictor of death.[87]

      To undergo PEA, the thromboemboli must be accessible, symptoms or hemodynamic abnormalities should be severe, and patients must be surgical candidates.[88] The role of PEA in early CTEPH is not defined—some recommend immediate intervention to prevent hemodynamic abnormalities and others suggest routine monitoring.[87]

      Before PEA, pulmonary angiography is essential to determine thrombi location. PEA is used for thromboemboli in the main, lobar, segmental, and some subsegmental pulmonary arteries.[89] It may not improve symptoms if the burden of disease is distal. This procedure has been described in detail elsewhere.[75,82,87,89] Briefly, after median sternotomy, cardiopulmonary bypass (CPB) is established to prevent collateral bleeding and ensure a clear surgical field. Profound hypothermia to 18-20°C is induced. An incision is made into the right PA and the endarterectomy plane is established[88]; if too deep, perforation may occur and if too shallow, PH will not resolve. This plane can be followed down to involved branches as necessary. Organized fibrous tissue is then removed. Given that the maximum cooling period is 20 minutes and PEA is usually bilateral, the right side is usually done first, the patient is reperfused, CPB is re-established, and then left PEA is performed.[88] Anticoagulation is usually started 4-8 h after PEA with IV unfractionated heparin. Warfarin can be restarted at days 8-14.[88] The role of other direct or "novel" anticoagulants is not established in this population.

b. Balloon Pulmonary Angioplasty

The role of BPA in CTEPH is not yet defined, given the limited outcomes data.[87,90] In select patients, it improves hemodynamics and 6MWD. There is no consensus yet on an optimal BPA population, but this procedure may be considered in patients who are inoperable, have distal disease, have post-PEA PH, or fail medical therapy.[87] Given that BPA is minimally invasive, it may also have a palliative role. It is contraindicated in patients with contrast allergies or severe renal dysfunction.

In BPA, internal jugular vein access is obtained. The procedure has been described in detail elsewhere.[91] Briefly, a sheath is inserted and a smaller introducer sheath is advanced through it into the main PA.[87] Heparin is given and selective pulmonary angiography is done. Intravascular ultrasound is used to determine vessel diameter for the correct balloon size. A guidewire is introduced until it crosses the clot, and then a balloon catheter is used to compress the thrombus and dilate the vessel. Generally, one BPA session can only target a few vessels, so multiple treatments may be needed. In early BPA studies, reperfusion pulmonary edema was not uncommon; however, rates of this complication have decreased as technique improves.

c. Medical Therapy

Medical therapy may be indicated in post-BPA/PEA CTEPH and nonintervenable candidates.[85,90] Riociguat is approved for both populations.[87] Of note, all inoperable patients should receive a second opinion at an expert CTEPH center, as definitions of surgical candidacy may differ between facilities and surgeons.

IV. Conclusions

PVD encompasses a spectrum of conditions with effects ranging from mild to severe. Significant improvements in diagnosis and therapy have been made, and patients benefit from a multidisciplinary approach. As research in this field continues, it is likely that therapeutic strategies will continue to rapidly evolve.

References

1. Pineda LA, Hathwar VS, Grant BJB. Clinical suspicion of fatal pulmonary embolism. *Chest.* 2001;120(3):791-795.
2. Torbicki A, Perrier A, Konstantinides S, et al. Guidelines on the diagnosis and management of acute pulmonary embolism: the Task Force for the Diagnosis and Management of Acute Pulmonary Embolism of the European Society of Cardiology (ESC). *Eur Heart J.* 2008;29(18):2276-2315.
3. Stein PD, Matta F, Musani MH, et al. Silent pulmonary embolism in patients with deep venous thrombosis: a systematic review. *Am J Med.* 2010;123(5):426-431.
4. Dalen JE, Alpert JS. Natural history of pulmonary embolism. *Prog Cardiovasc Dis.* 1975;17(4):259-270.
5. Rahimtoola A, Bergin JD. Acute pulmonary embolism: an update on diagnosis and management. *Curr Probl Cardiol.* 2005;30(2):61-114.
6. Tapson VF. Acute pulmonary embolism. *N Engl J Med.* 2008;358(10):1037-1052.
7. Horlander KT, Mannino DM, Leeper KV. Pulmonary embolism mortality in the United States, 1979–1998: an analysis using multiple-cause mortality data. *Arch Intern Med.* 2003;163(14):1711-1717.
8. Bělohlávek J, Dytrych V, Linhart A. Pulmonary embolism, part I: epidemiology, risk factors and risk stratification, pathophysiology, clinical presentation, diagnosis and nonthrombotic pulmonary embolism. *Exp Clin Cardiol.* 2013;18(2):129-138.
9. Goldhaber SZ, Elliott CG. Acute pulmonary embolism: part I. epidemiology, pathophysiology, and diagnosis. *Circulation.* 2003;108(22):2726-2729.
10. McIntyre KM, Sasahara AA. The hemodynamic response to pulmonary embolism in patients without prior cardiopulmonary disease. *Am J Cardiol.* 1971;28(3):288-294.
11. Konstantinides S, Torbicki A, Agnelli G, et al; The Task Force for the Diagnosis and Management of Acute Pulmonary Embolism of the European Society of Cardiology (ESC) Endorsed by the European Respiratory Society (ERS). 2014 ESC Guidelines on the diagnosis and management of acute pulmonary embolism. *Eur Heart J.* 2014;35(43):3033-3069.
12. Kholdani CA, Oudiz RJ, Fares WH. The assessment of the right heart failure syndrome. *Semin Respir Crit Care Med.* 2015;36(06):934-942.
13. Kholdani CA, Fares WH. Management of right heart failure in the intensive care unit. *Clin Chest Med.* 2015;36(3):511-520.
14. Jaff MR, McMurtry MS, Archer SL, et al. Management of massive and submassive pulmonary embolism, iliofemoral deep vein thrombosis, and chronic thromboembolic pulmonary hypertension. A scientific statement from the American Heart Association. *Circulation.* 2011;123(16):1788-1830.
15. Kucher N, Rossi E, De Rosa M, et al. Massive pulmonary embolism. *Circulation.* 2006;113(4):577-582.
16. Pollack CV, Schreiber D, Goldhaber SZ, et al. Clinical characteristics, management, and outcomes of patients diagnosed with acute pulmonary embolism in the emergency department: initial report of EMPEROR (Multicenter Emergency Medicine Pulmonary Embolism in the Real World Registry). *J Am Coll Cardiol.* 2011;57(6):700-706.
17. Goldhaber SZ. Echocardiography in the management of pulmonary embolism. *Ann Intern Med.* 2002;136(9):691-700.
18. Le Gal G, Righini M, Roy P, et al. Prediction of pulmonary embolism in the emergency department: the revised Geneva score. *Ann Intern Med.* 2006;144(3):165-171.
19. Wells PS, Anderson DR, Rodger M, et al. Derivation of a simple clinical model to categorize patients probability of pulmonary embolism: increasing the models utility with the SimpliRED D-dimer. *Thrombo Haemost.* 2000;83(3):416-420.
20. Konstantinides S, Tiede N, Geibel A, et al. Comparison of alteplase versus heparin for resolution of major pulmonary embolism. *Am J Cardiol.* 1998;82(8):966-970.
21. Jerjes-Sanchez C, Ramirez-Rivera A, de Lourdes Garcia M, et al. Streptokinase and heparin versus heparin alone in massive pulmonary embolism: a randomized controlled trial. *J Thromb Thrombolysis.* 1995;2(3):227-229.

22. Kasper W, Konstantinides S, Geibel A, et al. Management strategies and determinants of outcome in acute major pulmonary embolism: results of a multicenter registry. *J Am Coll Cardiol.* 1997;30(5):1165-1171.
23. Engelberger RP, Kucher N. Catheter-based reperfusion treatment of pulmonary embolism. *Circulation.* 2011;124(19):2139-2144.
24. Skaf E, Beemath A, Siddiqui T, et al. Catheter-tip embolectomy in the management of acute massive pulmonary embolism. *Am J Cardiol.* 2007;99(3):415-420.
25. Kuo WT. Endovascular therapy for acute pulmonary embolism. *J Vasc Interv Radiol.* 2002;23(2):167-179.e4.
26. Sobieszczyk P. Catheter-assisted pulmonary embolectomy. *Circulation.* 2012;126(15):1917-1922.
27. Dumantepe M, Teymen B, Akturk U, et al. Efficacy of rotational thrombectomy on the mortality of patients with massive and submassive pulmonary embolism. *J Card Surg.* 2015;30(4):324-332.
28. Poterucha TJ, Bergmark B, Aranki S, et al. Surgical pulmonary embolectomy. *Circulation.* 2015;132(12):1146-1151.
29. McFadden PM, Ochsner JL. Aggressive approach to pulmonary embolectomy for massive acute pulmonary embolism: a historical and contemporary perspective. *Mayo Clin Proc.* 2010;85(9):782-784.
30. Yavuz S, Toktas F, Goncu T, et al. Surgical embolectomy for acute massive pulmonary embolism. *Int J Clin Exp Med.* 2014;7(12):5362-5375.
31. Kearon C, Akl EA, Ornelas J, et al. Antithrombotic therapy for VTE disease: CHEST guideline and expert panel report. *Chest.* 2016;149(2):315-352.
32. Hoeper MM, Bogaard HJ, Condliffe R, et al. Definitions and diagnosis of pulmonary hypertension. *J Am Coll Cardiol.* 2013;62(25 suppl):D42-D50.
33. Fares WH. The other vascular beds in pulmonary arterial hypertension. Surrogates or associated? *Ann Am Thoracic Soc.* 2014;11(4):596-597.
34. Hoeper MM, Humbert M, Souza R, et al. A global view of pulmonary hypertension. *Lancet Resp Med.* 2016;4(4):306-322.
35. Bazan IS, Fares WH. Pulmonary hypertension: diagnostic and therapeutic challenges. *Ther Clin Risk Manag.* 2015;11:1221-1233.
36. Hoeper MM, Simon R. Gibbs J. The changing landscape of pulmonary arterial hypertension and implications for patient care. *Eur Respir Rev.* 2014;23(134):450-457.
37. McGoon MD, Benza RL, Escribano-Subias P, et al. Pulmonary arterial hypertension: epidemiology and registries. *J Am Coll Cardiol.* 2013;62(25 suppl):D51-D59.
38. Badesch DB, Raskob GE, Elliott CG, et al. Pulmonary arterial hypertension: baseline characteristics from the REVEAL registry. *Chest.* 2010;137(2):376-387.
39. Brown LM, Chen H, Halpern S, et al. Delay in recognition of pulmonary arterial hypertension: factors identified from the REVEAL registry. *Chest.* 2011;140(1):19-26.
40. McLaughlin VV, Archer SL, Badesch DB, et al. ACCF/AHA 2009 expert consensus document on pulmonary hypertension. A report of the American College of Cardiology Foundation task force on expert consensus documents and the American Heart Association developed in collaboration with the American College of Chest Physicians; American Thoracic Society, Inc; and the Pulmonary Hypertension Association. *J Am Coll Cardiol.* 2009;53(17):1573-1619.
41. Galiè N, Hoeper MM, Humbert M, et al. Guidelines for the diagnosis and treatment of pulmonary hypertension. *Eur Respir J.* 2009;34(6):1219-1263.
42. Galie N, Humbert M, Vachiery JL, et al. 2015 ESC/ERS guidelines for the diagnosis and treatment of pulmonary hypertension: the joint task force for the diagnosis and treatment of pulmonary hypertension of the European Society of Cardiology (ESC) and the European Respiratory Society (ERS): endorsed by: Association for European Paediatric and Congenital Cardiology (AEPC), International Society for Heart and Lung Transplantation (ISHLT). *Eur Heart J.* 2016;37(1):67-119.
43. Rosenkranz S, Preston IR. Right heart catheterisation: best practice and pitfalls in pulmonary hypertension. *Eur Respir Rev.* 2015;24(138):642-652.
44. Badesch DB, Abman SH, Simonneau G, et al. Medical therapy for pulmonary arterial hypertension: updated ACCP evidence-based clinical practice guidelines. *Chest.* 2007;131(6):1917-1928.

45. Tuder RM, Archer SL, Dorfmüller P, et al. Relevant issues in the pathology and pathobiology of pulmonary hypertension. *J Am Coll Cardiol.* 2013;62(25 suppl):D4-D12.
46. McLaughlin VV, Gaine SP, Howard LS, et al. Treatment goals of pulmonary hypertension. *J Am Coll Cardiol.* 2013;62(25 suppl):D73-D81.
47. Benza RL, Miller DP, Barst RJ, et al. An evaluation of long-term survival from time of diagnosis in pulmonary arterial hypertension from the REVEAL Registry. *Chest.* 2012;142(2):448-456.
48. Nickel N, Golpon H, Greer M, et al. The prognostic impact of follow-up assessments in patients with idiopathic pulmonary arterial hypertension. *Eur Respir J.* 2012;39(3):589-596.
49. Sauler M, Fares WH, Trow TK. Standard nonspecific therapies in the management of pulmonary arterial hypertension. *Clin Chest Med.* 2013;34(4):799-810.
50. McLaughlin VV, McGoon MD. Pulmonary arterial hypertension. *Circulation.* 2006;114(13):1417-1431.
51. Taichman DB, Ornelas J, Chung L, et al. Pharmacologic therapy for pulmonary arterial hypertension in adults: CHEST guideline and expert panel report. *Chest.* 2014;146(2):449-475.
52. Sitbon O, Humbert M, Jais X, et al. Long-term response to calcium channel blockers in idiopathic pulmonary arterial hypertension. *Circulation.* 2005;111(23):3105-3111.
53. Galiè N, Barberà JA, Frost AE, et al. Initial use of ambrisentan plus tadalafil in pulmonary arterial hypertension. *N Engl J Med.* 2015;373(9):834-844.
54. Benza RL, Miller DP, Gomberg-Maitland M, et al. Predicting survival in pulmonary arterial hypertension: insights from the registry to evaluate early and long-term pulmonary arterial hypertension disease management (REVEAL). *Circulation.* 2010;122(2):164-172.
55. Velázquez Martín M, Albarrán González-Trevilla A, Jiménez López-Guarch C, et al. Use of atrial septostomy to treat severe pulmonary arterial hypertension in adults. *Rev Esp Cardiol (Engl Ed).* 2016;69(01):78-81.
56. Reichenberger F, Pepke-Zaba J, McNeil K, et al. Atrial septostomy in the treatment of severe pulmonary arterial hypertension. *Thorax.* 2003;58(9):797-800.
57. Galiè N, Corris PA, Frost A, et al. Updated treatment algorithm of pulmonary arterial hypertension. *J Am Coll Cardiol.* 2013;62(25 suppl):D60-D72.
58. van der Linde D, Konings EE, Slager MA, et al. Birth prevalence of congenital heart disease worldwide: a systematic review and meta-analysis. *J Am Coll Cardiol.* 2011;58(21):2241-2247.
59. Bruce JT, Daniels C, Sood N. Management of atrial septal defect-related pulmonary hypertension using epoprostenol and percutaneous closure. *Chest.* 2010;138(4_MeetingAbstracts):6A.
60. Geva T, Martins JD, Wald RM. Atrial septal defects. *Lancet.* 2014;383(9932):1921-1932.
61. Baumgartner H, Bonhoeffer P, De Groot NMS, et al; The Task Force on the Management of Grown-up Congenital Heart Disease of the European Society of Cardiology (ESC). ESC guidelines for the management of grown-up congenital heart disease (new version 2010). *Eur Heart J.* 2010;31(23):2915-2957.
62. Warnes CA, Williams RG, Bashore TM, et al. ACC/AHA 2008 guidelines for the management of adults with congenital heart disease: a report of the American College of Cardiology/American Heart Association Task Force on practice guidelines (writing committee to develop guidelines on the management of adults with congenital heart disease). *Circulation.* 2008;118(23):e714-e833.
63. D'Alto M, Mahadevan VS. Pulmonary arterial hypertension associated with congenital heart disease. *Eur Respir Rev.* 2012;21(126):328-337.
64. Barst RJ, Ivy DD, Foreman AJ, et al. Four- and seven-year outcomes of patients with congenital heart disease–associated pulmonary arterial hypertension (from the REVEAL Registry). *Am J Cardiol.* 2014;113(1):147-155.
65. Mulder BJM. Not too old to be closed.... *Neth Heart J.* 2010;18(11):520-521.
66. Haworth SG. Pulmonary hypertension in the young. *Heart.* 2002;88(6):658-664.
67. Simonneau G, Robbins IM, Beghetti M, et al. Updated clinical classification of pulmonary hypertension. *J Am Coll Cardiol.* 2009;54(1 suppl):S43-S54.
68. Humbert M, Sitbon O, Chaouat A, et al. Pulmonary arterial hypertension in France: results from a national registry. *Am J Respir Crit Care Med.* 2006;173(9):1023-1030.
69. Savale L, O'Callaghan DS, Magnier R, et al. Current management approaches to portopulmonary hypertension. *Int J Clin Pract Suppl.* 2011;(169):11-18.

70. Golbin JM, Krowka MJ. Portopulmonary hypertension. *Clin Chest Med.* 2007;28(1):203-218.
71. Porres-Aguilar M, Altamirano JT, Torre-Delgadillo A, et al. Portopulmonary hypertension and hepatopulmonary syndrome: a clinician-oriented overview. *Eur Respir Rev.* 2012;21(125):223-233.
72. Saleemi S. Portopulmonary hypertension. *Ann Thorac Med.* 2010;5(1):5-9.
73. Martin P, DiMartini A, Feng S, et al. Evaluation for liver transplantation in adults: 2013 practice guideline by the American association for the study of liver diseases and the American society of transplantation. *Hepatology.* 2014;59(3):1144-1165.
74. Krowka MJ, Fallon MB, Mulligan DC, et al. Model for end-stage liver disease (MELD) exception for portopulmonary hypertension. *Liver Transpl.* 2006;12(12 suppl 3):S114-S116.
75. Lang IM, Madani M. Update on chronic thromboembolic pulmonary hypertension. *Circulation.* 2014;130(6):508-518.
76. Lang IM, Pesavento R, Bonderman D, et al. Risk factors and basic mechanisms of chronic thromboembolic pulmonary hypertension: a current understanding. *Eur Respir J.* 2013;41(2):462-468.
77. Tapson VF, Humbert M. Incidence and prevalence of chronic thromboembolic pulmonary hypertension: from acute to chronic pulmonary embolism. *Proc Am Thorac Soc.* 2006;3(7):564-567.
78. Fares WH, Heresi GA. Chronic thromboembolic pulmonary hypertension: a worldwide view of how far we have come. *Lung.* 2016;194(3):483-485.
79. Kim NH, Lang IM. Risk factors for chronic thromboembolic pulmonary hypertension. *Eur Respir Rev.* 2012;21(123):27-31.
80. Lang IM. Chronic thromboembolic pulmonary hypertension — not so rare after all. *N Engl J Med.* 2004;350(22):2236-2238.
81. Pengo V, Lensing AWA, Prins MH, et al. Incidence of chronic thromboembolic pulmonary hypertension after pulmonary embolism. *N Engl J Med.* 2004;350(22):2257-2264.
82. Hoeper MM, Mayer E, Simonneau G, et al. Chronic thromboembolic pulmonary hypertension. *Circulation.* 2006;113(16):2011-2020.
83. Tunariu N, Gibbs SJ, Win Z, et al. Ventilation-perfusion scintigraphy is more sensitive than multidetector CTPA in detecting chronic thromboembolic pulmonary disease as a treatable cause of pulmonary hypertension. *J Nucl Med.* 2007;48(5):680-684.
84. Auger WR, Kerr KM, Kim NH, et al. Evaluation of patients with chronic thromboembolic pulmonary hypertension for pulmonary endarterectomy. *Pulm Circ.* 2012;2(2):155-162.
85. McNeil K, Dunning J. Chronic thromboembolic pulmonary hypertension (CTEPH). *Heart.* 2007;93(9):1152-1158.
86. Kawakami T, Ogawa A, Miyaji K, et al. Novel angiographic classification of each vascular lesion in chronic thromboembolic pulmonary hypertension based on selective angiogram and results of balloon pulmonary angioplasty. *Circ Cardiovasc Interv.* 2016;9(10).
87. Hoeper MM, Madani MM, Nakanishi N, et al. Chronic thromboembolic pulmonary hypertension. *Lancet Respir Med.* 2014;2(7):573-582.
88. Klepetko W, Mayer E, Sandoval J, et al. Interventional and surgical modalities of treatment for pulmonary arterial hypertension. *J Am Coll Cardiol.* 2004;43(12 suppl):S73-S80.
89. Jamieson SW, Kapelanski DP, Sakakibara N, et al. Pulmonary endarterectomy: experience and lessons learned in 1,500 cases. *Ann Thorac Surg.* 2003;76(5):1457-1464.
90. Kim NH, Delcroix M, Jenkins DP, et al. Chronic thromboembolic pulmonary hypertension. *J Am Coll Cardiol.* 2013;62(25 suppl):D92-D99.
91. Mizoguchi H, Ogawa A, Munemasa M, et al. Refined balloon pulmonary angioplasty for inoperable patients with chronic thromboembolic pulmonary hypertension. *Circ Cardiovasc Interv.* 2012;5(6):748-755.

CHAPTER 22

Deep Vein Thrombosis

Robert R. Attaran, MD, FACC, FASE, FSCAI, RPVI

Key Points

- Venous thromboembolism is a common and sometimes devastating condition.
- In some cases, mechanical thrombus removal can be beneficial.
- The rate of recurrent DVT is high.
- Optimal duration of anticoagulation for DVT is controversial.
- Treatment of post-thrombotic syndrome should ideally address both venous obstruction and reflux.

I. Venous Thromboembolism

Venous thromboembolism (VTE) (deep vein thrombosis [DVT] and pulmonary embolism [PE]) is a common cause of mortality, morbidity, and loss of quality of life, particularly due to postthrombotic syndrome (PTS). This is a chronic condition of the leg that can result in pain, swelling, discoloration, and even ulceration, which occurs in at least 30% after DVT.[1] Rarely limb loss can occur through phlegmasia cerulean dolens. There are over 250,000 cases of VTE per annum in the United States alone.[2] Venous thrombosis is initiated by a combination of vessel injury, inflammation, hypercoagulability, and stasis. A first occurrence of VTE dramatically increases the risk of a subsequent one.

II. Venous Thromboembolism and Risk of Subsequent Recurrent Venous Thromboembolism

In a prospective cohort study, 355 patients with a first episode of DVT were followed for 8 years. Recurrent VTE occurred at 17.5% after 2 years and 24.6% after 5 years. PTS was reported in 22.8% after 2 years and 28% after 5 years.[3] The same investigators in a larger prospective cohort study of 1626 patients with VTE reported a recurrence of 11% at 1 year, 19.6% at 3 years, and 29.1% at 5 years.[4] Anticoagulation is effective at lowering recurrences but carries an increased risk of bleeding.[5]

III. Pharmacological Treatment

A. **Anticoagulation** Parenteral anticoagulation with a heparinoid followed by oral anticoagulation has been the mainstay of treatment for acute DVT. Anticoagulants help prevent thrombus propagation and embolization. Both vitamin K antagonists (VKAs) and non–vitamin K oral anticoagulants which are the novel oral anticoagulants (NOACs) have been used. An advantage of NOACs is the steady anticoagulation they provide (without the need for routine monitoring). They may also result in less intracranial bleeding than VKAs, although possibly more gastrointestinal bleeds as shown in some studies.[6,7]

B. **American College of Chest Physician Guidelines**

1. The required duration for anticoagulant therapy in DVT has been a contentious issue with significant variability in practice pattern. Some patients are maintained on

anticoagulation for years. The 2016 American College of Chest Physician Guidelines[8] made the following recommendations for anticoagulation in DVT:

- In patients with proximal DVT or PE, 3 months of anticoagulant therapy are recommended (Grade 1B). NOACs are preferred over VKAs.
- In proximal DVT or PE provoked by surgery or a transient risk factor, 3 months of anticoagulant therapy are recommended (Grade 1B).
- In proximal DVT of the leg or PE and cancer ("cancer-associated thrombosis"), low-molecular-weight heparin is recommended over oral anticoagulants. Anticoagulation should be extended beyond 3 months in those without a high bleed risk (Grade 1B).
- In unprovoked first proximal DVT or PE with low-moderate bleed risk, extended anticoagulant therapy beyond 3 months is suggested (Grade 2B).

In a second unprovoked proximal DVT or PE, extended anticoagulant therapy beyond 3 months is recommended with low bleed risk (Grade 1B) and moderate bleed risk (Grade 2B).

2. While anticoagulants prevent thrombus propagation, thrombolytics directly eliminate thrombus. One of the troublesome sequelae of DVT is PTS. DVT can acutely lead to elevated limb venous pressures and diminished venous outflow leading to inflammation, fibrosis, and valvular damage. This is particularly a concern if the DVT involves the venous outflow at the common femoral vein or even more proximal level (iliac vein or IVC). Thrombolysis can relieve the obstruction more rapidly than mere anticoagulation. A Cochrane review of randomized trials comparing thrombolysis against anticoagulation identified 17 trials ($n = 1103$). Thrombolysis reduced rates of PTS by a third and leg ulceration approximately a half, but there were more instances of bleeding (RR 2.23; 95% CI 1.41-3.52, $P = .0006$). There was no difference in mortality.[9]

C. Catheter-Directed Therapy

1. Systemic thrombolysis for DVT carries a significant bleed risk and has largely been superseded by catheter-directed therapy (CDT). With CDT, lower doses of thrombolytics are required and are often administered over a longer period. In addition to the availability of simple perfusion catheters, some available devices have a mechanical component that can help disrupt the thrombus.[10,11]
2. Two of the devices currently used for mechanical thrombectomy in the United States are AngioJet (Boston Scientific, Marlborough, MA) and EKOS (BTG, West Conshohocken, PA). AngioJet is a pharmacomechanical thrombectomy catheter.[12] Multiple high-velocity saline jets through orifices at the tip create a low-pressure zone using the Venturi-Bernoulli effect, resulting in dissociation of thrombus which is concurrently removed by suction. The power pulse function allows for local infusion of a thrombolytic agent (eg, 12-25 mg tissue plasminogen activator), while the suction function is stopped to prevent removal of the lytic.[12,13] With the AngioJet catheter tip positioned within the thrombus, power pulse lytic infusion can be run for approximately 90 minutes before the thrombectomy mode is reactivated and the tip manipulated up and down to retrieve thrombus.[14] The larger caliber AngioJet ZelanteDVT catheter (8F) is capable of removing thrombus more quickly.

3. **Trials**
   a. The EKOS device is an ultrasound-assisted lysis perfusion catheter. In vitro studies have demonstrated improved dispersion of tissue plasminogen activator into thrombus, when assisted by ultrasound.[15] The EKOS catheter is advanced into the venous thrombus and activated, infusing thrombolytics. The device is typically run for up to 24 hours before removal.[16]
   b. There are two randomized controlled trials comparing CDT with anticoagulation in DVT that merit discussion. In the TORPEDO trial 91 patients with proximal DVT received CDT in addition to anticoagulation, versus 92 patients who received anticoagulation only. The CDT devices included Trellis (Covidien, Plymouth, MN) and AngioJet (Boston Scientific, Marlborough, MA). Approximately 3rd of CDT patients also underwent venous balloon angioplasty and 3rd underwent venous stenting. The CDT group demonstrated significantly lower rates of recurrent VTE and PTS at 6 and 30 months.[11] CaVenT was a Norwegian multicenter trial that enrolled patients with acute iliofemoral DVT. In the CDT group (n = 101), a catheter perfused intravenous alteplase, and the control group (n = 108) received anticoagulation only. With CDT, iliofemoral vein patency was significantly higher at 65.9% versus 47.4% in the control group (P = .012). CDT led to an absolute risk reduction of 14.4% (NNT = 7) in PTS by Villalta score, at 24 months.[17] Five-year follow-up data of CaVenT continue to favor CDT over anticoagulation only.[18]
   c. Sponsored by the National Institute of Health, the ATTRACT trial has evaluated pharmacomechanical CDT in proximal DVT, enrolling 692 patients. The primary end point is rate of PTS on follow-up. Enrollment has been completed, and the study is currently in the follow-up phase.
      i. While there is some consensus that CDT should especially be considered for treating acute DVTs causing venous outflow obstruction (those involving the common femoral, iliac veins or IVC), more robust data are needed. The ATTRACT trial may help shed more light on this issue.
   d. Saha et al[19] have suggested the five-component "BLAST" mnemonic when assessing candidates for CDT. BLAST stands for Bleeding risk, Life expectancy, Anatomy of DVT, Severity of DVT, and Timing. Lysis is less desirable in thrombi that are older than 14 days, although some trials have included patients within 21 days.
      i. We believe that iliac stenting for venous outflow obstruction should be performed in addition to CDT for DVT, as it may enhance subsequent venous patency rates.[20]

IV. Superficial Venous Thrombosis of the Legs

A. **Presentation** Frequently, "superficial venous thrombosis" is also referred to as "superficial thrombophlebitis," signifying inflammation of superficial veins with thrombosis. It appears to be more common in older age, particularly in women.[21] Patients typically present with tender, erythematous legs along the region of affected veins. It can sometimes be mistaken for cellulitis, although infection is frequently not present. The affected veins may feel firm to palpation. Over time, pigmentation can develop.

B. **Etiologic Factors** Associated or etiologic factors include varicose veins, immobility, hypercoagulable states, surgery, intravenous access, pregnancy, malignancy, and estrogen therapy.[22] Karathanos[23] followed 97 patients with superficial thrombosis and varicose veins for a mean period of 55 months. Thirteen had a recurrence. There were higher rates of prothrombin gene (G20210A) mutation and dyslipidemia in those with recurrence.

C. **Clinical Diagnosis** Although superficial thrombosis is a clinical diagnosis, it may coincide with DVT.[24] It is therefore reasonable to consider venous duplex imaging to gauge its extent and to rule out deep vein involvement.

D. **Treatment** Superficial venous thrombosis has been treated in a number of ways including topical or oral nonsteroidal anti-inflammatory drugs (NSAIDs), aspirin, anticoagulants, and compression.[25] There is some evidence to support the role of NSAIDs as well as some anticoagulants in reducing recurrence, thrombus extension, or DVT. A 2013 Cochrane review noted a paucity of randomized controlled data for treatment modalities in superficial venous thrombosis. Prophylactic dose fondaparinux for 6 weeks appeared to show benefit by reducing thrombus extension.[26] It is our practice to ablate venous insufficiency and varicose veins in patients with a history of superficial venous thrombosis, particularly if more than one episode has occurred.

V. Isolated Below-the-Knee Deep Vein Thrombosis

A. History and Management

1. The infrapopliteal deep veins include the paired peroneal, anterior tibial, and posterior tibial veins, as well the gastrocnemius and soleal veins. Significant anatomic variability can exist. Isolated below-the-knee DVT, also referred to as isolated distal deep vein thrombosis (IDDVT), denotes thrombosis in any of the deep veins without involvement of the popliteal vein. Thrombotic involvement of the popliteal vein (or above) is referred to as proximal DVT.
2. The natural history of IDDVT is not clear, and therefore, its management is controversial. Between 23% and 59% of individuals diagnosed with DVT also have IDDVT.[27] Few studies have evaluated the natural history of IDDVT without anticoagulation. The CALTHRO study followed 59 patients with IDDVT. No anticoagulation was administered. After one week, proximal thrombus extension occurred in 3.1%.[28]

B. Risks of Recurrence

1. IDDVT may carry a lower risk of recurrence compared with proximal DVT.[29] However, chronic sequelae such as PTS can occur.[30]
2. A meta-analysis of (≥1 month therapy) anticoagulation trials for IDDVT suggested reduced rates of thrombus propagation and PE (odds ratio, 0.12; 95% confidence interval, 0.02-0.77; $P = .03$) and thrombus propagation (odds ratio, 0.29; 95% confidence interval, 0.14-0.62; $P = .04$).[31] However, the studies were small (126 patients treated with anticoagulation versus 328 controls), and many were judged to be of poor quality.

C. Recommendations

1. The International Consensus Statement on Prevention and Treatment of Venous Thromboembolism recommends 3 months of oral anticoagulants for patients with symptomatic IDDVT.[32]
2. The 2016 American College of Chest Physicians Guidelines[8] have identified a number of risk factors for IDDVT extension including D-dimer elevation, thrombus longer than 5 cm or in multiple sites, lack of reversible provoking factor, active cancer, history of VTE, inpatient status, and tibial or peroneal vein involvement. In patients without severe symptoms or risk factors for extension, they recommend serial imaging of the deep veins over anticoagulation (Grade 2C). Anticoagulation is recommended if the patient has severe symptoms.
3. Below-knee compression stockings should be worn and may have therapeutic benefit beyond reduction of edema and discomfort.[28]

VI. Indications for Hypercoagulable Workup

The evaluation and management of DVT in patients with thrombophilia is beyond the scope of this chapter. The American Society of Hematology provides a number of guidelines as part of its Choosing Wisely campaign to minimize unnecessary anticoagulation and testing.[33] In evaluating any patient with DVT, we seek the following information: whether the event was provoked or unprovoked, past medical history, history of miscarriages, family history, and medications. The following initial laboratory tests are obtained: complete blood count, peripheral blood smear, erythrocyte sedimentation rate and C-reactive protein, coagulation panel, basic metabolic panel, and urinalysis with microscopy. We typically test for a hereditary thrombophilia if one or more of the following criteria apply: the patient is young (age < 45 y), has a positive family history for VTE (age < 45 y), has recurrent VTE, and/or has unprovoked VTE.[34] However, screening all individuals with unprovoked VTE and their subsequent management are controversial.[35]

Owing to paucity of data and the inherent challenges of study implementation, it is difficult to define which populations should remain on anticoagulation indefinitely. Based on the current state of knowledge,[36–39] it is probably reasonable to offer indefinite anticoagulation in the following scenarios: 2 or more episodes of unprovoked VTE, unprovoked VTE and antithrombin deficiency, unprovoked massive PE, unprovoked cerebral or mesenteric vein thrombosis, and unprovoked VTE and two hereditary thrombophilias.

VII. Chronic Deep Vein Thrombosis

A. **Effects** Chronic disease of the deep veins can lead to PTS. Its harmful effects can be from a combination of obstruction, reflux, or both.[40] The reflux may also involve superficial veins. The severity of PTS is greatest among those with iliofemoral DVT, recurrent DVT, and older age.[1,41,42]

1. After a DVT the thrombus may resolve leaving minimal scarring. In many cases, however, the thrombus becomes more organized and fibrosis occurs within the vein, making the lumen narrower or occluded. Hardened cribriform synechiae formed from

endothelialized strands of residual thrombus can remain.[43,44] Collateral formation may occur. Stenosis or obstruction in a proximal vein results in venous stasis and hypertension more distally. Exercise and the use of the calf muscle pump are unable to lower venous pressures and ambulatory venous hypertension ensues.[43] Valvular dysfunction and venous dilatation can follow contributing to inflammation and edema in the affected limb.[45]

2. Approximately 75% of iliac veins are thought to develop obstruction after a DVT.[40,46] Over the past 10-15 years, angioplasty and stenting of the iliac veins has gained momentum as a therapy for chronic venous thrombosis and the symptoms of PTS. Raju[47] reviewed studies on iliac endovascular intervention (angioplasty and/or stenting) noting 3-5-year stent patency rates in the 74%-89% range among postthrombotic cases. Iliac intervention led to less edema, more venous ulcer healing, and pain relief. The studies did not report any cases of iatrogenic PE. A systematic review and meta-analysis[48] showed iliac vein stenting for both nonthrombotic and thrombotic iliac vein stenosis to be safe and efficacious, with technical success rates of approximately 95%, major bleeding up to 1.1%, PE up to 0.9%, and early thrombosis up to 6.8%. At 1-year follow-up, primary patency for postthrombotic patients was 79% and secondary patency was 94%.

B. **Treatment and Management** In patients with chronic DVT and disabling PTS, it is currently our practice to perform balloon angioplasty followed by stenting to fibrosed and/or stenosed iliac veins, but we rarely deploy currently available stents distal to the inguinal ligament owing to potential concerns over stent fracture and occlusion. If more distal venous segments are fibrosed and narrowed, balloon angioplasty alone (and occasionally venous atherectomy) can be used. After venous stenting in a postthrombotic patient, we prefer full-dose enoxaparin for the first month, after which the patient is transitioned to an oral anticoagulant for a further 5 months. There are no robust data on optimal anticoagulant strategy.

VIII. Imaging of Venous Thromboembolism

A. **Ultrasound** Ultrasound is the primary imaging modality for evaluation of venous thrombosis. Fresh thrombus can be anechoic,[49] but lack of vein compressibility with the ultrasound probe is diagnostic for DVT[50] as is the absence of color flow.[51] An abbreviated and simple test for leg DVT is the so-called two-point technique, where the common femoral region and popliteal veins are interrogated. More detailed protocols, sometimes referred to as "whole leg," are also available. The latter technique, although more complex and time-consuming, diagnoses IDDVTs that would otherwise be undetected with the two-point technique.[52]

Computed tomography (CT) venography can also be used to diagnose DVT and has high sensitivity (over 95%) and specificity (96%) with the added ability to better distinguish acute from chronic thrombus.[53,54] In our experience, it is a good tool particularly when evaluating iliac vein or IVC thrombosis. One challenge of CT venography is the proper timing of the image acquisition after contrast injection.

B. **Magnetic Resonance** Magnetic resonance (MR) venography is also a good tool for evaluation of DVT (particularly iliac and IVC) with high sensitivity and specificity and has the capability to distinguish fresh from residual thrombus.[55,56] Gadolinium may have the advantage of better venous phase distribution.

IX. Venous Thromboembolism and Risk of Subsequent Arterial Thrombosis

A. **Associated Disorders** VTE and arterial thrombotic diseases (eg, myocardial infarction [MI], ischemic stroke) have traditionally been regarded as separate disease entities, with different pathophysiology and therapy. There are, however, a number of well-known disorders characterized by both arterial and venous involvement, such as heparin-induced thrombocytopenia, antiphospholipid antibody syndrome, and myeloproliferative disorders. In addition, there is evidence to suggest that VTE may lead to increased arterial ischemic event rates.

B. **Trials and Studies**

1. A 20-year Danish population–based cohort study evaluated the risk of myocardial infarction and stroke among 25,199 patients with DVT and 16,925 patients with PE.[57] Patients with known cardiovascular disease were excluded. In the first year after the thrombotic event, compared with controls, DVT patients had a relative risk of 1.60 for MI (95% CI 1.35-1.91) and 2.19 for stroke (1.85-2.60). PE patients had a relative risk of 2.60 (2.14-3.13) for MI and 2.93 (2.34-3.66) for stroke. Relative risks did not differ significantly for those with provoked versus unprovoked VTE. The increased relative risk remained raised for the ensuing 20 years.
2. Another Scandinavian population–based study found an association between VTE and future arterial events in all woman and men aged <65 years, over a median follow-up of 12.2 years. Women with VTE had 3.3-fold higher risk of subsequent arterial disease; men under age 65 years had a hazard ratio of 2.06.[58]
   a. Hereditary thrombophilia or other hypercoagulable disorders may explain some of the increased arterial thrombotic disease after VTE.[59] In addition, there are a number of common factors that appear to predispose to both arterial and venous disease: platelet activation, higher clotting factor concentration, older age, smoking, obesity, inflammatory cytokines, and estrogens.[60]

In animal studies, VKA therapy results in arterial calcification.[61] In humans, prolonged VKA therapy appeared to be associated with (extracoronary) vascular calcification.[62]

X. The Potential Role of Statins in Venous Disease

A. **Jupiter Trial** In 2009, the Jupiter Trial evaluated rosuvastatin 20 mg in patients with elevated hsCRP (>2 mg/L) and made the observation that over a median follow-up of 1.9 years, the statin-treated group had lower rates of VTE (hazard ratio for rosuvastatin, 0.57; 95% confidence interval, 0.37-0.86; *P* = .007).[63]

B. Statin Therapy

1. An excellent systematic review by Rodriguez[64] discusses the data for statin therapy and its potential antithrombotic and anti-inflammatory roles. For example, IL-6–induced CRP is decreased by statins.[65] A 2009 meta-analysis[66] appears to support the potential role of statin therapy in the prevention of VTE.

2. In a murine DVT model, treatment of mice with daily statin reduced thrombus burden and DVT-induced venous scarring.[67] Venous scarring and valvular damage have been attributed to the development of PTS. Statins reduced platelet aggregation, tissue factor (TF), and myeloperoxidase.[67] In the same study, statin therapy also reduced TF levels within thrombus.

C. Platelet Recruitment Platelet recruitment and activity may also allow deep vein thrombus formation and extension.[68,69] Statins appear to limit cyclooxygenase-1 (COX-1) activation, while enhancing nitric oxide synthase, which can inhibit platelet activation and aggregation.[70]

D. Oral Anticoagulation In and of itself oral anticoagulation does not eliminate PTS, although the inability to anticoagulate raises the risk.[71] A clinical prospective randomized single-center open-label trial evaluated rosuvastatin in patients treated with low-molecular-weight heparins for DVT (n = 234). The treatment group received 5-10 mg daily rosuvastatin plus LMWH. The control group received LMWH only. After 3-months, D-dimer levels were not significantly different, but CRP levels were lower in the statin-treated group. The Villalta score for PTS was significantly lower in the statin group (3.45 ± 6.03 vs 7.79 ± 5.58, P = .035), and there was lower incidence of PTS in statin group (38.3% vs 48.5%, P = .019).[72] The major limitation of this trial was its open-label, single-center design.

XI. Summary

VTE is a disabling, potentially lethal disease with long-term sequelae and a high rate of recurrence. The current guidelines can help define the recommended duration of anticoagulation required. More studies are under way to determine the optimal treatment algorithm for an acute VTE as well as pharmaceutical therapies to reduce recurrence and disability.[73, 74]

References

1. Kahn SR, Shrier I, Julian JA, et al. Determinants and time course of the post-thrombotic syndrome after acute deep venous thrombosis. *Ann Int Med.* 2008;149:698-707.
2. Jaff MR, McMurtry MS, Archer SL, et al. Management of massive and submassive pulmonary embolism, iliofemoral deep vein thrombosis, and chronic thromboembolic pulmonary hypertension: a scientific statement from the American Heart Association. *Circulation.* 2011;123:1788-1830.
3. Prandoni P, Lensing AW, Cogo A, et al. The long-term clinical course of acute deep venous thrombosis. *Ann Int Med.* 1996;125(1):1-7.
4. Prandoni P, Noventa F, Ghirarduzzi A, et al. The risk of recurrent venous thromboembolism after discontinuing anticoagulation in patients with acute proximal deep vein thrombosis or pulmonary embolism. A prospective cohort study in 1,626 patients. *Haematologica.* 2007;92:199-205.

5. Linkins LA, Choi PT, Douketis JD. Clinical impact of bleeding in patients taking oral anticoagulant therapy for venous thromboembolism. *Ann Intern Med.* 2003;139:893-900.
6. Schulman S, Kearon C, Kakkar AK, et al. Dabigatran versus warfarin in the treatment of acute venous thromboembolism. *N Engl J Med.* 2009;361:2342-2352.
7. Sharma M, Cornelius VR, Patel JP, et al. Efficacy and harms of direct oral anticoagulants in the elderly for stroke prevention in atrial fibrillation and secondary prevention of venous thromboembolism: systematic review and meta-analysis. *Circulation.* 2015;132:194-204.
8. Kearon C, Akl EA, Ornelas J, et al. Antithrombotic therapy for VTE disease CHEST guideline and expert panel report. *Chest.* 2016;149(2):315-352.
9. Watson L, Broderick C, Armon MP. Thrombolysis for acute deep vein thrombosis. *Cochr Database Syst Rev.* 2014;1:CD002783.
10. Baekgaard N, Klitfod L, Broholm R. Safety and efficacy of catheter-directed thrombolysis. *Phlebology.* 2012;27(suppl 1):149-154.
11. Sharifi M, Mehdipour M, Bay C, et al. Endovenous therapy for deep venous thrombosis: the TORPEDO trial. *Catheter Cardiovasc Interv.* 2010;76(3):316-325.
12. Garcia MJ, Lookstein R, Malhotra R, et al. Endovascular management of deep vein thrombosis with rheolytic thrombectomy: final report of the prospective multicenter PEARL (Peripheral use of AngioJet Rheolytic Thrombectomy with a variety of catheter Lengths) registry. *J Vasc Interv Radiol.* 2015;26(6):777-785.
13. Cynamon J, Stein EG, Dym RJ, et al. A new method for aggressive management of deep vein thrombosis: retrospective study of the power pulse technique. *J Vasc Interv Radiol.* 2006;17:1043-1049.
14. Hager E, Yuo T, Avgerinos E, et al. Anatomic and functional outcomes of pharmacomechanical and catheter-directed thrombolysis of iliofemoral deep venous thrombosis. *J Vasc Surg Venous Lymphat Disord.* 2014;2:246-252.
15. Francis CW, Blinc A, Lee S, et al. Ultrasound accelerates transport of recombinant tissue plasminogen activator into clots. *Ultrasound Med Biol.* 1995;21:419-424.
16. Parikh S, Motarjeme A, McNanamra T, et al. Ultrasound-accelerated thrombolysis for the treatment of deep vein thrombosis: initial clinical experience. *J Vasc Interv Radiol.* 2008;19(4):521-528.
17. Enden T, Haig Y, Klow NE, et al. Long-term outcome after additional catheter-directed thrombolysis versus standard treatment for acute iliofemoral deep vein thrombosis (the CaVenT study): a randomised controlled trial: *Lancet.* 2012;379(9810):31-38.
18. Haig Y, Enden T, Grøtta O, et al. Post-thrombotic syndrome after catheter-directed thrombolysis for deep vein thrombosis (CaVenT): 5-year follow-up results of an open-label, randomised controlled trial. *Lancet Haematol.* 2016;3(2):e64-e71.
19. Saha P, Black S, Breen K, et al. Contemporary management of acute and chronic deep vein thrombosis. *Brit Med Bulletin.* 2016;117:107-120.
20. Mewissen M, Seabrook G, Meissner M, et al. Catheter-directed thrombolysis for lower extremity deep venous thrombosis: report of a national multicenter registry. *Radiology.* 1999;211:39-49.
21. Decousas H, Quere I, Presles E, et al. Superficial venous thrombosis and venous thromboembolism: a large, prospective epidemiologic study. *Ann Intern Med.* 2010;152:218-224.
22. De Maeseneer MGR. Superficial thrombophlebitis of the lower limb: practical recommendations for diagnosis and treatment. *Acta Chir Belg.* 2005;105:145-147.
23. Karathanos C, Spanos K, Saleptsis V, et al. Recurrence of superficial vein thrombosis in patients with varicose veins. *Phlebology.* 2016;31(7):489-495.
24. Leon L, Giannoukas AD, Dodd D, et al. Clinical significance of superficial vein thrombosis. *Eur J Vasc Endovasc Surg.* 2005;29:10-17.
25. Dua A, Patel B, Heller J, et al. Variability in the management of superficial venous thrombophlebitis among phlebologists and vascular surgeons. *Perspect Vasc Surg Endovasc Ther.* 2013;25:5-10.
26. Di Nisio M, Wichers IM, Middeldorp S. Treatment for superficial thrombophlebitis of the leg. *Cochrane Database Syst Rev.* 2013;(4):CD004982.

27. Palareti G, Schellong S. Isolated distal deep vein thrombosis: what we know and what we are doing. *J Thromb Haemost.* 2012;10:11-19.
28. Palareti G, Cosmi B, Lessiani G, et al. Evolution of untreated calf deep-vein thrombosis in high risk symptomatic outpatients: the blind, prospective CALTHRO study. *Thromb Haemost.* 2010;104(5):1063-1070.
29. Galanaud JP, Quenet S, Rivron-Guillot K, et al. Comparison of the clinical history of symptomatic isolated distal deep-vein thrombosis vs. proximal deep vein thrombosis in 11086 patients. *J Thromb Haemost.* 2009;7:2028-2034.
30. McLafferty RB, Moneta GL, Passman MA, et al. Late clinical and hemodynamic sequelae of isolated calf vein thrombosis. *J Vasc Surg.* 1998;27:50-56.
31. De Marino RR, Wallaert JB, Rossi AP, et al. A meta-analysis of anticoagulation for calf deep venous thrombosis. *J Vasc Surg.* 2012;56:228-237.
32. Nicolaides AN, Fareed J, Kakkar AK, et al. Prevention and treatment of venous thromboembolism- international consensus statement. *Int Angiol.* 2013;32:111-260.
33. Hicks LK, Bering H, Carson KR, et al. Five hematologic tests and treatments to question. *Blood.* 2014;124:3524-3528.
34. Lindhoff-Last E, Luxembourg B. Evidence-based indications for thrombophilia screening. *Vasa.* 2008;37(1):19-30.
35. Moll S. Thrombophilia: clinical-practical aspects. *J Thromb Thrombolysis.* 2015;39(3):367-378.
36. Bauer KA. The thrombophilias: well-defined risk factors with uncertain therapeutic implications. *Ann Intern Med.* 2001;135(5):367.
37. De Stefano V, Martinelli I, Mannucci PM, et al. The risk of recurrent deep venous thrombosis among heterozygous carriers of both factor V Leiden and the G20210A prothrombin mutation. *N Engl J Med.* 1999;341(11):801.
38. Heit JA, Cunningham JM, Petterson TM, et al. Genetic variation within the anticoagulant, procoagulant, fibrinolytic and innate immunity pathways as risk factors for venous thromboembolism. *J Thromb Haemost.* 2011;9(6):1133-1142.
39. National Clinical Guideline Centre (UK). *Venous Thromboembolic Diseases: The Management of Venous Thromboembolic Diseases and the Role of Thrombophilia Testing [Internet].* London: Royal College of Physicians (UK); June 2012.
40. Johnson BF, Manzo RA, Bergelin RO, Strandness DE. Relationship between changes in the deep venous system and the development of the post-thrombotic syndrome after an acute episode of lower limb deep vein thrombosis: a one- to six-year follow-up. *J Vasc Surg.* 1995;21:307-313.
41. Kahn SR. How I treat post-thrombotic syndrome. *Blood.* 2009;114:4624-4631.
42. Ziegler S, Schillinger M, Maca TH, et al. Post-thrombotic syndrome after primary event of deep venous thrombosis 10 to 20 years ago. *Thromb Res.* 2001;101:23-33.
43. Meissner MH, Moneta G, Bernand K, et al. The hemodynamics and diagnosis of venous disease. *J Vasc Surg.* 2007;46:4S-24S.
44. Rosfors S, Eriksson M, Leijd B, et al. A prospective follow-up study of acute deep venous thrombosis using colour duplex ultra- sound, phlebography and venous occlusion plethysmography. *Int Angiol.* 1997;16:39-44.
45. Coleridge Smith PD. Update on chronic-venous-insufficiency-induced inflammatory processes. *Angiology.* 2001;52(suppl 1):S35-S42.
46. Akesson H, Brudin L, Dahlström JA, et al. Venous function assessed during a 5-year period after acute iliofemoral venous thrombosis treated with anticoagulation. *Eur J Vasc Surg.* 1990;4:43.
47. Raju S. Best management options for chronic iliac vein stenosis and occlusion. *J Vasc Surg.* 2013;57(4):1163-1169.
48. Razavi MK, Jaff MR, Miller LE. Safety and effectiveness of stent placement for iliofemoral venous outflow obstruction: systematic review and meta-analysis. *Circ Cardiovasc Interv.* 2015;8(10):e002772.
49. Murphy TP, Cronan JJ. Evaluation of deep venous thrombosis: a prospective evaluation with ultrasound. *Radiology.* 1990;177:543-548.
50. Gornik HL, Sharma AM. Duplex ultrasound in the diagnosis of lower-extremity deep venous thrombosis. *Circulation.* 2014;129:917-921.

51. Cronan JJ, Dorfman GS. Advances in ultrasound imaging of venous thrombosis. *Semin Nucl Med.* 1991;21:297-312.
52. Goodacre S, Sampson F, Thomas S, et al. Systematic review and meta-analysis of the diagnostic accuracy of ultrasonography for deep vein thrombosis. *BMC Med Imaging.* 2005;5:6.
53. Baldt MM, Zontsich T, Stumpflen A, et al. Deep venous thrombosis of the lower extremity: efficacy of spiral CT venography compared with conventional venography in diagnosis. *Radiology.* 1996;200:423-428.
54. Thomas SM, Goodacre SW, Sampson FC, et al. Diagnostic value of CT for deep vein thrombosis: results of a systematic review and meta-analysis. *Clin Radiol.* 2008;63:299-304.
55. Sampson FC, Goodacre SW, Thomas SM, et al. The accuracy of MRI in diagnosis of suspected deep vein thrombosis: systematic review and meta-analysis. *Eur J Radiol.* 2007;17:175-181.
56. Tan M, Mol GC, Van Rooden CJ, et al. Magnetic resonance direct thrombus imaging differentiates acute recurrent ipsilateral deep vein thrombosis from residual thrombosis. *Blood.* 2014;124:623-627.
57. Sorensen HT, Horvath-Puho E, Pedersen L, Baron JA, Prandoni P. Venous thromboembolism and subsequent hospitalization due to acute arterial cardiovascular events: a 20-year cohort study. *Lancet.* 2007;370:1773-1779.
58. Lind C, Flinterman LE, Enga KF, et al. Impact of incident venous thromboembolism on risk of arterial thrombotic diseases. *Circulation.* 2014;129:855-863.
59. Roach RE, Lijfering WM, Flinterman LE, Rosendaal FR, Cannegieter SC. Increased risk of CVD after VT is determined by common etiologic factors. *Blood.* 2013;121:4948-4954.
60. Green D. Risk of future arterial cardiovascular events in patients with idiopathic venous thromboembolism. *Hematology.* 2009;1:259-266.
61. Price PA, Faus SA, Williamson MK. Warfarin causes rapid calcification of the elastic lamellae in rat arteries and heart valves. *Arterioscler Thromb Vasc Biol.* 1998;18:1400-1407.
62. Rennenberg RJ, van Varik BJ, Schurgers LJ, et al. Chronic coumarin treatment is associated with increased extracoronary arterial calcification in humans. *Blood.* 2010;115:5121-5123.
63. Glynn RJ, Danielson E, Fonseca FAH, et al. A randomized trial of rosuvastatin in the prevention of venous thromboembolism: the JUPITER trial. *N Engl J Med.* 2009;360;1851.
64. Rodriguez AL, Wojcik BM, Wrobleski SK, Myers DD, Wakefield TW, Diaz JA. Statins, inflammation and deep vein thrombosis: a systematic review. *J Thromb Thrombolysis.* 2012;33:371.
65. Arnaud C, Burger F, Steffens S, et al. Statins reduce interleukin-6-induced CRP in human hepatocytes: new evidence for direct anti-inflammatory effects of statins. *Arterioscler Thromb Vasc Biol.* 2005;25(6):1231.
66. Squizzato A, Galli M, Romualdi E, et al. Statins, fibrates, and venous thromboembolism: a meta-analysis. *Eur Heart J.* 2009;31(10):1248.
67. Kessinger CW, Kim JW, Henke PK, et al. Statins improve the resolution of established murine venous thrombosis: reductions in thrombus burden and vein wall scarring. *PLoS One.* 2015;10(2):e0116621.
68. Brill A, Fuchs TA, Chauhan AK, et al. von Willebrand factor-mediated platelet adhesion is critical for deep vein thrombosis in mouse models. *Blood.* 2011;117:1400-1407.
69. von Bruhl M-L, Stark K, Steinhart A, et al. Monocytes, neutrophils, and platelets cooperate to initiate and propogate venous thrombosis in mice in vivo. *J Exp Med.* 2012;209:819-883.
70. Pignatelli P, Carnevale R, Pastori D, et al. Immediate antioxidant and antiplatelet effect of atorvastatin via inhibition of Nox2. *Circulation.* 2012;126:92-103.
71. Van Dongen CJ, Prandoni P, Frulla M, Marchiori A, Prins MH, Hutten BA. Relation between quality of anticoagulant treatment and the development of the postthrombotic syndrome. *J Thromb Haemost.* 2005;3:939-942.
72. San Norberto EM, Gastambide MV, Taylor JH, García-Saiz I, Vaquero C. Effects of rosuvastatin as an adjuvant treatment for deep vein thrombosis. *Vasa.* 2016;45(2):133-140.

CHAPTER 23

May-Thurner Syndrome

S. Elissa Altin, MD and Gabriella Wilson, MD

I. Introduction

A. **History** May-Thurner syndrome (MTS) is a syndrome of venous outflow obstruction due to extrinsic compression by the arterial system against bony structures. In 1908, McMurrich first described isolated left lower extremity swelling due to left iliac vein compression. In this cadaver study, he observed that adhesions of the iliac veins were present in about one-third of the cadavers studied. Of these, the vast majority of adhesions attached to the iliofemoral vessels were present on the left side. This study thus proposed that adhesions could be a possible explanation for the left-sided predilection for iliofemoral thrombosis formation that Virchow first noted in 1851. Almost 40 years after McMurrich, Ehrich and Krumbhaar performed an autopsy study that revealed increased collagen and elastin deposition of the left common iliac vein, causing obstruction and possibly contributing to the increased prevalence of left-sided iliofemoral thrombosis.[1]

B. **Studies**

1. A hallmark study was conducted by May and Thurner in 1957 that proposed an anatomic variant as the underlying cause for increased prevalence of left-sided iliofemoral venous thrombosis. They evaluated 430 cadavers and noted that 22% of the cadavers exhibited compression of the left common iliac vein between the right common iliac artery and the fifth lumbar vertebra. They postulated that this anatomic abnormality could be an explanation for this side preference of iliofemoral deep vein thrombosis (DVT) first described by Virchow. They hypothesized that both pulsation and mechanical compression of the overlying right common iliac artery in these variants leads to focal stenosis of the wall of the underlying left common iliac vein. They referred to this area of stenosis as a "venous spur" and also proposed that this "spur" might play an instigative role in lower extremity venous outflow obstruction.[2]

2. The association between iliac vein compression and postthrombotic syndrome (PTS) was shown by Cockett et al in 1967.[3] They found that this anatomic variant may serve as both the main initiating factor in iliofemoral venous thrombus formation and the limiting factor in vessel recanalization after thrombosis. This study investigated 48 cases of postthrombotic iliac venous obstruction without inferior vena cava involvement and found that of these 48 cases, 39 were confined to the left leg. Of these, 33 showed the level of obstruction occurring at the junction where the right common iliac artery crosses the left common iliac vein.

C. **Setting of Iliac Vein Thrombosis** In the setting of iliac vein thrombosis, the vessel can either completely or incompletely recanalize. The subsequent thrombophlebitis triggers an acute inflammatory response within the vessel, which leads to scarring of the vein. This process drives recanalization and, in the majority of cases, results in incomplete recanalization. In this setting, adequacy of venous outflow depends on whether or not the body is able to develop sufficient collateral circulation. In the event of incomplete recanalization and inadequate collateral formation, the result is iliac vein obstruction manifesting clinically as PTS.

II. Epidemiology

A. May-Thurner Syndrome, Illiac Vein Compression Syndrome, or Cockett Syndrome

1. The presence of a compressed left common iliac vein by the overlying right common iliac artery is widely referred to as May-Thurner syndrome (MTS), although some refer to this anatomic variant as iliac vein compression syndrome or Cockett syndrome. MTS is most commonly seen in patients aged 20-40 years, disproportionately affecting females more than males. The autopsy studies of May and Thurner in the 20th century demonstrated left common iliac vein compression in 22% of cadavers, although the actual prevalence of this anatomic variant in the general population remains unknown.[4]
2. A study performed by Kibbe et al attempted to better define the prevalence of left common iliac vein compression in the asymptomatic population by performing a retrospective review of CT scans to determine the presence or absence of left iliac vein compression in patients without underlying evidence of or risk for iliac vein compression or DVT. Of the 50 CT scans reviewed in this group, mean left iliac vein compression was 35.5% ± 2.4%. Additionally, 24% of patient CT scans reviewed demonstrated at least 50% compression of the left iliac vein.[5]

B. May-Thurner Syndrome and Deep Vein Thrombosis MTS-associated DVT accounts for approximately 2%-3% of overall cases of lower extremity DVT, and MTS has only been diagnosed in 2%-5% of patients with venous disease of the lower extremity.[4,6] However, there are other studies that suggest a higher prevalence than this. In an MRI study of 24 patients with unilateral left lower extremity edema, 37% of these patients had evidence of MTS on magnetic resonance venography (MRV).[7] Another study on venous registry data found that in about 62% of patients with acute iliofemoral DVT, "spurlike lesions" were found.[8] This finding may suggest that the association of left-sided iliofemoral DVT with left common iliac vein compression is more common than previously thought.[9] The true association between MTS and lower extremity venous disease is not well defined and is likely underestimated.

III. Pathophysiology

MTS refers to extrinsic compression of the iliac venous system by an overlying iliac arterial vessel against the lumbar vertebrae. In the vast majority of cases, this involves compression of the left common iliac vein between the fifth lumbar vertebra and the overlying right common iliac artery.[4] However, other variants have been identified and include the right iliac artery compressing the inferior vena cava, right internal iliac artery compressing the right iliac vein, and left internal iliac artery compressing the left iliac vein. The compression and pulsation of the overlying artery causes increased deposition of elastin and collagen in the iliac vein wall and intimal proliferation, which leads to the formation of a "spur" that can cause complete or partial occlusion of the iliac vein. Over time, venous thrombosis may occur and without proper recanalization and development of collateral circulation, venous outflow obstruction and venous hypertension result.[3]

IV. Clinical Presentation

A. History

1. Patients with the anatomic variation underlying MTS are usually asymptomatic until thrombosis and venous outflow obstruction occur, usually in the second to fourth decades of life. The location of the symptoms is important to determine, as this suggests which vessels may be involved. If pain is the primary symptom, the patient should be prompted to localize the pain to the calf, thigh, groin, and/or pelvis. Additionally, when MTS and iliofemoral DVT are considered on the differential diagnosis, a full history should be taken to include the presence of any prior DVTs including location, age of occurrence, provoking factors, treatment course, and complications.[9] Finally, the history should also investigate any current risk factors for DVT, including recent surgery, prolonged immobilization, extended travel with prolonged motionlessness, hormone replacement therapy/oral contraceptive pill use, pregnancy, clotting disorder, malignancy, smoking, and obesity, as these risk factors have been implicated in MTS syndrome.
2. The clinical presentation is characterized by either acute thrombosis with unilateral edema or more chronic progressive left lower extremity edema and pain with development of chronic venous insufficiency. Lower extremity skin changes due to venous stasis may develop, such as hyperpigmentation, skin induration, and subcutaneous fat inflammation, consistent with lipodermatosclerosis.[4] As the venous outflow obstruction persists, patients may demonstrate signs of chronic venous insufficiency, including venous ulceration, varicose veins, and superficial venous thrombophlebitis. Additionally, those with longstanding venous outflow obstruction can also develop venous claudication. Finally, though rare, it is important to recognize that MTS can also present with complications, including pulmonary embolus and left common iliac vein rupture.[6] Suspicion for MTS should increase when a patient presents with a history concerning for DVT of the entire limb, primary complaints of venous claudication, and recurrent DVT in the same location.[9]

B. Physical Examination On physical examination, both lower extremities should be examined specifically for assessment of edema, erythema, tenderness, skin changes, varicose veins, and ulcers. Additionally, all lower extremity peripheral pulses should be palpated, and the pelvis and lower abdomen should be examined for the presence of varicose veins or any other changes consistent with chronic venous stasis. Following physical examination, duplex ultrasound can help determine compressibility of the common femoral vein with Doppler waveform phasicity to compare affected leg with unaffected.[9]

V. Diagnosis

A. Differential Diagnosis Clinical suspicion may lead a clinician to consider MTS on the differential diagnosis for unilateral lower extremity edema, but there are many conditions that may present similarly to MTS. Therefore, various imaging techniques have proven useful in both evaluating for the presence of iliac vein compression and also excluding other possible conditions that may mimic MTS. Currently color Doppler ultrasound (CDUS), conventional venography, computed tomography imaging (CT), magnetic resonance venography (MRV), and intravascular ultrasound (IVUS) are the most commonly used imaging techniques for evaluation of chronic venous insufficiency and possible MTS. These techniques differ in cost, invasiveness, and their ability to visualize the iliofemoral vessels, identify compression of the iliac vein, and rule out other causes of unilateral lower extremity edema. Although conventional venography remains the gold standard for diagnosis, these other modalities are noninvasive and clinically useful.

B. Imaging

1. Color Doppler Ultrasound

a. Although many imaging modalities are currently used in the workup of MTS, color doppler ultrasound (CDUS) is the most cost-effective and noninvasive imaging modality for evaluation of lower extremity superficial and deep veins and is therefore commonly used as a starting point for diagnostic imaging, with parameters described by Labropoulos et al. They investigated 37 patients with lower extremity swelling with or without pain using duplex ultrasound, venography, and IVUS to localize and diagnose venous stenosis and define criteria for diagnosis. Using a 2-4 MHz transducer to evaluate the iliac veins and inferior vena cava, an angle of insonation of $<60^\circ$ was applied in B-mode setting for comparison of vein diameter reduction. They found that a peak vein velocity ratio of >2.5 across the stenosis could most reliably predict the presence of a pressure gradient of 3 mm Hg, which represented a >50% reduction in luminal diameter. They identified the following parameters for diagnosis of central venous stenosis: mosaic color indicating poststenotic dilatation, abnormal Doppler signal at the site of stenosis, asymmetry of Doppler waveform of the affected extremity compared with unaffected extremity, poor flow augmentation, and low amplitude signals.[10]

b. Duplex ultrasound has been a mainstay in diagnostic workup for DVT and chronic venous insufficiency and is particularly useful for evaluation of the calf, popliteal, and femoral veins. In comparison, pelvic veins are more difficult to visualize with duplex due to bowel gas, body habitus, or location of the veins with respect to the bladder or adipose tissue. Additionally, CDUS can identify most cases of iliofemoral DVT by assessing for vessel patency but lacks the sensitivity to detect nonocclusive thrombosis of the common iliac vein and as a result may be insufficient to diagnose MTS.[11] In a prospective study quantifying the accuracy of duplex imaging in patients suspected of having DVT, duplex imaging could adequately assess the common and external iliac vein in only 47% of cases. For the external iliac vein alone, though, 79% of cases could be adequately assessed, underscoring the difficulty of visualizing the common iliac vein with CDUS within the pelvis.[12]

2. **Venous Phase CT and Magnetic Resonance Venography**
   a. CT imaging in the venous phase provides better visualization of the pelvic vessels in comparison with CDUS and is considered a sensitive and specific test for diagnosing iliofemoral thrombosis. CT is able to assess for vessel obstruction due to extrinsic compression within the pelvis not only from MTS, but also from malignancy, hematoma, or fibrosis as well. Limitations include visualization distortion in cases of chronic DVT where fibrosis within the vein may alter the vessel structure.[11] Additionally, CT imaging is costly, requires the use of IV contrast, is relatively contraindicated during pregnancy, and is technically difficult to time in the venous phase because of variations of cardiac output and the degree of stenosis.[9] Finally, degree of luminal compression may be affected by the patient's volume status, with dehydration overestimating degree of compression.
   b. MRV is another imaging technique that, similarly to CT imaging, provides improved visualization of the pelvic vessels. MRV is also comparable to CT scan in its ability to rule out extrinsic compression of the iliac veins and is considered superior at assessing the anatomy of the iliofemoral venous system. A primary advantage of MRV over CT venography is use of contrast agents that remain within the vascular system longer, eliminating the contrast timing difficulty encountered with venous phase CT imaging.[9] Additionally, enhancements including spin-echo imaging can evaluate inflammatory changes in the vessel wall that may help differentiate between acute and chronic thrombus.[13] MRV does share some limitations with CT scanning, including cost, contrast use, and availability. Also, vessels that demonstrate turbulent flow, such as areas above bifurcations, may be indistinguishable from filling defects on MRV. Finally, despite their high sensitivity and specificity, both MRV and CT imaging are limited by level of resolution, which in some instances may not be sufficient to pick up small spurs or subtle webs in the common iliac vein. Given these limitations, MRV seems to be more useful in patients with a low pretest probability of MTS who have mild disease.

3. **Contrast Venography** Invasive contrast venography allows direct visualization in the evaluation of iliac vein obstruction in suspected MTS and is the gold standard for diagnosis. This involves injection of dye via venous access (common femoral or popliteal) through a catheter with fluoroscopic visualization.[13] It can help identify the location and extent of occlusion or thrombosis, assess for any concomitant malformations, and assess the chronicity of the occlusion. Additionally, it allows for pressure measurement across a suspected stenosis via pullback gradient. Although there is no formal guideline in the literature on what degree of pressure gradient reflects a hemodynamically significant stenosis, most studies suggest that 2-3 mm Hg gradient is sufficient to cause symptoms.[9] Intervention is possible at the time of venography, including thrombolysis, balloon angioplasty, and stenting.[11]

4. **Intravascular Ultrasound** IVUS is a valuable adjunct to venography and may detect iliac venous outflow missed on conventional contrast venography. Using an IVUS catheter intraluminally, which is a specially designed catheter with a miniaturized ultrasound probe attached to the distal end, a 360° two-dimensional gray scale

ultrasound image can help to visualize the vessel lumen and vessel wall structure. It can detect the morphology and degree of stenosis at the lesion "spur" as well as be useful in sizing the vessel before any stent deployment.

IVUS offers improved visualization of intra- and extramural details, including external compression, trabeculation, frozen valves, and mural thickening as shown in a study by Neglen et al.[14] They assessed 304 limbs during balloon angioplasty and stenting for iliac vein compression, with IVUS as the standard, and found that venography had poorer sensitivity and negative predictive value (49%) to detect >70% stenosis. Given the absence of adequate hemodynamic testing for important venous obstruction, IVUS assessment is the best available tool for assessment of clinically significant stenosis.

VI. Treatment Options

Patients with MTS should only be treated if symptomatic. Treatment for MTS has evolved in recent years and is directed at relieving venous congestion to avoid PTS, venous ulceration, venous insufficiency, and venous claudication. Choice of initial strategy is dictated by the presence of coincident DVT for determination of the need for anticoagulation. In the absence of DVT, patients with CEAP class 1-3 disease are treated with conservative therapy with leg elevation and compression stockings. Patients with CEAP class 3 presentation and higher are reasonable candidates for invasive treatment to decrease venous hypertension after failure of conservative therapy. In the presence of DVT with concern for MTS, full-dose anticoagulation is indicated, although this is often insufficient. Catheter-directed or pharmacomechanical thrombolysis for reduction of clot burden may be necessary with mechanical relief of outflow obstruction. Historically, surgical procedures to relieve compression in MTS included autologous vein venovenous bypass, retroposition of the iliac artery with excision of the intraluminal spur with patch venoplasty, and tissue sling creation to mechanically elevate the right iliac artery. These open procedures have been variable in success. Endovascular advances with balloon angioplasty, stenting, and selective thrombolysis have improved outcomes relating to avoiding PTS.

A. **Noninvasive Treatment** Noninvasive options for treatment of MTS include primary prevention of the initial DVT in patients with known risk factors. However, in many patients, prevention of first DVT is not possible; therefore prevention of PTS is paramount. Therapeutic anticoagulation should be initiated once DVT is confirmed. Compression stockings may prevent progression to PTS by theoretically decreasing venous hypertension and reducing reflux. In one trial of 180 patients with proximal DVT on anticoagulation, one-half of patients developed postthrombotic sequelae at 5 years, with knee-high compression stockings applied for 2 years after DVT diagnosis reducing this rate by almost 50%.[15] The SOX trial, a multicenter randomized trial, enrolled 806 patients to active versus placebo compression. They found that incidence of PTS was 14.2% in the active compression group compared with 12.7% in the placebo group, suggesting based on this study that compression does not prevent PTS after proximal DVT.[16] Data for compression in MTS with DVT are extrapolated from patients with symptomatic proximal DVT, and it is reasonable to manage patients with therapeutic anticoagulation as well as 2 years of compression stockings. Unfortunately, there are patient-level barriers to adherence to compression, including cost and variable coverage by health insurance providers, difficulty applying stockings especially at higher compression, and patient discomfort wearing stockings especially in warmer climates.

1. **Surgical Management**
   a. Surgical options have had mixed success because of high rates of morbidity and variable patency rates. These options include contralateral saphenous vein graft bypass to the ipsilateral common femoral vein with creation of a temporary AV fistula (Palma crossover), division of right common iliac artery and relocation behind the left common iliac vein or inferior vena cava, and vein patch venoplasty with encasement of the left common iliac vein in ePTFE grafts after removal of intraluminal obstructions. These represent major surgeries with need for lifelong anticoagulation for patency and are only reserved for patients with the most severe PTS. Additionally, these surgical approaches to MTS treatment have not shown significant long-term improvement for patients from a symptomatic or functional standpoint. Jost et al looked at venous reconstructions with Palma procedure, ePTFE grafts, and patch venoplasty and showed primary and secondary patency rates of 54% and 62% at 3 years, with Palma procedures having the highest patency rate of 83% at 4 years and ePTFE bypass grafts showing 45% patency at 2 years.[17] In addition to variable patency rates, these procedures are associated with high operative risk largely based on patient-specific factors such as the presence of obstructive disease in the femoral vessels, presence of concurrent thrombosis, and caliber of the bypass graft.
   b. Combined surgical and endovenous management of iliofemoral DVT has been reported. Mickley and colleagues reported a series of 77 patients with acute iliac DVT who were treated with anticoagulation for 12 months and transfemoral venous thrombectomy with construction of temporary inguinal AV fistula. Of the patients who had left-sided thrombosis, half were found to have venous spurs on venogram. In the series, prior to 1994 those spurs were left untreated beyond oral anticoagulation with rethrombosis in 72% of patients compared with a 4% rate of recurrence in patients without spurs. In the stented group after 1994, only 1 out of the 8 patients experienced rethrombosis (13%).[18] This and other studies suggest that surgical thrombectomy of iliofemoral DVT alone may not be sufficient without relief of outflow obstruction associated with venous spurs via endovenous stenting.

2. **Endovenous Treatment Options**
   a. More recently, endovascular treatment strategies have become more successful for treatment of iliofemoral DVT and the underlying iliac vein compression. Although endovascular venoplasty dates back over 30 years, this was not explored in MTS until the 1990s when first case reports demonstrating successful management with stenting were published as a promising alternative to the existing disappointing medical and surgical strategies. In the mid-1990s,

the earliest case reports of stent placement as treatment of iliac vein compression were published. Berger and colleagues published one of these early case reports of a patient with MTS effectively treated with catheter-directed thrombolysis and subsequent stent placement, noting that balloon angioplasty alone was not sufficient to maintain patency likely owing to high elastic recoil of the fibrotic, compressed iliac vein. By 6 months' follow-up there was continued resolution of the patient's left leg edema with preserved stent patency by duplex ultrasound.[19] Three years later, an eight-case series of left iliac vein angioplasty in patients with symptomatic left iliac venous spur (defined as proximal DVT or PTS) showed immediate reduction in left leg circumference after stenting in all patients with 100% stent patency at 3-years follow-up.[20] This provided encouraging evidence for stenting as a viable first-line treatment option of iliac vein compression.

b. Subsequent studies have confirmed improved outcomes and high patency rates for MTS patients treated with endovascular stenting. Hartung and colleagues corroborated the use of stenting in patients with iliac vein occlusive disease in conjunction with surgical venous thrombectomy. This study followed up 29 patients who underwent thrombectomy with creation of an arteriovenous fistula and angioplasty with iliac vein stenting. Of these patients, 22 were found to have compression of the left common iliac vein by the right common iliac artery, 3 were found to have chronic left common iliac vein occlusion, 3 were found to have residual clot within the left common iliac vein, and 1 was found to have left external iliac vein compression by the left internal iliac artery. Of those patients treated with stenting, primary, assisted primary, and secondary patency rates at 1 year, 5 years, and 10 years were 79%, 86%, and 86%, respectively. Additionally, this stented group was shown to have high rates of valvular competence and low rates of rethrombosis.[21]

c. More recently, Liu et al in 2014 demonstrated a 93% primary patency rate at 1 year among 48 patients with iliac vein compression syndrome who received iliac vein stenting. This study also divided the patients into thrombotic versus nonthrombotic groups, both treated similarly with stenting, and found a dramatic reduction in reported pain in both groups as well as an 81.8% and 58.5% reduction in edema in the thrombotic and nonthrombotic groups, respectively.[22] Not only do these studies exhibit impressive patency rates for patients treated with stenting and catheter-directed thrombolysis (if applicable), but the latter offers some prognostic evidence, by demonstrating that thrombotic disease can have a negative impact on the degree of edema resolution with stenting.

d. The literature also supports use of catheter-directed thrombolysis in conjunction with stent placement in cases with concurrent thrombosis to promote stent patency and venous sufficiency. A study in 2010 investigated the patency rates in 30 patients with MTS and acute iliofemoral DVT who were treated with catheter-directed thrombolysis and stent placement. Follow-up CT venography was performed at various intervals and primary and secondary patency rates of 83.3%

and 90% at 1 and 5 years after treatment, respectively, were demonstrated. Park et al similarly showed primary patency rates after CDT and iliac vein stenting of 95.8% at 6 months, 87.5% at 12 months, and 84.3% at 24 months in 51 patients with symptomatic MTS.[23]

e. Randomized data for CDT in MTS do not yet exist; we can extrapolate from patients presenting with acute iliofemoral DVT. In the largest randomized controlled trial of CDT for deep venous thrombosis, the CAVenT study randomized 209 patients with first episode of acute DVT (<21 d duration) to standard therapy or standard therapy plus alteplase infusion. Absolute risk reduction was 14.4% of PTS at 24 months with the number needed to treat to prevent one episode of PTS of 7.[24] Five-year follow-up is available and shows absolute risk reduction of 28% and the number needed to treat to prevent one PTS case of 4.[25] Interestingly, quality-of-life scores did not differ significantly in either group. The soon to be published ATTRACT RCT trial evaluated outcomes of patients with femoropopliteal and iliofemoral DVT randomized to pharmacomechanical thrombolysis with anticoagulation versus anticoagulation alone. At 2 years, anticoagulation alone in the majority of patients is likely sufficient, and CDT was not shown to decrease PTS. Interestingly, they noted that CDT-treated patients had lower severity PTS and there was a nonsignificant trend toward less PTS in iliofemoral DVT patients receiving CDT, although the study was not powered for this (Society of Interventional Radiology 2017 Annual Scientific Sessions 4-9 March, Washington, DC, USA).

VII. Endovascular Approaches to Management of May-Thurner Syndrome

With evidence supporting newer endovascular approaches to management of MTS, consensus opinion recommends dividing patients into three categories based on clinical presentation with treatment strategies outlined in the sections that follow.

A. Iliac Vein Compression With Acute Deep Vein Thrombosis

1. The favored management for iliac vein compression with acute DVT currently involves anticoagulation possibly combined with additional thrombolysis or thrombectomy and outflow obstruction relief. The aim of treatment is to prevent pulmonary embolus, treat DVT and decrease symptoms associated with it, and prevent downstream complications including PTS. Catheter-directed thrombolysis allows for delivery of the thrombolytic agent directly to the clot, most and is effective when administered within 3 weeks of symptom onset. Anticoagulation is the mainstay of treatment with DVT. The addition of catheter-directed thrombolysis in iliofemoral DVT is more effective at clot removal and reduction of PTS sequelae than anticoagulation alone.[24] For more chronic DVT that has undergone fibrosis, direct injection of the thrombolytic agent may be insufficient to break up the clot, and mechanical thrombectomy may be required for more rapid clot debulking and faster recanalization.[26]

2. The addition of ultrasound pulsation to CDT accelerates fibrinolysis and decreases time of exposure to thrombolysis. An in vitro analysis of ultrasound-accelerated CDT found that using low-power, high-frequency microsonic energy can provide increased uptake and penetration of the thrombolytic agent into the thrombus, thus allowing improved total-clot lysis.[27] Grommes and colleagues evaluated safety and feasibility of ultrasound-accelerated CDT treatment in 12 patients with DVT who were treated with standard anticoagulation and compression stockings to avoid PTS. They found that ultrasound-accelerated thrombolysis resulted in >90% clot lysis in 85% of cases with only one case of bleeding at the catheter insertion site, with the major complication being pulmonary embolism secondary to mechanical disruption of the clot.[28] Recently announced results of the ACCESS PTS trial of 73 patients with iliofemoral DVT prospectively followed up after 3 months of conservative therapy who were treated with ultrasound-assisted thrombolysis and balloon angioplasty showed that there was significant improvement in Villalta scores of 34% at 30 days and 21% improvement in quality of life by VEINES-QOL (Society for Vascular Medicine 28th Annual Scientific Sessions 14-17 June, New Orleans, USA).

3. PTA alone without stent placement is associated with lower patency rates, with 73% recurrence rate of acute left-sided iliofemoral DVT in one study.[18] In another small study of 21 patients, 18 received iliac stenting after CDT and 3 received PTA alone after CDT. All of the three patients treated with PTA alone showed recurrent thrombosis.[29] A retrospective study of 36 patients who received iliofemoral venous stenting for chronic venous hypertension showed a patency rate of 78% at 2 years, with higher rates in MTS patients compared with lower rates in patients with thrombophilias.[30] These signals in the literature suggest that stents are effective at reestablishing the normal caliber of the vessel, preventing compression, and disrupting any venous spurs present from chronic vein compression.

4. After stent placement, anticoagulation is continued, with duration of anticoagulation necessarily determined by the clinical context. In the case of unprovoked DVT, recommended treatment is usually a for minimum of 3 months, with lifelong anticoagulation indicated for patients with certain underlying hypercoagulable conditions or complications.[11] There are no studies to date comparing optimal type and duration of anticoagulation strategies after endovenous intervention for DVT. Antiplatelet agents are prescribed routinely following stenting, but there are no data supporting efficacy on stent patency versus bleeding risk in these cases.[9,31]

5. In summary for acute DVT and iliac vein compression, the Society for Interventional Radiology and Society of Vascular Surgery recommend early thrombus removal (catheter-based or open thrombectomy based on patient-specific factors and local expertise) in patients with acute iliofemoral DVT <14 days duration with low bleeding risk and good functional status, especially if there is limb-threatening venous ischemia. Routine placement of inferior vena cava filters in conjunction with CDT is not endorsed and is only to be determined on a patient-based level. Finally, they recommend the use of self-expanding metallic stents for any obstructive iliac outflow lesions after thrombus removal.[32]

B. Iliac Vein Compression With Postthrombotic Syndrome

1. Selected patients with established PTS benefit from stent recanalization of occluded iliac veins. Historically, surgical venous bypass had been used to provide symptomatic outflow relief with variable patency rates. Endovenous techniques of direct recanalization with balloon venoplasty and stenting with decreased periprocedural risk and improved patency rates have supplanted surgical techniques as first-line therapies. Several studies suggest improvement in PTS symptoms, healing venous ulcers, and improved quality of life with outflow obstruction relief via stenting. In a retrospective series of 36 patients with symptomatic iliocaval venous stenosis, occlusion, or venous compression, patients were divided into two groups: those with MTS and those without. Of the 22 patients with MTS, 18 had successful angioplasty and stenting with or without CDT with symptomatic improvement in 94% and a decrease in CEAP score in 83%.[33]

2. In 2007, Neglén and colleagues published a prospective study of 982 patients without acute thrombosis who received iliofemoral venous stents. They were divided into "thrombotic" and "nonthrombotic" cohorts, where the "thrombotic" group included any patients with history of prior DVT or postthrombotic changes evident on imaging. Patients underwent venous Doppler, venography, and IVUS to diagnose obstructive iliac vein lesions defined as >50% stenosis and were then stented. There was a significant reduction in pain score from 55% to 11% after stenting with a reduction of leg swelling score from 44% to 18%. Additionally, at 5-years follow-up, stented patients exhibited a 58% rate of ulcer healing. Although there were various etiologies to explain chronic venous obstruction in this patient subset, IVUS findings suggested that about half of the "nonthrombotic" group had underlying compression of the external iliac vein by the internal iliac artery, suggesting applicability of this study to MTS patients to support stenting in the setting of PTS.[31]

C. Iliac Vein Compression With Symptomatic Nonthrombotic Chronic Venous Insufficiency

1. Patients with MTS can exhibit venous obstruction owing to compression of the common iliac vein without evidence of active or prior DVT. Their presenting symptom may be venous hypertension, with sequelae of chronic venous insufficiency, edema, pain, and venous ulceration. In selected patients with moderate to severe symptoms, there may be symptomatic benefits from stenting of the iliac outflow obstruction. In fact, these patients may receive the largest benefit from stenting, evidenced by superior long-term patency rates compared with patients with PTS treated with stenting.[30] In 2012, Kaichuang Ye et al performed a retrospective study of 205 patients with nonthrombotic iliac vein compression lesions treated with stenting and found a primary patency rate of 98% at 1 year.[34]

2. In these patients, shared decision-making between the patient and the provider is necessary, especially in the case of young patients who will have years of poststenting follow-up and possibility for long-term restenosis. Conservative therapy with compression is always first-line treatment followed by determination of whether invasive treatment is warranted by the clinical picture.

D. Treatment Strategy Summary

To summarize treatment strategies for MTS, a consolidated approach to MTS incorporates the use of noninvasive and invasive therapies based on the individual risk-benefit profile after diagnostic confirmation. Currently, initiation of treatment for MTS is only indicated in patients who are symptomatic (CEAP 4-6 or CEAP 3 with massive painful edema not alleviated by compression).[6] Upon symptom onset, the use of graduated compression stockings is highly recommended as the initial step in management. Additionally, patients with MTS may exhibit some degree of superficial venous reflux, in which case ablation of the greater saphenous vein may provide relief. The decision to proceed to more invasive treatment options depend on presentation with severe symptoms or hemodynamically significant venous outflow obstruction or collateral vessel formation present on venogram. Although newer endovenous interventions are minimally invasive in comparison with the open surgical bypass procedures that were once more routinely performed for MTS, they still carry risks that must be discussed with each patient carefully in a process of shared decision-making. Goals of therapy should be discussed to include symptomatic and functional improvement, as well as the prevention of complications such as recurrent thrombosis, pulmonary embolism, and PTS.[9]

VIII. Determinants of Stent Patency

A. **Endovenous Intervention With Balloon Angioplasty and Stenting** Endovenous intervention with balloon angioplasty and stenting for management of MTS has greatly improved symptomatic and functional outcomes for patients. Initial concerns for stent patency due to low-flow venous system have not been shown in the literature, with patency rates greater than 95% in some studies discussed above. Patency rates in patients without DVT are significantly greater as outlined above than in those with thrombosis. Although high patency rates seem similar in multiple studies, there are very little data defining the factors relating to long-term patency. Neglen and Raju evaluated restenosis in MTS patients (324 limbs) treated with stenting at 42-months after stent placement. Only 23% of limbs had no restenosis, 61% had >20% restenosis, and 15% had >50% in-stent restenosis. There was significantly more restenosis in cases where there was coincident thrombotic disease. They concluded that the presence of thrombosis, underlying thrombophilia, and lesions requiring longer stents extending past the inguinal ligament were associated with higher risks of in-stent recurrent stenosis.[35] Knipp and his colleagues published a retrospective chart review in 2007 that used a Cox proportional risk model to analyze patency rates after stent treatment. This study reported that in their relatively small sample of 58 patients, male gender, age under 40 years, and history of recent trauma predicted decreased primary patency rates. In fact, without any of these risk factors, patency rates in their study were 94.4% and 63% at 1 and 5 years after stent placement, respectively. In the event of two or more risk factors, however, patency rates decreased to 28.6% and 14.3% at 1 and 2 years, respectively.[36]

B. **Recurrent Stenosis** Among patients who experience recurrent stenosis, the majority of cases occur in the early months postintervention with luminal patency preserved in long-term follow-up. Jeon and colleagues evaluated 30 patients with acute iliofemoral DVT secondary to MTS diagnosed by CT venography and treated with CDT and stenting. Follow-up CT venography was performed for primary patency with the finding that 4 patients suffered in-stent thrombosis and one with stent collapse at the first CT follow-up within the first year. Overall stent patency was 83% and 90% at 1 and 5-years follow-up.[37]

IX. Follow-up

As yet, there are no formal guidelines to guide long-term management and follow-up for MTS patients after endovenous stenting. However, it is generally agreed that patients should be given dual antiplatelet therapy for at least 4 weeks after stent placement to prevent stent thrombosis (usually aspirin 81 mg daily and clopidogrel 75 mg daily). After short term dual antiplatelet treatment, the patient may continue on either aspirin or clopidogrel indefinitely, although there are no studies comparing the type or duration of appropriate antiplatelet agents after venous stenting; these regimens are adapted from arterial stenting studies. Patients who present with acute DVT are anticoagulated for 3 months for unprovoked DVT or longer for thrombophilias or recurrent DVT. Although designated follow-up intervals have not been established, most practitioners follow MTS patients with periodic duplex ultrasonography of the iliofemoral veins to assess for patency. Generally, neither CT venogram nor conventional venography with IVUS is necessary for follow-up unless the patient has recurrent symptoms or new signs of venous occlusion or thrombosis.[38]

X. Summary

In summary, MTS patients should be treated first-line with compression and anticoagulation in the setting of DVT. In the case of severe symptoms and failure of conservative therapy, severe symptoms and failure of conservative therapy and provides excellent long-term patency. Medical therapy poststenting includes anticoagulation for DVT if present with short-term dual antiplatelets followed by single antiplatelet treatment thereafter.

References

1. Cerquozzi S, Pineo GF, Wong JK, Valentine KA. Iliac vein compression syndrome in an active and healthy young female. *Case Rep Med.* 2012;2012:786876. doi:10.1155/2012/786876.
2. May R, Thurner J. The cause of the predominantly sinistral occurrence of thrombosis of the pelvic veins. *Angiology.* 1957;8(5):419-427. doi:10.1177/000331975700800505.
3. Cockett FB, Thomas ML, Negus D. Iliac vein compression.–Its relation to iliofemoral thrombosis and the post-thrombotic syndrome. *Br Med J.* 1967;2(5543):14-19.
4. Mousa AY, AbuRahma AF. May-Thurner syndrome: update and review. *Ann Vasc Surg.* 2013;27(7):984-995. doi:10.1016/j.avsg.2013.05.001.
5. Kibbe MR, Ujiki M, Goodwin AL, Eskandari M, Yao J, Matsumura J. Iliac vein compression in an asymptomatic patient population. *J Vasc Surg.* 2004;39(5):937-943. doi:10.1016/j.jvs.2003.12.032.

6. Kalu S, Shah P, Natarajan A, Nwankwo N, Mustafa U, Hussain N. May-Thurner syndrome: a case report and review of the literature. *Case Rep Vasc Med.* 2013;2013:740182. doi:10.1155/2013/740182.
7. Wolpert LM, Rahmani O, Stein B, Gallagher JJ, Drezne AD. Magnetic resonance venography in the diagnosis and management of May-Thurner syndrome. *Vasc Endovascular Surg.* 2002;36(1):51-57. doi:10.1177/153857440203600109.
8. Mewissen MW, Seabrook GR, Meissner MH, Cynamon J, Labropoulos N, Haughton SH. Catheter-directed thrombolysis for lower extremity deep venous thrombosis: report of a national multicenter registry. *Radiology.* 1999;211(1):39-49. doi:10.1148/radiology.211.1.r99ap4739.
9. Birn J, Vedantham S. May-Thurner syndrome and other obstructive iliac vein lesions: meaning, myth, and mystery. *Vasc Med.* 2015;20(1):74-83. doi:10.1177/1358863X14560429.
10. Labropoulos N, Borge M, Pierce K, Pappas PJ. Criteria for defining significant central vein stenosis with duplex ultrasound. *J Vasc Surg.* 2007;46(1):101-107. doi:10.1016/j.jvs.2007.02.062.
11. Shebel ND, Whalen CC. Diagnosis and management of iliac vein compression syndrome. *J Vasc Nurs.* 2005;23(1):10-17; quiz 18-19. doi:10.1016/j.jvn.2004.12.001.
12. Messina LM, Sarpa MS, Smith MA, Greenfield LJ. Clinical significance of routine imaging of iliac and calf veins by color flow duplex scanning in patients suspected of having acute lower extremity deep venous thrombosis. *Surgery.* 1993;114(5):921-927.
13. Carpenter JP, Holland GA, Baum RA, Owen RS, Carpenter JT, Cope C. Magnetic resonance venography for the detection of deep venous thrombosis: comparison with contrast venography and duplex Doppler ultrasonography. *J Vasc Surg.* 1993;18(5):734-741.
14. Neglen P, Raju S. Intravascular ultrasound scan evaluation of the obstructed vein. *J Vasc Surg.* 2002;35(4):694-700.
15. Prandoni P, Lensing AW, Prins MH, et al. Below-knee elastic compression stockings to prevent the post-thrombotic syndrome: a randomized, controlled trial. *Ann Intern Med.* 2004;141(4):249-256.
16. Kahn SR, Shapiro S, Wells PS. Compression stockings to prevent post-thrombotic syndrome: a randomised placebo-controlled trial. *Lancet.* 2014;383(9920):880-888. doi:10.1016/S0140-6736(13)61902-9.
17. Jost CJ, Gloviczki P, Cherry KJ, et al. Surgical reconstruction of iliofemoral veins and the inferior vena cava for nonmalignant occlusive disease. *J Vasc Surg.* 2001;33(2):320-327; discussion 327-328. doi:10.1067/mva.2001.112805.
18. Mickley V, Schwagierek R, Rilinger N, Gorich J, Sunder-Plassmann L. Left iliac venous thrombosis caused by venous spur: treatment with thrombectomy and stent implantation. *J Vasc Surg.* 1998;28(3):492-497.
19. Berger A, Jaffe JW, York TN. Iliac compression syndrome treated with stent placement. *J Vasc Surg.* 1995;21(3):510-514.
20. Binkert CA, Schoch E, Stuckmann G, et al. Treatment of pelvic venous spur (May-Thurner syndrome) with self-expanding metallic endoprostheses. *Cardiovasc Intervent Radiol.* 1998;21(1):22-26.
21. Hartung O, Benmiloud F, Barthelemy P, Dubuc M, Boufi M, Alimi YS. Late results of surgical venous thrombectomy with iliocaval stenting. *J Vasc Surg.* 2008;47(2):381-387. doi:10.1016/j.jvs.2007.10.007.
22. Liu Z, Gao N, Shen L, et al. Endovascular treatment for symptomatic iliac vein compression syndrome: a prospective consecutive series of 48 patients. *Ann Vasc Surg.* 2014;28(3):695-704. doi:10.1016/j.avsg.2013.05.019.
23. Park JY, Ahn JH, Jeon YS, Cho SG, Kim JY, Hong KC. Iliac vein stenting as a durable option for residual stenosis after catheter-directed thrombolysis and angioplasty of iliofemoral deep vein thrombosis secondary to May-Thurner syndrome. *Phlebology.* 2014;29(7):461-470. doi:10.1177/0268355513491724.
24. Enden T, Sandvik L, Klow NE, et al. Catheter-directed venous thrombolysis in acute iliofemoral vein thrombosis–the CaVenT study: rationale and design of a multicenter, randomized, controlled, clinical trial (NCT00251771). *Am Heart J.* 2007;154(5):808-814. doi:10.1016/j.ahj.2007.07.010.
25. Enden T, Haig Y, Klow NE, et al. Long-term outcome after additional catheter-directed thrombolysis versus standard treatment for acute iliofemoral deep vein thrombosis (the CaVenT study): a randomised controlled trial. *Lancet.* 2012;379(9810):31-38. doi:10.1016/S0140-6736(11)61753-4.

26. Vedantham S, Vesely TM, Parti N, Darcy M, Hovsepian DM, Picus D. Lower extremity venous thrombolysis with adjunctive mechanical thrombectomy. *J Vasc Interv Radiol.* 2002;13(10):1001-1008.
27. Francis CW, Blinc A, Lee S, Cox C. Ultrasound accelerates transport of recombinant tissue plasminogen activator into clots. *Ultrasound Med Biol.* 1995;21(3):419-424.
28. Grommes J, Strijkers R, Greiner A, Mahnken AH, Wittens CH. Safety and feasibility of ultrasound-accelerated catheter-directed thrombolysis in deep vein thrombosis. *Eur J Vasc Endovasc Surg.* 2011;41(4):526-532. doi:10.1016/j.ejvs.2010.11.035.
29. Kim JY, Choi D, Guk Ko Y, Park S, Jang Y, Lee DY. Percutaneous treatment of deep vein thrombosis in May-Thurner syndrome. *Cardiovasc Intervent Radiol.* 2006;29(4):571-575. doi:10.1007/s00270-004-0165-7.
30. Titus JM, Moise MA, Bena J, Lyden SP, Clair DG. Iliofemoral stenting for venous occlusive disease. *J Vasc Surg.* 2011;53(3):706-712. doi:10.1016/j.jvs.2010.09.011.
31. Neglen P, Hollis KC, Olivier J, Raju S. Stenting of the venous outflow in chronic venous disease: long-term stent-related outcome, clinical, and hemodynamic result. *J Vasc Surg.* 2007;46(5):979-990. doi:10.1016/j.jvs.2007.06.046.
32. Meissner MH, Gloviczki P, Comerota AJ, et al. Early thrombus removal strategies for acute deep venous thrombosis: clinical practice guidelines of the society for vascular surgery and the American venous forum. *J Vasc Surg.* 2012;55(5):1449-1462. doi:10.1016/j.jvs.2011.12.081.
33. DeRubertis BG, Alktaifi A, Jimenez JC, Rigberg D, Gelabert H, Lawrence PF. Endovascular management of nonmalignant iliocaval venous lesions. *Ann Vasc Surg.* 2013;27(5):577-586. doi:10.1016/j.avsg.2012.05.024.
34. Ye K, Lu X, Li W, et al. Long-term outcomes of stent placement for symptomatic nonthrombotic iliac vein compression lesions in chronic venous disease. *J Vasc Interv Radiol.* 2012;23(4):497-502. doi:10.1016/j.jvir.2011.12.021.
35. Neglen P, Raju S. In-stent recurrent stenosis in stents placed in the lower extremity venous outflow tract. *J Vasc Surg.* 2004;39(1):181-187. doi:10.1016/S0741.
36. Knipp BS, Ferguson E, Williams DM, et al. Factors associated with outcome after interventional treatment of symptomatic iliac vein compression syndrome. *J Vasc Surg.* 2007;46(4):743-749. doi:10.1016/j.jvs.2007.05.048.
37. Jeon UB, Chung JW, Jae HJ, et al. May-Thurner syndrome complicated by acute iliofemoral vein thrombosis: helical CT venography for evaluation of long-term stent patency and changes in the iliac vein. *AJR Am J Roentgenol.* 2010;195(3):751-757. doi:10.2214/AJR.09.2793.
38. Rajachandran M, Schainfeld RM. Medical and interventional options to treat pulmonary embolism. *Curr Cardiol Rep.* 2014;16(7):503. doi:10.1007/s11886-014-0503-6.

CHAPTER 24

Superficial Venous Disease of the Legs and Treatment

Robert R. Attaran, MD, FACC, FASE, FSCAI, RPVI

Key Points

- Reflux of the great saphenous veins is the leading cause of superficial venous insufficiency in the lower extremity.
- Edema, restless legs, hyperpigmentation, pain, and venous ulcers are among the symptoms of venous reflux.
- Radiofrequency ablation, laser ablation, mechanochemical ablation (MOCA), and sclerotherapy are undertaken for closure of refluxing veins not responding to traditional therapies such as compression.

I. Introduction

Venous insufficiency and varicose veins are very common, affecting more than 40% of men and 70% of women in their 60s.[1] In addition to being unsightly, in many cases they can lead to aching, edema, pruritis, stasis dermatitis, lipodermatosclerosis, and even ulceration.[2,3] They can affect quality of life and be disabling.[4] The leading cause of superficial venous insufficiency in the legs is great saphenous vein (GSV) reflux.[5] For centuries, compression therapy has been used as the mainstay of venous disease therapy. In addition, numerous surgical techniques have been adopted. These include avulsion (phlebectomy) of varicosities, saphenous vein stripping, and ligation of the saphenofemoral junction (SFJ).[6] Over recent years many surgical options have been replaced by minimally invasive techniques with lower complications, faster recovery, and comparable success rates. These include thermal ablation, for example, laser and radiofrequency, and nonthermal ablation, for example, nontumescent nonthermal (NTNT) techniques (foam sclerotherapy, mechanochemical ablation, and cyanoacrylate glue). The current US and UK guidelines (American Venous Forum/Society of Vascular Surgery and the National Institute for Health and Care Excellence) recommend endovenous thermal ablation in preference to surgical treatment for saphenous vein incompetence.[7,8] These nonsurgical techniques are less invasive, safer, and require less convalescence time. There are few strong contraindications to venous ablation, but they include pregnancy and femoral/popliteal vein occlusion.[9] In this chapter, we review the contemporary endovascular and approaches to treat superficial venous disease.

II. Compression Therapy

A. Compression Stockings

1. Regardless of the pathophysiology, reflux or obstruction, the mainstay of therapy in venous disease remains compression.[10] Compression stockings are utilized as they are thought to compensate for increased ambulatory venous pressure, for prevention of deep and superficial vein thrombosis, reduction in inflammation, swelling and pain. In addition to various forms of stocking, compression can be provided with bandages as well as pneumatic devices.

2. Conrad Jobst made the observation that hydrostatic pressures in a pool relieved venous insufficiency symptoms. The applied pressure was greater with depth, and in the 1950s he developed compression stockings to emulate them.[11]
   a. The ankle venous pressure represents the weight of the column of blood leading up to the right atrium. While low in the supine position, ankle venous pressures rise closer to 80-100 mm Hg upon standing. When venous valves are healthy, the use of the calf pump dramatically reduces this pressure.
   b. In venous insufficiency, compression stockings can help improve venous return and reduce ambulatory venous pressure[12,13] in part by using a Starling gradient that favors edema resolution.[14]

B. C5/C6 Disease

1. For C5/C6 disease (healed or active venous ulcer) two Cochrane reviews have reported lower ulcer recurrence with compression therapy. Compression noncompliance is associated with lower ulcer healing and greater recurrence.[10,15] Higher pressure compression may work better than medium compression to prevent recurrence.[15]

2. El-Sheika's[16] systematic review of randomized control trials on posttreatment compression found seven suitable for analysis. Three studies were surgical, two used sclerotherapy, and two endovenous laser ablation (EVLA). Heterogeneity in study quality and duration of compression made meta-analysis difficult. No specific conclusions could be drawn about efficacy or optimal duration of compression therapy.

   Two studies suggested that longer compression resulted in less postprocedural pain. Bakker et al[17] randomized patients undergoing EVLA of the GSV to 2 versus 7 days of compression stockings (35 mm Hg). At 1-week follow-up, the 7-day compression group reported less pain and better physical function. Another similarly designed prospective study noted a small but significant reduction in pain scores when compression was worn after EVLA.[18] These studies did not demonstrate any difference in procedural success or ablative efficacy.

C. **Evidence** The evidence for compression therapy is discussed in more detail in a review by this chapter's author.[19]

III. Laser Ablation

A. **Endovenous Laser Ablation** Endovenous laser ablation (EVLA) was initially described by Boné and Navarro[20,21] using an 810 nm diode laser. Using ultrasound guidance, a laser fiber (with or without a sheath) is inserted into the GSV at typically the knee level and advanced toward the SFJ. Local anesthetic was initially used but has now been superseded by tumescent anesthesia (saline, lidocaine, bicarbonate, and epinephrine). The activated laser fiber heats the vein and generates steam bubbles. It is withdrawn at a steady rate along the vein. In animal models, fiber temperatures in excess of 1000°C have been recorded.[22]

B. **Endovenous Laser Ablation Treatment** The treatment results in the thrombosis, gradual necrosis, and shrinkage of the treated vein.[23] Postprocedure compression is recommended. Successful closure rates, based mostly on observational studies, have been in the range of 90%-98%.[24,25]

Various laser fiber wavelengths have been developed, which typically focus energy for absorption by either red blood cells or water. A 1470 nm wavelength laser, for example, targets water. The 810 and 980 nm wavelengths target hemoglobin. The water-focused higher wavelength lasers may result in less discomfort and bruising.[26]

C. **Endovenous Laser Ablation Complications** Complications of EVLA, similar to radiofrequency ablation (RFA), include ecchymosis, hematoma, skin burns, nerve injury (the saphenous nerve courses close to the GSV below the mid-calf and the sural nerve courses close to the small saphenous vein (SSV) distally), and endothermal heat–induced thrombosis (EHIT).[27]

IV. Radiofrequency Ablation

A. **VNUS Closure System** Use of heat from radiofrequency energy to ablate the GSV was first described by Goldman[28] using the VNUS Closure System (Sunnyvale, CA). A sheath was inserted into the saphenous vein in the knee region, through which the radiofrequency fiber was advanced more proximally to the saphenofemoral junction. The electrode tip element generated local heat (85°C) which burned the vein wall. The original protocol involved slow steady pullback of the catheter. To facilitate vein emptying and occlusion, the procedure was performed in reverse Trendelenburg and compression bandaging was applied.[29]

B. **Medtronic ClosureFast Device**

1. The current iteration is the Medtronic ClosureFast device (Minneapolis, MN) (Fig. 24.1). For saphenous vein ablation it comes with a 3- or 7-cm heating element, reaching 120°C. Each vein segment is treated for 20 seconds before the fiber is repositioned to the adjacent segment. The procedure is performed with tumescent anesthesia, administered around the vein and typically within the saphenous fascia. Our usual practice is to add 250 mg (25 mL) 1% lidocaine with epinephrine (1:100,000) plus 2.5 mL of 8.4% sodium bicarbonate to a bag of 500 mL saline (after discarding approximately 25 mL of saline). This creates a 500 mL bag of 0.05% lidocaine solution. The tumescent anesthetic is typically refrigerated before administration. The net effect is to create local anesthesia, a heat sink as well as vasoconstriction, improving contact of the heating element with the vein. In our experience, bicarbonate reduces the discomfort of the injections. The tumescent anesthesia can also be used to ensure the saphenous vein is at least 1 cm deep to the dermis, to prevent skin burns with thermal ablation. It can also help create separation from nerves in certain locations.

2. Patients are recommended to wear compression stockings for up to 2 weeks postablation. There is no strong evidence that compression improves the efficacy of thermal ablation, but it may lower discomfort.[16,17,30]

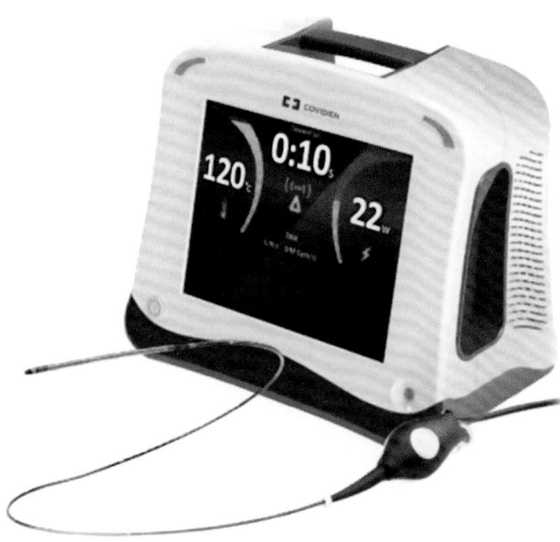

FIGURE 24.1: The Medtronic ClosureFast radiofrequency ablation device (fiber and generator). Used with permission by Medtronic© 2019.

3. Five-year follow-up data for radiofrequency ablation of the GSV (295 GSVs in 225 patients) found occlusion rates of 92%, with 95% free of reflux and only six patients reporting ongoing symptoms.[31] Symptoms and quality of life scores improve dramatically after ablation.[32–34]

C. Radiofrequency Ablation Complications

1. The range of RFA complications and their rates are similar to EVLA.[27,35] EHIT is rare with meticulous technique. Lawrence et al[36] (Fig. 24.2) describe a classification system for EHIT based on extent of bulging and deep vein involvement. From 500 patients undergoing RFA to the GSV, thrombus bulging into the femoral vein was seen in 2.6%. Even without anticoagulation, all thrombi retracted to the SFJ at approximately 16-day follow-up, with no cases of deep vein thrombosis (DVT).
2. In our laboratory, it is common practice to anticoagulate EHIT types 4-6, ie, in any cases where thrombus extends into the deep venous system. For types 4 and 5 we repeat ultrasound imaging in 1-2 weeks and stop anticoagulation if the thrombus has become flush at the SFJ. With type 6, anticoagulation is administered longer, for up to 3 months.

D. Endothemal Heat–Induced Thrombosis With Ablation A similar evaluation and classification system has been proposed for EHIT with ablation of the SSV.[37] After RFA of the SSV in 80 limbs, 3% experienced EHIT, with thrombus extension into the popliteal vein. No occlusive DVTs occurred. Similar to EHIT with GSV, we anticoagulate patients with any thrombus extension into the popliteal vein. If there is thrombus bulge into the popliteal vein without occlusion, we normally anticoagulate for 1-2 weeks and repeat imaging. We stop anticoagulation if the thrombus has become flush at the saphenopopliteal junction.

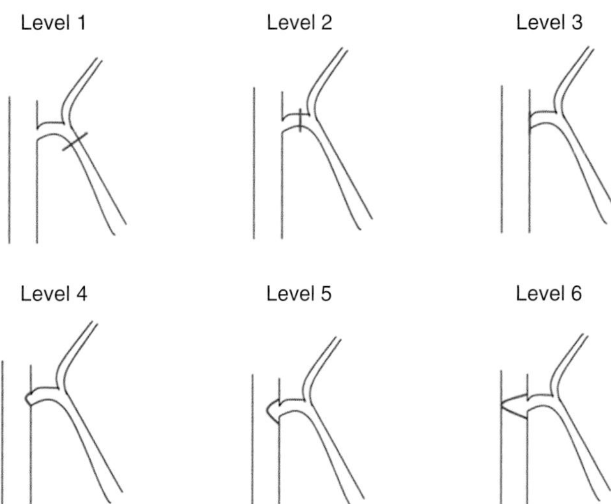

FIGURE 24.2: Classification of endothermal heat–induced thrombosis (EHIT). Level 1: thrombus distal to the level of the superficial epigastric vein. Level 2: closure with thrombus extension flush with the orifice of the epigastric vein. Level 3: closure with thrombus extension flush with the saphenofemoral junction. Level 4: closure with thrombus bulging into the common femoral vein. Level 5: closure with proximal thrombus extension adherent to the adjacent wall of the common femoral vein past the saphenofemoral junction. Level 6: closure with proximal thrombus extension into the common femoral vein, consistent with a deep vein thrombosis (DVT). EHIT levels 1-3 are typically not anticoagulated. From Lawrence PF, Chandra A, Wu M. Classification of proximal endovenous closure levels and treatment algorithm. *J Vasc Surg*. 2010;52:388-393.

V. Mechanochemical Ablation

Mechanochemical ablation (MOCA) combines abrasion of venous endothelium by a rapidly rotating metal element with chemical ablation by sclerotherapy.

A. **ClariVein Device** MOCA (Fig. 24.3) with the ClariVein device (Vascular Insights, Quincy, MA) was approved by the FDA in 2015 and is also approved in Europe. Saphenous vein access is obtained through a 4-Fr sheath, through which the device is advanced close to the GSV. Typically, the procedure is commenced 2 cm distal to the SFJ or the superficial epigastric vein. The metallic tip of the device rotates at approximately 3,500 RPM. Sclerosants can be injected through the metallic via a syringe loaded on the device handle. As this action is performed, the device is withdrawn slowly at a rate of approximately 1 cm, every 7-10 seconds. It is recommended to apply manual compressive pressure especially with vein diameters of 1 cm or greater. As with other nonthermal technologies, no tumescent anesthesia is required. Owing to the lack of anesthesia, the patient can feel discomfort particularly if the wire tip catches a valve. In those cases, local lidocaine anesthetic can be given or the wire tip can be resheathed, withdrawn slightly and restarted. Patients are advised to pump their foot or better still walk around, immediately after the MOCA procedure. Compression wrapping is applied.

B. **Mechanochemical Ablation Versus Radiofrequency Ablation** In a prospective head-to-head comparison of MOCA versus RFA (total $n = 119$), at 1-month follow-up, 83% of the MOCA group and 92% of the RFA group demonstrated complete GSV closure. In 9% of the MOCA group only the proximal GSV was occluded. Procedural pain scores were lower in the MOCA group. Quality of life score improvements were equivalent in the two groups. One limitation of this study was the sizable loss to follow-up.[38] The completed study findings were published more recently.[39] About 170 patients were randomized to MOCA versus RFA, with similar findings as Bootun et al.[38] Most treated veins (86%) were GSVs; the remainder (14%) were small saphenous veins (SSVs). Of these, 74% underwent concurrent phlebectomy. Six-month follow-up was completed in 71%. At 6 months, MOCA demonstrated complete or proximal GSV occlusion in 87%, versus 93% for RFA. Venous clinical severity scores showed equivalent improvement.[39]

VI. Sclerotherapy

A. **Varicose Veins** Sclerotherapy of varicose veins has been used in various formulations, for decades.[40] It results in vein thrombosis, fibrosis, and atrophy. Sclerotherapy can be applied to any size vein from telangiectasia to large veins such as the GSV.[41] Two of the leading sclerosants available are polidocanol and sodium tetradecyl sulfate (STS). Both belong to the detergent class. The recommended strengths of polidocanol are 1% in large varicose veins, 0.5% in reticular veins, 0.5% or lower in telangiectasia (spider veins). For STS, 1%-1.5% in large varicose veins, 0.5%-1% in reticular veins, and approximately 0.2%-0.3% in telangiectasia. For the first sclerotherapy session, we would recommend lower dosages to gauge patient response.

B. **Liquid or Foam Application** Sclerosants can be applied as a liquid or foam. Foam is considered more effective in larger caliber veins[41,42] as it displaces more venous blood and the sclerosant bubbles allow for better sclerosant contact with the venous endothelium. Both air and carbon dioxide have been used to generate foam. A simple way to generate foam is the Tessari technique that uses two syringes and a three-way stopcock.[43] Typically an air-to-liquid ratio of 4:1 is created by vigorously flushing the two syringes back and forth.

C. Liquid or Foam Application With Ultrasound Guidance

1. Sclerotherapy can be applied using ultrasound guidance. For large caliber veins such as the GSV, past data have shown foam sclerotherapy to be inferior to RFA, EVLA, and surgical stripping.[44,45] Darvall et al[46] followed 351 patients (479 limbs) after ultrasound-guided foam sclerotherapy for varicose veins. At 5-year follow-up 81.2% were evaluated. An estimated 15.3% had required retreatment. High satisfaction scores as well as improved symptoms scores were reported.

2. While there is no definitive evidence that compression therapy improves the success of sclerotherapy for telangiectasis, some small studies suggest it may reduce pigmentation.[47,48]

D. Varithena

1. Varithena, a proprietary canister system to generate and dispense 1% polidocanol foam is available from BTG International (London, UK) (Fig. 24.4). The foam has a gas-to-liquid ratio of approximately 7:1 and appears to have greater stability than physician-compounded foam. The gas is a combination of O_2 and CO_2.

2. Using ultrasound guidance, a sheath is placed into the vein of interest. A catheter is then advanced through the vein, typically at least 3 cm distal to the SFJ, and aspirated. The leg is elevated. An ultrasound probe can be used to monitor the foam entering the GSV and can also be used to compress over the SFJ. The catheter can be withdrawn as the foam is injected through it. Typically, compression is applied thereafter and leg elevation is maintained for 10 minutes. Compression wraps or stockings are applied and the patient is advised to walk right away. The maximum recommended foam dosage per session is 15 mL and each canister contains approximately 45 mL.

3. Varithena was approved by the FDA in 2013 based on the findings of the VANISH Phase III studies. VANISH-1 showed improved patient-reported venous symptom scores at 8-weeks with acceptable safety.[49] In VANISH-2, 232 patients received 0.5%-1% polidocanol (Varithena) microfoam. By duplex ultrasound, 84.7% showed "response" to treatment at 8 weeks. A duplex response was defined as the elimination of SFJ reflux and/or complete occlusion of the GSV and/or accessory veins identified as incompetent at baseline. Sixty percent reported some adverse event, mainly retained coagulum, phlebitis, and pain. Common femoral vein thrombus extension occurred in 3.9% and proximal DVT in 2.6% with Varithena. Most of these adverse events were mild or moderate. Varithena was shown to improve symptom and appearance scores at 8 weeks. No neurologic events were reported in the treatment group.[50]

4. Varithena has also been evaluated as an adjunct to endovenous thermal ablation. Vasquez et al[51] randomized 117 patients receiving RFA or EVLA to also receive 0.5% polidocanol (n = 39), 1% polidocanol (n = 40), or placebo (n = 38). The patients had GSV incompetence and visible varicosities. The study drug could be used above and below the knee for visible varicosities, incompetent regions of the GSV system or tortuous areas of the saphenous trunk not treated with thermal ablation. The patients were blinded for all interventions and polidocanol randomized cases were double-blinded. The combined thermal and polidocanol treated group showed improved appearance at 8 weeks.

VII. Cyanoacrylate

A. Application

1. To date, numerous forms of cyanoacrylate glue (CAG) have been used in medicine, for example as the skin adhesive Dermabond (Ethicon, Somerville, NJ),

as a sealant in intracranial arteriovenous malformations and pelvic and gastric varices.[52,53] VeClose (n-butyl-2-cyanoacrylate), a form of CAG, with greater viscosity and faster polymerization (originally developed by Sapheon (Morrisville, NC) and acquired by Medtronic (Minneapolis, MN) is available for closure of incompetent saphenous veins. After vein occlusion the polymer is slowly absorbed leading to granuloma formation and vein fibrosis.[54] VeClose was FDA approved in 2015 and has also been approved in Europe. Each device kit comes with CAG, catheter, guidewire, dispenser gun, dispenser tips, and syringes (Fig. 24.3).

2. After placement of a 5Fr introducer sheath into the GSV, the delivery catheter is advanced 4-5 cm caudal to the SFJ. The proximal GSV is compressed with ultrasound guidance as CAG is injected, and then compressive pressure is applied. The catheter is withdrawn 3 cm before another injection is given and compression reapplied, and so on. We recommend at least 30 seconds of compressive pressure after each administration. Ultrasound is used to confirm GSV occlusion. There is no need for compression wraps postprocedure.

B. **eSCOPE Study** In the prospective eSCOPE study (*n* = 70) CAG demonstrated a 93% closure rate at 12-months. Postprocedural phlebitis was noted in 8.5%.[55] In another study (*n* = 108), at 3 months CAG demonstrated 99% GSV closure rates by ultrasound.[56] The 2-year results of the eSCOPE trial showed VenaSeal GSV closure rates of 94.3% compared with 94% with ClosureFast RFA.[55] In the WAVES study, 50 patients with incompetent GSVs, SSVs, and/or accessory saphenous veins (diameters up to 20 mm) were treated with VensSeal cyanoacrylate closure. At 1 month, all treated veins were occluded by duplex ultrasound and venous symptom scores were improved. Postprocedure phlebitis was noted in 20%.[57]

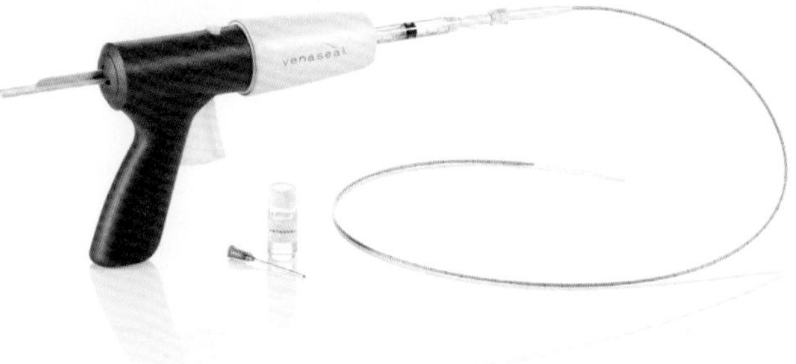

FIGURE 24.3: The VenaSeal cayanoacrylate glue device. Used with permission by Medtronic© 2019.

VIII. Comparison Studies

A. Radiofrequency Ablation Versus Endovenous Laser Ablation

1. Sydnor et al[58] performed a prospective randomized study to compare RF ablation with EVLT with 980 nm diode laser for GSV reflux. The RF group experienced significantly less postprocedure pain and bruising. Over a 1-year follow-up symptom relief was equivalent as was overall patient satisfaction.

B. Ultrasound-Guided Foam Sclerotherapy Versus Endothermal Ablation Davis et al[59] reviewed all randomized controlled trial literature up to January 2015. Six publications were identified with variable inclusion criteria and methodologies. Anatomical GSV closure rates were higher with thermal technologies (RFA and EVLA). Patient-reported quality of life scores, however, did not significantly differ. Foam sclerotherapy was more economical.

C. Cyanoacrylate Glue Versus Endovenous Laser Ablation Bozkurt et al[60] randomized 310 patients to CAG (n = 154) versus EVLA (n = 156) for ablation of the GSV as the primary end point. Patients with C2-C4b disease were included. The CAG was the VariClose Vein Sealing System (Biolas, Ankara, Turkey). The EVLA was a 1470 nm fiber. There was significantly shorter operative time and procedural pain with CAG. In addition, there was less ecchymosis and no cases of paresthesia in CAG, versus 7 cases of temporary or permanent paresthesia with EVLA. Twelve-month GSV closure rates were 95.8% with CAG and 92.2% with EVLA. Both groups experienced improved venous symptoms scores (Venous Clinical Severity Score and Aberdeen Varicose Vein Questionnaire), with no significant difference between the two scores.

References

1. Brand FN, Dannenberg AL, Abbott RD, Kannel WB. The epidemiology of varicose veins: the Framingham study. *Am J Prev Med.* 1988;4:96.
2. Magnusson MB, Nelzén O, Risberg B, Sivertsson R. A color Doppler ultrasound study of venous reflux in patients with chronic leg ulcers. *Eur J Vasc Endovasc Surg.* 2001;21:253.
3. Weiss RA, Weiss RA. Resolution of pain associated with varicose and telangiectatic leg veins after compression sclerotherapy. *J Dermatol Surg Onc.* 1990;16:333.
4. Phillips T, Stanton B, Provan A, et al. A study of the impact of leg ulcers on quality of life: financial, social, and psychologic implications. *J Am Acad Dermatol.* 1994;31(1):49-53.
5. Labropoulos N, Leon M, Nicolaides AN, et al. Superficial venous insufficiency: correlation of anatomic extent of reflux with clinical symptoms and signs. *J Vasc Surg.* 1994;20(6):953-956.
6. Lees TA, Beard JD, Ridler BM, et al. A survey of the current management of varicose veins by members of the Vascular Surgical Society. *Ann Roy Coll Surg Engl.* 1999;81(6):407-417.
7. Gloviczki P, Comerota AJ, Dalsing MC, et al. The care of patients with varicose veins and associated chronic venous diseases: clinical practice guidelines of the Society for Vascular Surgery and the American Venous Forum. *J Vasc Surg.* 2011;53(5 suppl):2S-48S.
8. *Varicose Veins: Diagnosis and Management.* NICE Guidelines [CG168]: National Institute for Health and Clinical Excellence; 2013. https://www.nice.org.uk/guidance/cd168.

9. Kilnani NM, Grassi CJ, Kundu S, et al. Multi-society consensus quality improvement guidelines for the treatment of lower-extremity superficial venous insufficiency with endovenous thermal ablation from the Society of Interventional Radiology, Cardiovascular Interventional Radiological Society of Europe, American College of Phlebology, and Canadian Interventional Radiology Association. *J Vasc Interv Radiol.* 2010;21:14-31.
10. O'Meara S, Cullum N, Nelson EA, et al. Compression for venous leg ulcers. *Cochrane Database Syst Rev.* 2012;11:CD000265.
11. Bergan JJ. Conrad Jobst and the development of pressure gradient therapy for venous disease. In: Bergan JJ, Yao JS, eds. *Surgery of the Veins.* Orlando: Grune & Stratton; 1985:529-540.
12. Ludbrook J. *Aspects of Venous Function in the Lower Limbs.* Springfield, IL: Charles Thomas; 1966.
13. Partsch B, Partsch H. Calf compression pressure required to achieve venous closure from supine to standing positions. *J Vasc Surg.* 2005;42(4):734-738.
14. Nehler MR, Moneta GL, Woodard DM, et al. Perimalleolar subcutaneous tissue pressure effects of elastic compression stockings. *J Vasc Surg.* 1993;18:783.
15. Nelson EA, Bell-Syer SE. Compression for preventing recurrence of venous ulcers. *Cochrane Database Syst Rev.* 2014;9:CD002303.
16. El-Sheikha J, Carradice D, Nandhra S, et al. Systematic review of compression following treatment for varicose veins. *Brit J Surg.* 2015;102(7):719-725.
17. Bakker NA, Schieven LW, Bruins RMG, et al. Compression stockings after endovenous laser ablation of the great saphenous vein: a prospective randomized controlled trial. *Eur J Vasc Endovasc Surg.* 2013;46(5):588-592.
18. Elderman JH, Krasznai AG, Voogd AC, et al. Role of compression stockings after endovenous laser therapy for primary varicosis. *J Vasc Surg Venous Lymphati Disord.* 2014;2:289-296.
19. Attaran RR, Ochoa Chaar CI. Compression therapy in venous disease. *Phlebology.* 2016;32(2):81-88. pii:0268355516633382. [Epub ahead of print].
20. Navarro L, Min RJ, Bone C. Endovenous laser: a new minimally invasive method of treatment for varicose veins – preliminary observations using an 810nm diode laser. *Dermatol Surg.* 2001;27(2):117-122.
21. Boné C. Tratamiento endoluminal de las varices con laser de Diodo. Estudio preliminar. *Rev Patol Vasc.* 1999;5:35-46.
22. Weiss RA. Comparison of endovenous radiofrequency versus 810 nm diode laser occlusion of large veins in an animal model. *Dermatol Surg.* 2002;28(1):56-61.
23. Proebstle TM, Sandhofer M, Kargl A, et al. Thermal damage of the inner vein wall during endovenous laser treatment: key role of energy absorption by intravascular blood. *Dermatol Surg.* 2002;28:596-600.
24. Min RJ, Kailnani N, Zimmet SE. Endovenous laser treatment of saphenous vein reflux: long-term results. *J Vasc Interv Radiol.* 2003;14:991-996.
25. Proebstle TM, Gul D, Lehr HA, et al. Infrequent early recanalization of greater saphenous vein after endovenous laser treatment. *J Vasc Surg.* 2003;38:511-516.
26. Kabnick LS. Outcome of different endovenous laser wavelengths for great saphenous vein ablation. *J Vasc Surg.* 2006;43:88-93.
27. Dexter D, Kabnick L, Berland T, et al. Complications of endovenous lasers. *Phlebology.* 2012;27(suppl 1):40-45.
28. Goldman MP. Closure of the great saphenous vein with endoluminal radiofrequency thermal heating of the vein wall in combination with ambulatory phlebectomy: a preliminary 6-month follow-up. *Dermatol Surg.* 2000;26(5):452-456.
29. Chandler JG, Pichot O, Sessa C, et al. Treatment of primary venous insufficiency by endovenous saphenous vein obliteration. *Vasc Surg.* 2000;14(3):201-214.
30. Palfreyman SJ, Michaels JA. A systematic review of compression hosiery for uncomplicated varicose veins. *Phlebology.* 2009;24(suppl 1):13-33.

31. Proebstle TM, Alm BJ, Göckeritz O, et al. Five year results from the prospective European multicentre cohort study on radiofrequency multisegment thermal ablation for incompetent great saphenous veins. *Brit J Surg*. 2015;102(3):212-218.
32. Goldman MP, Amiry S. Closure of the great saphenous vein with endoluminal radiofrequency thermal heating of the vein wall in combination with ambulatory phlebectomy: 50 patients with more than 6-month follow-up. *Dermatol Surg*. 2002;28(1):29-31.
33. Merchant RF, Pichot O, Myers KA. Four-year follow-up on endovascular radiofrequency obliteration of great saphenous reflux. *Dermatol Surg*. 2005;31:129.
34. Sybrandy JE, Wittens CH. Initial experiences in endovenous treatment of saphenous vein reflux. *J Vasc Surg*. 2002;36:1207.
35. Marsh P, Price BA, Holdstock J, et al. Deep vein thrombosis (DVT) after venous thermoablation techniques: rates of endovenous heat-induced thrombosis (EHIT) and classical DVT after radiofrequency and endovenous laser ablation in a single centre. *Eur J Vasc Endovasc Surg*. 2010;40:521-527.
36. Lawrence PF, Chandra A, Wu M. Classification of proximal endovenous closure levels and treatment algorithm. *J Vasc Surg*. 2010;52:388-393.
37. Harlander-Locke M, Jimenez JC, Lawrence PF, et al. Management of endovenous heat-induced thrombus using a classification system and treatment algorithm following segmental thermal ablation of the small saphenous vein. *J Vasc Surg*. 2013:1-6.
38. Bootun R, Lane TR, Dharmarajah B, et al. Intra-procedural pain score in a randomised controlled trial comparing mechanochemical ablation to radiofrequency ablation: the Multicentre Venefit™ versus ClariVein® for varicose veins trial. *Phlebology*. 2016;31(1):61-65. doi:10.1177/0268355514551085. Epub 2014 Sep 5.
39. Lane T, Bootun R, Dharmarajah B, et al. A multi-centre randomised controlled trial comparing radiofrequency and mechanical occlusion chemically assisted ablation of varicose veins – final results of the Venefit versus Clarivein for varicose veins trial. *Phlebology*. 2017;32(2):89-98. pii:0268355516651026. [Epub ahead of print].
40. Linser P. Über die konservative behandlung der varicen. *Med Klin*. 1916;12:897-902.
41. Rabe E, Otto J, Schliephake D, et al. Efficacy and safety of great saphenous vein sclerotherapy using standardized polidocanol foam (ESAF): a randomized controlled multicenter clinical trial. *Eur J Endovasc Vasc Surg*. 2008;35:238-245.
42. Yamaki T, Nozaki M, Iwasaka S, et al. Comparative study of duplex-guided foam sclerotherapy and duplex-guided liquid sclerotherapy for the treatment of superficial venous insufficiency. *Dermatol Surg*. 2004;30:718-722.
43. Tessari L, Cavezzi A, Frullini A. Preliminary experience with a new sclerosing foam in the treatment of varicose veins. *Dermatol Surg*. 2001;27:58-60.
44. Biemans AA, Kockaert M, Akkersdijk GP, et al. Comparing endovenous laser ablation, foam sclerotherapy, and conventional surgery for great saphenous varicose veins. *J Vasc Surg*. 2013;58:727-734.
45. Rasmussen LH, Lawaetz M, Bjoern L, et al. Randomized clinical trial comparing endovenous laser ablation, radiofrequency ablation, foam sclerotherapy and surgical stripping for great saphenous veins. *Br J Surg*. 2011;98:1079-1087.
46. Darvall KA, Bate GR, Bradbury AW. Patient-reported outcomes 5-8 years after ultrasound-guided foam sclerotherapy for varicose veins. *Br J Surg*. 2014;101:1098-1104.
47. Weiss RA, Sadick NS, Goldman MP, et al. Post-sclerotherapy compression: controlled comparative study of duration of compression and its effects on clinical outcome. *Dermatol Surg*. 1999;25:105-108.
48. Nootheti PK, Cadag KM, Magpantay A, et al. Efficacy of graduated compression stockings for an additional 3 weeks after sclerotherapy treatment of reticular and telangiectatic leg veins. *Dermatol Surg*. 2009;35:53-58.
49. King JT, O'Byrne M, Vasquez M, et al. Treatment of truncal incompetence and varicose veins with a single administration of a new polidocanol endovenous microfoam preparation improves symptoms and appearance. *Eur J Vasc Endovasc Surg*. 2015;50(6):784-793.
50. Todd KL, Wright DI. The VANISH-2 study: a randomized, blinded, multicenter study to evaluate the efficacy and safety of polidocanol endovenous microfoam 0.5% and 1.0% compared with placebo for the treatment of saphenofemoral junction incompetence. *Phlebology*. 2014;29(9):608-618.

51. Vasquez M, Gasparis AP; Varithena Investigator Group. A multicenter, randomized, placebo-controlled trial of endovenous thermal ablation with or without polidocanol endovenous microfoam treatment in patients with great saphenous vein incompetence and visible varicosities. *Phlebology*. 2017;32(4):272-281.
52. Quinn J, Wells G, Sutcliffe T, et al. A randomized trial comparing octylcyanoacrylate tissue adhesive and sutures in the management of lacerations. *JAMA*. 1997;277(19):1527-1530.
53. Pollak JS, White RI. The use of cyanoacrylate adhesives in peripheral embolization. *J Vasc Interv Radiol*. 2001;12(8):907-913.
54. Vinters HV, Galil KA, Lundie MJ, et al. The histotoxicity of cyanoacrylates. A selective review. *Neuroradiology*. 1985;27:279-291.
55. Proebstle TM, Alm J, Dimitri S, et al. The European multicenter cohort study on cyanoacrylate embolization of refluxing great saphenous veins. *J Vasc Surg Venous Lymph Disord*. 2015;3(1):2-7.
56. Morrison N, Gibson K, McEnroe S, et al. Randomised trial comparing cyanoacrylate embolization and radiofrequency ablation for incompetent great saphenous veins (VeClose). *J Vasc Surg*. 2015;61(4):985-994.
57. Gibson K, Ferris B. Cyanoacrylate closure of incompetent great, small and accessory saphenous veins without the use of post-procedure compression: initial outcomes of a post-market evaluation of the VenaSeal System (the WAVES Study). *Vascular*. 2017;25(2):149-156. doi:10.1177/1708538116651014. [Epub ahead of print].
58. Sydnor M, Mavropoulos J, Slobodnik N, et al. A randomized prospective long-term (>1 year) clinical trial comparing the efficacy and safety of radiofrequency ablation to 980 nm laser ablation of the great saphenous vein. *Phlebology*. 2017;32(6):415-424. pii:0268355516658592. [Epub ahead of print].
59. Davies HOB, Popplewell M, Darvall K, et al. A review of randomized controlled trials comparing ultrasound-guided foam sclerotherapy and endothermal ablation for the treatment of great saphenous veins. *Phlebology*. 2016;31(4):234-240.
60. Bozkurt AK, Yilmaz MF. A prospective comparison of a new cyanoacrylate glue and laser ablation for the treatment of venous insufficiency. *Phlebology*. 2016;31(1 suppl):106-113.

Index

Note: Page numbers in *italics* denote figures; those followed by "t" denotes tables.

B

D

E

F

G

H

I

J

L

M

N

O

P

Q

R

S

T

U

V